Designing and Teaching Fitness Education Courses

Innovative Ideas and Practical Solutions for Secondary Schools

Jayne D. Greenberg, EdD
Nichole D. Calkins, EdD
Lisa S. Spinosa, MSEd

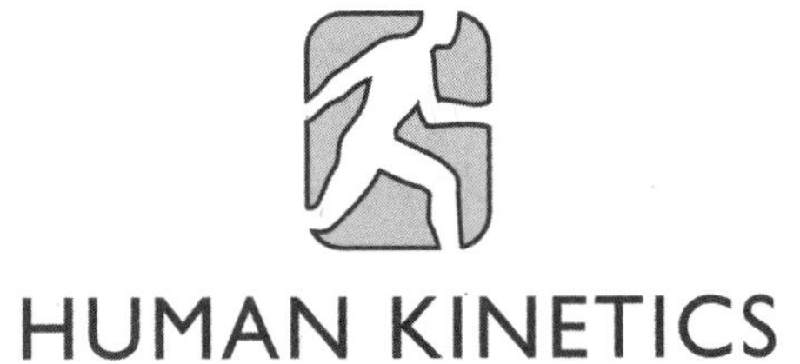

Library of Congress Cataloging-in-Publication Data

Names: Greenberg, Jayne Debra, author. | Calkins, Nichole D., 1979- author. | Spinosa, Lisa S., 1962- author.
Title: Designing and teaching fitness education courses / Jayne D. Greenberg, Nichole D. Calkins, Lisa S. Spinosa.
Description: Champaign, IL : Human Kinetics, Inc., 2022. | Includes bibliographical references and index.
Identifiers: LCCN 2021011726 (print) | LCCN 2021011727 (ebook) | ISBN 9781718200265 (paperback) | ISBN 9781718200272 (epub) | ISBN 9781718200289 (pdf)
Subjects: LCSH: Physical education and training--Study and teaching. | Physical education and training--Curricula.
Classification: LCC GV361 .G735 2022 (print) | LCC GV361 (ebook) | DDC 796.071--dc23
LC record available at https://lccn.loc.gov/2021011726
LC ebook record available at https://lccn.loc.gov/2021011727

ISBN: 978-1-7182-0026-5 (print)

Acquisitions Editor: Scott Wikgren; **Developmental Editor:** Jacqueline Eaton Blakley; **Managing Editor:** Anne E. Mrozek; **Copyeditor:** Amy Pavelich; **Proofreader:** Leigh Keylock; **Indexer:** Nancy Ball; **Permissions Manager:** Dalene Reeder; **Graphic Designer:** Denise Lowry; **Cover Designer:** Keri Evans; **Cover Design Specialist:** Susan Rothermel Allen; **Photograph (cover):** Danny Palomba; **Photographs (interior):** Photos in chapters 9-14, courtesy of Danny Palomba, except for photos on p. 215 (bottom), p. 216 (top), p. 219 (top L, middle L), p. 221 (bottom), p. 232 (middle), p. 234 (bottom), p. 235 (top L, bottom), and p. 237 (bottom), which are courtesy of Nichole Calkins; figures 2.4, 7.7, 7.12, and 7.13, courtesy of Jayne Greenberg; chapter 1 photo and figures 7.6, 7.11, and 8.5, copyright Human Kinetics; figures 7.8-7.10, courtesy of Nichole Calkins; other photos as noted in text; **Photo Asset Manager:** Laura Fitch; **Photo Production Manager:** Jason Allen; **Senior Art Manager:** Kelly Hendren; **Illustrations:** © Human Kinetics, unless otherwise noted; **Printer:** Sheridan Books

Printed in the United States of America 10 9 8 7 6 5 4 3 2 1

The paper in this book is certified under a sustainable forestry program.

Human Kinetics
1607 N. Market Street
Champaign, IL 61820
USA

United States and International
Website: **US.HumanKinetics.com**
Email: info@hkusa.com
Phone: 1-800-747-4457

Canada
Website: **Canada.HumanKinetics.com**
Email: info@hkcanada.com

E8171

CONTENTS

PREFACE

Fitness education teaches students the knowledge, skills, and values needed to benefit from a physically active lifestyle and is critical to the health and well-being of all students. Therefore, it is an integral component of every quality physical education program. However, as important as fitness education is to overall student development and achievement of physical literacy, there are many barriers to successful implementation, such as large classes, lack of equipment, access to the weight room, and professional development. Additionally, some teachers find it challenging to incorporate fitness instruction into the already crowded class time dedicated predominately to sport and movement skill instruction and development. To provide assistance and solutions to these real-life issues, this book provides physical education teachers with innovative ideas, ready-to-use teacher and student resources, and instructional strategies for implementing effective fitness education courses.

The approach of this book is to provide fitness instruction activities that are appropriate for all students enrolled in physical education, which is embedded in all sports, rather than sport-specific fitness instruction. The thought process behind this approach is that the fit student can participate in a variety of activities at an overall higher level of proficiency, and, best of all, the activities and exercises presented require *no equipment*. For the physical education student, this approach will also lead to feelings of elevated health and wellness in hopes of leading healthy and fit lifestyles and adhering to participation in lifelong activities.

The authors and contributors to this book have a vast array of combined experiences, including teaching at the elementary school, middle school, senior high school, and university and college levels in urban, suburban, and rural settings; serving as a school site administrator; holding physical education administrative positions at the regional and district levels; and holding certification in strength and conditioning and personal training. Drawing on our experience as teachers and administrators, we are excited to present innovative ideas and practical scenarios that work in diverse settings and various class sizes. Thus, the reader (student or professional) gains both the theory and practical application behind implementing an innovative, quality fitness education program as part of their overall physical education curriculum.

This book is divided into three major sections, each representing a major component inherent in fitness education programs. Since many physical education teachers integrate fitness education into their general physical education instructional standards, this book is intended to delineate the components inherent in a quality and effective fitness education program.

Part I, *Foundations of Fitness Education*, includes seven chapters and takes a theoretical look at fitness education while presenting practical and necessary content knowledge describing what fitness education is; the importance of fitness education in a comprehensive, standards-based physical education curriculum; pedagogical considerations; nutrition; wellness; consumer issues; and the general components of fitness education—all of which enable the physical education teacher to achieve the goals and objectives of the physical education program directly affecting student learning. Through the lens of the *personal side of fitness education*, we further take a deep dive into the factors that address social and emotional learning; behavior modification principles and adherence to fitness activities; Social Cognitive Theory; classroom management issues; student safety; and equity, diversity, inclusion, and social justice.

Part II, *Fitness Elements and Lesson Plans*, focuses on the various components of fitness education: flexibility, muscular strength and endurance, and cardiorespiratory fitness. Each fitness component includes specific chapters that comprise overall instruction followed by *upper-body, core*, and *lower-body activities* that support and produce student-learning outcomes. The inclusion of anatomical figures illustrating the activity, along with student photos, videos, routines, and circuits, will provide for complete, easy to implement lesson plans for each activity. The flow of each chapter enables a systemic process of planning, designing, and implementing a quality standards-based instructional fitness education program.

Part III, *Extending Fitness Education*, was designed as an extension to the physical education program, enabling students to participate in community-wide fitness and activity events. This provides students an opportunity to transition from class to community events which will further support the development of lifelong fitness habits. Training progressions are recommended for the students to challenge themselves to participate in local fun runs, the one-mile, 5K runs, or even half and full marathons. The book concludes with pacing guides for semester planning, which assist teachers in mapping out the topics and content to ensure that all components, goals, standards, and outcomes are achieved by the end of the semester, as well as to ensure curricular continuity in school districts where there is a high mobility rate.

It should be noted that, throughout this book, all activities are aligned with the National Standards in Physical Education and Grade-Level Outcomes. Emphasis is placed on program development, how to plan for the essential components of a fitness education program, how to align the fitness education instructional program with the overall strategic initiatives of your physical education program, and how the school environment can serve as the hub of a Comprehensive School Physical Activity Program and the Whole School, Whole Community, Whole Child.

In addition to the content just outlined, we have included a variety of lesson plans and printable handouts online in HK*Propel* to assist in expanding your instructional opportunities. Many of these are referred to within the chapters. See the card at the front of the print book for your unique HK*Propel* access code. For ebook users, reference the HK*Propel* access code instructions on the page immediately following the book cover.

We are hopeful that this book and accompanying HK*Propel* resources serve as perpetual resources to provide you with the instructional materials and opportunities to implement a school site fitness education program for secondary school students.

ACKNOWLEDGMENTS

The authors would like to recognize and thank many individuals for their expertise and input during the preparation of this book. Your contributions will have an everlasting impact, through this important work, on providing quality fitness education programs that enable all students to embrace lifelong physical activity habits.

The authors extend a heartfelt thanks to the team at Human Kinetics for their assistance, support, patience, and guidance in making this book possible. In particular, a special thanks is extended to Scott Wikgren, acquisitions editor; Jacqueline Blakley, developmental editor; Amy Pavelich, copyeditor; Anne Mrozek, managing editor; Denise Lowry, graphic designer; Dalene Reeder, permissions manager; and Leigh Keylock, proofreader, for their expertise and attention to detail during the writing, editing, and revision process.

The authors would like to recognize the following individuals for providing guidance, content, and technical support:

- Dr. Michael Marge and Dr. Dorothy Marge, who are scholars, professors, researchers, technical advisors, and strong advocates for improving the health and quality of life of children and adults with disabilities
- Dr. Lauren Lieberman, a distinguished service professor at State University of New York College at Brockport
- Dr. Karen Rickel, the department chair for kinesiology, sport management, and sport and athletic administration at Gonzaga University and a strong advocate for cultural diversity in physical activity and sport opportunities
- Frankie Ruiz, running coach and international race director
- Dr. Jenifer Thorn, the director of the health and human performance program at Keiser University

The authors would like to recognize the teachers from Miami-Dade County Public Schools who provided content, lesson plans, circuits, and routines:

- Sheryl A. Henderson, Palm Springs Middle School
- Cesar Lacasi, Felix Varela Senior High School

The authors wish to thank the following individuals from various educational institutions and community-based organizations for providing models for the photos of fitness activities and exercises, as well as the models themselves who participated in these photo shoots:

- Teresa Skinner for coordinating the athletes from ParaSport Spokane, Dr. Karen Rickel for coordinating the students from Cheney Public and Spokane Public Schools, Alice Busch for coordinating the student from Pride Prep, Stacie Holcomb and Sharon Ruiz for coordinating the students from Trinity Catholic School, and Pete Hanson for coordinating the students from St. Aloysius Gonzaga Catholic School
- Students from Gonzaga University: Alexis Lee, Logan Graves, Reina Rover, Taryn Hilts-Hoskins, Samantha Beeman, Jazmine Redmon, Mia Kline, Neal Calimlim, Jared Jackson, Darcy Woodward, and Gideon Davis
- Athletes from ParaSport Spokane: Jackson Atwood, Hannah Dederick, Elizabeth Floch, Mike Lucas, Sophie Hunter, Bob Hunt, Phillip Croft, Isaiah Rigo, and Amberlynn Weber
- Students from Cheney Public and Spokane Public Schools: Madi Rickel, Skylar Branson, Kennedy Smith, Braxton Hinton, Benjamin Smith, and Carissa Hinton
- Student from Pride Prep: Johanna Schuele-Van Aken
- Students from Trinity Catholic School: Jared Arias, Jonah Keller, Giancarlo Lentes, and Kameron Pitts
- Students from St. Aloysius Gonzaga Catholic School: Karolina Flanagan and Haydin B.
- Students from Independent Schools in Florida: Xavier S., Tiffany S., Anthony S., and Jordan S.

And a very special thank you to Danny Palomba from the Gonzaga University School of Education for being the photographer for all of the photos and videos in chapters 9 through 14.

HOW TO USE HK*PROPEL*

Designing and Teaching Fitness Education Courses includes access to a rich online resource designed to make it easy and straightforward to develop a fitness education course and incorporate fitness education into your physical education program. Full of ready-to-use documents and multimedia content, this resource is an incredibly valuable teaching supplement. Material is organized in a variety of ways to help you find what you need in a way that works for you:

- By book chapter
- By week (following an 18-week course)
- By type of content (videos, PowerPoint presentations, pacing guides, handouts)

See the card at the front of the print book for your unique HK*Propel* access code. For ebook users, reference the HK*Propel* access code instructions on the page immediately following the book cover.

In HK*Propel* you will find all of the following:

- **Video demonstrations and technique photos.** In chapters 9 through 14 of the book, stretches and strength exercises are described and illustrated so that you can lead students to execute them with correct technique. Short video clips in HK*Propel* reinforce correct technique and clearly demonstrate for students how the stretches and exercises should be done.

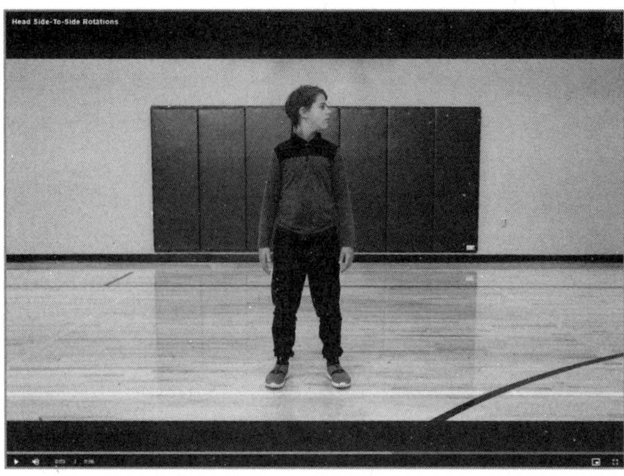

- **Pacing guides.** Chapter 17 of the book includes 18 pacing guides, which show exactly how to integrate fitness education into your curriculum, outlining the following for each week of an 18-week course:
  - Topics and chapters addressed
  - Standards and grade-level outcomes addressed
  - Objectives
  - Class discussion topics
  - Class activities
  - Assessments and student assignments
  - Teaching strategies and tips
  - Instructional tools
  - Vocabulary
  - Online resources

  Each week's pacing guide is available in chapter 17 of the book and in HK*Propel*, and a template is included that you can download and customize for your own class.

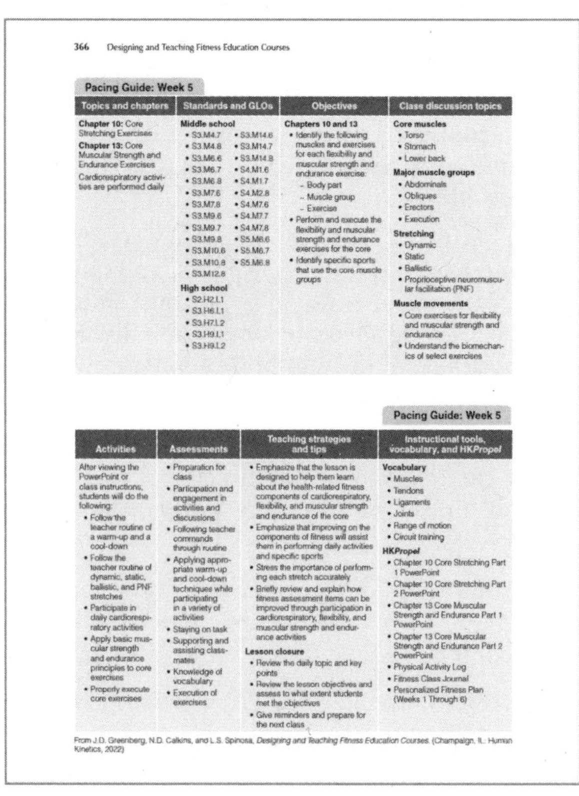

366 Designing and Teaching Fitness Education Courses

Pacing Guide: Week 5

Topics and chapters	Standards and GLOs	Objectives	Class discussion topics
Chapter 10: Core Stretching Exercises **Chapter 13:** Core Muscular Strength and Endurance Exercises Cardiorespiratory activities are performed daily	**Middle school** • S3.M4.7 • S3.M14.6 • S3.M4.8 • S3.M14.7 • S3.M6.6 • S3.M14.8 • S3.M6.7 • S4.M1.6 • S3.M6.8 • S4.M1.7 • S3.M7.6 • S4.M2.8 • S3.M7.8 • S4.M7.6 • S3.M9.6 • S4.M7.7 • S3.M9.7 • S4.M7.8 • S3.M9.8 • S5.M6.6 • S3.M10.6 • S5.M6.7 • S3.M10.8 • S5.M6.8 • S3.M12.8 **High school** • S2.H2.L1 • S3.H6.L1 • S3.H7.L2 • S3.H9.L1 • S3.H9.L2	**Chapters 10 and 13** • Identify the following muscles and exercises for each flexibility and muscular strength and endurance exercise: – Body part – Muscle group – Exercise • Perform and execute the flexibility and muscular strength and endurance exercises for the core • Identify specific sports that use the core muscle groups	**Core muscles** • Torso • Stomach • Lower back **Major muscle groups** • Abdominals • Obliques • Erectors • Execution **Stretching** • Dynamic • Static • Ballistic • Proprioceptive neuromuscular facilitation (PNF) **Muscle movements** • Core exercises for flexibility and muscular strength and endurance • Understand the biomechanics of select exercises

Pacing Guide: Week 5

Activities	Assessments	Teaching strategies and tips	Instructional tools, vocabulary, and HK*Propel*
After viewing the PowerPoint or class instructions, students will do the following: • Follow the teacher routine of a warm-up and a cool-down • Follow the teacher routine of dynamic, static, ballistic, and PNF stretches • Participate in daily cardiorespiratory activities • Apply basic muscular strength and endurance principles to core exercises • Properly execute core exercises	• Preparation for class • Participation and engagement in activities and discussions • Following teacher commands through routine • Applying appropriate warm-up and cool-down techniques while participating in a variety of activities • Staying on task • Supporting and assisting classmates • Knowledge of vocabulary • Execution of exercises	• Emphasize that the lesson is designed to help them learn about the health-related fitness components of cardiorespiratory, flexibility, and muscular strength and endurance of the core • Emphasize that improving on the components of fitness will assist them in performing daily activities and specific sports • Stress the importance of performing each stretch accurately • Briefly review and explain how fitness assessment items can be improved through participation in cardiorespiratory, flexibility, and muscular strength and endurance activities **Lesson closure** • Review the daily topic and key points • Review the lesson objectives and assess to what extent students met the objectives • Give reminders and prepare for the next class	**Vocabulary** • Muscles • Tendons • Ligaments • Joints • Range of motion • Circuit training **HK*Propel*** • Chapter 10 Core Stretching Part 1 PowerPoint • Chapter 10 Core Stretching Part 2 PowerPoint • Chapter 13 Core Muscular Strength and Endurance Part 1 PowerPoint • Chapter 13 Core Muscular Strength and Endurance Part 2 PowerPoint • Physical Activity Log • Fitness Class Journal • Personalized Fitness Plan (Weeks 1 Through 6)

From J.D. Greenberg, N.D. Calkins, and L.S. Spinosa, *Designing and Teaching Fitness Education Courses*. (Champaign, IL: Human Kinetics, 2022)

• **Reproducible forms.** Fifty-seven handouts—assessments, worksheets, rubrics, assignments, and more—are ready to use in your class. Download and print any of these forms as needed.

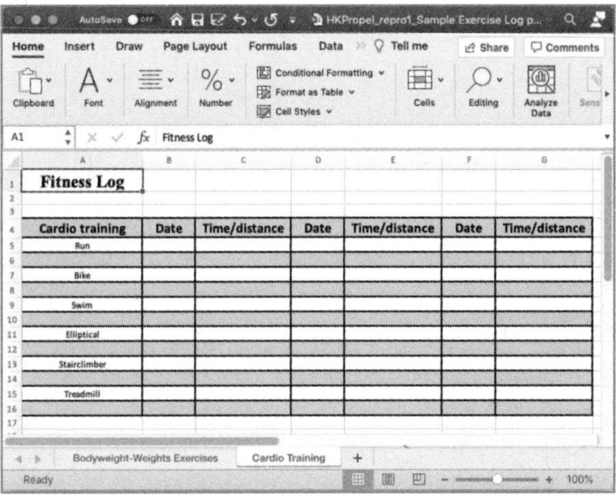

Purpose: To assess the class climate in order to determine the current state of motivation, respect, engagement, and sense of belonging in this class. This survey helps the teacher understand wh

have the most

Directions: Th

how you feel a

between teache

you feel when

you feel about

Reflection

1. What is

2. What c

positive learnin

Class Climate Survey

Name: ____________ **Class Period:** ______ **Date:** _______

1	In this class, how often do you feel a positive energy to learn and engage?	Almost never	Once in a while	Sometimes	Frequently	Almost always
2	How often are you excited to participate in activities in this class?	Almost never	Once in a while	Sometimes	Frequently	Almost always
3	In this class, how often does the behavior of other students **hurt or negatively** impact your learning?	Almost never	Once in a while	Sometimes	Frequently	Almost always
4	How often are students respectful to each other in this class?	Almost never	Once in a while	Sometimes	Frequently	Almost always
5	How often do you feel like you belong in this class?	Almost never	Once in a while	Sometimes	Frequently	Almost always
6	How often do others encourage you to do your best in this class?	Almost never	Once in a while	Sometimes	Frequently	Almost always
7	In this class, how often do you worry about being embarrassed or judged by others?	Almost never	Once in a while	Sometimes	Frequently	Almost always

• **PowerPoint presentations.** Twenty-four PowerPoint presentations are available to help you as you teach the content of this book's chapters. The presentations also include book illustrations, photos, and links to streaming videos to help students understand concepts and techniques.

A Guided Fitness Goal

- When setting a SMART fitness goal, you want to consider how long you have to train.
- The number of weeks you have to train determines all the other factors in the SMART framework.
- Consider how much improvement is physically possible in the total number of training weeks.

Time-bound: I have ______ weeks to train before the next fitness assessment. My current fitness assessment score is: ________.

Realistic: I am writing a realistic goal based upon the amount of improvement that I could expect if I gave 100% effort on my pretest, if I follow the principles of training, and if I commit to engaging in the recommended FITT prescription for the fitness component I have selected. It is realistic for me to improve my score by ______ in ____ weeks of training.

Part I

Foundations of Fitness Education

CHAPTER 1

Introduction to Fitness Education

Chapter Objective

After reading this chapter, you will be able to describe what fitness education is and why it is an essential component in a physical education program. You will understand why promoting lifelong physical activity is a priority for adolescents and a major public health concern, know how to implement fitness education in any secondary school physical education course, and be able to assist students in understanding the importance of being physically active for their life span.

Key Concepts

- Regular physical activity prevents numerous chronic diseases and enhances social, emotional, physical, and mental well-being.
- Fitness education is an inclusive, evidence-based, standards-based curriculum and instructional approach that focuses on teaching the knowledge, skills, and values that lead to lifelong health and fitness.
- Fitness education emphasizes college or career readiness through the promotion of lifetime physical activity.
- A three-step backward design approach can be used to plan fitness education learning experiences.

INTRODUCTION

Regular physical activity during adolescence provides numerous immediate and long-term health benefits. For children and adolescents aged 6 to 17 years, the recommended physical activity guidelines consist of participating in 60 minutes or more of moderate- to vigorous-intensity physical activity every day and then at least three days per week doing muscle-strengthening and bone-strengthening activities (Centers for Disease Control and Prevention, 2020; U.S. Department of Health and Human Services, 2018). Unfortunately, most adolescents are not moving enough to experience the physical, mental, and social and emotional health benefits of regular physical activity. An estimated 80 percent of adolescents aged 11 to 17 years do not meet the recommended 60 minutes of daily physical activity, compromising their current and future health (Guthold, Stevens, Riley, & Bull, 2019). Worldwide, physical inactivity has been identified as a leading risk factor for premature death as it increases the risk of cancer, heart disease, stroke, and diabetes by 20-30% (World Health Organization, 2021). Youth who do not engage in sufficient levels of physical activity are at a greater risk for prematurely developing type 2 diabetes, cardiovascular disease, osteoporosis, and certain types of cancers (Hruby & Hu, 2015; Reilly & Kelly, 2011). Chronic disease risk factors such as obesity, high blood pressure, and metabolic syndrome start developing in childhood (Hallal, Victoria, Azevedo, & Wells, 2006). Since adolescent physical activity behaviors typically track into adulthood, establishing healthy physical activity behaviors during childhood and adolescence is an effective way to prevent chronic diseases.

The prevalence of youth physical inactivity and obesity pose serious implications for future public health by placing a substantial burden on health care systems (Sanyaolu et al., 2019). Both the health and academic benefits students gain from a quality physical education program have long been established. Cardiovascular diseases are the leading cause of death worldwide: A person dies from heart disease roughly every 37 seconds in the United States (Centers for Disease Control and Prevention, 2020). The average age of a first heart

Benefits of Regular Physical Activity for Adolescents

Physical Benefits

- Improved sleeping habits, increased energy to perform everyday activities (Master et al., 2019)
- Maintaining a healthy weight, reduced risk for obesity (Sanyaolu, Okorie, Qi, Locke, & Rehman, 2019)
- Improved cardiorespiratory fitness, muscular fitness, and bone health that reduces future risk for developing chronic diseases like heart disease, type 2 diabetes, osteoporosis, and cancer (Booth, Roberts, & Laye, 2012)

Mental and Academic Benefits

- Improved brain functioning and cognitive ability (e.g., attention, memory, and information processing) (Donnelly, Hillman, Castelli, Etnier, Lee, Tomporowski, Lambourne, & Szabo-Reed, 2016; Logan, Raine, Drollette, Castelli, Khan, Kramer, & Hillman, 2020)
- More positive academic behaviors such as enhanced memory, on-task behavior, attention control, faster task performance, and greater academic achievement (Budde et al., 2008; Centers for Disease Control and Prevention, 2010; Fedewa & Ahn, 2011; Chaddock-Heyman, Erickson, Voss, Knecht, Pontifex, Castelli, Hillman, & Kramer, 2013; Hillman et al., 2014; Donnelly et al., 2016; Logan et al., 2020)

Social and Emotional Benefits

- Fewer symptoms of anxiety and depression (Philippot, Meerschaut, Danneaux, Smal, Bleyenheuft, & De Volder, 2019)
- More effectively managing and tolerating stress (Bland, Melton, Bigham, & Welle, 2014)
- Better self-esteem (Ahmed, Walter, Rudolph, Morris, Elayaraja, Lee, & Randles, 2017)

attack is 65 for men and 72 for women, but it has become much more common over the last 10 years for individuals under the age of 40 to suffer a heart attack due to poor lifestyle choices in adolescence and early adulthood (American College of Cardiology, 2019). The risk of early onset heart disease increases substantially if an individual has poor cardiorespiratory fitness, is obese, and engages in very little physical activity from age 15 to age 30, as that is an accumulation of 15 years of excessive workload on a poor-conditioned heart. Regular physical activity and maintaining an appropriate weight are necessary to support the long-term health of the body systems, specifically the cardiovascular system. In addition, physical activity provides immediate mental and emotional benefits, such as improved brain functioning and reduced anxiety.

More health benefits can be accrued when adolescents consistently engage in specific forms of activity at sufficient intensities and durations. School-based physical education plays an imperative role in the effort to increase youth physical activity, as it is the only sure opportunity for the majority of school-aged youth to both learn about and engage in physical activity (Institute of Medicine, 2013). Physical education is an academic subject that teaches the knowledge and skills to engage in physical activity and exercise while also providing opportunities for students to perform physical activity and exercise. *Physical activity* is defined as "any bodily movement that is produced by the contraction of skeletal muscle and that substantially increases energy expenditure" (Centers for Disease Control and Prevention, 2017). *Exercise* is "a type of physical activity that involves planned, structured, and repetitive bodily movement done to maintain or improve one or more components of physical fitness" (Centers for Disease Control and Prevention, 2017). Physical activity includes exercise as well as other movement activities, such as playing recreational sports or games, working, traveling on foot or bicycle, and doing household chores (see figure 1.1). Knowing what type of activity, how intensely to be active, and how long to exercise to accrue the benefits is a function of physical education, specifically fitness education.

Fitness education, a component of a physical education program, teaches students the knowledge and skills needed to benefit from a physically active lifestyle. This chapter describes what fitness education is, why it is a necessary part of physical education, and how to implement it in a secondary physical education program.

PHYSICAL EDUCATION AND FITNESS EDUCATION: WHAT IS THE DIFFERENCE?

Goals, objectives, and outcomes describe the purpose of programs and help educators develop meaningful learning experiences for students. In education, we use goals, objectives, and outcomes to plan what to teach and what to assess to determine the success of the program. Figure 1.2 illustrates the differences between goals, objectives, and outcomes. *Goals* describe what the program intends to do. They typically are broad statements that provide a general direction and the expected long-term effects. *Objectives* specify how to accomplish the program goals by describing what will be taught in the program. They tend to be teacher-focused statements that detail what the instructor intends for students to learn in the course. *Student learning outcomes (SLOs)* are learner-focused statements that describe what the students will be able to do at the end of the program. SLOs are observable, measurable, and written in student-friendly language so that students understand what is expected of them. SLOs can be written as course outcomes, project outcomes, or unit outcomes. Physical education and fitness education programs share a similar goal—to develop individuals who engage in a lifetime of physical activity—but fitness education has more

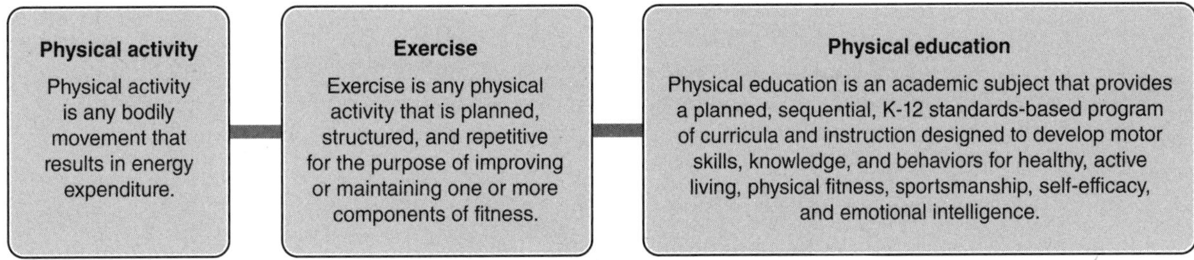

Figure 1.1 Defining physical activity, exercise, and physical education.

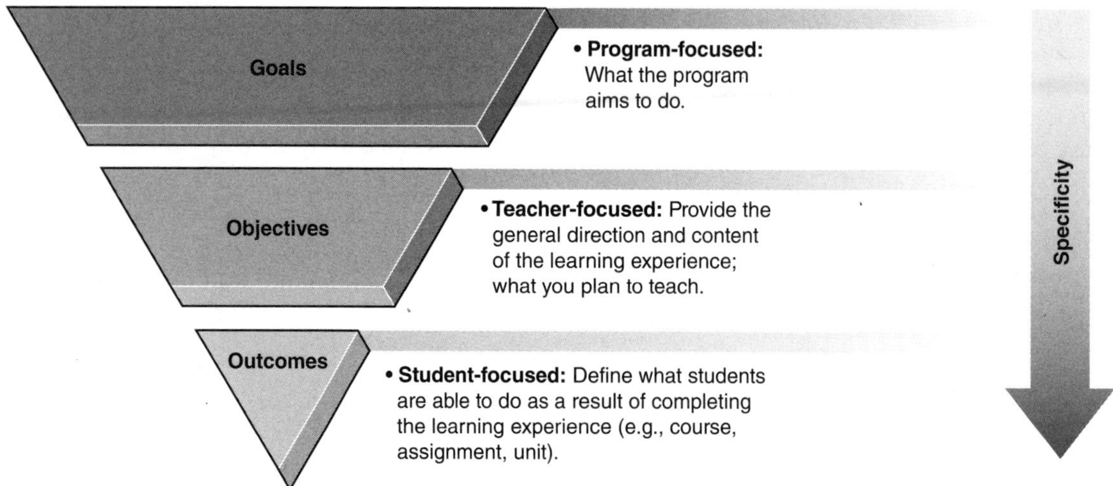

Figure 1.2 Program goals, objectives, and outcomes.
Adapted by permission from DePaul University. Teaching Commons https://resources.depaul.edu/teaching-commons/teaching-guides/course-design/Pages/course-objectives-learning-outcomes.aspx. Permission Granted: Joseph Oliver, DePaul University.

specific objectives and outcomes related to one part of a physical education program.

Physical Education

A physical education program provides students with learning experiences to develop motor skills, knowledge, and behaviors for healthy active living, physical fitness, appropriate sports behavior, self-efficacy, and emotional intelligence (SHAPE America, 2015). Its primary goal is to develop physically literate students who have the competence, confidence, and desire to engage in physical activity for a lifetime (SHAPE America, 2014). *Physical literacy* is defined as "the ability to move with competence and confidence in a wide variety of physical activities in multiple environments that benefit the healthy development of the whole person" (Mandigo, Francis, Lodewyk, & Lopez, 2012). The National Standards for K-12 Physical Education (see The National Standards for K-12 Physical Education sidebar) and their accompanying *grade-level outcomes (GLOs)* provide a framework of what to teach in a physical education program to produce physically literate individuals. These standards describe what students should know and be able to do as a result of participating in a physical education program. These standards are objectives for a comprehensive physical education program, as they describe the subject matter content and skills that teachers intend to cover. The GLOs that accompany each standard are SLOs that define age appropriate and developmentally appropriate outcomes for students to demonstrate their achievement of the standards.

The National Standards for K-12 Physical Education

- *Standard 1.* The physically literate individual demonstrates competency in a variety of motor skills and movement patterns.
- *Standard 2.* The physically literate individual applies knowledge of concepts, principles, strategies, and tactics related to movement and performance.
- *Standard 3.* The physically literate individual demonstrates the knowledge and skills to achieve and maintain a health-enhancing level of physical activity and fitness.
- *Standard 4.* The physically literate individual exhibits responsible personal and social behavior that respects self and others.
- *Standard 5.* The physically literate individual recognizes the value of physical activity for health, enjoyment, challenge, self-expression, and/or social interaction.

Physical education is the process through which sport, fitness, outdoor pursuits, dance, aquatics, games, and gymnastics are used by physical educators to teach students how to be physically active. *Physical education* is an umbrella term that can be further broken down into different components: sport education, fitness education, personal and social responsibility education, movement education, and outdoor education (Greenberg & LoBianco, 2020). A comprehensive physical education program will provide students with opportunities to learn how to engage in a variety of physical activities and the components of physical education. Each physical education component has different pedagogical approaches or curriculum models to guide its curriculum and instruction. Physical education *curriculum models* are theme-based frameworks with distinct characteristics that help educators organize content into meaningful patterns to deliver coherent instruction. These models identify how specific objectives and learning outcomes can best be achieved through aligning objectives, content, physical activities, and teaching methods (Kirk, 2013). As you can see in table 1.1, curriculum models can guide the design of physical education curriculum by organizing learning experiences around specific objectives. Each curriculum model also emphasizes the learning associated with some standards more than others. Table 1.1 lists only a few of the physical education curriculum models to show that a physical education program comprises different types of learning experiences.

Fitness Education

Fitness education is a component of a comprehensive physical education program and a curriculum model that focuses on teaching students how and why to achieve and maintain good health-related physical fitness (SHAPE America, 2017). The goal of fitness education is to help students acquire the knowledge, skills, and values necessary to adopt a physically active lifestyle and to develop physical activity habits and other healthy lifestyle behaviors that lead to health and wellness (SHAPE America, 2012).

Figure 1.3 shows the content objectives that specify what will be taught in a fitness education program. Although the objectives of fitness education encompass all of the five National Standards for K-12 Physical Education, it is predominantly

Table 1.1 Physical Education Component Curriculum Models and Objectives

Curriculum model	Emphasized standard and sample program objectives	Sample textbook resources
Fitness education	Emphasized standard: 3 • Develop physical competency to be able to perform moderate-to-vigorous physical activity. • Acquire an understanding of the health-related components of fitness and the relationship of fitness to health.	Corbin, C., LeMauier, G., & Lambdin, D. (2014). *Fitness for life middle school* (2nd ed.). Champaign, IL: Human Kinetics. Corbin, C.B., Castelli, D.M., Sibley, B.A., & Le Masurier, G.C. (2022). *Fitness for life* (7th ed.). Champaign, IL: Human Kinetics.
Outdoor education	Emphasized standard: 1 • Develop an understanding of ecological processes. • Develop physical competence in outdoor activities that take place in the natural environment, such as fishing, hiking, backpacking, and stand-up paddle boarding.	Gilbertson, K., Bates, T., McLaugling, T., & Ewert, A. (2006). *Outdoor education: Methods and strategies.* Champaign, IL: Human Kinetics.
Personal and social responsibility education	Emphasized standard: 4 • Take responsibility for personal well-being and for supporting the well-being of others. • Value respect, effort, cooperation, and helping others.	Hellison, D. (2011). *Teaching personal and social responsibility through physical activity* (3rd ed.). Champaign, IL: Human Kinetics.
Sport education	Emphasized standard: 2 • Develop physical competency to execute motor skills in game situations. • Develop game sense: the knowledge of using technical and tactical skills during game-play. • Value the culture and contributions of sport.	Siedentop, D., Hastie, P., & van der Mars, H. (2020). *Complete guide to sport education* (3rd ed.). Champaign, IL: Human Kinetics.

centered on the mastery of National Standards 3 and 5, as those standards most directly relate to developing knowledge and skills, while 1, 2, and 4 emphasize the skills and strategies that students can use in achieving and maintaining health-enhancing fitness levels. Fitness education is characterized by a curricular and instructional approach that

- teaches a conceptual understanding of health-related fitness,
- provides opportunities for students to engage in lifetime physical activity during class time, and
- helps students develop self-management skills to maintain healthy behaviors (SHAPE America, 2012).

Fitness education is more than getting students fit through the performance of fitness activities like running on the track, doing push-ups, or conducting fitness assessments. It includes an educational component that connects physical activity to health-related outcomes—essentially teaching a cause-and-effect relationship of regular physical activity and good health. A comprehensive scope of fitness education concepts can be found in a guidance document published by SHAPE America titled *Instructional Framework for Fitness Education in Physical Education*. This document provides a framework to develop fitness education curriculum, as it defines the subject matter that has been identified as the essential knowledge and skills to include in fitness education. It also includes learning benchmarks for specific grade levels to help you understand if your students are developing the knowledge and skills they need to achieve lifelong physical activity. The Instructional Framework for Fitness Education sidebar shows the domains and subdomains from the guidance document highlighted as key curricular components that identify what to teach in fitness education.

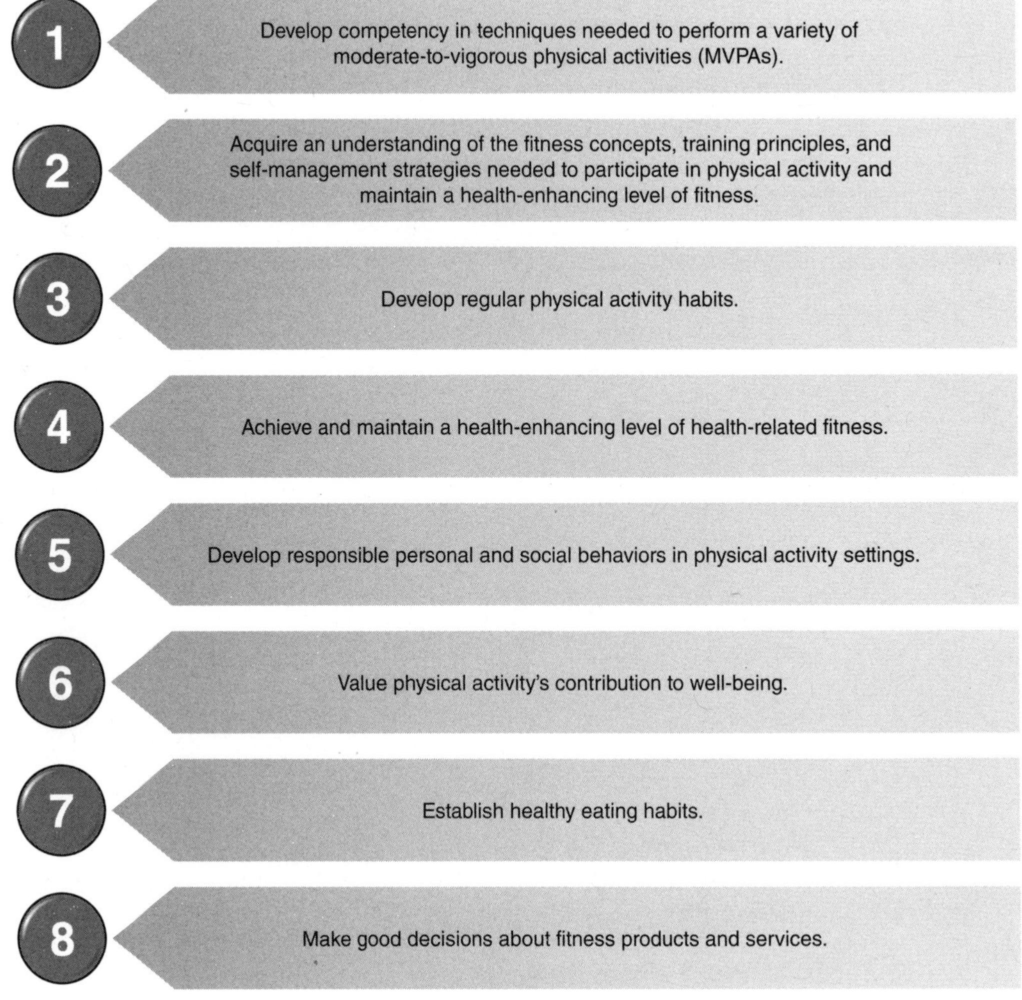

Figure 1.3 Fitness education program objectives.
Based on SHAPE America (2012).

Instructional Framework for Fitness Education

Technique. Demonstrate competency in techniques needed to perform a variety of moderate-to-vigorous physical activities (MVPAs).

- Technique in developing cardiovascular fitness
- Technique when developing muscle strength and endurance activities
- Technique in developing flexibility
- Safety techniques

Knowledge. Demonstrate understanding of fitness concepts, principles, strategies, and individual differences needed to participate in and maintain a health-enhancing level of fitness.

- Benefits of physical activity and dangers of physical inactivity
- Basic anatomy and physiology
- Physiological responses to physical activity
- Components of health-related fitness
- Training principles (overload, specificity, progression) and workout elements
- Application of the FITT (frequency, intensity, time, type) principle
- Factors that influence physical activity choices

Physical activity. Participate regularly in fitness-enhancing physical activity.

- Physical activity participation (e.g., aerobic, muscle strength and endurance, bone strength, flexibility, enjoyment [social and personal], meaning)
- Create an individualized physical activity plan
- Self-monitor physical activity and adhere to a physical activity plan

Health-related fitness. Achieve and maintain a health-enhancing level of health-related fitness.

- Physical fitness assessment (including self-assessment) and analysis
- Set goals and create a fitness improvement plan
- Work to improve fitness components
- Self-monitor and adjust plan
- Achieve goals

Responsible personal and social behaviors. Exhibit responsible personal and social behaviors in physical activity settings.

- Social interaction and respecting differences
- Self-management
- Personal strategies to manage body weight
- Stress management

Values and advocates. Value fitness-enhancing physical activity for disease prevention, enjoyment, challenge, self-expression, self-efficacy, and social interaction and allocate energies toward the production of healthy environments.

- Value physical activity
- Advocacy
- Fitness careers
- Occupational fitness needs

Nutrition. Strive to maintain a healthy diet through knowledge, planning, and regular monitoring.

- Basic nutrition and benefits of a healthy diet
- Healthy diet recommendations
- Diet assessment
- Plan and maintain a healthy diet

Consumerism. Access and evaluate fitness information, facilities, products, and services.

- Differentiate between fact and fiction regarding fitness products
- Make good decisions about consumer products

(SHAPE America, 2012)

WHY FITNESS EDUCATION?

Over the past 40 years, more physical education programs have started implementing fitness education, especially with the introduction of the Comprehensive School Physical Activity Program (CSPAP) as a national framework for physical activity and physical education in schools (Corbin, Kulinna, & Yu, 2020). However, there is still a pressing need to increase access to high-quality fitness education in secondary schools (Raghuveer, Hartz, Lubans, Takken, Wiltz, Mietus-Snyder, Perak, Baker-Smith, Pietris, & Edwards, 2020). This is evidenced by factors such as the low physical activity rates among youth, high obesity rates, and the inadequate health-related fitness knowledge that secondary students possess (Williams, Phelps, Laurson, Thomas, & Brown, 2013). Physical activity habits, healthy body composition, and healthy cardiorespiratory fitness are all by-products of health-related fitness knowledge (Thompson & Hannon, 2012; Williams et al., 2013). It is apparent that our youth are not receiving the learning experiences needed to develop the knowledge to improve their health and fitness. In most secondary physical education programs in the United States, a traditional multi-activity, sport-based approach to delivering physical education continues to dominate (Ennis 2014). The multi-activity approach has a one-size-fits-all philosophy and focuses almost exclusively on developing sports-based skills for a variety of sport activities (Kirk, 2013). Also termed *exposure curriculum*, this model favors breadth over depth so that students develop a basic understanding of the different skills and rules associated with multiple sports. The activities selected in this approach typically are based upon teacher preferences, class size, and equipment availability. Although there are many positive benefits to a sport education curriculum (Siedentop, Hastie, & van der Mars, 2019), unless combined with fitness education, it does not directly address overall health-related fitness or lifestyle behaviors.

Unfortunately, in some instances, this teaching approach appears to contribute to negative attitudes toward physical education and physical activity, specifically for less-skilled students who are embarrassed by their lack of competence (Bernstein, Phillips, & Silverman, 2011; Capel & Blair, 2007). Students will disengage in physical education class if they are not interested in the sports taught and most likely will not develop a physically active lifestyle, as they are unable to make any connections between their physical education experience and regular physical activity habits. Educators should avoid using a multi-activity approach and instead use a multi-model approach to physical education (Quay & Peters, 2008). *Multi-model* means that teachers use more than one curriculum model to deliver a physical education program. The models presented in table 1.1 have defined pedagogical approaches that intentionally influence a student's learning experience around a central theme. Several reasons for including fitness education as a primary component in secondary physical education are presented next.

Fitness Education Is for Everyone

A philosophy that guides the curricular and instructional choices in fitness education is the HELP philosophy: Health for Everyone for a Lifetime in a Personal Way (Corbin, Kulinna, & Sibley, 2020). The implication for physical education teachers is to focus on helping every student achieve health-related fitness through activities that are matched to their needs. Fitness education is for everyone regardless of age, gender, ethnicity, skill level, ability, disability, or cultural background. In fact, fitness education is necessary for everyone to understand how they can develop a healthy lifestyle that leads to attaining health-enhancing fitness and numerous health benefits.

Students with disabilities need quality fitness education to enhance their ability to function independently and reduce their risk for obesity and associated diseases. Individuals with disabilities are four times more likely to develop health-related conditions, such as obesity, heart disease, stroke, and diabetes, due to a lack of physical activity (Yun & Beamer, 2018). Children and adolescents with disabilities tend to participate in significantly fewer skills-based physical activities, such as sports-oriented lessons or participation on sports teams, compared to peers without disabilities, which further limits their opportunities for activity (Ross, Smit, Yun, Bogart, Hatfield, & Logan, 2020). Fitness education provides students with disabilities the resources for continual participation in health-enhancing activity because its central goal is to *HELP* students learn how to achieve health-enhancing fitness in a personalized way. The fitness activities in part II describe modifications and accommodations for students with disabilities or any student who is unable to perform the activity as described.

Youth athletes who regularly participate in sports are also in need of fitness education. Recent research has stated that many youth athletes, specifically males, have poor health-related fitness levels, as compared to the general population, and are at increased risk for sports injury, health issues, and decreased sports performance (Pfeifer, Sacko, Ortaglia, Monsma, Beattie, Goins, & Stodden, 2019). A common assumption is that sports practices provide enough physical activity for students to attain the benefits of health-related fitness, but that assumption appears to be inaccurate, as 44 percent of male athletes and 37 percent of female athletes do not meet the minimum health standards for cardiorespiratory fitness, and 50 percent of male athletes and 22 percent of female athletes do not meet the minimum health standards for muscular endurance (Pfeifer et al., 2019). The knowledge and skills necessary for attaining health-related fitness are not by-products of participating in sports; they must be intentionally taught and developed through fitness education learning experiences.

Fitness Education Is Evidence Based

Using evidence based methods means identifying the best available research and combining it with other factors (e.g., knowledge of students, engaging methods, cultural competency) to deliver the best possible education for students. Effective physical educators use curricula, resources, and strategies that have demonstrated the ability to achieve positive outcomes. Research has shown that fitness education can increase physical activity during class time and positively affect physical activity behaviors into adulthood (Kulinna, Corbin, & Yu, 2018; Lonsdale, Rosenkranz, Peralta, Bennie, Fahey, & Lubans, 2013).

What is considered usual teaching practice in physical education is best described by skill development and game-play (Lonsdale et al., 2013). Historically, physical education has been skill-and-drill instruction and practice for various sports followed by competitive games. Many physical education teachers have realized that this type of instruction is not working for many of their students and have attempted other types of instruction to increase engagement in physical activity during class time. A review and meta-analysis of 13 physical education interventions found that 24 percent more active learning time occurred for students when teachers made a deliberate attempt to increase the time spent in moderate-to-vigorous physical activity (MVPA) (Lonsdale et al., 2013). Some interventions used fitness education teaching strategies (e.g., activity selection, class organization, and instructional practices) to increase MVPA, and others infused fitness activities by supplementing lessons with more intense activities. Increasing MVPA in physical education offers the greatest potential for increasing students' physical, mental, social, and emotional health benefits. When you intentionally select activities and design learning tasks that promote MVPA, you are helping students to develop health-enhancing fitness.

Kulinna et al. (2018) investigated the physical activity habits of adults who participated in a yearlong fitness education course that emphasized the conceptual understanding of health-related fitness and physical activity and found that 68 percent of females and 86 percent of males were meeting the national guidelines for MVPA 20 years after graduation, compared to a nationally representative sample in which only 50 percent of females and 52 percent of males met the MVPA guidelines. Also, no males and 5 percent of females from the conceptual physical education (CPE) course reported being physically inactive, compared to 25 percent and 27 percent of the representative sample. In addition,

> about 56% of respondents indicated that they remembered content from the class, 50% indicated that they still used the information, 47% indicated that they found the class useful after graduation, and 92% indicated that they currently consider themselves to be well informed about fitness and physical activity. (Kulinna et al., 2018, p. 929)

Adults who had completed the CPE course in high school were less likely to be inactive and significantly more likely to engage in the recommended levels of MVPA, indicating the value of teaching students the knowledge and skills of lifelong physical activity.

Fitness Education Is Standards Based

Standards-based refers to using established learning standards (national, state, or locally adopted physical education standards) as the academic expectations for the course or grade level. The national physical education standards are founded on motor-development research, which guides educators in designing and delivering age appropriate and developmentally appropriate learning experiences. Some school districts may have a policy that requires curriculum to be standards based as part of an adoption process. Program effectiveness is often determined by students demonstrating competency of the standards. As mentioned previously, the targeted standards in fitness education are as follows (SHAPE America, 2014):

- *Standard 3.* The physically literate individual demonstrates the knowledge and skills to achieve a health-enhancing level of physical activity and fitness.
- *Standard 5.* The physically literate individual recognizes the value of physical activity for health, enjoyment, challenge, self-expression, and/or social interaction.

When educators deliver standards-based curriculum, they are ensuring that students are acquiring the knowledge and skills necessary to develop physically active lifestyles and that instruction is not based on teacher preference. In addition, following fitness education standards means that educators don't just deliver intense exercise sessions and grade students on fitness assessments. The standards emphasize the process of developing a physically active lifestyle, not just the product of physical fitness.

Fitness Education Emphasizes College and Career Readiness

Fitness education prepares students to be college and career ready more than any other component of physical education. College students report that stress is the number one impediment to their academic performance (Frazier, Gabriel, Merians, & Lust, 2019). Stress, anxiety, and depression are the actors that most often hinder a college student's ability to succeed. Therefore, teaching successful stress-management strategies, a component of fitness education, will benefit students' ability to cope with the increased stresses of college life.

In addition, the research on the relationship of health-related fitness and physical activity and worker productivity is mounting. The economic cost associated with poor health and worker productivity is estimated to cost U.S. employers more than US$530 billion each year (Integrated Benefits Institute, 2018). Many companies are investing in worksite wellness programs because studies are showing a direct correlation between healthy, fit workers and increased profits from greater productivity and fewer health care costs (Mattke, Liu, Caloyeras, Huang, Van Busum, Khodyakov, & Shier, 2013). By achieving and maintaining a health-enhancing fitness and physical activity, students improve their occupational productivity, which makes them more career ready.

Addressing the importance of a physically active lifestyle with students in reference to career readiness further provides the physical education teacher with the opportunity to discuss potential careers outside of the sport, health, and wellness industries. Careers that promote a physically active lifestyle across the lifespan include careers in the trades industry, such as construction workers, landscapers, electricians, and pipefitters; careers in the protective services, which include military, law enforcement, firefighters, paramedics, park rangers, and select government agency employees; careers in agriculture, which include farming, livestock, beekeeping; careers in the medical field, including physicians, nurses, orderlies; and careers in the travel industry, including hotel, airport, bus, and rail positions. Table 1.2 shows SHAPE America's benchmarks for grades 6 to 8 and grades 9 to 12 for occupational fitness needs.

Fitness education prepares students to be college or career ready by teaching the knowledge and skills to

- improve brain functioning and cognitive performance through physical activity,
- improve their occupational productivity by achieving and maintaining health-enhancing fitness and physical activity,
- reduce medical costs associated with chronic diseases and health conditions related to physical inactivity,
- employ stress-management techniques, and
- apply personalized strategies that result in enhanced energy by ensuring adequate sleep, meeting nutritional needs, and maintaining a healthy weight.

Through effective fitness education curriculum and instruction, students will gain the confidence and competence to care for their own health and fitness. Quality fitness education experiences will support students' ability to develop physical competence, apply conceptual understanding of health-related fitness, develop a physically active lifestyle, attain and maintain health-related fitness, develop responsible and social behaviors, and establish healthy nutrition and consumer behaviors. Each of these elements of fitness education is important in producing physically literate students who can independently engage in health-enhancing behaviors throughout their life.

Table 1.2 Instructional Framework for Fitness Education in Physical Education: Occupational Fitness Needs

Descriptor	Grades 6-8 benchmark	Grades 9-12 benchmark
Occupational fitness needs	Discuss components of health- and skill-related fitness necessary for successful and safe performance in various occupations.	• Create a fitness/wellness plan for sedentary careers that one could use to maintain health-related fitness. • Analyze components of health- and skill-related fitness necessary for successful and safe performance in various occupations. • Identify questions to ask potential employers about their support of healthy lifestyles.

Based on SHAPE America (2012).

IMPLEMENTING FITNESS EDUCATION

There is no one right way to implement fitness education. The defining features of fitness education include a curricular and instructional approach that

- teaches a conceptual understanding of health-related fitness,
- provides opportunities for students to engage in lifetime physical activity during class time, and
- helps students develop self-management skills to maintain healthy behaviors (SHAPE America, 2012).

Fitness education can be implemented in different ways to match your teaching context as long as it adheres to its defining features. How you implement fitness education will depend on various factors, such as available time, access to resources, age of students, students' skill level, how many days per week you see your students, the course delivery mode, and your confidence in using specific approaches. Fitness education is successful when students learn and can apply the knowledge and skills for achieving and maintaining health-related fitness and lifelong physical activity.

If you have never used a fitness education approach, it can be overwhelming to think about changing your current practice, and you may be unsure about how to start. At this point, you may have a general idea of what the content or curriculum of fitness education includes, but you may not be clear as to what to do with that content. Figure 1.4 suggests a backward design curriculum planning sequence to begin developing your students' fitness education experience. Backward design planning starts with the desired results or end product and then works backward to plan everything that will help students meet the desired results (Wiggins & McTighe, 2005). For fitness education, this process works well because the focus is on learning fitness education outcomes as the primary goal that can be accomplished through a variety of physical activities.

Step 1: Identify the Desired Results

Outcomes: What do you want students to learn?

Fitness education goal. I want students to learn the knowledge, skills, and values necessary to adopt a physically active lifestyle and how to develop physical activity habits and other healthy lifestyle behaviors that lead to health and wellness.

A fitness education curriculum is a written plan that identifies the content to be taught, the standards it aligns to, the objectives to teach, the SLOs to meet the objectives, and units and lessons that will help students learn the knowledge and skills to meet the goal of fitness education (SHAPE America, 2015). It identifies what you want students to learn and the desired results of their learning. So far, we have provided resources to help you complete this step by identifying the goal of fitness education and listing several fitness-education teaching objectives (see the Instructional Framework for Fitness Education sidebar on page 9) that you can use to create SLOs matched to your specific situation. It may not be possible for you to teach all eight of those objectives well due to time constraints. The number of days per week, the number of minutes per class, and the required number of courses for credit dictate the total amount of time in a student's physical education experience for grades 6 to 12.

After you have identified the program objectives, you will develop course outcomes. The course outcomes specify what students will learn and be able to do as a result of the program. They are the products of learning that provide evidence that the objectives were achieved. You can then create unit, project, or lesson outcomes that further detail what students will learn. The student learning outcomes (SLOs) are a way to communicate to students what

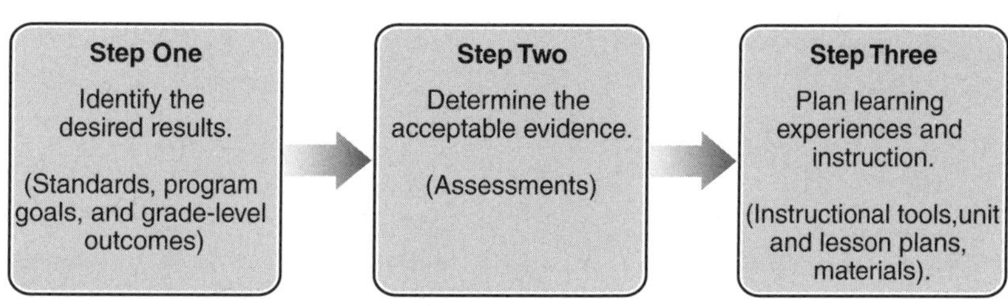

Figure 1.4 A backward design approach to fitness education planning.

they will learn and what they must do to demonstrate their learning.

Additionally, since fitness education is a component of the total physical education program, there are other objectives that will be included in a course. This is especially true at the middle school level, as the major emphasis is on developing the skills and knowledge of tactics and strategies to engage in games and sports (SHAPE America, 2014). As shown in table 1.3, the majority of the physical education GLOs are in standard 1 for middle school. At the middle school level, fitness education may complement sport education, as students at this level are developing the physical competence and tactical knowledge to engage in a variety of physical activities. A strategy for effectively teaching fitness education objectives may be to embed fitness education into all of the sport or activity units rather than teaching a two-week fitness education unit in which you superficially cover a lot of content. You don't want to simply cover information, but rather teach so that students have the opportunity to learn, understand, retain, and apply the concepts. This can be done by integrating fitness and sports concepts into each lesson so that students are learning health-related fitness concepts that align with improved performance in that sport or activity. Table 1.4 shows an example of how fitness education objectives can be embedded into sport or activity units. For example, to achieve the technique objective, the instructor can select stretches, resistance-training exercises, and skill-related component activities that match the sport's or activity's demands; to meet the fitness knowledge objective, the instructor can focus on how skills-related and health-related components work together to improve performance in that sport or activity.

At the high school level, there is a special emphasis on standard 3 and outcomes that prepare students to participate in self-directed physical activity in adulthood (SHAPE America, 2014). Nearly all of the high school grade-level outcomes are associated with demonstrating competency in health-related fitness activities, developing personalized physical activity plans, or understanding the value of physical activity. There is a de-emphasis on learning game-play strategies and on tactics and technique in sports-based skills. Therefore, at the high school level, fitness education should be the primary focus, and, if necessary, another curriculum model may complement the fitness education objectives. The high school standards are divided into two levels (SHAPE America, 2014):

- *Level 1.* Minimum knowledge and skills for college and career readiness
- *Level 2.* Knowledge and skills that are desirable for college and career readiness

Table 1.5 shows an example of how high school courses can organize several of the fitness education objectives for a level 1 and level 2 course.

The district you teach in or will teach in may have an established curriculum guide with curriculum maps that identify the grade-level or course objectives and student learning outcomes. If this

Table 1.3 The Number of Secondary Physical Education Grade-Level Outcomes

The National Physical Education Standards		Number of grade-level outcomes	
The physically literate individual . . .		Middle school grades 6-8	High school grades 9-12
1	Demonstrates competency in a variety of motor skills and movement patterns.	24	3
2	Applies knowledge of concepts, principles, strategies, and tactics related to movement and performance.	13	4
3	Demonstrates the knowledge and skills to achieve and maintain a health-enhancing level of physical activity and fitness.*	18	14
4	Exhibits responsible personal and social behavior that respects self and others.	7	5
5	Recognizes the value of physical activity for health, enjoyment, challenge, self-expression, and/or social interaction.*	6	4
Total GLOs for each grade level		68	30

*The emphasized standards in fitness education.

Adapted by permission from Iowa Department of Education Guidance, *Guidance for Physical Education Standards.* https://educateiowa.gov/sites/files/ed/documents/Guidance%20for%20Physical%20Education%20Standards.pdf

Table 1.4 Middle School Fitness Education Objective Planning Example

	September to November	December to February	March to June
Targeted fitness education concepts and objectives	**6th grade Activities: soccer and lacrosse**	**7th grade Activities: tennis and badminton**	**8th grade Activities: hiking and rowing**
Engages in regular physical activity: develops regular physical activity habits	Participates in a variety of lifetime recreational team sports, outdoor pursuits, or dance activities (S3.M5.6)	Participates in a variety of lifetime dual and individual sports, martial arts, or aquatic activities (S3.M5.7)	Participates in a self-selected lifetime sport, dance, aquatic, or outdoor activity outside of the school day (S3.M5.8)
Fitness knowledge: develops understanding of fitness concepts, principles, strategies, and individual differences needed to participate and maintain a health-enhancing level of fitness	• Identifies the components of skill-related fitness (S3.M7.6) • Identifies major muscles used in selected physical activities (S3.M14.6)	• Distinguishes between health-related and skill-related fitness (S3.M7.7) • Describes how muscles pull on bones to create movement in pairs by relaxing and contracting (S3.M14.7)	• Compares and contrasts health-related fitness components (cardiovascular endurance, muscle strength, muscle endurance, flexibility, and body composition) (S3.M7.8) • Designs and implements a warm-up/cool-down regime for a self-selected physical activity (S3.M12.8)
Fitness technique: develops competency in techniques needed to perform a variety of moderate-to-vigorous physical activities (From Fitness Instructional Framework)	Demonstrates correct techniques and methods of stretching, resistance training, and cardiorespiratory fitness training that correspond to performance in invasion games such as soccer, lacrosse, and basketball	Demonstrates correct techniques and methods of stretching, resistance training, and cardiorespiratory fitness training that correspond to performance in racquet sports such as tennis, badminton, and pickleball	Demonstrates correct techniques and methods of stretching, resistance training, and cardiorespiratory fitness training that correspond to performance in outdoor pursuits such as hiking, rowing, and skiing
Responsible personal and social behaviors: develops responsible personal and social behaviors in physical activity settings	Exhibits personal responsibility by using appropriate etiquette, demonstrating respect for facilities, and exhibiting safe behaviors (S4.M1.6)	Exhibits responsible social behaviors by cooperating with classmates, demonstrating inclusive behaviors, and supporting classmates (S4.M1.7)	Accepts responsibility for improving one's own level of physical activity and fitness (S4.M2.8)

is the case, review the curriculum map to see if fitness education objectives are included. Some school systems may have intentionally developed a K-12 scope and sequence for fitness education and mapped out the objectives for each grade level, while others may not have organized that component of the physical education program, instead designing curricula around sports or activity-based units. If you find that your courses require you to teach specific sports or activities with no mention of fitness education objectives, you can reference the table 1.4 example as a way to embed fitness education objectives and outcomes into those courses.

Figure 1.5 summarizes the process in step 1. The fitness education objectives presented in figure 1.3 represent the underlying concepts of benefitting from a physically active lifestyle. Each objective represents an important skill, concept, or attitude that students must learn and apply to optimize their health. These objectives encompass the three learning domains of physical education: psychomotor, cognitive, and affective (SHAPE America, 2014). Students are demonstrating movement competency with technique (psychomotor), understanding of concepts with knowledge of fitness (cognitive), and developing of positive attitudes toward physical activity (affective). Each learning domain and corresponding objectives contribute to the development of the knowledge, skills, and values of a physically active lifestyle.

Two resources for creating developmentally appropriate SLOs for your fitness education course

Table 1.5 High School Fitness Education Objective Planning Example

Targeted fitness education concepts and objectives	9th grade Personal Fitness Fitness activities: circuit training, yoga, jogging, kickboxing	10th grade Lifestyle Fitness Activities: student-selected lifetime activities
Engages in regular physical activity: develops regular physical activity habits	Participates several times a week in a self-selected lifetime activity, dance, or fitness activity outside of the school day (S3.H6.L1)	Creates a plan, trains for, and participates in a community event with a focus on physical activity (e.g., 5K, triathlon, tournament, dance performance, cycling event) (S3.H6.L2)
Fitness knowledge: develops understanding of fitness concepts, principles, strategies, and individual differences needed to participate and maintain a health-enhancing level of fitness	Calculates target heart rate and applies that information to personal fitness plan (S3.H10.L1)	Adjusts pacing to keep heart rate in the target zone, using available technology (e.g., pedometer, heart rate monitor), to self-monitor aerobic intensity (S3.H10.L2)
Fitness technique: develops competency in techniques needed to perform a variety of moderate-to-vigorous physical activities (From Fitness Instructional Framework)	Demonstrates correct techniques and methods of stretching, resistance training, and cardiorespiratory fitness training that correspond to performance in fitness activities such as yoga, kickboxing, and body-weight resistance training	Demonstrates correct techniques and methods of stretching, resistance training, and cardiorespiratory fitness training that correspond to performance in self-selected activities that relate to life and career goals
Fitness assessment and program planning: supports achieving and maintaining a health-enhancing level of health-related fitness	Designs a fitness program including all components of health-related fitness, for a college student and an employee in the learner's chosen field of work (S3.H12.L1)	Analyzes the components of skill-related fitness in relation to life and career goals and designs an appropriate fitness program for those goals (S3.H12.L2)
Values physical activity: promotes the value of physical activity	Analyzes the health benefits of a self-selected physical activity (S5.H1.L1)	Chooses an appropriate level of challenge to experience success and desire to participate in a self-selected physical activity (S5.H2.L2)

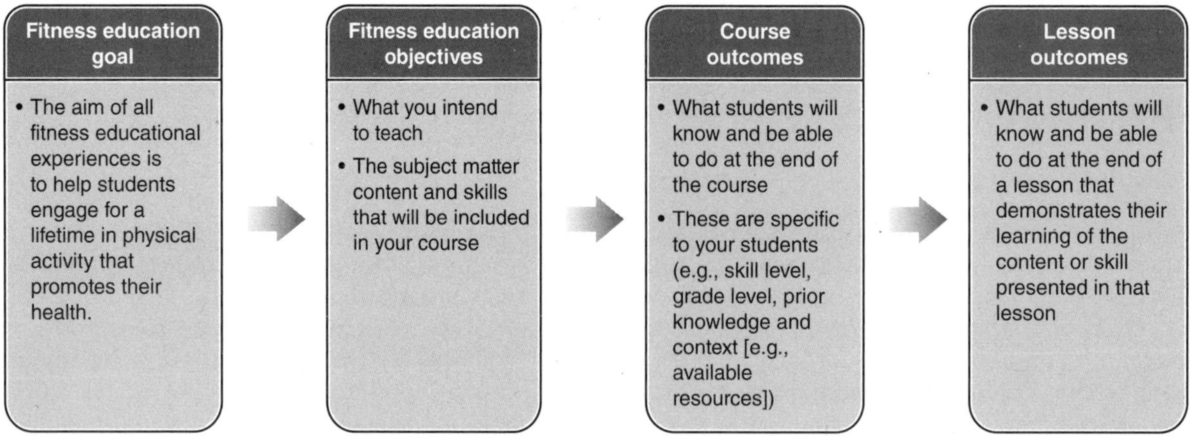

Fitness education goal
- The aim of all fitness educational experiences is to help students engage for a lifetime in physical activity that promotes their health.

→

Fitness education objectives
- What you intend to teach
- The subject matter content and skills that will be included in your course

→

Course outcomes
- What students will know and be able to do at the end of the course
- These are specific to your students (e.g., skill level, grade level, prior knowledge and context [e.g., available resources])

→

Lesson outcomes
- What students will know and be able to do at the end of a lesson that demonstrates their learning of the content or skill presented in that lesson

Figure 1.5 Step 1: Identify the desired results.

are the GLOs from the SHAPE America K-12 National Physical Education Standards and the learning benchmarks in the *Instructional Framework for Fitness Education in Physical Education* guidance document. Once you have defined the SLOs, you will determine how students will demonstrate their proficiency, which is in step 2.

Step 2: Determine the Acceptable Evidence of Learning

Assessment: How will students (and the teacher) know if they are learning?

Once you have defined the learning outcomes, you will determine how students will demonstrate their proficiency. Assessments are how educators gather evidence about a student's level of achievement and then make inferences based on that data. Assessments are generally classified into two types: *formative* and *summative*. Formative assessments are assessments for learning and inform the student and teacher about the student's progress toward meeting outcomes. Formative assessments are not graded, as they are intended to guide future instruction. Summative assessments are assessments of learning. They evaluate student learning at the end of a unit or course. Summative assessments show how much one has learned as a result of the unit or course. They are used for calculating a student's grade for a course. Since summative assessments are evaluations of student learning and impact grading, they are what you will need to create or select in this step. All of the learning experiences that you design (step 3) will prepare students to demonstrate their proficiency on a summative assessment. Since fitness education includes the psychomotor, cognitive, and affective domains, you may decide to create a summative assessment for each one. Each learning domain will require a different type of assessment, such as demonstrating movements, understanding concepts, or demonstrating attitudes and behaviors. Table 1.6 provides an example for how you can align learning domains, your fitness education teaching objectives, and an assessment appropriate for that domain.

In addition, fitness testing is a valuable assessment tool for meeting fitness education outcomes. Because students' fitness scores should not be used to grade students, they are formative assessments (SHAPE America, 2017). Fitness tests provide information on a student's progress toward achieving health-enhancing fitness. They are used to detect any potential health risks, as our levels of physical fitness relate to how well our body systems are functioning. Fitness tests will fit into two learning domains: psychomotor, as they require correct technique to perform the movement patterns, and cognitive, as students will analyze their scores and then develop fitness plans to improve or maintain components of their health-related fitness. Without the cognitive piece attached to a fitness test, they serve very little purpose because students will not understand what their scores mean in relationship to their health. Chapter 7 provides more detail on best practices for assessment strategies in fitness education.

Course Delivery Modes and Assessments

Your course delivery mode will play a role in how you design course assessments. Course delivery can be defined by the level of technology integration and the amount of synchronous (real-time) interaction between the instructor and students. Figure 1.6 shows a continuum of modes based on how much technology is used to deliver instruction. In the face-to-face (FTF) and web-enhanced modes, all instruction is delivered FTF in real-time with web-enhancements, providing students with online resources to enhance their learning. In a flipped classroom, all classes are delivered FTF in real-time, but the expectation is that students watch videos and interactive lessons accessed online in advance of class so that class time involves less direct instruction and more collaborative learning. In a blended or hybrid course, there are fewer FTF meetings, as part of them are replaced with online meetings. Online meetings may be synchronous or asynchronous (no real-time interaction).

Table 1.6 Learning Assessments in Fitness Education

Learning domain	Fitness education objective	Sample assessments
Psychomotor: physical movement, coordination, and use of motor skills	Develop competency in techniques needed to perform a variety of moderate-to-vigorous physical activities	• Students demonstrate five correct body-weight squats • Rubric that includes the critical elements of the technique for the movement
Affective: behaviors, emotions, feeling, motivation, and attitudes	Develop responsible personal and social behaviors in physical activity settings	• Students complete a written self-assessment reflection on how they are demonstrating personal and social responsibility in the class • Rubric that includes the required criteria for the reflection
Cognitive: knowledge and understanding of concepts, principles, and strategies	Acquire an understanding of the fitness concepts, training principles, and the self-management strategies needed to participate and maintain a health-enhancing level of fitness	• Students develop a personalized fitness plan using the FITT framework and principles of training • Rubric that includes the required criteria for the plan

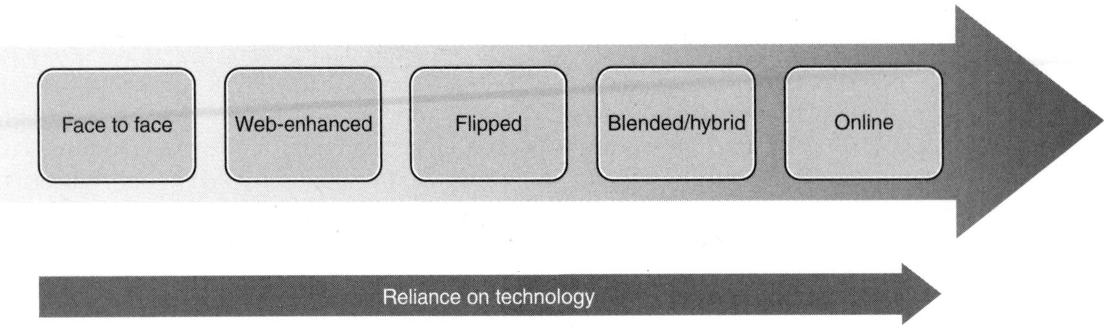

Figure 1.6 Continuum of course delivery modes.

Adapted from Bates, T. (2001). La Cyberformation dans l'enseignement supérieur: développement de stratégies nationales. IIEP/UNESCO. IIEP/UNESCO Publishing. Used with permission from IIEP/UNESCO

In a completely online model, there are no FTF meetings, and teachers may choose to use a blend of synchronous meetings and asynchronous work.

Assessments can be similar in all delivery modes, but their design may differ. For example, in an online course, a teacher may require students to upload videos of themselves performing exercises so that they can evaluate their technique. The technique checklist will remain the same, and the student having to demonstrate the skill stays the same, but there are more instructional steps involved when a student has to create and upload a video. When teachers have less FTF time, they may design assessments differently so they can provide more meaningful feedback.

Step 3: Plan Learning Experiences and Instruction

Design: How will the teacher design curriculum and deliver instruction?

Designing the learning experiences involves selecting the activities that you will use to teach the outcomes. The activities may be more sport- or fitness-oriented depending on the course objectives and outcomes. The following questions can help you plan the content and delivery of fitness education learning experiences:

- What are the students learning today?
- Why are they learning it?
- How will they learn it?
- How will they show they learned it?
- How will I organize and present the content so that it is relevant and meaningful to students?
- What routines and procedures will I implement to maximize active learning time?
- What teaching methods will I use to deliver instruction (e.g., direct instruction, peer feedback, guided discovery)?

It is especially important with fitness education to consider how you will teach the cognitive concepts while also maximizing the opportunity for students to engage in MVPA. If content knowledge is not organized into meaningful patterns or connected to the physical activity experience in a relevant way, then students are likely to forget it and won't be able to apply that knowledge in different physical activity settings (Haidar, 1997). This means you do not want to give students worksheets on nutrition to take home and complete to check off that you covered nutrition if there is no connection to what you are doing in the class.

If you are teaching in a face-to-face setting, you will have to decide how to organize teaching cognitive concepts and the corresponding physical activities. In a hybrid model, students could access the cognitive content online and complete learning tasks prior to engaging in the physical activity sessions so that in-class sessions are devoted to applying the content learned online through physical activity. If an online course is in a synchronous format, the teacher must decide how real-time class sessions will be structured, whether they will consist of delivering the cognitive concepts or having students perform physical activity. Chapter 3 provides details on how teachers can use effective instructional strategies for each of these structures.

In FTF classes, there are two common options for delivering the cognitive portion of the course: a conceptual physical education (CPE) structure or a mini-lectures structure. Table 1.7 provides an example of both. CPE is a fitness education curriculum model that uses a textbook, classroom sessions, and physical activity sessions to teach concepts and skills (Corbin, Kulinna, & Sibley, 2020). Students are taught conceptual fitness content in a classroom-based setting and then apply those concepts in a physical activity setting. It may seem counterproductive to have students in a classroom setting when we are trying to increase their physical activity, but the time spent in learning the cognitive concepts yields more physical activity later in life, so the long-term benefits outweigh the short-term loss of activity time (Corbin, Kulinna, & Sibley, 2020). The mini-lecture option is when teachers deliver all of the content and instruction in the physical activity setting. The lectures can be performed right before or at the end of the lesson, depending on how the content relates to the physical activity. You will be most successful if you select a system, communicate that system to students, and commit to the system. This means that you do not haphazardly select a few days out of the month to cover content or that you deliver cognitive content instruction only when it is convenient. Students may complain about having to do classwork in physical education, but as the instructor, you must set the tone that fitness education is about learning to enhance their health and that classroom-based sessions help them understand the process of achieving health-related fitness. You must emphasize that both the cognitive portion and the physical activity portion are equally important to their learning and health. Chapter 3 describes how you can best develop a system to deliver instruction based upon your course delivery mode and context.

In designing learning experiences, you will create learning outcomes from the objectives that define what students will know and be able to do. The learning experience delivers the content to students. It is how you align all of the tasks in a single class session to the student learning outcomes. The next section provides several examples of course outcomes and student learning outcomes for each of the fitness education objectives.

Objective 1: Technique Competency

Develop competency in techniques needed to perform a variety of moderate-to-vigorous physical activities.

Physical competence, also termed *motor skill competence,* refers to the proficiency of movement skills and patterns that allow an individual to participate in a wide range of physical activities. Physical competence is the underlying mechanism needed to perform a variety of moderate-to-vigorous physical activities that lead to developing adequate health-related fitness across the life span (MacDonald, 2015). Locomotor skills, such as running, skipping, and hopping; object-control skills, such as throwing, catching, and kicking; and stability skills, such as twisting and bending, are foundational for engaging in a variety of games and activities. Children learn these fundamental motor skills so that the skills can be refined into more-specific movement patterns as children age, which allows them to participate in sports or fitness-specific activities. At the secondary level, this includes demonstrating competency in health-related fitness activities, such as appropriate technique in resistance-training exercises, methods of stretching, and aerobic-fitness activities. Learning proper exercise technique is necessary for engaging in physical activity that promotes physical fitness and reduces the risk of injury. A student's level of physical competence greatly affects her ability to meet physical activity guidelines (Belanger et al., 2018). Students with low physical competence lack options for engaging in select physical activities. Therefore, a fitness education program needs to ensure that students develop the physical competence to perform a variety of physical activities so they have options to choose from.

A personal fitness course for ninth-graders that meets the technique competency objective might have the following sample elements:

Course outcome. Students will demonstrate appropriate technique in resistance-training body-weight and free-weight exercises.

Lesson outcome. Students will be able to perform five consecutive body-weight squats with correct technique and form.

Table 1.7 Examples of Fitness Education Instructional Delivery

Options	Monday	Wednesday	Friday
CPE model: alternating classroom and activity sessions	Location: classroom Topics: benefits of cardiorespiratory fitness, how to calculate target heart rate zone	Location: track Activity: interval training	Location: gym Activity: circuit training
Mini-lectures (5-10 min of cognitive instruction before physical activity)	Location: gym Topic: benefits of cardiorespiratory fitness Activity: circuit training	Location: gym and track Topic: how to calculate target heart-rate zone Activity: interval training	Location: gym Topic: assessing cardiorespiratory fitness Activity: Progressive Aerobic Cardiovascular Endurance Run (PACER)

Assessment. Skills performance checklist of critical elements.

Lesson plan elements. Demonstrate skill; self-assessment using body-weight squat checklist; peer feedback using body-weight squat checklist; teacher feedback using body-weight squat checklist.

What does this mean? Students will demonstrate the correct mechanical movements of the body-weight squat (skill cues), and they will perform those movements in rhythm and under control. They will use the skill cues checklist to self-assess and peer-assess, and then when they feel competent, they will demonstrate for the teacher.

Objective 2: Knowledge

Acquire an understanding of the fitness concepts, principles, strategies, and individual differences needed to participate and maintain a health-enhancing level of fitness.

A lack of knowledge of health-related fitness concepts may be a contributing factor to physical inactivity and obesity in adolescents. Several studies have shown that adolescents lack physical fitness and activity knowledge and have misconceptions about what constitutes healthy behaviors (Zhu, Haegele, & Sun, 2019). Secondary students with higher knowledge scores self-report greater participation in physical activity outside of school, so understanding health-related fitness concepts contributes to greater physical activity levels (Thompson & Hannon, 2012). Examples of health-related fitness knowledge include knowing how to train the components of health-related fitness using exercise prescription and planning principles and knowing the benefits of physical activity, the consequences of living a sedentary lifestyle, and the physiological effects of exercise.

Fitness education attempts to develop higher-order or conceptual understanding of health-related fitness concepts so that students can apply the knowledge in various situations and settings. This cognitive understanding provides an opportunity for students to design, evaluate, and apply knowledge to meet their health needs, not just to recall, identify, or describe concepts. A high school physical education course may be the only opportunity for some students to learn how to maintain health-related fitness throughout adulthood, so understanding how and why to maintain health-enhancing fitness across the life span is vital to improving health-related outcomes.

A personal fitness course for sixth-graders that meets the knowledge objective might have the following sample elements:

Course outcome. Students will demonstrate knowledge of how to train for the components of health-related fitness.

Lesson outcome. Students will describe how to apply the FITT framework to train for muscular endurance.

Assessment. Fill in the FITT framework with activities to train for muscular endurance.

Lesson plan elements. Direct instruction on the application of FITT to muscular endurance; think-pair-share to compare muscular endurance to cardiorespiratory fitness; written sheet on FITT and muscular endurance.

What does this mean? Students will write out what they need to do each week in order to attain a health-enhancing level of muscular endurance.

Objective 3: Physical Activity Habits

Develop regular physical activity habits.

The current levels of physical inactivity are partially due to having physical activity engineered away through labor-saving devices, increased motor vehicle transportation, and a greater reliance on screens for work and leisure. Adolescents spend an average of eight hours a day in sedentary behaviors inside and outside of school (Lou, 2014). Sedentary behavior, especially prolonged periods of sitting, is a major risk factor for health consequences such as cardiovascular disease and diabetes. Too much sitting and too little exercise are actually separate risk factors for chronic diseases (Biddle, Bennie, Bauman, Chau, Dunstan, Owen, Stamatakis, & van Uffelen, 2016). Sitting for more than six hours per day can increase the risk of death by 19 percent, compared with sitting less than three hours per day regardless of one's exercise habits (Patel, Maliniak, Rees-Punia, Matthews, & Gapstur, 2018). Developing a physically active lifestyle involves more than exercising at the gym for an hour a day; it means incorporating more movement and less sitting into one's daily life. Fitness education promotes physical activity behavior by helping students to explore and participate in leisure-time physical activity and understand the importance of incorporating physical activity breaks during prolonged periods of sitting.

A personal fitness course for seventh-graders that meets the physical activity habit objective might have the following sample elements:

Course outcome. Students will participate in regular physical activity.

Lesson outcome. Students will participate in 60 minutes of physical activity three times a week outside of physical education class.

Assessment. A written journal of what they did on each day and for how long.

Lesson plan elements. Direct instruction on the benefits of physical activity, small-group discussion on ways to be active outside of physical education; explanation of the journal due at the end of the week; exit ticket on their plan and a commitment to be physically active for the week.

What does this mean? Students will plan at the beginning of the week to get 60 minutes of physical activity on at least three different days. Students will track their physical activity outside of physical education class and submit the journal at the end of the week.

Objective 4: Health-Related Fitness

Achieve and maintain a health-enhancing level of health-related fitness.

Physical activity benefits one's health, but only exercise can influence one's physical fitness. As mentioned previously, exercise is a type of structured and planned physical activity that intentionally improves one or more components of physical fitness. To maintain a health-enhancing level of physical fitness, one must consistently adhere to an exercise program that incorporates the principles of training. Achieving health-related fitness involves knowing how to design a personalized fitness program, how to progress it over time, and how to maintain the motivation to exercise on a regular basis. As part of the personalized fitness-planning process, students analyze their current health-related fitness through physical fitness assessments in order to set goals and create a fitness improvement plan. Assessing fitness is key to identifying areas in need of improvement and provides data for developing a realistic and effective fitness plan.

A personal fitness course for 10th-graders that meets the health-related fitness objective might have the following sample elements:

Course outcome. Students will design a personalized fitness plan to achieve health-enhancing fitness in all of the health-related components of fitness.

Lesson outcome. Students will analyze their current level of cardiorespiratory fitness and write a Specific, Measurable, Achievable, Realistic, and Time-Bound goal (SMART) to improve or maintain a health-enhancing level of cardiorespiratory fitness.

Assessment. Mile fitness test, PACER test, and a cardiorespiratory fitness SMART goal sheet.

Lesson plan elements. Review the healthy fitness-zone times for the mile run; commit to putting forth full effort and maintaining a personalized pace throughout the run; find a running buddy who has similar goals to challenge each other during the run; engage in appropriate warm-up and dynamic stretching; complete the mile run; engage in appropriate cool-down and static stretching; analyze scores compared to healthy fitness zones; complete the SMART goal sheet for improving or maintaining cardiorespiratory fitness health.

What does this mean? Students will self-assess their level of cardiorespiratory fitness. They will challenge themselves to overcome physical and motivational obstacles for giving full effort. They will encourage peers to give their best effort. They will write a goal for maintaining or improving their current level of cardiorespiratory fitness.

Objective 5: Responsible Personal and Social Behaviors

Develop responsible personal and social behaviors in physical activity settings.

Personal responsibility involves taking care of one's well-being and accepting responsibility for one's personal health and fitness behaviors. Every person needs effective self-management skills to be able to cope with stress, interact with others, and develop positive habits. Self-management skills include time-management, stress-management, and behavior-monitoring strategies. In order to achieve a healthy body composition, a student may choose to monitor both physical activity and nutrition behaviors to ensure a balance of calories. If that student wants to engage in more physical activity to increase calorie expenditure, then he will have to manage his time to be able to devote more minutes to physical activity. Fitness education teaches behavior modification principles and how students can develop good fitness habits through self-management strategies.

Social responsibility involves demonstrating adaptive and positive behaviors while interacting with others of varying skills, abilities, and cultural backgrounds. Physical activity settings often require that individuals follow rules for fair and safe play, use equipment respectfully, and cooperate with teammates. Social skills include communication, collaboration, and emotional control. Adolescents are more likely to engage in physical activity that involves some form of play with peers, and the companionship provided by friends during physical activity often increases their positive emotions toward physical activity (Salvy et al., 2009). Teaching students how to positively interact with

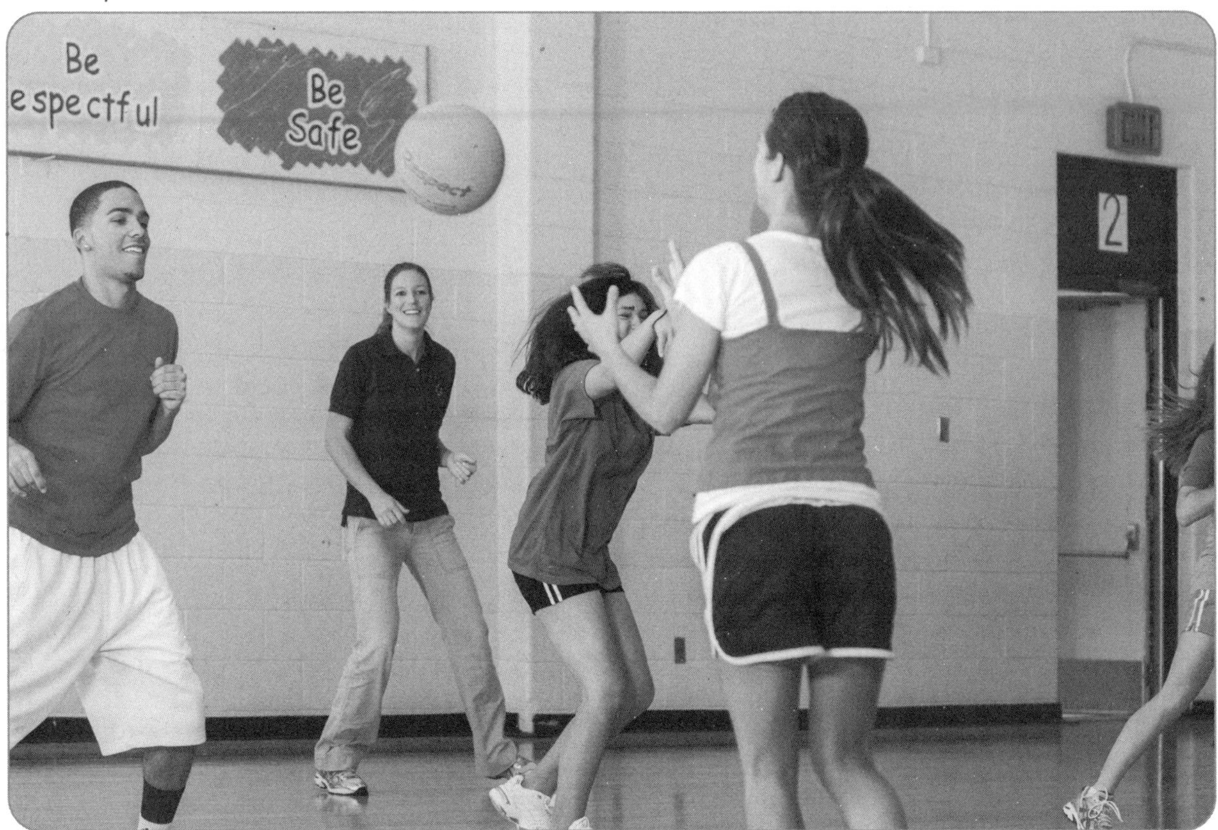

Physical activity settings are conducive to the development of social responsibility in adolescents as they interact respectfully and cooperatively.

others and build relationships through activity is an important piece for sustaining adolescent motivation to engage in physical activity.

A personal fitness course for seventh-graders that meets the personal and social responsibility objective might have the following sample elements:

Course outcome. Students will exhibit responsible personal and social behaviors by using appropriate etiquette, following safety guidelines, demonstrating inclusive behaviors, and respectfully cooperating with others.

Lesson outcome. Students will demonstrate inclusive behaviors by supporting classmates during a game of sitting volleyball.

Assessment. An exit ticket that provides evidence of how they demonstrated inclusive behaviors and an example of how they supported a classmate during the game.

Lesson plan elements. Direct instruction on the teamwork element of sitting volleyball; explanation on how communication in volleyball affects performance; instruct students on the expectations of the game and that the focus is on communication and supporting teammates; play sitting volleyball; think-pair-share to compare and contrast sitting and standing volleyball fitness and teamwork components; exit ticket on inclusive behaviors and peer support.

What does this mean? Students will analyze how a game of sitting volleyball can be more inclusive to everyone than a game of standing volleyball. Students will participate in a Paralympics activity to develop respect for others of differing abilities (e.g., it is just as physically challenging but in different ways). Students will reflect on their ability to demonstrate inclusive behaviors and support their teammates.

Objective 6: Valuing Physical Activity

Value physical activity's contributions to well-being.

Despite the overwhelming evidence of the importance of physical activity and exercise, only one in five high school students fully meet the physical activity guidelines for aerobic and muscle-strengthening activities (Centers for Disease Control and Prevention, 2020b). With so few meeting the recommendations, physical educators must support students in increasing their motivation to engage in physical activity and exercise. Motivation is a force that influences our behaviors—those influences are often determined by what we value. Youth need to value physical activity's outcomes to make it a priority in their lives (Teixeira, Carraça, Markland, Silva, & Ryan, 2012). Fitness education addresses the social and emotional, mental, and occupational ways that physical activity can contribute to one's well-being. While disease prevention can be highly motivating for adults, it may not be as motivational for adolescents. Youth may find more value in physical activity outcomes, such as having fun, socializing, and improving appearance, so emphasizing those outcomes through physical activity experiences may lead to greater participation levels.

Self-efficacy is the belief one has the ability to succeed in specific situations or accomplish a task (Bandura, 1977). Self-efficacy is most often influenced by past performance and observation. Succeeding in the past and seeing others succeed at the task can instill more confidence in a student. When activities are personalized to deliver the appropriate amount of challenge, students will be more likely to succeed and develop the confidence to continue on to the next challenge.

Adolescents' attitudes toward sports, exercise, and fitness predict their future physical activity behavior (Graham, Sirard, & Neumark-Sztainer, 2011). When youth experience pleasure in physical activity, they develop more positive attitudes toward it and choose to engage in it more consistently and into adulthood (Graham, Sirard, & Neumark-Sztainer, 2011). Employing creative and innovative strategies that allow youth to explore how they most enjoy physical activity is imperative to experiencing the value of physical activity.

A personal fitness course for 10th-graders that meets the valuing physical activity objective might have the following sample elements:

Course outcome. Students will recognize the value of participating in regular physical activity.

Lesson outcome. Students will analyze the physical, mental, and social and emotional benefits of a self-selected physical activity.

Assessment. Students will write a reflection on how their choice of physical activity affects their physical, mental, and social and emotional health.

Lesson plan elements. Think-pair-share on which physical activities are most enjoyable; small-group discussions on how certain physical activities affect physical health differently; relate types of exercise to health-related components (e.g., muscular endurance, flexibility, cardiorespiratory fitness); explanation on how to write the reflection for self-selected physical activity.

What does this mean? Students will evaluate how their choice of physical activity benefits them. Through discussions, students will come to understand how different types of activities benefit them in different ways and the importance of engaging in a variety of physical activities to obtain the most health benefits.

Objective 7: Nutrition

Establish healthy eating habits.

Nutrition is an important element of fitness education, as dietary habits influence body composition and energy levels. Calories are the fuel our bodies use for energy and are necessary to engage in physical activity. When students make healthy eating choices, they are improving their chances to be able to engage in a more active lifestyle. In addition, diet plays a role in preventing chronic diseases such as obesity, diabetes, and osteoporosis, the same way that physical activity does. Neglecting to discuss the interconnectedness of dietary habits and physical activity habits to achieving physical fitness goals may discourage some students from continuing with activity. Specifically, if students try to lose weight by exercising and not modifying their eating habits, they will experience very little success. This may lead to participating in less physical activity because it is not helping them to reach their goal. Understanding how nutrition and exercise go hand in hand for improving sports performance and modifying body composition can support students in making healthy choices for both behaviors. As youth age, they become more independent and start making their own food choices, so they need the knowledge of how to select food and beverages that will lead to the best health outcomes. Nutrition education will be discussed more comprehensively in chapter 5.

A personal fitness course for eighth-graders that meets the nutrition objective might have the following sample elements:

Course outcome. Students will be able to describe the relationship between poor nutrition and health risk factors.

Lesson outcome. Students will compare beverages to make a healthy choice.

Assessment. Students rate the health of a beverage by comparing nutritional content—show the teacher in class the ratings.

Lesson plan elements. Direct instruction on reading the nutritional label on a beverage; explain the importance of analyzing drinks for sugar content; discuss benefits of beverages with calcium and potassium content; small-group activity to compare four to five different beverages and discuss how healthy they are; engage in a "Capture the Healthy Drink" game; have teams show how they organized their drinks into health categories.

What does this mean? Students will analyze the nutritional content of 15 to 20 different beverages. They will look at how much sugar, calcium, potassium, and other vitamins or minerals are in different beverages. Students will engage in physical activity while comparing nutrition labels. Students will be able to defend their rationale for their healthy beverage ratings using the nutrition facts label.

Objective 8: Consumerism

Make good decisions about fitness products and services.

Fitness education also teaches students how to distinguish between fact and fiction regarding nutritional and physical activity products. There are many misconceptions around the best weight-loss or muscle-building strategies, and acting on those misconceptions can lead to harmful outcomes for students. Making informed decisions about products and programs is a skill that can reduce potential harmful side effects and support lifelong nutrition and physical activity habits.

A personal fitness course for ninth-graders that meets the consumer education objective might have the following sample elements:

Course outcome. Students will be able to analyze health and fitness information, products, and services to make decisions that support good health outcomes.

Lesson outcome. Students will distinguish between fact and fiction about weight-loss and weight-gain methods.

Assessment. Quiz over key concepts related to calories and weight-management strategies.

Lesson plan elements. Direct instruction on appropriate weight-management strategies; students review several different websites that promote products related to weight management; take a quiz to demonstrate their ability to distinguish between fact and fiction from the website contents.

What does this mean? Students will analyze media sources, use of fact and fiction to sell weight-management products. Students will be able to identify what products and services can best support their health.

FITNESS EDUCATION BARRIERS AND SOLUTIONS

Even if you believe that fitness education is best for your students and their future health, there are several challenges you may face in the form of institutional, personal, and student-related barriers to implementing effective fitness education (Jenkinson & Benson, 2010). Your ability to overcome these barriers will impact the success of your fitness education program. Table 1.8 lists common barriers to implementing fitness education and potential solutions. The subsequent chapters of this text provide more details on how to use the solutions presented.

Institutional barriers are factors that teachers may not have direct control over because of the way that the institution or system is structured. These barriers, such as the facility you teach in and how much time you have per class, may never change. However, it is possible to devise solutions to these challenges through innovative teaching strategies. For example, many programs lack funding to purchase physical education equipment, and the teacher has no control over the budget. Teachers can use lessons and instructional methods that help students have a meaningful experience without the use of equipment.

Teacher-related barriers are personal factors that you have direct control over, such as your confidence, content knowledge, pedagogical content knowledge, and motivation. Your content knowledge is your understanding of the subject matter that you teach. Pedagogical content knowledge (PCK) is your ability to teach that subject matter so that students comprehend it (Shulman, 1986). PCK involves your ability to provide appropriate feedback, differentiate instruction, and manage student behaviors. Fitness education will require different PCK than sport education or other components of a physical education program. In fitness education, you must be able to teach content related to developing habits, training adaptations to exercise, applying training principles, and program-planning design in such a way that students are motivated and capable of living a physically active lifestyle. In order to help students develop personalized fitness plans, you need to understand and be able to demonstrate how to adapt and modify exercises for students with disabilities. The greater your PCK is, the greater your capacity to match learning tasks with students' abilities and provide constructive feedback (Ward, 2016). Other personal factors may include your motivation and confidence to implement fitness education. These may be influenced by how much time you have to make curricular changes, the perceived amount of

Table 1.8 Barriers to Delivering Fitness Education

Types of barriers	Common barriers	Potential solutions
Institutional	• Lack of facilities (suitable teaching spaces) • Budget constraints to purchase equipment • Lack of time (too much to teach) • Limited academic value—others don't see the value of fitness education	• Facility rotations (coordinating with other teachers or administrators to schedule activities in different teaching spaces based on need) • Activities with minimal equipment required • Define scope and sequence for maximal learning on fewer objectives • Evidence-based curricular and instructional approaches that produce positive health outcomes
Teacher-related	• Lack of content knowledge • Limited pedagogical knowledge (instructional strategies) • Difficulty engaging students • Inefficient classroom management strategies	• Professional development • Published educational books and professional resources • A universal design for learning approach
Student-related	• Lack of interest in physical activity • Lack of motivation to perform fitness activities • Past negative experiences with physical education • Influences of peers • Lack of confidence in ability to succeed • Lack of skill or technique	• Class management • Student-interest survey • Appropriate practices • Cooperative learning • Task-oriented climate

Reprinted by permission from J.D. Greenberg and J.L. LoBianco, *Organization and Administration of Physical Education: Theory and Practice* (Champaign, IL: Human Kinetics, 2020).

effort and energy it will require, how students might perceive fitness education, and how valuable you believe it to be. The central purpose of this textbook is to reduce your personal barriers in delivering fitness education at the secondary level by providing you with the knowledge and resources that you need for successful program implementation and enhanced student fitness gains.

Student-related barriers are factors that interfere with the students' ability to fully engage in lessons. They include attitudes toward physical activity, skill levels, and beliefs about physical education that have been shaped by previous experiences. Overcoming student barriers involves getting to know your students: their interests, fears, needs, and preferred ways of engaging in the course. When you know your students, you can adapt your teaching style to best support their learning style. Such an inclusive teaching practice is often referred to as a *universal design for learning (UDL)* approach. In UDL, teachers proactively plan varied instructional strategies and multiple ways for students to engage and to express their learning (Lieberman, Grenier, Brian, & Arndt, 2020). Teachers do not expect students to adapt to their teaching; they adapt their teaching to their students. Many of the student-related barriers can be reduced by creating a positive learning environment, providing choice of activities, increasing students' level of autonomy, and exhibiting a caring and compassionate attitude (Bryan & Solomon, 2012).

ROLES AND RESPONSIBILITIES IN FITNESS EDUCATION

As the physical education teacher, you have several responsibilities to ensure that students have a positive fitness education experience and learn the knowledge and skills necessary for developing a healthy and active lifestyle. First and foremost, you must protect students' physical and social and emotional health. There are always inherent physical risks with engaging in exercise, such as strained muscles, sprained ankles, heat exhaustion, and bruised knees. In addition, poor social skills and poor motor skills are risk factors for becoming bullied in physical education class (Bejerot, Edgar, & Humble, 2011). Both the risks of injury and victimization can be minimized through proper planning and effective classroom management. Chapter 4 describes management strategies to help you create a safe and positive learning environment. The Responsibilities of a Fitness Education Teacher sidebar lists several responsibilities of a physical education teacher teaching fitness education to ensure that students are physically active

Responsibilities of a Fitness Education Teacher

- Keep the program student centered; give students choice; allow them to take ownership over their learning and voice what they value.
- Maximize class time through effective organization of equipment and student groupings.
- Design lessons that provide for maximum participation and engagement in MVPA for at least 50 percent of class time.
- Focus on teaching the process of physical activity and not just the product of physical fitness.
- Design learning experiences that effectively teach health-related fitness knowledge and provide opportunities for students to independently demonstrate their understanding of fitness concepts.
- Model and promote healthy lifestyle behaviors through words and actions.
- Consistently monitor student behavior and performance and provide immediate and constructive feedback when necessary.
- Keep students motivated and encouraged to keep reaching their goals.

during class, learn fitness concepts, and develop healthy habits.

When physical education teachers provide a class environment where all students feel safe and respected, develop an open and transparent communication system with the physical education teacher, are provided with maximum physical activity time in the class period, and receive quality instruction and encouragement, then the intended program outcome of students becoming more knowledgeable, skilled, and physically fit will be achieved.

CONCLUSION

Fitness education is an important part of a comprehensive physical education program designed to help students acquire the knowledge, skills, values, and behaviors to benefit from a lifetime of physical activity. Adolescents need to engage in regular physical activity to reduce their risk of developing chronic diseases later in life, as well as to enjoy the immediate cognitive and stress-relieving benefits. Fitness education is an inclusive, evidence-based, standards-based curriculum and instructional approach that will prepare students for college or career readiness through its focus on both the process of physical activity and the product of health-enhancing fitness.

This chapter presented a backward design approach to planning fitness education learning experiences in which educators start with the desired results or outcomes of the program, develop assessment for and of learning, and then design learning experiences that will lead to the desired results. There are several barriers to implementing a quality fitness education program, and educators can overcome these with innovative lesson design and teaching methods. The chapters to follow provide you with the knowledge and resources that you need to overcome the barriers and deliver quality fitness education in secondary physical education programs.

Review Questions

1. Compare and contrast the goals and objectives of physical education, physical activity, and fitness education.
2. Describe how individual fitness goals can be achieved through fitness assessment.
3. Identify the physical, cognitive, and social and emotional benefits of participating in regular physical activity.
4. Explain which fitness education objectives focus primarily on the psychomotor domain and which objectives focus on the cognitive domain.
5. Explain how self-esteem and social responsibility can be learned through fitness education.

Visit HK*Propel* for additional material related to this chapter.

CHAPTER 2

Fitness Components and Training Principles

Chapter Objective

After reading this chapter, you will understand the differences between health-related and skill-related fitness components and how each relates to overall physical fitness, understand the principles of training, understand how the FITT framework is used to prescribe exercise, understand the benefits of a HIIT program, provide examples of how the principles of training influence a fitness education training program, and employ best teaching practices that enhance student learning and comprehension.

Key Concepts

- Skill-related fitness and health-related fitness components both contribute to a student's overall fitness level.
- The FITT framework should be used in applying the basic fitness education program at all levels.
- Principles of training including specificity, individuality, overload, progression, variation, and regularity should be taught for students to comprehend components of a fitness education training program.
- Training methods and adaptations contribute to cardiorespiratory fitness.
- Accommodations and modifications are recommended so that all activities and instructional materials can be adjusted and delivered to all students in the class.

INTRODUCTION

An effective fitness education course prepares students to develop their own individual exercise plans, based on their fitness assessment results, and to execute their plans by applying fitness-training principles. Understanding and using fitness-training principles is necessary for improving and maintaining a health-enhancing level of fitness.

The foundation to developing an effective fitness education course is the ability of the physical education teacher to teach students how to apply fitness-training principles to develop their individualized exercise plans through their lesson design and curriculum delivery. Chapter 1 discussed the benefits of a fitness education program, physical activity, and physical fitness, but reaping those benefits requires the student to gain a cognitive understanding of what needs to be done to attain them. Knowing how to design and implement a fitness education program is an essential skill for assisting students in achieving a health-enhancing level of fitness. This chapter provides an overview of the fundamental concepts of fitness program design: the components of physical fitness, basic training principles, and exercise-training planning for student fitness gains.

THE COMPONENTS OF PHYSICAL FITNESS

Physical fitness is the capacity of your body systems to complete physical tasks without excessive fatigue. When all of your body systems are operating efficiently, you can perform physical activities with more sustainable energy over longer periods of time. Physical fitness is multidimensional in that it consists of numerous components with each one contributing to the health of the body systems (e.g., cardiovascular, respiratory, muscular, skeletal, nervous) in a unique way (see table 2.1). Those components are typically classified into two general categories: health related and skill related.

The five health-related components of fitness—*cardiorespiratory endurance, muscular strength, muscular endurance, flexibility,* and *body composition*—influence how well your body systems operate. These fitness components are considered to be health markers, as they are clear predictors of chronic disease, disability, and premature death (Henriksson et al., 2020). For example, low levels of cardiorespiratory endurance and a high body fat percentage increase the risk for cardiovascular diseases, cancer, and type 2 diabetes. In addition, these components relate to one's ability to function

Table 2.1 The Components of Physical Fitness

Component		Definition
Health related	Body composition	The relative amounts of muscle, fat, bone, and other vital parts of the body
	Cardiorespiratory endurance	The ability of the circulatory and respiratory system to supply oxygen during sustained physical activity
	Muscular strength	The ability of muscle to exert force
	Muscular endurance	The ability of muscle to continue to perform without fatigue
	Flexibility	The range of motion available at a joint
Skill related	Power	The ability to exert muscle force quickly
	Reaction time	The ability to react quickly to one of your senses recognizing a stimulus
	Coordination	The ability to use senses, such as sight and hearing, together with body parts in performing motor tasks smoothly and accurately
	Speed	The ability to perform a movement within a short period of time
	Agility	The ability to rapidly change the position of the body with speed and accuracy
	Balance	The ability to maintain equilibrium when moving or in a static position

From U.S. Department of Health and Human Services (2010).

in everyday life, as daily tasks such as climbing stairs, standing up, and carrying groceries require a minimum amount of strength and endurance to perform. We can measure and monitor these components to determine if we are on a path to a high quality of life or if we need to modify our physical activity habits to reduce our risk for disease and long-lasting injuries.

Skill-related or performance-related fitness components refer to how efficiently the body moves, typically within the context of a sport. The skill-related components of physical fitness are power, speed, reaction time, coordination, balance, and agility. These components are often measured to predict how well a person may perform in a given sport or athletic competition and can be used to make training decisions for improving athletic performance (National Strength and Conditioning Association, 2015).

However, it should be also noted that, although power is most often referenced as a skill-related component of fitness (ACSM, 2018) and defined "as the ability of the neuromuscular system to produce the greatest amount of force in the shortest amount of time" (Pavlovic, 2018), as well as related to bone health in youth and enhancing muscular strength in adults (IOM, 2012; Corbin & LeMasurier, 2014), some consider power to be a combination of both health-related and skill-related fitness.

A physically fit individual possesses a healthy standard of all the health-related fitness components, plus is capable of efficient movement when participating in physical activity. Each of the health-related and skill-related fitness components uniquely influence one's physical health, yet they all advance athletic performance and health outcomes in some way. Many of the health-related fitness components are also necessary for enhancing athletic performance in various sports. For example, soccer players with higher cardiorespiratory-endurance fitness levels perform more effectively on the field than those with lower levels (Jemni, Prince, & Baker, 2018). Muscular strength is foundational for sports that require power production, such as football, soccer, netball, and basketball, whereas leg strength can help athletes sprint faster and jump higher. Flexibility and body composition greatly affect performance in gymnastics, diving, and wrestling.

Improving skill-related components doesn't only affect one's ability to perform in sports, but it can also have a positive impact on health-related fitness. Many individuals find more enjoyment in engaging in sport activities, such as playing lacrosse, pickleball, and golf, rather than in fitness-focused activities, which include cycling, running, and resistance training. Enjoyment of movement typically equates to longer and more consistent exercise sessions and a greater likelihood of enhancing health-related fitness components. Body composition, in particular, will be positively influenced through increased calorie expenditure. Additionally, as student-athletes become more coordinated and agile and develop quicker reaction times, they can create fast-paced games with extended rallies as exhibited in tennis, badminton, and volleyball, promoting greater cardiorespiratory endurance. A student may never choose to run on a track after graduation, but she may play a sport for an hour, creating a similar positive outcome on cardiorespiratory endurance. However, engaging in an hour of sport activity does require a higher level of skill-related components than running on a track. By possessing functional levels of the skill-related components, individuals increase their options for engaging in a variety of physical activities across their life span.

Since physical fitness is multidimensional, knowing how to train each of the components and their relationship to health and performance are critical curricular topics in fitness education. *Exercise prescription* is the process for making decisions about how to train the fitness components. Students learn how to prescribe themselves the right kind and amount of exercise to achieve the level of physical fitness that they desire.

THE BASIC PRINCIPLES OF TRAINING

Since the development of fitness education and exercise training programs are embedded in physiological sciences, it is important for the physical education teacher to gain a higher-order understanding of how the physiology of exercise impacts student fitness gains for the purpose of teaching students how to apply the knowledge and skills necessary to achieve health-enhancing levels of fitness.

Exercise produces acute or immediate physical responses in the body systems, such as an increased heart rate, increased rate of breathing, and activation of additional muscle fibers. When an individual consistently engages in exercise, those acute responses result in *training adaptations.* Training adaptations are how the body physiologically changes to meet the demands of exercise. Examples of adaptations include increased muscle mass, decreased body fat percentage, and increased energy to perform exercise. Different exercises elicit different responses, so a fitness education program must consider what types of exercises will produce the desired training adaptations. Described next are several basic training principles that guide how to design fitness programs to create the desired physiological adaptations, which include the *principles of specificity, individuality, overload, progression, variation,* and *regularity*.

As the physical education teacher, attention should be based on the individual student in the application of training principles. It is important to note that not all students start at the same fitness level and not all students will end up at the same fitness level. Careful consideration should be placed on how active the student was before entering your class, how motivated the student is to improve her own level of fitness, and how inclusive you develop your lesson plans to ensure that students with disabilities are engaged with the fitness activities delivered throughout the course.

Specificity

The very first step in designing a fitness plan is to identify a specific training goal. A program designed to improve sports performance will look different than a program focused on health outcomes such as losing weight or reducing high blood pressure. Therefore, decisions regarding the types of exercises and training methods will be dependent on the specific purpose of the educational program, and the desired outcomes of the student.

The principle of specificity states that the type of demand that is placed on the body dictates the type of adaptation that will occur. An individual must perform the appropriate frequency, intensity, time, and type of exercise to achieve the desired result. Variations in each of those variables will create a distinct training adaptation. How often, how long, and how hard I train will impact how my body systems change in response to exercise. Running shorter distances at a faster speed creates different training adaptations than running longer distances at slower speeds. Lifting lighter weights at a faster speed and with more repetitions will create a different training adaptation than lifting heavier weights at a slower speed with fewer repetitions.

The first question to answer in the fitness planning process is: What do I want to accomplish by implementing this fitness plan? Students may be very clear about what they want to accomplish, such as increase their quickness on the basketball court, jump higher, or do more pull-ups. Some students may not have goals until after they assess their fitness and are made aware of an area of growth. As mentioned in chapter 1, fitness assessments are key to knowing the state of one's physical health and are essential in prescribing the appropriate amount of exercise to improve fitness. In this way, the principles of specificity and individuality, described next, work together to help students formulate appropriate fitness plan goals.

Examples of how to apply specificity in fitness planning include:

- *Which specific fitness component will I focus on?* Examples: cardiorespiratory endurance, muscular strength, or flexibility
- *What specific movement patterns will I train?* Examples: jumping, throwing, or sprinting
- *What specific muscle groups will I target?* Examples: quadriceps, biceps, or deltoids
- *What specific energy system will I train?* Phosphagen, an immediate energy source; anaerobic, explosive short-term energy without oxygen; or aerobic, an energy system that uses oxygen used for longer periods of exercise at a lower intensity

An individual with multiple goals, such as decreasing mile time and improving upper-body muscular endurance, will require different fitness plans for each of these components. Examples of such plans are described later in the chapter.

Individuality

The *individuality* principle states that training programs must be customized for the individual based on his needs, goals, and responses to exercise. There is no one-size-fits-all fitness program. Each person has different fitness levels, genetic potential, exercise experience, body limitations, access to equipment, and motivation levels. In adolescence, heredity and maturation greatly affect students' fitness levels and how they respond to exercise even if they are the same age. Students may have contraindications to exercise, conditions that increase the risk of injury when engaging in some form of activity, that prevent them from participating in certain activities. For example, exercises that cause hyperflexion, such as deep squats or the standing toe-touch stretch, are contraindicated for students with Down syndrome because of their tendency to have joint hypermobility, which increases their risk for dislocation (Winnick & Porretta, 2017). Once any contraindications are identified, the teacher can work with the student to select developmentally appropriate activities that reduce the risk for injury. Therefore, making all students perform the same workout in a class session without accounting for individuality can be hazardous to students' health. The following are questions to answer to apply the individuality principle:

- What is my current fitness level for each component of fitness?
- What equipment, if any, do I have access to?
- Do I have any physical limitations in performing exercises?
- What physical activities do I like to do?

Overload

Fitness assessment establishes a baseline or starting point in program design and is essential for applying the overload principle. The overload principle states that a person must increase the workload or intensity, either in the cardiorespiratory, muscular, or skeletal systems that the body is accustomed to in order for adaptations to occur. To improve a component of fitness, a person must do more than her baseline. By stressing the body with more than it has done in the past, the body will react by causing physiological changes to handle that workload the next time it occurs. Keeping the same intensity will result in a plateau, a point when progress stops, as the body systems have adjusted to those demands and don't need to exert more effort. Examples of applying the overload principle include:

- Lifting heavier weights
- Increasing the number of exercises performed
- Decreasing the rest time in between exercises
- Increasing the amount of time spent in sessions

Progression

The principle of progression emphasizes the need to gradually and systematically overload to bring about the desired improvements. Achieving higher levels of fitness or performance cannot occur without overload; however; there is a balance to increasing exercise intensity. Overloading too quickly can lead to injury, and overloading too slowly can stunt improvement. Rest and recovery are vital in progression, as training hard without adequate recovery time can lead to overtraining. Overtraining symptoms include excessive fatigue, constantly sore muscles, decreased performance, depression, and chronic injuries. Recommendations for applying the progression principle include the following:

- Increase only one variable at a time (frequency, intensity, or time).
- Start low and go slow.
- If excessive fatigue or soreness occurs, lower intensity.
- Master the correct form with the load before adding more.
- Plan a recovery day.
- Keep a fitness log of progressions.

Examples of exercise progressions will be demonstrated in part II, chapters 8 through 15, and in the routines that follow each respective chapter.

Variation

Individuals who follow the same fitness plan over an extended period of time will reach a point where it is extremely difficult to see any improvement or stay motivated. The principle of variation must be applied in fitness programs to yield more consistent gains. Variation denotes consistently changing aspects of your workout while maintaining progressive overload.

Consequences associated with neglecting the principle of variation include boredom, plateauing, and repetitive stress injuries. Not only may someone grow bored by doing the exact same exercises over and over again, but one also may acquire a repetitive stress injury (RSI). RSIs occur from overusing certain muscles and joints without adequate rest time. For example, RSIs in the shoulder joint are common in wheelchair basketball players, as they repetitively use pushing motions to propel themselves. To combat this issue, a training program needs to vary movement patterns by emphasizing pulling movements more than pushing movements to help promote a balanced shoulder joint that is less prone to injury (Athletics for All, n.d.).

Examples of how to apply the principle of variation include the following:

- Use different types of aerobic activities, such as swimming, running, biking, rowing, and arm cycling.
- Adjust resistance training sets and repetitions after three to five weeks. For example, instead of always using 3 sets of 10 for every exercise, do 2 sets of 15 or 4 sets of 8.
- Incorporate different resistance training exercises for similar movement patterns, such as incline or decline push-ups instead of regular push-ups.
- Engage in cross-training and avoid sport specialization to use muscle groups in different ways.

Regularity

Once a fitness program is established and implemented, the regularity principle must be applied. The principle of regularity states that fitness training adaptations are not permanent and that individuals must exercise on a regular basis to maintain fitness levels. Inconsistent training will limit potential fitness gains, and extended sedentary behavior will result in a loss of fitness improvement. "Use it or lose it" is a true saying in this case, as fitness improvements cannot be "stored" for later use. If cardiorespiratory training is reduced, the acquired training adaptions can be retained for several months, but if all training stops, or detraining, any gains will typically be reversed within two to four weeks (Neufer, 1989). Gains in muscular strength can be maintained for three to four weeks of detraining, but then gradually disappear if retraining doesn't start (McMaster, Gill, Cronin, & McGuigan, 2013).

EXERCISE FITNESS PLANNING: DESIGNING THE TRAINING TO FITT THE GOAL

FITT is an acronym used for assigning the right type of exercise plan that incorporates the four essential program design elements: *Frequency, intensity, time,* and *type* and the basic training principles for each component of fitness. As mentioned previously, each of the program design variables can be manipulated to create a specific training adaptation. FITT provides a framework that teachers can use to help students answer the question, "Does my training FITT my goal?" When students design their workout sessions using the FITT framework (see table 2.2), they will be applying the principles of specificity, individuality, and overload to their workout sessions (see table 2.3). Answering the questions listed in the FITT framework after two to four weeks can then incorporate the principles of progression and variation, as responses to the questions may change if students are regularly following their fitness plans.

Fitness professionals have established recommended exercise prescriptions using the Exercise is Medicine initiative by the American College of Sports Medicine (ACSM) to achieve health-enhancing fitness for various age groups using the FITT frameworks. These prescriptions can further be used as starting points to help students design personalized fitness plans that will improve the different components of fitness. The basic FITT prescriptions for adolescents and adults to achieve a healthy standard for each of the health-related

Table 2.2 The FITT Framework

Program design element	Question
Frequency	How often should I train this week to meet my goal?
Intensity	How hard do I need to work this week to meet my goal?
Time	How long should I train for each session this week to meet my goal?
Type	What exercises should I do each session this week to meet my goal?

Adapted from Klavora (2018).

Table 2.3 Sample Applications of FITT Guidelines

Fitness component	FITT guidelines
Cardiorespiratory endurance	F—most days of the week I—60%-70% of maximal heart rate T—60 min T—walking, jogging, biking, swimming, rowing
Muscular fitness	F—2-3 days per week with rest days between I—body resistance training weight that allows for 8-15 reps, 1-3 sets T—no specified time, part of getting 60 min of physical activity daily T—body weight
Flexibility	F—at least 3 days per week or more I—stretching to mild discomfort, backing off slightly, then holding T—holding each stretch for 10-30 sec (repeat 4-5 times) T—static stretching that targets major muscles and tendons

Adapted from SHAPE America (2020, p.49).

components of fitness are described in each of the subsequent sections.

Cardiorespiratory Endurance

Your level of cardiorespiratory endurance demonstrates how well the circulatory and respiratory systems can deliver oxygen to the muscles during physical activity (see figure 2.1). These two systems have to work together to supply all parts of the body with oxygenated blood. The respiratory system brings in oxygen to the body through breathing and then moves it to the alveoli and blood in the capillaries of the lungs. That oxygen is then transferred to the left atrium of the heart and from there to the left ventricle, which pumps oxygenated blood to the rest of the body. Deoxygenated blood is then circulated back to the heart and enters the right atrium, and the blood is then passed into the right ventricle, which pumps deoxygenated blood to the lungs.

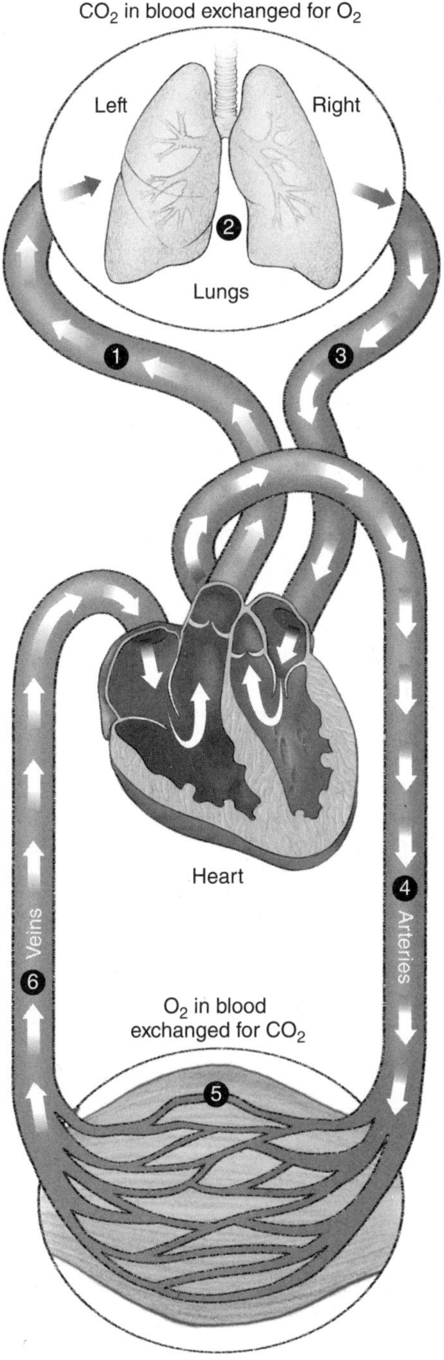

Figure 2.1 Circulation of blood.

The more oxygen that you can use, the longer that you can perform activity before fatigue sets in. Maximal oxygen uptake ($\dot{V}O_2$max), also termed *aerobic capacity*, is the maximal rate of oxygen that can be used during intense exercise. $\dot{V}O_2$max testing is the most acceptable measure of cardiorespiratory fitness; however, it is not realistic to use this assessment in a school setting due to the required equipment and time constraints. In place of a $\dot{V}O_2$max laboratory test, the mile run and the 20-meter shuttle run (FitnessGram PACER test) can be used as valid estimates of cardiorespiratory fitness in adolescents (Batista, Romanzini, Castro-Piñero, & Vas Ronque, 2017). Chapter 7 provides details on using different fitness assessments to determine cardiorespiratory fitness levels in the physical education setting. Aerobic capacity is dependent upon how well the respiratory system can bring oxygen into the body and how fast the heart can pump oxygenated blood to the rest of the body. A higher $\dot{V}O_2$max equals a greater capacity to perform physical activity because your body can efficiently pump and use oxygen longer before your energy is maxed out and you have to stop. *Cardiac output*, the total volume of blood pumped through the circulatory system in one minute, is a major limiting factor in prolonged physical activity. A greater cardiac output means more blood can be delivered to the body at a faster rate. Cardiac output is primarily controlled by the number of times the heart beats per minute and stroke volume, the amount of blood that is pumped with each beat. It can be improved through aerobic training.

Training Methods and Adaptations

Cardiorespiratory endurance can be improved by performing aerobic exercise of sufficient intensity and duration. Sufficient intensity means that the circulatory and respiratory systems are overloaded through aerobic activity that is above the baseline. *Aerobic* exercise is any activity that requires oxygen as an energy source and uses large muscle groups continuously and in a rhythmic nature, such as swimming, walking, or cycling. *Anaerobic* exercise, on the other hand, involves quick bursts of energy and is performed at maximum capacity for a short time, such as jumping or sprinting.

A major training adaptation that occurs by engaging in aerobic exercise that overloads the circulatory system is an increased stroke volume. *Stroke volume* is how much blood is pumped out of the left ventricle with each beat, and it is affected by the strength of each contraction, known as *contractility*. The left ventricle becomes stronger through exercise and is able to pump more blood with each beat. Physiologically, the heart becomes a more efficient pump because a larger stroke volume means that your heart needs fewer beats to distribute blood throughout the body. Eventually, this adaptation will lower the *resting heart rate* (RHR), which is the number of heartbeats per minute while at rest. A lower RHR decreases the overall workload on the heart since it is not working as hard to pump blood throughout the body. Maintaining a lower RHR over time greatly reduces the risk of heart disease and premature death, which is one way that cardiorespiratory training contributes to improving one's quality of life (Jouven et al., 2009). Students can take their RHR to determine if they are in healthy range. After the age of 10, normal RHR ranges are between 60 to 100 beats per minute, with the average adolescent RHR at 78 beats per minute (Ostchega, Porter, Hughes, Dillon, & Nwankwo, 2011). Elite athletes may have an RHR between 40 to 60 beats per minute, indicating that they have highly efficient circulatory and respiratory systems. To find your RHR, count your pulse for 60 seconds, or 30 seconds, and multiply by 2, right after you wake up and before you get out of bed in the morning.

Benefits of Aerobic Exercise

Engaging in consistent aerobic exercise has been shown to

- decrease blood pressure,
- improve cognitive performance and memory function,
- reduce risk for chronic diseases (cardiovascular diseases, cancer, stroke, and diabetes), and
- decrease rates of depression and anxiety.

FITT Prescription for Cardiorespiratory Endurance

The recommended FITT prescription for adolescents and adults performing aerobic exercise is outlined in table 2.4. The session frequency and time are determined by the intensity of the activity performed. The greater the intensity of the aerobic exercise, the less time and fewer days are required to accrue the training adaptation benefits. To maximize aerobic gains in adolescents, it is recommended to use a mixed intensity approach (Faigenbaum, Lloyd, Oliver, & ACSM, 2020). Such an approach is typically referred to as *high-intensity interval training* (HIIT), and involves shorter durations of higher intensities followed by periods of rest or low-intensity exercise. Training

Table 2.4 FITT Prescription for Cardiorespiratory Endurance

	Adolescents (≥ 11 years)[a]	Adults[b]
Frequency	Three or more sessions per wk of vigorous activity	Three or more sessions per wk, depending on time and intensity of activity
Intensity	Most sessions should be moderate to vigorous ≥ 75% HRR (heart rate reserve)	Relative intensity is the level of effort required to do an activity. Relative intensity can be estimated using a scale of 0 to 10, where sitting is 0 and the highest level of effort possible is 10. Moderate-intensity activity is a 5 or 6. Vigorous-intensity activity begins at a level of 7 or 8
Time	Session duration 5-60 min dependent on intensity and baseline fitness	The equivalent of at least 150 min of moderate-intensity aerobic activity each week or 75 min of vigorous-intensity activity
Type	Structured or unstructured intervals of high-intensity work ranging from < 10 sec to 4 min Activities that can be performed at a high intensity intermittently with lower intensity and that are enjoyable to perform, such as playing games or sports, biking, and running	Aerobic activities that move the large muscle groups in a rhythmic manner for a sustained period of time; examples include running, brisk walking, bicycling, playing basketball, dancing, arm cycling, cross-country skiing, and swimming

[a]Adapted from Faigenbaum, Lloyd, Oliver (2020).

[b]Adapted from U.S. Department of Health and Human Services (2018), 57-58.

that involves longer durations at lower intensities is referred to as *continuous training*. Studies have shown that children and adolescents, including overweight and obese youth, respond more favorably psychologically and physiologically to HIIT exercise than other types of aerobic training, such as continuous training (Delgado-Floody, Espinoza-Silva, García-Pinillos, & Latorre-Román, 2018; Garcia-Hermoso, et al., 2016). HIIT is much more time efficient than other forms of aerobic training while also stimulating greater gains in aerobic capacity and decreasing blood pressure and body fat percentage to a greater extent.

Exercising at the appropriate intensity is essential to attaining the training benefits of cardiorespiratory training. The following list is three methods that can be used to help students monitor their aerobic exercise intensity to determine if they are safely creating an overload effect.

1. *Measuring heart rate.* One way to gauge intensity is by measuring your heart rate to see if you are in an overload range. This method is especially useful if students can use heart rate monitors or if they are able to count their pulse during activity. The heart rate reserve method (HRR), as shown in The Heart Rate Reserve (HRR) Method for Finding Target Heart Rate Zone sidebar is a formula for calculating a target heart rate zone based upon the student's age and current level of heart health as measured through RHR.
2. *Breathing rate.* When engaged in activity, students can simply speak out loud and the intensity of the activity can be determined by how uncomfortable it is to talk while exercising. If you can talk but not sing during the activity, that is considered moderate-intensity activity, and if you will not be able to say more than a few words without pausing for a breath or stopping the activity, then that is considered vigorous-intensity activity (Centers for Disease Control and Prevention, 2020).
3. *Rating of perceived exertion (RPE).* RPE measurements estimate intensity by self-reporting the degree of physical strain that one is feeling during the activity using a pre-established scale. The Children's OMNI Scale of Perceived Exertion (figure 2.2) has pictures and verbal cues that allow students to explain through pictures or cues attached to pictures how high they perceive their intensity to be. The picture version of these scales can be extremely useful with students for whom English is their second language or students with speech or communication disorders. Scores of 4 to 6 are considered moderate intensity, while scores above 7 would be vigorous intensity.

The Heart Rate Reserve (HRR) Method for Finding Target Heart Rate Zone

- Step 1: Determine resting heart rate (RHR).
- Step 2: Calculate your maximum heart rate (MHR); 220 – your age = MHR
- Step 3: Subtract your RHR from your MHR and then multiply it by the recommended target heart rate zones (THRZs) for your intensity.

Recommended zones: Moderate = 40%-59% HRR, Vigorous = 60%-89% HRR

(MHR – RHR) × 0.40 + RHR = Low end of THRZ

(MHR – RHR) × 0.59 + RHR = High end of THRZ

Example for determining a moderate intensity THRZ for an 18-year-old student with a resting heart rate of 73 bpm.

220 – 18 = 202

[(202 – 73) × 0.40] + 73 = 124 Low end of THRZ

[(202 – 73) × 0.59] + 73 = 149 High end of THRZ

His THRZ would be between 124 and 149 beats per minute during aerobic exercise.

Note: One way to determine if you are in your THRZ if you do not have a heart rate monitor is by counting your pulse immediately after performing the activity. A recommended way to check pulse is to count for 10 seconds and then multiply by 6.

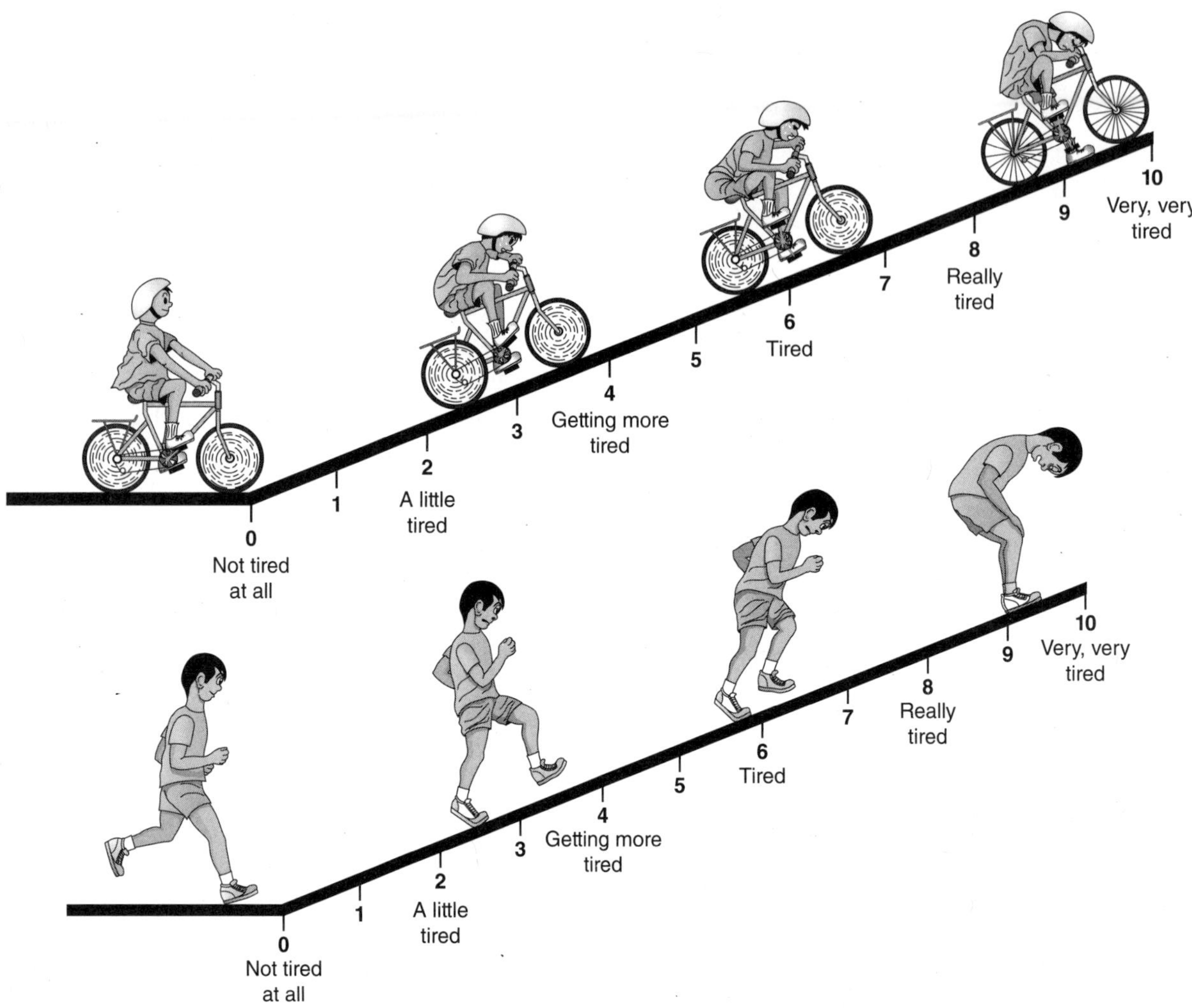

Figure 2.2 Children's OMNI Scale of Perceived Exertion.

Reprinted from R. Robertson, *Perceived Exertion for Practitioners: Rating Effort With the OMNI Pictures System* (Champaign, IL: Human Kinetics, 2004), 145, 146. By permission of R. Robertson.

Muscular Fitness: Strength, Endurance, and Power

Muscular fitness defines your ability to use your muscles to perform work against a resistance. There are three separate yet interrelated components of muscular fitness: muscular strength, muscular endurance, and power. *Muscular strength* is the ability to exert maximum force in order to overcome a resistance in a single effort. Having a high level of muscular strength means that when loads are heavy, you can generate enough force to move the load, such as lifting a heavy box from the floor to the bed of a truck. One's level of strength can be determined through tests such as the one-repetition max (1-RM) lift on bench press or squat, if you are performing resistance training using weights. Power is the ability to exert force in the shortest period of time. It is essentially high-speed strength, as you are exerting high force while contracting at a high speed. Power, a skill-related component, is heavily used in sport performance such as when spiking a volleyball, pitching a fastball, or throwing a shot put. It can be measured through tests such as the vertical jump and power clean, if weights are being used. *Muscular endurance* is the ability of muscle to continue to contract against a submaximal resistance without fatigue. Sports like swimming, rock-climbing, and cycling require high levels of muscular endurance as do jobs such as landscaping or construction when you may need to shovel loads of dirt repeatedly over a period of time. Tests for muscular endurance include the push-up and curl-up assessments, as they are performed in a continuous manner for several seconds to several minutes without a rest period while maintaining proper technique.

Training Methods and Adaptations

To improve muscular fitness levels, an increased stress must be applied to skeletal muscles through resistance training. *Resistance training* is any physical activity that causes the muscles to work against an external resistance. Examples of resistance-training modalities include conditioning with your own body weight exercises, free weights, weight machines, elastic bands, or implements such as kettlebells, medicine balls, or sandbags. A common misconception is that resistance training requires the use of heavy weights and is primarily for sport performance. There are different types of resistance-training methods, such as weightlifting, powerlifting, or bodybuilding, that require the use of specialized equipment and heavy loads. However, resistance training to develop functional levels of muscular strength and endurance is vital across one's lifespan and necessary to reduce the risk of disease and disability. Adolescents need to engage in resistance training to improve bone-mineral density, and adults need to engage in resistance training to avoid muscular atrophy. Failure to engage in weight-bearing exercises may put adolescents at risk for developing long-term bone-health complications, such as osteoporosis. Muscular atrophy is a reduction in the size of a muscle; it can be a partial or a complete wasting away of muscle and occurs with aging and a sedentary lifestyle.

Regular resistance training creates two major types of physiological adaptations to skeletal muscle: neural adaptations and structural changes to muscle fibers. At the start of a resistance-training program, the first adaptation is an improved ability of the nervous system to activate and coordinate more muscle fibers. Muscles become more efficient at the movement patterns because the fibers have learned how to work together through a nerve–muscle connection to create more force for those movements. After the neural adaptations occur, structural changes to the muscle fibers are dependent upon the intensity of the resistance, maturational status, and genetic potential.

There are two main types of muscle fibers in the body: type I, slow-twitch fibers, which use oxygen efficiently and are best suited for long-duration, low-intensity activity; and type II, fast-twitch fibers, which produce powerful bursts of strength at high speeds and fatigue quickly. Each person typically has a balance of type I and type II, but some people are born with more of one type than the other, which predisposes them to be better at long-duration activities such as marathons or powerful, high-speed activities such as sprinting or powerlifting. When training type I fibers, the resistance is lower and the repetitions are higher, which can create the structural adaption of increased capillaries to the muscle fibers so that more oxygen can be delivered to the working muscles. When training type II fibers, the resistance is higher, the repetitions are lower, and the structural adaptation of hypertrophy, or enlargement of the muscle fibers, can occur. Strength gains through hypertrophy typically don't happen until after six to eight weeks of training and are also impacted by maturation status. Prior to puberty, adolescents' ability to increase strength through hypertrophy may be limited due to the reliance on hormonal responses for muscle growth.

Benefits of Resistance Training

Although resistance training increases muscular strength through the use of free weights, weight machines, or body weight, the physical education teacher who may not have access to weight equipment should focus on increasing muscular strength solely through the use of body weight without any equipment. Engaging in consistent and developmentally appropriate resistance training has been shown to:

- enhance bone-mineral density and improve skeletal health,
- reduce body fat and increase lean muscle mass,
- improve motor skill performance (e.g., throwing, running, jumping) and reduce sport-related injury risk,
- reduce risk for chronic diseases: osteoporosis, cardiovascular diseases, arthritis, and diabetes,
- help maintain functional independence to perform daily self-care activities,
- improve postural control and reduce risk for back and join pain, and
- improve psychological health (e.g., self-esteem, self-efficacy, overall mood).

FITT Prescription for Muscular Fitness

Each component of muscular fitness (i.e., strength, endurance, power) can be improved by following a resistance-training program that modifies the FITT variables according to one's training age and experience, strength levels, and personal goals. Keep in mind that a resistance-training program does not require the use of equipment to gain the benefits, as body-weight exercises can meet the recommendations. There are minimum recommendations for adolescents and adults to engage in weekly resistance training to improve the health-related components of muscular strength and endurance. These recommendations are listed in table 2.5 and are considered what is necessary to maintain a healthy skeletal and muscular system to avoid the risk of osteoporosis, a bone disease, and to have enough muscular fitness and be able to engage in daily life activities.

Table 2.5 FITT Prescription for Muscular Strength and Endurance

	Children and Adolescents[a]	Adults[b]
Frequency	At least 3 days per week with rest days in between	Engage in activities that strengthen the muscles at least 2 days a week
Intensity	Activities that make muscles do more work than usual activities of daily life Overloading the major muscle groups to feel a resistance	1-3 sets of 8-12 repetitions per activity Complete each set of repetitions to the point where it's hard for you to do another repetition without help
Time	No specified duration, just part of getting 60 min of physical activity daily	No set time for muscular-strengthening sessions. Time depends upon how long it takes to complete exercises that work all the major muscle groups
Type	Muscle and bone-strengthening physical activities that are structured resistance activities (e.g., weight training, push-ups, planks) or unstructured (e.g., climbing trees, monkey bars, skipping)	Resistance activities, such as body-weight exercises, resistance bands, or weight-training exercises that work all the major muscle groups of your body—legs, hips, back, chest, abdomen, shoulders, and arms

[a]Adapted from U.S. Department of Health and Human Services (2018), 49-52.
[b]Center for Disease Control and Prevention (2020).

The resistance or the amount of weight lifted for a specific exercise determines the intensity for muscular fitness. The assigned weight or load is typically expressed as a percentage of the 1-RM or a repetition range. A 1-RM means that the student can successfully perform only one repetition of an exercise. Due to safety concerns associated with supervision and appropriate technique, as well as time constraints, the 1-RM test may not be prudent in a school-based setting. An alternate method for determining appropriate intensity can be to use goal-based repetition ranges. This means that the repetitions are assigned based upon the goal of the student and his training status. Students calculate the appropriate weight for their exercise based upon performing the assigned number of repetitions. Therefore, if the goal is to complete 10 repetitions, through trial and error, the student could find the weight that allows him to complete 10 so that on the 10th rep, he could not complete another repetition. Determining appropriate load is especially important for those with strength-training goals. If the goal is six repetitions and you could complete 15 reps with the weight you are using, then you are not training for strength because the load is not heavy enough to create the training adaptation of increased muscle size. Table 2.6 shows how a training goal impacts the assigned intensity of a resistance-training program. As you can see, students with goals of improving muscular endurance would lift lighter loads for more repetitions than students with goals of improving strength or power.

Regardless of the training goal, a resistance-training program must follow the progression principle, especially for adolescents just starting a resistance program. Table 2.7 shows how FITT can be adjusted based upon *training age*. A youth's training age is the length of time that she has consistently followed a resistance-training program. Training age impacts what adaptations can occur through resistance training as well as how proficient that each student would be in the movement patterns related to different lifts. The longer a person has been training, the less she will see strength improvements from neural adaptations since those occur in the first six to eight weeks of training.

Table 2.6 Assigning Resistance-Training Intensity Based on Training Goal

Training goal	Load (% 1-RM)	Goal repetitions	Sets
Power	75-90	1-5	3-5
Strength	85-100	1-6	2-6
Hypertrophy	67-85	6-12	3-6
Endurance	≤ 67	≥ 12	2-3

Adapted by permission from J.M. Sheppard and N.T. Triplett, "Program Design for Resistance Training," in *Essentials of Strength Training and Conditioning*, 4th ed., edited by G.G. Haff and N.T. Triplett (Champaign, IL: Human Kinetics, 2016), 458, 463.

Table 2.7 Recommendations for Resistance-Training Progressions

Training status	Beginner	Basic	Intermediate	Advanced
Training age	< 2 months Just starting	2-6 months	6 months-1 year	≥ 1 year
Frequency	1-3 sessions per week with 2-3 days of recovery between sessions	2-3 sessions per week with 2-3 days of recovery between sessions	2-4 sessions per week with 2 days of recovery between sessions	2-5 sessions per week with 1-2 days of recovery between sessions
Volume and recovery	1-2 sets of 8-12 reps with 1-min rest between sets	1-2 sets of 8-12 reps with 1-2-min rest between sets	2-3 sets of 4-8 reps with 2-3-min rest between sets	3-5 sets of 2-8 reps with 2-5-min rest between sets
Intensity	Body weight or 50%-70% 1-RM	60%-80% 1-RM	70%-80% 1-RM	85%-95% 1-RM
Type	One exercise for each major muscle group	One exercise for each major muscle group	Two exercises for each major muscle group	8-10 exercises utilizing the major muscle groups that are selected for sport-specificity

Adapted from R. Lloyd et al., *UKSCA Position Statement: Youth Resistance Training,* UK Strength and Conditioning Association 26 (2012): 26-39; National Strength and Conditioning Association (2016).

The most important factor in advancing the intensity is the individual's ability to perform the exercise with proper technique. External loads should not be used until form is perfected. That is why there needs to be an emphasis on body weight–resistance training for youth because developing the correct movement patterns is fundamental to effective resistance training and injury prevention. Many students want to lift heavy weights, but they lack the ability to move their muscles and joints through the full range of motion because they don't have the neural adaptations from practicing the correct form. Allowing students to engage in heavy resistance training without ensuring they have proper technique increases the risk for injury and liability in the physical education classroom. For this reason, it is recommended that the physical education teacher focuses only on examples of body weight–resistance-training exercises.

Strength-training exercises for the upper body, core, and lower body, including the muscle groups activated in each exercise, can be found in chapters 12 through 16. These detailed lesson and activities should be used as a guide in designing activities to improve a student's muscular fitness.

Flexibility

Flexibility, another component of health-related fitness, is the ability of your joints to move through a full range of motion (ROM). ROM is the degree of movement that occurs at a joint. Maintaining an optimal ROM in all joints is fundamental in a fitness program, as it helps our bodies to move efficiently and effectively. Muscular discomfort and stiffness can negatively impact our ability to perform a variety of movement skills. As examples, a tight lower back can cause pain when bending over or walking downstairs; stiff neck muscles can hinder driving because it is hard to turn the head side to side; and a volleyball serve or a push-up can be hard to perform if the shoulder joint is stiff. We may shy away from physical activity if movement causes discomfort, or we may have to lower our intensity levels to avoid sustaining an injury, like a strain, if our muscles are overly stiff and tight.

Many factors can influence one's flexibility: activity level, disease, age, sex, body composition, and joint structure. The less we move, the less our joints go through a full ROM, and inactivity makes the connective tissues stiffer. Body composition can inhibit ROM, as excessive body fat or bulky muscles can block a joint's path of movement. Younger individuals tend to be more flexible, as there is a gradual loss of elasticity in our muscles as we age. Conditions such as arthritis and tendinitis can reduce ROM in joints. Females are generally more flexible than males due to differences in tendon properties (Kato et al., 2005). The structure of the joint, bones, ligaments, tendons, and muscles dictates the possible ROM available at a joint.

Synovial joints, the most common types of joint in the body, are found between bones that move against each other such as the shoulder, hip, elbow, and knee; produce several ranges of movement in the body; and each type of joint has a specific movement or function. These are flexion and extension; abduction and adduction; circumduction; rotation;

supination and pronation; dorsiflexion and plantar flexion; protraction and retraction; depression and elevation; excursion; superior rotation and inferior rotation; and opposition and reposition.

Types of synovial joints include pivot joint, which allows for rotational movements; hinge joint allows for flexion and extension; condyloid joint allows for biaxial movements, such as forward and backward or side to side, and are found in the metacarpal joints; saddle joint; also biaxial, allowing for flexion and extension and abduction and adduction notably in the thumb; plane joint, or gliding joint, allowing for inversion and eversion of the foot and lateral flexion of the vertebral column; and the ball and socket joint, multiaxial, allowing for flexion and extension, abduction and adduction, circumduction, and medial and lateral rotation movements, such as shoulder and hip joints. For example, the knee, a hinge joint, can only move forward and backward, while the shoulder, a ball-and-socket joint, can rotate in all directions. Figure 2.3 shows different types of joints and the movements they afford.

While many of these factors are uncontrollable, a joint's ROM is most affected by the elastic and plastic properties of the muscle and tendons attached

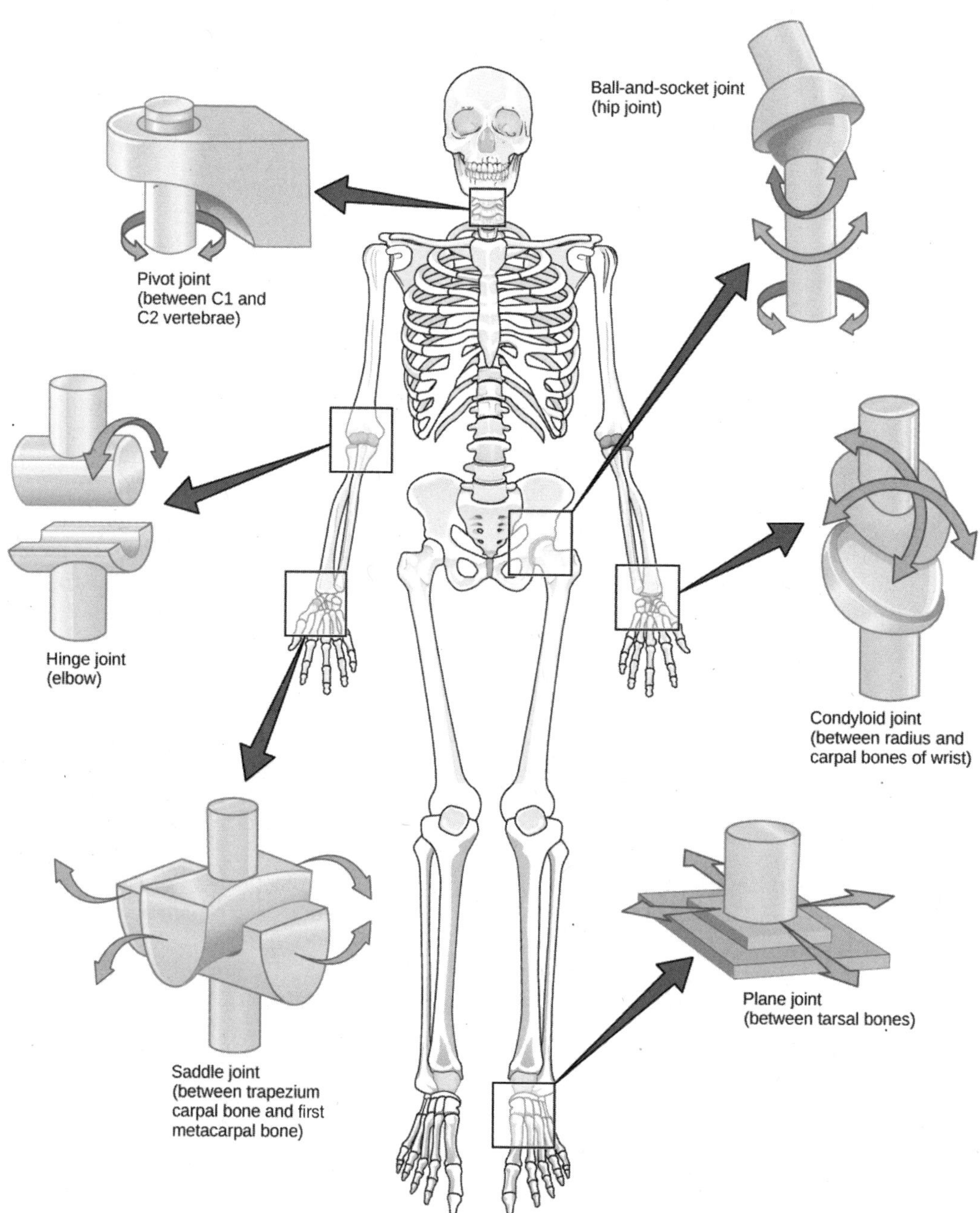

Figure 2.3 Different types of joint movements.

to it, which can be altered through stretching (Hedrick, 2012). Stretching puts parts of the body into positions with the intent of lengthening or elongating the muscles and connective tissues around the joints. There are different stretching methods that can be used in a flexibility plan to increase one's ROM. These methods must be used on various muscle groups as flexibility is joint specific, which includes the muscles, tendons, and ligaments of the engaged joints. To assess flexibility requires different assessments, such as the shoulder stretch, the trunk lift, and the sit-and-reach test, because each one measures ROM at different joints.

As an example, the shoulder flexibility test as part of the FitnessGram test battery, which will be discussed further in chapter 7, is a simple evaluation of flexibility and mobility of your shoulder joint (see figure 2.4). Also known as the modified Apley test, it is used to assess the range of motion (ROM) of your shoulder, including flexion and extension. The muscles engaged in the shoulder stretch test are the rotator cuff muscle group, including supraspinatus, infraspinatus, teres minor, and subscapularis (Quinn, 2019).

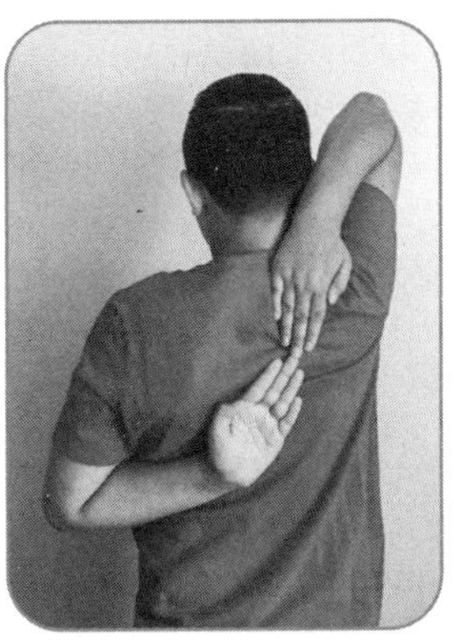
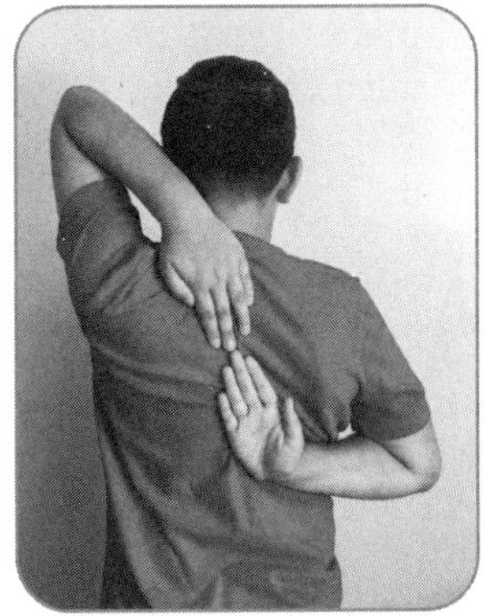

Figure 2.4 Student doing the shoulder stretch.

Training Methods and Adaptations

Since some level of flexibility is needed to perform everyday activities, as well as physical activity and sports competition, incorporating flexibility exercises into physical education lessons is extremely important. The most commonly used modes of stretching used to increase flexibility are static stretching, dynamic stretching, proprioceptive neuromuscular facilitation (PNF), and ballistic stretching.

Static stretching is a slow, constant, and controlled movement in which an end position in held for 10 to 30 seconds (ACSM, 2018). The muscles are slowly elongated, and the student holds a static position at the point of tension, but not pain, for the duration of the stretch. Static stretches can be active or passive. Passive static stretching is when you relax the muscle and an external force is applied to assist in the stretch. The external force, such as a partner or a bench, will hold the body part in place so that the muscle can be stretched against that force. Active static stretching is when there is no application of an outside force. You relax the muscle, and the only force comes from the opposing muscle that is being stretched, such as when you lift your abdomen off the ground to perform a trunk lift. Static stretching is usually performed as part of your post exercise or activity cool-down.

Dynamic stretching is actively moving a joint through its full ROM. In this type of stretching, the joint is moved in a controlled manner, avoiding any bouncing or jerking motions, while gradually increasing the speed and ROM as the movement is repeated several times. Muscles remain active during the entire stretch as opposed to static stretching when they are held stationary. An example of dynamic stretching for the shoulders is performing arm circles. One starts slowly making small arm circles and then gradually increases the size of the circles and the speed of the movement until the shoulder goes through its complete ROM (Schroeder & Alencar, 2017). Dynamic stretching is most often used before a training session and should prepare the body for similar movement patterns that will be performed during a training session.

Proprioceptive neuromuscular facilitation (PNF) is a form of stretching that involves alternating an active isometric contraction with a passive static stretch in a sequence to achieve a greater ROM. This type of stretching generally requires a partner to effectively perform both of the muscle actions. There are numerous forms of PNF, but all tend to involve some type of contract-and-relax method (Garber, et al., 2011). One such form, the hold-relax technique, starts with a 10-second passive stretch applied by a partner, and that action is followed by a six-second isometric contraction in which the student actively holds the leg in place by pushing against the partner's resistive force (Jeffreys, 2016). Once the contraction is released, the partner applies another passive stretch to be held at tension for 30 seconds, but hopefully a little farther than before because of a response in the muscles known as autogenic inhibition (Jeffreys, 2016). The autogenic inhibition response causes a temporary reduction in the tension of a muscle allowing for a further stretch, which is why this form of stretching is thought to create the most gains in static ROM (Page, 2012). Care must be taken when peers are assisting in PNF stretching to avoid any potential injury from overstretching or using improper technique.

Ballistic stretching involves using rapid, high-speed bouncing-type movements. This type of stretching uses the momentum of a body part to try and force it beyond its normal ROM. Ballistic stretching is not recommended as a form of flexibility training in the physical education setting. The degree of stretch and force applied with bouncing is difficult to control, and vigorously pushing muscles and tendons to stretch beyond their limits increases the risk for injury. Students should be highly discouraged from engaging in any stretching activity that uses rapid, jerky motions to try and reach past the point of tension or mild discomfort in a muscle.

The training adaptations that occur with consistent stretching are that the joint connective tissues, tendons, and ligaments can assume a greater length. Muscles have elastic properties that allow them to be stretched like elastic, but they return to their original state after the stretch. Ligaments and tendons have elastic and plastic properties, which means that they can maintain an elongated state after being stretched and don't have to go back to their original state (Jeffreys, 2016). Individuals who want greater flexibility or need it for sport performance, such as gymnasts, will need to engage in more frequent and intense stretching sessions. However, muscles can be overstretched, possibly leading to hypermobility or joint laxity, which can increase the risk for ankle sprains, knee injuries, shoulder instability, and other musculoskeletal injuries (Parrot & Zhu, 2013). To avoid these potential problems, students do not need to perform excessive stretching beyond a functional ROM.

Benefits of Flexibility Training

Flexibility training has several important benefits that cannot be overlooked or taken for granted. Engaging in consistent flexibility training has been shown to

- increase a joint's functional ROM, making physical activity easier,
- improve posture,
- improve performance in sports-related activities,
- release muscle tension, and
- decrease risk of injuries.

FITT Prescription for Flexibility

The recommended FITT prescription for any age group to perform flexibility exercises is outlined in table 2.8. ROM can be immediately improved after stretching, but more permanent gains in ROM have been shown to require a minimum of two to three times a week of flexibility exercises for three to four weeks (ACSM, 2018). Again, flexibility is joint specific, so ROM improvements will only occur in the joints that are being stretched on a regular basis.

The timing of when to perform flexibility exercises is critical to reaping the most benefits. First, flexibility training should be performed after a warm-up that increases core body temperature. If intense stretching occurs when the muscles are cold, there is a greater risk of damaging the muscles and connective tissues. A general warm-up of five minutes with activities such as jogging, cycling, or rolling can increase heart rate, blood flow, and the temperature of the muscles so that they are more pliable. Following a general warm-up, students should engage in dynamic stretching. Dynamic stretching should consist of movement patterns that are similar to the exercise or sport session that will follow. Dynamic stretching prepares the students both mentally and physically for the training session by gradually increasing the intensity of activities.

Static stretching is best performed post-workout. It has been found that performing static stretching prior to training sessions can reduce strength endurance, power performance, reaction time, and running speed for up to one hour after stretching (Faigenbaum, 2012). ROM can be increased more when the muscles are warm, so the best time to do static stretching is after exercise. Static stretching

Table 2.8 The FITT Prescription for Flexibility

Frequency	Perform flexibility exercises with each workout session, as part of a warm-up or cool-down A minimum of 2-3 days a week
Intensity	Stretching to a mild pulling in the muscle, as far as comfortable without pain
Time	Hold static stretches for 10-30 seconds Repeat each stretch 3-5 times so that it is held for a total of 60 seconds
Type	Performing stretches for each of the major muscle groups when muscles are warm (either after a warm-up or at the end of a workout)

Based on American Heart Association, *Flexibility Exercises (Stretching)* (2018). www.heart.org/en/healthy-living/fitness/fitness-basics/flexibility-exercise-stretching

post exercise can help to calm the body by reducing heart rate and breathing rate, restoring muscles to their resting length, and reducing muscle spasms (Hedrick, 2012). Using static stretching at the end of the session can be especially important for students in a physical education class who may need to decompress and gain emotional control before going to another class.

Body Composition

Body composition describes the percentage of fat mass versus nonfat mass (e.g., muscle mass, body water, bone mass) in your body. Body fat percentage is a measurement of body composition telling what proportion of your total weight is fat. Body composition is different than the other health-related components of fitness in that it is not demonstrated or assessed through movement. However, it is similar to all the other health-related components in that it is modifiable through physical activity, it influences how well the body systems operate, and it is a health marker that indicates one's risk for developing various diseases and conditions.

A healthy body composition is one in which your health is not impaired by excessive fat, too little fat, or a negative distribution of body fat. Too low of a body fat percentage compromises health, as the body needs an essential amount of fat to perform various functions related to regulating body temperature, shock absorption, and utilizing different body nutrients, such as the fat-soluble vitamins A, D, E, and F. Too high of a body fat percentage, defined as being overweight or obese based upon the proportion of fat, has negative effects on health by increasing the risk for heart disease, stroke, diabetes, osteoarthritis, and many types of cancer. Having excess fat around the abdominal area, known as visceral fat, is also associated with a high risk for many chronic diseases, regardless of the total amount of body fat. Therefore, the location of excess fat, not just the amount of fat, can negatively impact one's health.

Body composition standards have been established to show what ranges of body fat percentages are considered adequate for healthy living and disease reduction. Table 2.9 shows the recommended body fat percentages based upon age and gender that help to identify if adolescents are at risk for metabolic syndrome (Laurson, Eisenmann, & Welk, 2011). *Metabolic syndrome* consists of a collection of health-related factors, such as increased blood pressure; high triglyceride levels; insulin resistance; and poor cholesterol levels that directly increase the risk of heart disease, type 2 diabetes, and premature death (Al-Hamad & Raman, 2017). Youth who are in the needs improvement category are at a moderate risk for metabolic syndrome, while youth in the needs improvement health risk category are likely to have metabolic profiles that increase the risk of developing diseases (Plowman & Meredith, 2013). Adolescents in the very lean category may be at risk for conditions that impair growth and decrease energy levels, as they may not have enough essential fat for basic body functioning. Methods of assessing body composition will be found in chapter 7.

There are a number of factors that influence body composition and what is deemed healthy for an individual. First, during childhood and adolescence, the body is still developing into a mature form, so height and weight are changing at a rapid

Table 2.9 FitnessGram Body Composition Standards: Percent Body Fat

	Males				Females			
Age	Very lean	Healthy fitness zone	Needs improvement	Needs improvement health risk	Very lean	Healthy fitness zone	Needs improvement	Needs improvement health risk
12	≤ 8.3	8.4-23.6	≥ 23.7	≥ 35.9	≤ 12.6	12.7-26.7	≥ 26.8	≥ 35.5
13	≤ 7.7	7.8-22.8	≥ 22.9	≥ 35.0	≤ 13.3	13.4-27.7	≥ 27.8	≥ 36.3
14	≤ 7.0	7.1-21.3	≥ 21.4	≥ 33.2	≤ 13.9	14.0-28.5	≥ 28.6	≥ 36.8
15	≤ 6.5	6.6-20.1	≥ 20.2	≥ 31.5	≤ 14.5	14.6-29.1	≥ 29.2	≥ 37.1
16	≤ 6.4	6.5-20.1	≥ 20.2	≥ 31.6	≤ 15.2	15.3-29.7	≥ 29.8	≥ 37.4
17	≤ 6.6	6.7-20.9	≥ 21.0	≥ 33.0	≤ 15.8	15.9-30.4	≥ 30.5	≥ 37.9
>18	≤ 6.9	7.0-22.2	≥ 22.3	≥ 35.1	≤ 16.4	16.5-31.3	≥ 31.4	≥ 38.6

Adapted by permission from S. Going and M. Hingle, "Body composition," in *Physical Best*, 4th ed., edited by J. Conkle (Champaign, IL: Human Kinetics, 2020), 138, 139; Adapted by permission from Cooper Institute, *FitnessGram/Activitygram Test Administration Manual*, 5th ed. (Dallas TX: Cooper Institute, 2017), 86, 87.

rate. This is why there are standards for each year during adolescence, which is different than adults, as they are based upon typical growth and development patterns (Centers for Disease Control and Prevention, 2017). Next, females need more essential fat for normal reproductive health and hormone function, so their body fat percentages tend to be higher than males. Genetics also plays a part in body composition, specifically in how body fat is distributed. The largest role in determining body composition is behavioral factors such as physical activity and eating habits, which at a young age are heavily influenced by the environment, as parents and the school setting often dictate the food available and the amount of activity that is possible. Since body weight is primarily impacted by the difference between calories consumed and calories expended, good nutrition and physical activity habits are necessary to achieving a healthy body composition. When teaching body composition, it is important for students to understand the factors that they have control over and then provide them with the education and resources to monitor and manage their body composition. Chapter 5 describes healthy weight-management strategies for adolescents.

TRAINING METHODS FOR THE COMPONENTS OF FITNESS

As you will see throughout this book, various training methods used are contingent on the fitness component that you are trying to improve. Each training method will have a significant impact on your fitness outcome, should be relevant to your fitness goals and objectives, and should be specific in nature. Here, we'll explore two methods, high-intensity interval training and functional training, in greater depth.

High-Intensity Interval Training (HIIT)

A training method that can effectively and efficiently improve multiple components of physical fitness in a single session is the HIIT method. As mentioned previously, HIIT is characterized by brief, repeated bursts of intense exercise followed by periods of rest or low-intensity exercise. It has been shown to be one of the most effective ways to improve cardiorespiratory endurance and metabolic functioning, as well as physical performance in sports (Buchheit & Laursen, 2013). The main goal of the HIIT protocol is to repeatedly exercise close to one's $\dot{V}O_2max$ to elicit the cardiovascular training adaptations. HIIT is most frequently used in aerobic training sessions, but the protocol of high intensity followed by active or passive recovery can be used to structure a variety of lessons in the physical education setting. HIIT can also benefit muscular fitness and skill-related components of fitness and improve body composition through increased calorie expenditure from high-intensity activity.

As shown in table 2.10, any physical education lesson, whether it is fitness or sports-focused, could implement the HIIT protocol. Keys to implementing HIIT effectively are to show students the plan and have them monitor their intensity levels. Knowing the set time frame for exerting near-maximal energy increases the motivation to fully engage because they know there will be a rest period. After several bouts of exercise, the instructor can have students gauge their intensity using one of the methods described in the Cardiorespiratory Endurance section to determine if they are working hard enough to achieve the benefits.

Students, specifically less-conditioned students, can also learn better pacing strategies for exerting their energy when the work intervals are shorter. Having students play soccer for 15 minutes may not elicit very many fitness benefits because students may put in low-to-moderate intensity effort due to the length of time. However, creating a small-sided game with fewer students and for a shorter period of time changes the intensity dynamics. Students are not able to "hide" in the game, so their ability to fully engage increases, and their belief in being able to work hard for three minutes as opposed to 15 minutes may increase effort.

There are a number of variables that HIIT protocols can manipulate, such as the recovery-time duration, the mode of exercise, the exercise duration, the intensity levels, the total time spent in a session, and the number of interval repetitions. The following are three key recommendations to implement HIIT safely and effectively in the physical education class setting.

First, select an appropriate work-to-rest ratio. If rest periods are too short, students will not be able to put forth a quality effort on the subsequent interval, and they will fatigue too quickly to receive the fitness benefits. Also, if rest periods are too long, then the body systems are not overloaded, and there is less possibility for fitness improvement. Rest periods can be active, such as walking or jogging to the next station, or passive, such as drinking water while sitting down.

The recommended work-to-rest ratio depends on how intense the activity is. If students are doing

Table 2.10 Examples of Lessons Using a HIIT Structure

Fitness circuit	Cardio interval training	Small-sided games	Sports training
30-sec push-ups	10-sec sprint	3-min soccer game	1-min defensive slides
30-sec rest	50-sec walk	3-min rest	2-min rest
30-sec air squats	15-sec sprint	3-min soccer game	1-min cone dribbling drill
30-sec rest	75-sec walk	3-min rest	2-min rest
30-sec jumping jacks	20-sec sprint	3-min soccer game	1-min continuous lay-ups
30-sec rest	100-sec walk	3-min rest	2-min rest

interval training that is close to $\dot{V}O_2max$ (75 to 90 percent HRR), then the work-to-rest ratio is 1:1. Therefore, if they are exercising for 30 seconds, then they rest for 30 seconds. If they are doing high-intensity training and operating at their maximal capacity, then the recommended work-to-rest ratio is 1:5; now, a work session of 30 seconds requires a recovery of 2 minutes and 30 seconds (Reuter & Dawes, 2016).

A strategy may be to have students select the intensity of their intervals that best matches their current fitness and motivation levels. Less-fit students may need longer recovery periods or shorter work periods when first starting a fitness program. Based upon how the lesson is structured, you could set the intervals at a 1:2 work-to-rest ratio, but then allow students to select the duration of the work interval and their options could be:

15 seconds work: 30 seconds recovery

20 seconds work: 40 seconds recovery

30 seconds work: 60 seconds recovery

Secondly, select the appropriate frequency of HIIT. Since HIIT is so much more intense and fatiguing than other forms of exercise, there is a greater chance of injury and burnout. It would not be recommended to do multiple days of HIIT training in a week. A proper progression would be to start with one HIIT session each week and then progress up to two or three but spreading the sessions out so they are not consecutive sessions.

And thirdly, do not compromise technique for intensity. A common problem when utilizing fitness circuits in interval training is that students may use improper technique when going all out. Remind students about the importance of maintaining proper technique throughout the entire interval and that reducing the intensity to perform the exercise correctly is more important than trying to get a higher heart rate.

Additional lessons and activities that utilize the concepts and training methods described here and in the physical education setting can be found in chapters 8 and 15.

Functional Training

Another training method that educators can use to improve health- and skill-related components of fitness is functional training. Functional training is a method in which exercises are selected based upon how well they mimic the movement patterns that you wish to improve. You are essentially trying to improve your functional capacity to perform movements that you need to do in daily life. Movement patterns can differ for individuals based upon their participation in sports; their job requirements; and ways they have to move throughout the day, such as biking to school, walking up and down flights of stairs in an apartment building, and maneuvering through doorways in a wheelchair.

In resistance training, the focus tends to be on developing specific muscle groups for either strength, power, or endurance. But, in functional training, the focus is on performing movements and that may require developing strength, flexibility, balance, and coordination in multiple planes of motion. For example, in playing basketball, to perform a layup, a player has to stabilize on one leg while also rotating the upper body toward the backboard. Performing a layup requires balancing on one leg. Functional training means that basketball players would be performing exercises that have them balancing on one leg so that they can improve those movement patterns that are specific to their sport. Table 2.11 shows an example of how some exercises would be more functional for people who have to balance on one leg as part of their everyday life or sport performance. While the other exercises are not bad, they simply are not as helpful in developing the strength, balance, and flexibility that is needed to improve the functional capacity of stabilizing on one leg. The less-functional exercises might be a way to progress to the more-functional exercises, but a goal should be

Table 2.11 The Continuum of Functional Exercises for One-Leg Movement Patterns

Less functional ←		→ More functional
Leg extension machine	Back squat	Single-leg split squat
Sitting hamstring stretch	Standing hamstring stretch	Single-leg forward reach

Adapted from Boyle (2016).

to make the training as close to the performance movement patterns as possible.

Physical educators can incorporate the skill-related components of fitness into the physical education setting through functional training. The benefits of this training are that it can improve the health-related components of fitness while also improving the skill-related components of fitness. An example of improving agility, reaction time, coordination, and cardiorespiratory endurance could be to have students pair up with a tennis ball on the baseline. One partner can toss the tennis ball somewhere between the baseline and half-court, and the other partner has to catch it before it bounces twice. This drill can be repeated several times so that students' heart rates increase, but, at the same time, they are working on reacting, using hand–eye coordination and agility. This drill would be more functional to any sport that requires those skill-related components than simply having students run sprints up and down the court.

CONCLUSION

A well-designed fitness program is necessary to achieving a health-enhancing level of physical fitness. The health-related components of fitness are health markers that can be measured and monitored to improve quality of life and reduce risk for disease and disability. Each of those components–cardiorespiratory endurance, muscular strength and endurance, flexibility, and body composition–requires knowledge of exercise prescription and the basic training principles, including specificity, individuality, overload, progression, variation, and regularity, in order to effectively design an exercise program that will enhance health and fitness gains.

Through an understanding of the training methods for the components of fitness, instruction should also be delivered to introduce the students to the difference between health-related fitness and skill-related fitness and the connectedness of the two in the improvement of sports-skill development. Educators can also maximize physical education time and increase the fitness benefits to students by incorporating exercise prescription principles and strategies, such as HIIT and functional fitness, into their lessons. Educators can also maximize physical education time and increase the fitness benefits to students by incorporating exercise prescription principles and strategies, such as HIIT, into their lessons.

Review Questions

1. Explain the differences between the health-related and skill-related components of fitness.
2. Describe each of the elements of the FITT framework.
3. Explain how you would you use the principles of training to improve cardiorespiratory endurance.
4. Explain why the principle of specificity is important to muscular fitness and flexibility-training program design.
5. Describe the benefits of using HIIT as a training method.

Visit HK *Propel* for additional material related to this chapter.

CHAPTER 3

Curricular and Instructional Considerations in Fitness Education

Chapter Objective

After reading this chapter, you will be able to design an instructional framework for delivering fitness education curriculum in your courses. You will be able to describe a variety of teaching strategies to engage learners in the affective, cognitive, and psychomotor learning domains in online, hybrid, and face-to-face course delivery modes. You will understand how to modify fitness activities and instructional methods to make them accessible to all students. You will understand how to provide feedback that motivates students to improve.

Key Concepts

- Designing an effective fitness education instructional framework will result in low management time, high rates of active student engagement, and greater learning gains.
- Appropriate teaching strategies maximize student learning by organizing the delivery of the instruction so that the teacher and learner roles are well defined in performing the learning task.
- A universal design for learning approach (UDL) involves designing learning experiences so that all students can access the content, regardless of their ability, and proactively designing flexible learning paths.
- Using effective feedback can motivate students to improve future performances more than evaluative grading practices.

INTRODUCTION

The content or curriculum is the driving force in fitness education. The "what" you teach in fitness education was clearly established in chapter 1: the knowledge, skills, and values necessary to achieve health-enhancing fitness and developing behaviors that promote lifetime physical activity. Since health-related fitness concepts are based upon scientific principles, the content will be constant across various physical education programs, but how you teach fitness education will be adaptable to your situation. Chapter 1 described a lack of content knowledge and limited pedagogical content knowledge (PCK) as teacher-related barriers to delivering fitness education. Throughout this chapter, providing you with specific knowledge and skills, you will be able to design learning experiences that increase students' health-related fitness knowledge as you begin to understand what students need to know to achieve and maintain a health-enhancing level of fitness. In addition, you will be able to effectively deliver instruction developed through PCK to organize it in a coherent way, use relevant teaching strategies, make modifications to accommodate diverse learners, and provide feedback that motivates and helps students to improve.

CONTENT KNOWLEDGE AND PEDAGOGICAL CONTENT KNOWLEDGE

Through a progression, chapter 1 described the content of a fitness education curriculum and how you can create student learning outcomes that increase students' health-related fitness knowledge and levels of physical activity. Chapter 2 provided you with a fundamental knowledge base of fitness program design principles and basic anatomy and physiology concepts so that you understand why students must engage in specific types of fitness training. This relevant knowledge will assist you in designing developmentally appropriate fitness-training sessions. Achieving health-related fitness is only possible when students incorporate the principles of training in their fitness activities.

Chapters 8 to 15 will describe the content knowledge necessary to teach correct technique for various fitness-related activities. Since learning in fitness education most often occurs through engaging in physical activity, you must be able to select appropriate exercises, demonstrate proper form, and intervene with corrective feedback when you identify errors. Proper form reduces excessive pressure on joints or muscles that may contribute to injury, and proper technique helps you to target the specific muscle groups you want to work on. Proper form and technique are keys to injury prevention and achieving desired results. Your ability to instruct, modify, and provide feedback on various exercises is not only important for delivering fitness education content but also a form of risk management.

Limited PCK is a barrier to high-quality fitness education because simply knowing the subject matter does not mean that you can translate it into student learning. Some subject matter experts have difficulty helping others understand the content because they do not know how to use instructional methods that accommodate learners' needs. Higher PCK means that you are able to more effectively teach the subject matter to a diverse population of students because you can match learning tasks, teaching strategies, and feedback to the students' skills and abilities (Ayvazo & Ward, 2011). The purpose of this chapter is to increase your PCK for delivering fitness education curriculum by describing how to

- design an instructional framework that organizes the fitness education curriculum,
- employ a variety of teaching strategies to engage diverse learners,
- modify learning tasks to appropriately challenge and progress students, and
- provide feedback that motivates and helps students to improve.

DESIGNING AN INSTRUCTIONAL FRAMEWORK

Fitness education is a curriculum model that articulates what to teach, but not necessarily how to teach it, so you must determine an appropriate instructional model for delivering the curriculum. Instructional models and frameworks describe a cohesive pattern of instructional planning and instructional delivery that effectively promote learning outcomes (Metzler, 2011). Models provide a structure for how students receive the content, engage in the content, and interact with the teacher and their peers in the learning experiences. An effective instructional structure will result in low management time, high rates of active student engagement, and greater learning gains. In addition, adhering to consistent instructional routines may help students feel a sense of security and predictability which can reduce stress and anxious feelings about performing in class, particularly for students who have experienced trauma (Ellison, Walton-Fisette, & Eckert, 2019). Instructional models will utilize different teaching strategies in their approach to student learning. Teaching strategies are your plans for how you will engage the learner and communicate the learning tasks during a lesson. Your instructional framework helps you to align appropriate teaching strategies with curricular goals to maximize student learning.

Three instructional frameworks that can be used in fitness education are presented in table 3.1. Each of these frameworks provides a different structure for delivering fitness education content based upon the learning domains that they prioritize and the curricular components that they emphasize. Despite their different approaches, a common characteristic that all three share is a focus on developing self-management skills. The instructional framework that you choose will be determined by your students' developmental readiness and how you believe that they will best learn the content based upon your instructional capacity and the available resources (e.g., time, technology, and curricular materials).

Each of these frameworks can be used in any of the course delivery modes discussed in chapter 1 (e.g., online, hybrid, face to face). The following section summarizes key features and describes considerations for implementation in the different course delivery modes. The recommended teaching strategies listed with each of the instructional frameworks are explained more fully later in the chapter.

For the completely online mode, there are suggestions for both asynchronous and synchronous learning experiences. The assumption with the synchronous recommendations is that you are able to provide a live option for your students via Zoom, Microsoft Team, Google Hangout, or whichever

Table 3.1 Fitness Education Instructional Frameworks

Instructional framework	Learning domain priorities	Fitness education emphasis
Conceptual physical education instructional approach	1. Cognitive 2. Psychomotor 3. Affective	Conceptual understanding of health-related fitness knowledge
Personalized system of instruction	1. Psychomotor 2. Cognitive 3. Affective	Mastery of fitness activity technique and health-related fitness concepts
Personal and social responsibility model	1. Affective 2. Cognitive 3. Psychomotor	Values, attitudes, and personally and socially responsible behaviors

Increasing Parent–Teacher Communication in Online Teaching

- Provide a weekly schedule of the live synchronous meeting times and the learning tasks that students are to complete.
- Email or post the schedule at the same time (e.g., Sunday at 3:00 p.m.) so that parents know when and where they can access it. Suggest that parents review it with their child to make a weekly plan for attending the class sessions or completing the assigned learning tasks. Explain how students who cannot attend the live sessions will engage with the content.
- Include in your weekly schedule a section on parent support tips that explains how parents can best assist their child with the learning tasks. This might include filming the child performing an exercise, engaging in some form of physical activity with them, asking parents if they would be willing to have their child teach them a new exercise to practice their peer-teaching skills, or discussing fitness-related topics.
- If emailing the parents directly, possibly send them some questions they can use to quiz their students along with the answers so that the parents have the same information you have. Provide them with teacher resource tools to help students prepare for upcoming tests, quizzes, or projects.

video communication system your district supports. While synchronous sessions are beneficial for building community, providing meaningful feedback, and engaging students in the content, they may be challenging for some students to attend due to lack of access to technology at the assigned time (e.g., multiple students in one household, parents needing devices for work, no quiet space to work). For this reason, it is important to be flexible and offer recorded options or alternative means of engagement for students who cannot attend live. In addition, there will be a greater need for increased parent–teacher communication in the online delivery mode, as parents often take on the role of a co-teacher by assisting with a daily schedule, acting as a tutor, and monitoring their child's progress. The more information that you can relay to parents about the expectations of the course, the more likely they will be able to support their child in completing the tasks. The Increasing Parent–Teacher Communication in Online Teaching sidebar provides several ideas for how to involve parents in the online teaching process.

Conceptual Physical Education Approach

As mentioned in chapter 1, conceptual physical education (CPE) is a common curricular delivery method in fitness education. The instructional approach of CPE involves teachers delivering health-related fitness content in a classroom setting using a textbook and then engaging students in physical activity sessions that use the cognitive content (Corbin, Hodges Kulinna, & Sibley, 2020). Table 1.6 in chapter 1 provided examples of instructional delivery ideas according to a CPE and mini-lecture approach. A critical feature in these approaches is that physical activity sessions are specifically chosen to align with the cognitive con-

Table 3.2 A Conceptual Physical Education Instructional Approach Example

Weekly topic	Classroom sessions	Physical activity sessions
Components of physical fitness	• Health-related components • Skill-related components • Purpose of fitness testing	• Introduction to health-related fitness-testing protocols
Fitness principles	• Elements of a workout: warm-up, workout, cool-down • FITT framework • Principles of training	• Conducting warm-ups • Dynamic stretching
Flexibility	• Benefits of flexibility • Basic anatomy of skeletal and muscular systems • FITT for flexibility	• Static stretching • Flexibility fitness testing pre-assessments
Cardiorespiratory fitness	• Benefits of cardiorespiratory fitness • Basic anatomy of circulatory and respiratory systems • FITT for cardiorespiratory fitness • Target heart rate zone • Types of aerobic training	• Cardiorespiratory fitness testing pre-assessments • Interval training • HIIT training • Continuous training
Resistance training	• Benefits of resistance training • Basic anatomy of muscular and skeletal systems • FITT for muscular fitness • Muscular strength versus muscular-endurance training	• Muscular fitness testing pre-assessments • Body-weight training exercises: upper body • Flexibility exercises for upper body • Body-weight training exercises: lower body and core • Flexibility exercises for lower body and core
Program design	• Goal-setting • Creating a personal fitness plan and routine	• Fitness routines: Tabata, circuit training
Stress management	• Benefits of exercise and physical activity on mental and social well-being	• Yoga
Body composition and nutrition	• Maintaining a healthy weight • Food for fuel • Hydration	• Training for a community event
Physically active for life	• Physical activity monitoring • Physical activity plan	• Training for a community event

cepts. You want to connect what students learn in the classroom—the what and why—with the physical activity sessions—the how. Table 3.2 shows an example of how to structure an instructional delivery system using a CPE approach, followed by table 3.3, which provides CPE implementation considerations.

Personalized System of Instruction Approach

A personalized system of instruction (PSI) model is a very effective approach for fitness education because of its ability to individualize instruction. Research studies have shown using the PSI model in high school fitness education courses can improve students' health-related fitness knowledge and help them engage in physical activity for more than 50 percent of class time (Hannon, Holt, & Hatten, 2008; Prewitt, Hannon, Colquitt, Brusseau, Newton, & Shaw, 2015). In a PSI model, student learning is self-paced, as the content and skills are predetermined and presented in units of instruction either on an online platform or in a written workbook. This requires teachers to produce all of the learning tasks up-front, but then it also frees them to be able to provide more individualized support to students. Teachers spend less of class time delivering whole-group instruction, as the learning tasks are described in the written materials. The pre-organized tasks allow for students to work independently and move at a faster pace if they already have experience with some of the content or move at a slower pace if they need more time to master the skills and content. Students must demonstrate mastery of learning benchmarks for each unit of instruction before progressing to the next unit. The teacher takes on more of a facilitator role by monitoring students' progress, providing supports when needed, and then assessing students' work at the learning benchmarks. Table 3.4 summarizes several of the major design characteristics of the PSI instructional model.

Table 3.3 Conceptual Physical Education Instructional Implementation Considerations

Course mode delivery	Instructional Implementation Considerations
Completely online	**Asynchronous time:** Physical activity sessions: Students engage in physical activity on their own time following either teacher-guided directions for activity or a personalized fitness plan. Students may film videos of their form on various fitness activities and upload for teacher review. ***Recommended teaching strategies:*** *Self-instructional learning* **Synchronous time:** Classroom sessions: The teacher delivers cognitive content that precedes the teacher-directed or self-directed physical activity sessions students engage in asynchronously. The teacher demonstrates proper form and technique for required fitness activities or shows students how to access videos to help them learn new fitness activities. ***Recommended teaching strategies:*** *Discussion strategies, direct instruction, cognitive strategies*
Hybrid	**Asynchronous online time:** Classroom sessions: Students complete the cognitive learning tasks as they are presented on the platform, such as watching exercise-technique videos, watching teacher-recorded presentations, or reading written material. Students can prepare their part of a cooperative-learning task by reading content or watching videos on the assigned teaching to present during FTF class time. ***Recommended teaching strategies:*** *Inquiry-guided learning, self-directed learning, direct instruction* **FTF time:** Students engage in physical activity sessions and psychomotor learning tasks that are connected to the cognitive content they are learning online. The asynchronous content has prepared them to actively engage in the class with less time devoted to direct instruction of activities. ***Recommended teaching strategies:*** *Station teaching, reciprocal coaching, cooperative-learning tasks*
Face to face	On Mondays, Wednesdays, and Fridays, students are in the gymnasium or fitness center engaging in physical activity sessions. ***Recommended teaching strategies:*** *Station teaching, reciprocal coaching, cooperative-learning tasks* On Tuesdays and Thursdays, students are in a classroom setting learning health-related fitness concepts that they will apply in the physical activity sessions. Direct instruction of concepts typically occurs in the classroom to increase activity time in the gymnasium or fitness center. ***Recommended teaching strategies:*** *Cognitive strategies, direct instruction discussion strategies, inquiry-guided learning*

Table 3.4 Major Design Characteristics of the PSI Instructional Model

PSI design characteristics	Characteristic description
Learning tasks that are in written form	All or the majority of learning tasks are presented in written or media form and are sequenced in a coherent order that students can follow without much teacher guidance. Students can independently access the learning tasks online or in a personal workbook.
Self-paced progression	Students complete all the tasks at a pace that allows them to become competent. Their progress is tracked and tangible, as it is displayed in their personal workbook.
Self-assessment	Students engage in multiple forms of self-assessment, which allows for immediate detection and correction of errors.
High rate of activity time	Most of class time is spent in individualized subject-related practice and activity time.
Mastery-based learning	The emphasis is on learning the content and skills well and not just moving on to the next thing. Students cannot move on until they have mastered the learning benchmark.
Personalized feedback	Since students are working independently, the teacher has more opportunities to provide personalized feedback related to the students' cognitive and physical abilities.
Reduced classroom management	There are minimal lectures or whole-group demonstrations resulting in less time spent on management procedures. The workbook or online platform manages the instruction of the learning tasks.

Adapted, by permission from S. Prewitt et al. "Implementation of a Personal Fitness Unit Using the Personalized System of Instruction Model," *The Physical Educator* 72 (2015): 382-402.

Successful implementation of PSI has several student prerequisites, such as: Students can read and follow written directions, make wise decisions about their practice time, and assume responsibility for their own learning. If you believe that many students would have difficulty with written material and lack the maturity to pace their own learning, then PSI may not be a good instructional framework to use. However, if you must teach a completely online course in which many students cannot access your synchronous meeting times, then this model would be extremely beneficial, as students could pace their own learning. However, every effort should be made to conduct one-on-one synchronous meetings with individual students based upon an agreed on time to ensure learning gains continue.

Table 3.5 shows an example of how instructional units in a PSI framework could be sequenced, followed by table 3.6, which provides implementation considerations. While PSI is self-paced, there also needs to be a suggested time frame for completing each unit to assist students in maintaining a pace that will fit within the time frame of the course. The suggested time frame holds them accountable to using class time wisely so they are not falling too far behind. You can create such a time frame based upon an estimated number of hours it takes to complete the tasks in each unit and how many hours per week the students have the physical education class. For example, if a student has not completed the first three units after five weeks of the course, that can be a warning sign that he is either disengaged from the course or struggling to understand the content and hasn't reached out for help yet. You can offer the student additional supports to help him get back on track. The goal of PSI is for students to demonstrate mastery of the identified learning benchmarks at a self-determined pace with teachers providing individualized support so students master the required content and skills.

Teaching Personal and Social Responsibility Approach to Fitness Education

The teaching personal and social responsibility (TPSR) model emphasizes students learning how to take responsibility for their own health and well-being and for contributing to the well-being of others. It is both a curriculum and instructional framework that prioritizes the affective domain and embeds the importance of values, attitudes, and responsible behavior into the content and instruction. Using TPSR as an instructional framework for fitness education means that you are framing the curriculum so that students take responsibility for their personal fitness and understand how they can support others in developing healthy lifestyles. This model aligns well with the goals of fitness education because of its strong emphasis on empowering students by teaching self-control, self-direction, and self-motivation. A premise of

Table 3.5 An Example PSI Fitness Education Instructional Framework

Unit topic	Unit components	Learning benchmarks (unit assessments)
• Unit 1: Components of physical fitness • Content hours: 3 • Suggested time frame: 1 week	• Health-related components • Skill-related components • Exercise versus physical activity	Content exam over components of physical fitness (cognitive assessment)
• Unit 2: Fitness principles • Content hours: 6 • Suggested time frame: 2 weeks	• FITT framework • Principles of training • Elements of a workout (warm-up, workout, cool-down)	Quiz on FITT concepts Quiz on principles of training
• Unit 3: Program design • Content hours: 5 • Suggested time frame: 2 weeks	• Fitness assessment • Goal-setting • Creating a fitness plan and routine • Types of fitness-training routines	Documentation of fitness assessment scores (psychomotor assessment) Submit a personal fitness SMART goal sheet using current fitness assessment data (cognitive assessment)
• Unit 4: Cardiorespiratory fitness • Content hours: 5 • Suggested time frame: 2 weeks	• Benefits of cardiorespiratory fitness • Basic anatomy of circulatory and respiratory systems • Training adaptations with aerobic exercise • Target heart rate zone • FITT and principles of training for cardiorespiratory fitness	Submit a FITT plan for cardiorespiratory fitness based upon current fitness data (cognitive assessment) Quiz on basic anatomy of circulatory and respiratory systems (cognitive assessment)
• Unit 5: Resistance training • Content hours: 8 • Suggested time frame: 4 weeks	• Benefits of resistance training • Basic anatomy of muscular and skeletal systems • FITT for muscular fitness • Training adaptations using the principles of training for resistance training • Form and technique for a variety of body-weight exercises for upper body, lower body, and core	Demonstrate 2 lower-body, 2 upper-body, and 2 core resistance-training exercises using correct form (psychomotor assessment) Quiz on training adaptations using the principles of training for resistance training (cognitive assessment) Submit a FITT plan for muscular fitness based upon current fitness data (cognitive assessment)
• Unit 6: Flexibility • Content hours: 5 • Suggested time frame: 2 weeks	• FITT for flexibility • Form and technique for a variety of flexibility exercises for upper body, lower body, and core	Demonstrate 2 lower-body, 2 upper-body, and 2 core flexibility-training exercises using correct form (psychomotor assessment) Submit a FITT plan for flexibility based upon current fitness data (cognitive assessment)
• Unit 7: Body composition and nutrition • Content hours: 4 • Suggested time frame: 1 week	• Weight management • Developing a personal nutrition plan • Food as fuel	Weekly food journal and reflection (cognitive assessment) Quiz on nutrients (cognitive assessment)
• Unit 8: Physically active for life • Content hours: 4 • Suggested time frame: 1 week	• Stress management • Benefits of exercise and physical activity on mental and social well-being • Physical activity community resources	Physical activity in the community assignment

Table 3.6 PSI Instructional Implementation Considerations

Course mode delivery	Instructional implementation considerations
Completely online	**Asynchronous time:** Students complete the learning tasks as they are presented on the platform, such as watching exercise-technique videos, reading written material, completing quizzes, or engaging in fitness-training sessions. Students reach out to instructor for assistance on tasks. ***Recommended teaching strategies:*** *Inquiry-guided learning, self-instructional learning* **Synchronous time:** The teacher can meet with students in small groups or one-on-one in a live session to discuss progress on the tasks and respond to student questions. Teachers can schedule times for students to demonstrate mastery of the learning benchmarks before moving into the next instructional unit. ***Recommended teaching strategies:*** *Self-instructional learning, discussion strategies (if meeting in small groups)*
Hybrid	**Asynchronous online time:** Students complete the cognitive learning tasks as they are presented on the platform, such as watching exercise-technique videos, reading written material, and completing online quizzes. Students reach out to instructor for assistance on tasks. ***Recommended teaching strategies:*** *Self-instructional learning* **FTF time:** Students engage in the physical activity and psychomotor learning tasks of the workbook. The teacher has organized spaces and equipment so that students don't have to wait and can engage in their individualized physical activities safely and effectively. The teacher may work to pair or group students according to their progress so that students can complete physical activities together as a pair or in a small group. ***Recommended teaching strategies:*** *Self-instructional learning, station teaching (self-directed)*
Face to face	Students begin class by reading the tasks in their workbook. The teacher has organized spaces and equipment so that students don't have to wait and can engage in their individualized physical activities safely and effectively. The teacher monitors students' progress and verifies mastery of the learning benchmarks tasks as necessary. For the class closure, the teacher can bring the class together to debrief key concepts. Students may be paired or grouped to discuss exercise strategies they are using. ***Recommended teaching strategies:*** *Self-instructional learning, station teaching (self-directed), discussion strategies*

this model is that students will become empowered when they recognize that they have control over how they treat other people, how much they learn, how they will handle adversity, and their fitness behaviors and use that control for the betterment of their personal health and the health of others (Hellison, 2011). When using TPSR as an instructional framework, there are two main resources that you can use in the instructional design and delivery: the learning experience components and the responsibility levels.

Learning Experience Components

Five components are recommended for each TPSR lesson (shown in the following list) (Hellison, 2011). Teachers use these components for instructional planning of the content and as the format for delivering each learning experience. This format allows for teachers to deliver both the fitness education content as well as the TPSR content, which is described in the responsibility levels (see table 3.7). Table 3.8 shows how the learning experience components can be utilized in different course delivery modes.

Relational time. Build personal relationships with the students and focus on connecting with students to learn their strengths and weaknesses and how to best support them. This part of the session can happen at different points during the session based upon when teachers are best able to interact with students without disrupting the session.

Awareness talk. This starts the class session; the teacher delivers a message to the class about personal and social responsibility and how it relates to the learning outcomes for that class session. The purpose of the talk is to help students to become more self-aware of their personal and social behaviors and how to make good decisions. The levels presented in table 3.7 provide the themes for awareness talks (e.g., self-control, resilience, leadership).

Physical activity. This takes up the majority of each session and is when students can demonstrate TPSR through physical activity opportunities. Providing some type of choice in the physical activity can help students to feel empowered and thus encourage self-responsible behaviors.

Group meeting. This is a class discussion centered on evaluating how well the session went. It is a group process in which both students and the teacher can express concerns and suggest solutions for meeting the learning outcomes. Students can share personal success stories or give a positive shout-out to a peer.

Reflection time. After the group meeting, students will evaluate their decisions and actions during the session. The focus of this reflection is on how well the student as an individual performed so that she can continue to monitor her behavior and set appropriate goals for herself.

Levels of Responsibility

Teachers can use the five levels of responsibility described in table 3.7 to design learning experiences that provide students with opportunities to develop and demonstrate personally and socially responsible behaviors. The levels can be themes or topics for the awareness talks throughout a course so that students progress in their behaviors and are able to demonstrate responsibility outside of the classroom environment.

As you can see, there are multiple ways that you can deliver fitness education. Each framework presents a different approach to the content, and one framework may match your context better than another. Table 3.9 lists several student characteristics that may match to a fitness education instructional approach more than the others.

Table 3.7 TPSR Responsibility Levels Applied to Fitness Education

Level	Student behaviors	Application to fitness education
I: Respecting others	• Demonstrates self-control by avoiding distracting behavior that hinders others' ability to learn • Controls temper and avoids negative talk, such as put-downs or vulgar language • Engages with peers in the class and does not exclude anyone from activities	• Recognizes that everyone has different levels of physical fitness • Does not demean others for their fitness performance • Demonstrates a positive attitude when paired or grouped with students of differing skill or ability
II: Participation and effort	• Exhibits self-motivation by actively engaging in the tasks • Participates in new tasks and does not sit out or refuse to cooperate • Perseveres through difficult tasks and doesn't quit	• Challenges self to improve health-related fitness by striving to give best effort in every activity and not simply going through the motions • Does not complain about trying new activities or having to do activities of high intensity • Uses positive self-talk and other strategies to maintain motivation in fitness activities
III: Self-direction and being on task	• Shows initiative by setting short- and long-term goals that include demonstrating responsible behavior in various situations • Displays an ability to self-start and self-direct; teacher does not have to give reminders to get started on the task or to continue with a task • Demonstrates resiliency and resourcefulness by not allowing obstacles to interfere with the ability to perform the task and reach goals	• Stays on task even if peers display off-task behavior, such as in a fitness station • Holds self accountable for setting SMART fitness goals, and then does what it takes to achieve them (inside and outside of class) • Does not quit because an activity is too difficult; instead, modifies the tasks to create the appropriate level of challenge
IV: Helping others and leadership	• Takes on leadership roles in formal and informal settings to help accomplish tasks • Encourages and supports others to give their best effort	• Volunteers to lead group fitness activities • Provides motivational and constructive feedback to peers • Offers to tutor or help a peer that may not understand the fitness content or activity
V: Transfer beyond the classroom	• Strives to be a positive role model through responsible behavior • Uses values and skills from class in all aspects of life • Attempts to make a social contribution by becoming involved in the community	• Engages in health-enhancing behaviors outside of the classroom • Invites friends or family members to engage in physical activity • Encourages others outside of the classroom to choose healthy lifestyle behaviors

Table 3.8 TPSR Instructional Implementation Considerations

Course mode delivery	Instructional implementation considerations
Completely online	**Asynchronous time:** Physical activity time and reflection time: Students engage in teacher or self-directed physical activity sessions on their own time and then complete their reflections after engaging in the group meetings. ***Recommended teaching strategies:*** *Self-instructional strategies, cognitive strategies (writing prompts in reflection journal)* **Synchronous time:** Awareness talks, group meetings, and relational time: The teacher meets with students in small groups in live sessions to present the awareness talks and conduct the group meetings. The teacher engages students in different discussion-based activities to make personal connections with the students. ***Recommended teaching strategies:*** *Discussion strategies, direct instruction, cooperative-learning tasks*
Hybrid	**Asynchronous online time:** Awareness talks: Students watch or read an awareness talk message to prepare to discuss the topic in class. Students prepare part of a cooperative lesson by reading content or watching videos on assigned teaching topic. Students will complete their reflection after the FTF session and set behavior goals for the next session. ***Recommended teaching strategies:*** *Direct instruction, cognitive strategies, self-instructional strategies* **FTF Time:** Physical activity time, group meetings, and relational time: The teacher focuses on making personal connections with students, has students engage in a cooperative fitness activity, and conducts a group meeting. ***Recommended teaching strategies:*** *Station teaching, discussion strategies, cooperative-learning tasks, reciprocal coaching*
Face to face	The teacher uses all five components of the TPSR learning experience by delivering an awareness talk, having students engage in a cooperative fitness activity, conducting a group meeting, and then instructing students to self-reflect in their writing journal. ***Recommended teaching strategies:*** *Station teaching, discussion strategies, cooperative-learning tasks, reciprocal coaching, cognitive strategies (writing prompts in a reflection journal)*

Table 3.9 Fitness Education Instructional Approaches and Student Characteristics

Instructional approach	Student characteristics
CPE	Students have very little content knowledge on how to achieve health-related fitness; lack maturity to self-pace; and may have varied literacy skills and fitness levels that can be accommodated for in the classroom and physical activity setting.
PSI	Students in the course have very different fitness levels—some very physically fit and others with very low fitness, but the majority of students have good literacy skills and can self-regulate their learning.
TPSR	A majority of students thrive in social settings or they need to establish good support systems for continued engagement in physical activity. Other classes in the school use a value or responsibility-level system similar to TPSR that students are accustomed to and respond well to.

EMPLOYING A VARIETY OF TEACHING STRATEGIES

Teaching strategies are the methods that you use each class session to engage students in the content so they can meet the learning outcomes. They organize the delivery of the instruction so that the teacher and learner roles are well defined in performing the learning task. Not all fitness education objectives can be taught effectively with the same teaching strategies since they encompass learning in the cognitive, affective, and psychomotor domains. You will want to utilize a variety of teaching strategies in your fitness education program to help students develop different skills in each domain. The three instructional frameworks presented previously recommended specific teaching strategies matched to the frameworks' key features and the course delivery mode. The following section explains these strategies so that you understand how to use them in delivering your fitness education program.

A common mistake in implementing teaching strategies is not clearly explaining the student's role in the learning task. It is important to explain the structure of the learning task and what the student needs to do to ensure that she is maximizing active learning time. Chances are you will use several strategies more than once throughout a course, so you can reduce management time by clearly explaining and displaying the expectations of each teaching strategy so that they become an automatic response. When creating expectations for your teaching strategies, think through what students need to know to maximize their time and effort in performing the task, such as how they will be grouped, how long the activity will last, which resources they will need, and the learner responsibilities. There are several examples of how to communicate the expectations of various teaching strategies in the next section.

Station Teaching or Task-Teaching

Description. Students are organized into groups and assigned to start at a station. Each station has its own objective with learning task directions. Stations are typically timed so that students rotate through each station that has an allocated space and equipment. The tasks at each station can be teacher-directed or student-directed. Teacher-directed would include specific instructions on what to perform at each station. Student-directed would allow for students to have more choice over the tasks within the parameters of the station (e.g., time, space, equipment).

Learning domain. This is primarily used for psychomotor tasks, but you can create cognitive or affective tasks for stations.

Teacher role. Set up the designated space and equipment for each station, provide directions for tasks at each station, demonstrate station tasks as necessary, monitor students' performance during station work, and provide feedback on performance.

Student role. Pay attention to visuals and task directions at each station to correctly perform the activity, perform the task at each station, and ask for modifications or clarification if unable to perform tasks at each station.

Considerations for online delivery. This would not be a teaching strategy to use in a completely online course, as there is no need to share equipment or allocate space.

Considerations for hybrid delivery. Teachers can have students prepare for engaging in the stations during FTF time by watching skill videos or reading skill cues cards prior to class. In this mode, the directions to the stations and the instruction for what is expected at each station could occur asynchronously online so that students know how to perform each station. This way active learning time is maximized so that students engage in the station tasks the whole FTF instead of watching demonstrations to activities at the beginning of the FTF session.

Teachers could have students prepare their own fitness activities to do at each station ahead of time by providing the number of stations, the focus of the station, and the equipment available at each station so that students bring a plan to class for what to do at each station.

Considerations for face-to-face delivery. Directions and presentations for each station are provided at the start of class. It is recommended that you have predetermined groups for each station and that they are chosen in a meaningful way, such as by interest, ability, or behavioral management concerns, for example. During class, random groups can also be selected by friends or by commonalities, such as birth months.

Reciprocal Coaching or Peer Feedback

Description. Students work together in pairs to observe and provide feedback to each other using a teacher-generated performance criteria checklist. One student performs the task while the other observes and evaluates, and then the students switch roles. The teacher monitors the students and talks to the peer evaluator rather than the participant if an error is demonstrated. This strategy helps students become proficient in analyzing performances, providing feedback, and developing communication skills.

Learning domain. This can incorporate all domains: psychomotor for performing a fitness activity, affective for receiving feedback and providing constructive feedback, and cognitive for analysis of a peer's performance.

Teacher role. Provide direct instruction on the task to perform, provide direct instruction on how to peer-evaluate the task, provide performance criteria sheets for evaluators to use, monitor students performing task and peers providing feedback, and make suggestions to peer evaluator rather than participant on how to correct the form.

Student role. Both watch and listen to how to perform and how to evaluate the task, perform the task and receive peer feedback, analyze a peer's performance, and provide feedback using the established performance criteria.

Considerations for online delivery. This strategy can be used in a live synchronous session as follows:

Step 1. The teacher demonstrates a fitness activity.

Step 2. The teacher explains the performance criteria checklist and how to evaluate the activity using skill cues.

Step 3. The teacher has students practice evaluating the activity by performing or showing an incorrect performance. Students practice identifying the error(s) using the performance criteria checklists. The teacher works to determine if students are capable of identifying errors and models how to deliver appropriate feedback.

Step 4. The teacher assigns partners and places students into breakout rooms. Every student has access to the performance criteria checklist.

Step 5. Peers perform the fitness activity as directed and evaluate each other's performance using the checklist.

Step 6. The teacher brings all students back to the main session and conducts a group meeting with questions and answers on performing and evaluating the activity. The teacher conducts another demonstration for students to practice identifying errors, possibly using an example of a common error that students demonstrated during practice time. The teacher can ask for a student volunteer to conduct the evaluation or have all students type into a chat box their evaluation responses.

Considerations for hybrid delivery. Have students perform steps 1 to 3 prior to class by providing an online lesson with videos. Steps 4 to 6 can be conducted in the FTF session.

Considerations for face-to-face delivery. The same steps can be utilized in an FTF session. If students have access to video technology and are mature enough to use it appropriately, you can have the peer evaluators record the performance, and then the evaluator can provide the feedback to the student while they both watch the video together, pausing the video to point out any errors or to show examples of excellent form.

Inquiry-Guided Learning

Description. Inquiry-guided learning uses seeking answers to questions as the process to learn new knowledge, solve a problem, or formulate an opinion. This process provides an opportunity for students to explore concepts they are interested in. Questions can be teacher- or student-driven. Once the question is identified, students first gather and organize relevant information; then, they interpret and analyze it; after that, they evaluate and draw conclusions; and, then, they communicate their answers to an audience. In the fitness education context, this strategy could be used with the cognitive content in either of the following ways:

- *Structured inquiry.* You provide the students with a fitness question to answer and a list of reliable resources to use to answer the question.
- *Sample structured inquiry.* How can exercise and physical activity improve mental health?
- *Guided inquiry.* You provide students with a broad fitness topic and a list of resources related to the fitness topic. Then, students develop a question that they would like to research the answer to.
- *Sample guided inquiry topic.* Creating the best fitness plan

Once students have completed the inquiry process they can communicate their answers in a variety of ways, such as through written assignments, verbal discussions, or presentations.

Learning domain. This is primarily cognitive, but it may include affective if the inquiry involves working together as a team.

Teacher role. Provide the directions for the inquiry, model to students how to research answers, and provide support to students who need help finding evidence-based answers.

Student role. Investigate or develop a question, use research methods and evidence-based reasoning to answer the question, and present the answer in the format as directed.

Considerations for online delivery. Students can submit their answers to the inquiry as a written assignment, share it verbally in a synchronous live session to the class or in small groups, or record a presentation and then upload it (presentations may be viewed by the teacher only or by peers in a discussion thread).

Considerations for hybrid delivery. Students can work on conducting their research during their asynchronous online time and then present their question and response in a small group or class discussion during the FTF class time.

Considerations for face-to-face delivery. Students may work in pairs or small groups to research or design a question to research. Each student may select a different resource to read or watch to answer the question, and then the members together can create a response using the information from the different resources.

Discussion Strategies

Description. Discussion strategies require students to communicate with others. These strategies can be used for developing connections, such as getting to know other students in the class, or for furthering understanding by verbally processing information and hearing different perspectives from peers rather than just from the instructor. They can be brief, spontaneous discussions, such as think-pair-share and turn-and-talk, in which students turn to a partner in class to discuss for a few minutes an assigned topic. They can also be planned, in-depth discussions, such as a Socratic seminar (read an assigned text and come to class with prepared questions to discuss) or numbered discussions, in which students prepare their discussion points prior to class.

Learning domain. The domain is primarily cognitive and affective.

Teacher role. Create an open-ended question for students to discuss. Select a discussion strategy and group students in an appropriate way, keeping in mind that the larger the group is, the more difficult it will be for all students to share their responses. Establish norms for the discussion and monitor students' adherence to the norms. Debrief the discussion. To engage students in a discussion strategy, prepare them with the prompt, "When I have you do think-pair-share, this is the process" and the following steps:

Step 1. I will pose a question. You will have one minute to silently think about your response.

Step 2. You will pair up with your assigned partner in the designated area.

Step 3. Partner A will share first. Discuss your responses for two minutes and together formulate a "gold medal" response.

Step 4. Be prepared to share your gold medal response with the class.

Student role. Follow the norms for engaging in the discussion, such as no put-downs, no interrupting, and staying on topic. Listen and be prepared to build upon, challenge, summarize, or clarify other students' responses.

Considerations for online delivery. When delivering a presentation in a live session, teachers can put students into breakout rooms to do a think-pair-share with a discussion question. You can use a format such as numbered discussions as shown in the Discussion Strategy: The Numbered Discussions Expectations sidebar so that students are prepared to discuss their assigned questions prior to the live session.

Considerations for hybrid delivery. Students can prepare for a discussion during the asynchronous

Discussion Strategy: The Numbered Discussions Expectations

Teacher Role

1. Step 1. Assign four discussion questions for students to answer.
2. Step 2. Organize students in groups of four, assigning each student with a number from one to four.

Student Role

1. Step 1. Bring your prepared discussion responses to class.
2. Step 2. The first member in the group starts the discussion by sharing his response to discussion question 1.
3. Step 3. The second member then shares her response, making some connection to or challenging the first member's response. This is either agreeing and confirming the answer or disagreeing and explaining why.
4. Step 4. The third member continues with the process by sharing his response and refers to how his response relates to the responses of the first two members.
5. Step 5. The fourth member repeats the process and then summarizes the key differences and similarities between all of the members' responses.

Note: The process can be repeated so that the fourth member starts the discussion for the second question, and then the first member summarizes the key differences and similarities.

time by reading assigned material and developing responses to the questions. Since students may have a longer period of time to prepare their responses, using the Socratic seminars or numbered discussions format may work well during the FTF time.

Considerations for face-to-face delivery. In this mode, you can use brief discussion strategies, such as think-pair-share and turn-and-talk, so that students are processing and debriefing the content that you have presented. These strategies can be used as a formative assessment to see if students have questions regarding the content. You can do a check for understanding by calling on several partner groups to share their responses to determine if you need to clarify any misunderstandings. You can also use the Socratic seminars or the numbered discussions, along with the following debriefing suggestions:

- First, have groups debrief their responses to the whole class.
- Next, have the second members of each group rotate groups.
- Then, have the second member share his summarized responses with his new group.
- Next, have the other members of each group clarify, build upon, or challenge the new member's responses.
- Finally, have the second members return to their original group and share out the other groups' ideas.

Cognitive Strategies

Description. Cognitive strategies are designed for using your mind to solve a problem or complete a task. These strategies are intended to help students activate prior knowledge, link new information to prior knowledge, and retain new knowledge. Cognitive strategies will help students learn information so that they can explain, discuss, and describe their learning in either written, verbal, or media formats. Examples of cognitive strategies include summarizing or paraphrasing content, creating graphic organizers, comparing and contrasting topics, taking notes, creating acronyms to remember concepts, self-quizzing, writing prompts, and solving problems. Teachers can present problems for students to solve in either a guided-discovery or a divergent-style problem method. *Guided-discovery* problem-solving is when there is a single correct response and the teacher guides the learner or group of learners through a series of questions to discover the answer (Rink, 2020). A *divergent-style* problem is when there is no single correct response, and the learner or group of learners can develop multiple ways to solve the problem (Rink, 2014). These strategies typically are teacher-directed and are used to determine students' understanding of the subject matter after they have read or listened to content information. The Fitness Education Cognitive Strategy Examples sidebar shows examples of different ways that students could demonstrate their understanding of cognitive concepts.

Learning domain. The priority is cognitive; these strategies are intended to help students learn and apply the cognitive content taught in fitness education.

Teacher role. Create the task and explain the cognitive strategy; model to students how to use the strategy if necessary (it is recommended to use a different topic so as to show how to do it but not give answers with the current topic); analyze student responses to determine if there is a need to reteach concepts; and ask students higher-order questions to get them to think more critically about their responses.

Student role. Work to complete the task as effectively as possible and ask for clarification of information if necessary.

Considerations for online delivery. These are the most user-friendly strategies in an online format because they can easily be done asynchronously. Self-check quizzes and writing prompts after reading a section of text or watching an online presentation are examples of cognitive strategies that work well in the online format. They are also a very quick way that teachers can determine if students are understanding the content, as teachers can review data from a self-quiz or responses to writing prompts to see if a majority of students struggled with the same question.

There are several online teaching resources that use gamification to engage students in recalling information in a game-type format. You can create individual or group challenges using the interactive quiz platform Kahoot, or a Jeopardy-style quiz game such as Factile. If there is access to technology by both the teacher and the student, you can use these resources in any of the course delivery modes.

Considerations for hybrid delivery. Any of the listed cognitive strategies in the Fitness Education Cognitive Strategy Examples sidebar would work well in the hybrid mode. The sample exit ticket would work best in an FTF format and could also be modified to be a verbal exit ticket (instead of written) by having students point to where the muscle is located and then demonstrate two repetitions of an exercise that targets that muscle group.

Considerations for face-to-face delivery. If you are delivering a presentation during the class session, you can use these strategies to check for student understanding. After you present content for 5 to 10 minutes or before you switch concepts, have

Fitness Education Cognitive Strategy Examples

Sample Self-Check Quiz Questions

1. If I do a set of squats and a set of curl-ups, what muscle groups am I missing in my workout?
   a. Deltoids and abdominals
   b. Abdominals and quadriceps
   c. Biceps and pectoralis major
   d. Hamstrings and gluteus maximus
2. As a 15-year-old, which of the following resting heart rates indicates a well-conditioned heart?
   a. 130 bpm
   b. 85 bpm
   c. 40 bpm
   d. 25 bpm

Writing Prompt Examples

1. Explain the principle of specificity in fitness program design and tell why it is important to incorporate in order to achieve a health-enhancing level of physical fitness.
2. Why does having a healthy level of cardiorespiratory fitness reduce your risk for heart disease?
3. Identify a career you are interested in pursuing. Explain how your level of physical fitness could impact your performance in that career.
4. What barriers do you face when trying to maintain a healthy body composition?

Problem-Solving Examples

- *Guided discovery.* Can Elena make push-ups at a 30-second fitness station more challenging so that she improves her muscular strength? (Once students have their answer, the teacher can guide them through a series of follow-up questions that has them explain the rationale for their answer. For example, if students answered "no," a follow-up question would be "What would Elena need to do to improve her muscular strength at a 30-second fitness station?")
- *Divergent style.* Sean is a player on the school's wheelchair basketball team, and he wants to start strength training to improve his performance. What upper-body resistance-training exercises would you recommend that he perform, and why?

Sample Exit Ticket

1. Draw a picture that shows where the hamstring muscle is located.
   a. Name and label on your picture the opposing muscle group.
   b. Draw and label a picture of an exercise that targets the hamstring.
   c. Draw and label a picture of an exercise that targets the opposing muscle group of the hamstring.

students engage in a cognitive strategy, such as completing a quick two-question self-quiz of the content or paraphrasing the information on a slide. Having students complete an exit ticket at the end of the class session is a way to formatively assess their understanding before your next class session.

Cooperative Strategies

Description. Cooperative strategies require small groups of students to work together on a common task. These strategies foster communication, promote knowledge sharing, and enhance collaborative problem solving. Informal cooperative tasks are short, impromptu activities that do not require preparation and can be completed in a few minutes. Formal cooperative tasks are structured activities that require each group member to play an active role in accomplishing the goal. These tasks involve more in-depth planning and may take several class sessions to be completed. An example of a formal cooperative task is the jigsaw technique where students are put into groups and become experts on an assigned topic. Each group is assigned a different topic or segment of material, and the students work together to learn as much as possible about their topic. The students are then rearranged into new groups where one member from each expert team teaches the material to the other group members. This then becomes peer teaching where each member of the new group is the only one that is an expert on that topic.

Learning domain. The primary focus is the affective domain, but strategies will require either cognitive or psychomotor learning tasks as well.

Teacher role. Organize appropriate groups, explain directions, and provide resources to complete the task. Monitor groups to ensure all group members are engaged and answer questions as they arise.

Student role. Communicate respectfully with group members and work collaboratively as a team. Fulfill the role that you have been assigned in the group (e.g., leader, recorder, speaker) to the best of your ability.

Considerations for online delivery. Informal or formal cooperative-learning tasks can be used for community building in an online format. Students can be assigned to groups and then put into breakout rooms to complete the tasks. Students can work on formal, cooperative-task research during asynchronous learning time, and then you can conduct the group activity during the live synchronous time.

Considerations for hybrid delivery. The jigsaw technique would work well in a hybrid mode. Students can be assigned to their expert groups prior to FTF, and they can conduct research on their assigned

Informal Cooperative-Learning Tasks for Online Delivery

- *Indoor scavenger hunt.* Students have to find a list of items in their house (e.g., soup can, paper plate, laundry basket, etc.). Members work together to get the most items as quickly as possible. Once they have items, the group members have to create a fitness activity to use with each of the items and relate that activity to a health-related fitness component (e.g., laundry-basket shoulder presses).
- *Website scavenger hunt.* Create a list of questions from reliable health and fitness websites such as Centers for Disease Control and Prevention, ChooseMyPlate.gov, Mayo Clinic, American Heart Association, and American Diabetes Association. Students have to work together to find the responses to the questions in the fastest time.

Sample Formal Cooperative-Learning Task: Jigsaw Personal Training

- Step 1. Create multiple groups of three to four students in each group. Each group is assigned the role of Upper Body Coach, Lower Body Coach, or Core Coach.
- Step 2. Explain the objective of the activity, for example: The objective of this activity is to complete a total body workout in 15 minutes using no equipment other than a bleacher, step, or sturdy chair. Each coach must design a five-minute workout that uses at least two flexibility exercises, three resistance-training exercises, and one vigorous exercise that gets the heart rate up for their assigned body section. You will coach your peers in your five-minute workout acting as their personal trainer. At the end of the session, you will all evaluate the total workout using the muscle group handout. You will determine which muscle groups you worked during the exercises and identify any muscle groups that were neglected in your workout.
- Step 3. Provide time for the expert groups to work together to design a five-minute workout. You can tell students that not all workouts have to be the same and that each coach may have to differentiate the workout for their clients.
- Step 4. Rearrange the groups so that there is one of each coach in the new groups of three.
- Step 5. Have students complete the jigsaw by delivering their personal training session.
- Step 6. Have students evaluate their workout with a muscle diagram handout.
- Step 7. (Optional) Students can return to their expert groups with their evaluation sheets and share how effective their workouts were at targeting different muscle groups.

topic asynchronously. In the first FTF session, the expert groups can share their ideas and formulate their peer-teaching lesson. In the second FTF session, the expert groups are then divided into new groups, and they teach their lesson to the new group. See the Sample Formal Cooperative-Learning Task: Jigsaw Personal Training sidebar for directions for a fitness education jigsaw activity.

Considerations for face-to-face delivery. Cooperative strategies can often be used at the beginning of a course as a way for students to get to know each other through social interaction. You can create activities that have students depending upon each other to achieve a goal and inspiring each other to perform better. The Sample Informal Cooperative-Learning Task for Face-to-Face Delivery: Keep It Up sidebar provides an example of a cooperative task that encourages social interaction, requires students to depend on each other, and facilitates communication.

Self-Instructional Learning

Description. Self-instructional strategies require that the teacher has established the content and the tasks beforehand. The tasks are sequenced and include written materials or media formats, such as videos. Students follow the task directions and then ask for feedback or clarification as they need it.

Learning domain. Self-instructional learning is primarily cognitive and psychomotor. Since students are rarely interacting with peers and rarely with the teacher, the affective domain is typically not targeted with this strategy.

Teacher role. Prepare all of the tasks and materials in advance. Provide directions on how to access the materials. Create performance criteria checklists or rubrics for students to be able to self-evaluate their work. Monitor students' progress of the tasks.

Student role. Follow the tasks in sequential order. Read the directions carefully and ask clarifying questions. Complete all tasks as described using the performance criteria checklists to evaluate work.

Considerations for online delivery. One way to teach proper form for health-related fitness activities is to record demonstrations of various exercises or have pictures of the movement stages and provide performance criteria checklists with skill cues to accompany the videos. Students can record themselves performing the activity and compare it to the

Sample Informal Cooperative-Learning Task for Face-to-Face Delivery: Keep It Up

- Step 1. Create and organize groups into different spaces. It is recommended that no more than six students are to be in one group. Each group will need one beach ball or one balloon.
- Step 2. Give the directions for the activity, for example: In Keep It Up, the objective is to accumulate the highest number of consecutive hits in a two-minute time frame by keeping the beach ball [or balloon] in the air. You will count how many consecutive hits you get without the ball touching the ground, going out of bounds [designate what out of bounds would be], or someone hitting it twice in a row. If one of those three things happens, the team must start the count over.

Note: Allow three rounds of play, making each round more difficult from the last with a specific challenge. The following are some ideas for the different rounds (create challenges based upon the grade level and ability of your students):

- Bump or set like a volleyball.
- Every student spins 360 degrees every time you make a signal.
- Only use one arm (students must keep their dominant arm at their side).
- Play the whole round rotating between sitting and standing. Call out the different positions every 15 to 30 seconds.

In between rounds, give students time to strategize as a team to discuss how they will face the upcoming challenge. You will state before each round what the challenge will be, and then the teams must communicate about how they will complete that challenge to get the most consecutive hits. You may assign a different person in each group to be a captain for the various rounds so that different team members make the group decision about the strategy to use or watch to see who steps up as a leader in each group. After each round or at the end of the class, ask the winning teams which strategy worked the best for them to get the most consecutive hits.

performance criteria checklist and demonstration model to assess their exercise form. Students can then submit a recording or demonstrate in a live session the proper form for the exercise.

Considerations for hybrid delivery. In the asynchronous time, students can design personal fitness plans using teacher-generated templates. You can create prerecorded videos or written instructions for how to write a fitness plan. The students would then perform the fitness plan during the FTF class time. As the students are performing their fitness routines, the teacher can walk around monitoring form and asking students questions related to their plan. Sample questions include:

- Why did you select this exercise as part of your fitness plan?
- How can you make this exercise more challenging? It appears to be very easy for you.
- What would happen if you narrowed your stance and placed your hands closer together when performing that exercise?

Considerations for face-to-face delivery. Students can have a list of tasks to complete, such as perform a side plank, a good morning, and a triceps dip. Once students have practiced those three skills and are confident that they can execute the proper form, then they can ask the teacher to watch them as they perform the movements. The teacher then signs off on those tasks so the students can move on to the next skills.

Students can create and engage in a personal fitness plan utilizing templates as described in the hybrid delivery mode. Students with similar fitness plans may be grouped together to challenge each other to perform certain exercises at greater intensities (e.g., a push-up challenge, a sprinting challenge, a medicine ball throw challenge).

Direct Instruction

Description. Direct instruction comprises explicit, guided instructions that teachers deliver to students in a structured and sequenced manner. Typically, this involves the presentation of cognitive content by teachers in a lecture or demonstration format. It is one of the most effective strategies for teaching new content by presenting the new material in small steps and providing guided practice after each step.

Learning domain. This teaching approach uses the cognitive domain. It is typically combined with other approaches that may incorporate the affective or psychomotor domains. For example, teachers may use direct instruction for a portion of the class and then use discussion strategies or reciprocal coaching strategies after delivering the content.

Teacher role. Develop a presentation with clear learning outcomes that provides clear and detailed instructions. Prepare probing questions to ask during the presentation to check for student understanding of the content. Incorporate other strategies, such as discussion or cognitive strategies, to engage students in the content.

Student role. Actively listen while the teacher is presenting information. Engage in guided practice as directed. Ask questions if information needs more clarification.

Considerations for online delivery. A benefit of the online learning format is that you can create lecture videos or demonstrations that students can view on their own and re-watch on demand. To keep students engaged in the content, it is recommended to segment prerecorded lectures into chunks that are shorter than six minutes (Guo, Kim, & Rubin, 2014). This means that you should create three to four mini-lectures to deliver a 20-minute presentation to avoid students becoming passive listeners in the learning process. For example, instead of having a longer lecture on the broad topic of cardiorespiratory fitness, you could have several short mini-lectures on segments of that topic: the benefits of cardiorespiratory fitness, training adaptations to aerobic exercise, and the FITT framework for cardiorespiratory fitness with checks for understanding at the end of each segment.

Considerations for hybrid delivery. In this mode, you can create prerecorded lectures for students to watch prior to arriving at FTF class. These lectures can include cognitive content that they need to be able to apply in the classroom or directions on the physical activity that will be conducted in the next session. Conversely, you could provide the cognitive lessons in class, and the students could do the physical activity exercises at home.

Considerations for face-to-face delivery. This teaching approach is helpful when introducing cognitive concepts to students for the first time. However, it is not recommended to use this as the only teaching approach in a class session. Integrate other teaching strategies along with your lecture to keep students engaged. Direct instruction will be more successful if instruction is scripted in a clear and logical sequence with a defined objective of the most essential material. This strategy will typically be used prior to teaching a new fitness activity, such as how to execute proper form for the shoulder stretch. Guided practice most often follows a segment of direct instruction so that teachers can monitor students' performance to determine if they understood the instruction.

These teaching strategies are designed to engage students in the content by defining the teacher's and students' roles in the learning process. Some teaching strategies are more effective in teaching psychomotor objectives, while others are more cognitive-focused. Regardless of the teaching strategy you select, you will have to plan for a diverse group of learners by designing learning-task modifications for students who need variations to be able to learn the content and perform the skills.

MODIFYING LEARNING TASKS: A UNIVERSAL DESIGN FOR LEARNING APPROACH

In fitness education, as well as in physical education in general, it is best to use a universal design for learning (UDL) approach in your instructional planning to create an inclusive environment. A UDL approach means that *before* delivering the lesson, you think through how all students can perform the fitness activities and how all students can learn the cognitive content. Instead of trying to make multiple modifications during your lesson, you design the learning experiences to reduce potential learning barriers (Lieberman, Grenier, Brian, & Arndt, 2020). Learning barriers occur when the environment, instruction, or task do not allow for a student to engage in the content. An example of an *environmental* learning barrier is if a student in a wheelchair could not access a fitness space because it is too small to maneuver to. An example of an *instructional* learning barrier is if a student with a learning disability cannot process auditory information very well, and no supports, such as written directions with pictures or demonstrations, are provided when delivering instruction. An example of a *task* learning barrier is making an activity too challenging for a student to physically perform correctly and not allowing modifications, such as only having students perform standard push-ups for the push-up assessment and not allowing a modified version. UDL involves planning learning experiences so that all students can access the content regardless of their ability and proactively designing flexible learning paths (Lieberman et al., 2020). Flexible learning paths include offering a variety of ways to demonstrate proficiency of the learning outcomes rather than one fixed way so as to not exclude a student based upon a physical or cognitive limitation.

In fitness education, a majority of the content includes learning how to perform exercises to enhance health-related fitness. Having the content knowledge to know how to modify exercises by providing accessible and challenging movement patterns is necessary to create an inclusive environment and to be able to challenge students to improve their health-related fitness. Fitness activities in chapters 8 through 15 further provide specific modifications for specific exercises. Accessible movement patterns are not too technically demanding for students and can be adapted with basic modifications such as those shown in the How to Modify Body-Weight Exercises sidebar. In addition, they do not require specialized equipment, which can be difficult for all students to access, so the use of body-weight exercises may be the most accessible movement patterns for many students in a physical education class.

As an example, in a fitness station, if you create a task of performing 10 push-ups and five students lack the strength to perform one correct push-up, another student has an elbow injury that restricts repetitive elbow flexion, and another student uses a wheelchair—what happens? A task of 10 push-ups automatically excludes the student who cannot bend his elbow repetitively and the student using the wheelchair. Ten push-ups become a task barrier to those students. Therefore, how can you provide multiple means of engagement so that all of your students can perform a task with the same purpose as 10 push-ups? In this case, the purpose of 10 push-ups is to develop muscular strength in the upper body, specifically the chest muscles, and the triceps muscles somewhat, while also strengthening the lower back, abdominal muscles, and shoulder muscles, as they are stabilizer muscles needed to execute good form. In a UDL approach, you would label the task "Exercises That Target Upper Body and Core" to allow for student choice rather than limiting the task as 10 push-ups.

Allow students to select the type of exercise that they can do that best challenges themselves by providing options and teaching them how to select the best option. At a station with the task of "Exercises That Target Upper Body and Core," students can select from the options listed in table 3.10. Students who cannot do isotonic exercises because of joint problems can select isometric exercises; a student who is in a wheelchair and has to perform exercises from a seated position may use some equipment to provide resistance. Students who want a more challenging workout can perform clap push-ups at the station to increase strength and power. While all of the exercise options listed in table 3.10 do not work the exact same muscles in the same way, they are similar in function to strengthen many of the same muscle groups as those required in a standard push-up.

How to Modify Body-Weight Exercises

1. *Change body position.* Changing the angle of your body changes the intensity. Exercises done in a plank position become easier when your body is in a more upright position, and they become more difficult when your body is parallel to the ground. Using a wall or a bench to elevate yourself when doing push-ups or planks helps to decrease the challenge.
2. *Reduce or increase impact.* Adding a jumping motion such as a squat jump instead of a body-weight squat to an exercise will increase intensity. To reduce impact, do not have students hit the ground with force for any type of movement (e.g., running, jumping jacks, line-hops). Reducing impact is especially important for students with Osgood-Schlatter disease (knee pain and inflammation that occurs during growth spurts), over-use injuries like shin splint and plantar fasciitis, or obesity (the excess body weight already stresses joints, and more impact increases the risk of developing joint problems).
3. *Reduce the range of motion.* It's best to use the full range of motion of an exercise, but due to injury or reduced strength, a student may not be able to perform exercises in her full range of motion. Isometric exercises involving muscular contractions without movement, such as a plank or wall sit, not only can improve muscle strength, especially in stabilizing muscles but also can eliminate painful movement in joints. Isotonic exercises involve muscular contractions when a body part is moved or the muscles go through a range of motion, such as when performing a squat or push-up.
4. *Reduce or increase stability.* Reducing the stability of an exercise means that you have fewer points of contact with a surface. Reduced stability makes an exercise more challenging, and increased stability will decrease the intensity. Performing a one-arm push-up versus a two-arm push-up or a single-leg squat versus a double-leg squat increases the intensity or load on the moving body part. Lifting an arm or leg off the ground in the plank position increases the challenge of the plank.
5. *Reduce or increase speed.* Increasing the speed of cardiorespiratory fitness activities such as jumping jacks, arm cycling, mountain climbing, or jumping rope increases the intensity. Students with poor fitness levels can still perform those movement patterns, but at a much slower pace until their cardiorespiratory fitness improves.

Students can choose an acceptable level of challenge if there are choices for how they can participate in an activity. Any number of students may come to class tired, sore, or injured at any point, and, by providing different intensity options, you reduce their ability to simply opt out because they "can't do it." You have now made movement patterns more accessible to students in your class by providing flexible learning paths and allowing for multiple means of engaging in the task without changing the purpose of the task.

Not only must fitness activities be accessible, but so must your instruction. As you develop learning tasks for cognitive concepts, determine how you can plan multiple means of instruction so that all students understand the task and how they will be evaluated. For example, if students have difficulty with attention control and working memory, you will want to break instruction into small steps and deliver the instructions right before they perform the task. Because many physical activities require sequential actions, it may be helpful to create task sheets that outline the steps of completing a task in order. Using a format of Step One, Step Two, Step Three for both the skill cues of performing a fitness activity as well as the directions for completing a learning task may be helpful to students with cognitive impairments who benefit from consistent formatting that minimizes distracting information. The Instructional Modifications for Fitness Education sidebar shows ways that you can accommodate students with different information-processing needs through instructional modifications.

UDL is a learning-experience design approach where you attempt to eliminate learning barriers;

Table 3.10 Station Task: Exercises That Target Upper Body and Core

Less challenging ⟷ More challenging					
Body-weight isotonic exercises	Wall push-up	Incline push-up	Push-up	Decline push-up	Plyometric or clap push-up
Seated isotonic exercises	Chest press movements, no load	Chest press with resistance band (Pick level of resistance.)		Chest press with medicine ball (Pick lighter or heavier ball.)	
Isometric exercises	Incline plank	High plank	Low plank	Plank up-downs	Plank with alternating leg lifts

Instructional Modifications for Fitness Education

- Repeat verbal cues in different ways using examples that students can connect with—such [as] "The movement is the same as zipping up a coat zipper."
- Provide demonstrations of fitness activities using pictures or modeling actions. Try to use models that are the same size as the students. Show activities in a whole-part manner before breaking [them] down into parts.
- Do not give directions for all of the learning experiences for the whole sessions at the beginning of class. Only provide directions one task at a time and then provide directions for the next task after that one is completed.
- Break instruction into smaller steps with less information. For example, only provide instruction to three fitness stations instead of six. Have all students practice at those three stations before providing instructions to the next three.
- Physically assist a student to get in the right position and perform the movement if the student allows physical touch.
- Establish consistent routines and transitional cues so that students have assigned spaces to report when you signal a transition time. It may be difficult for students to hear you or see your lips move if you are giving instruction from the other side of the gym, so create routines for how students will be grouped when you give instruction.
- Utilize a buddy system by pairing students with a peer [who] can relay information in a different way or repeat information again after the instructions have been given.

Source: Lieberman, L.J. & Houston-Wilson, C. (2018). *Strategies for inclusion* (3rd ed.) Champaign IL: Human Kinetics.

however, you cannot plan for every modification a student may need, so you will need to differentiate instruction during the learning experiences to further support student learning and achievement. Differentiated instruction is responsive teaching: You respond to student needs as you see them in the moment (Donnelly, Mueller, & Gallahue, 2017). You may need to differentiate the task during a session because you recognize that a student or a small group of students are not progressing toward meeting the learning outcomes. As a teacher, you need to continuously monitor students' performance and conduct formative assessments to know if students need differentiated instruction. The need to differentiate psychomotor tasks is often visible, as you can see if the student is unable to demonstrate proper form for the skill; the differentiated instruction may be to modify body position through physical assistance. You may not know if you need to differentiate instruction for cognitive tasks if you are not collecting formative data on students' content knowledge and ability to apply the cognitive concepts. Students must understand the principles of training to design an effective personal fitness plan. Assessing their understanding and differentiating your instruction to support them in learning that content is vital to achieving fitness education objectives.

THE INSTRUCTIONAL DELIVERY PROCESS

This chapter has primarily focused on the instructional design process: the planning that must occur prior to you actually delivering the lesson. Figure 3.1 shows an instructional delivery process for your planned learning experience. This will be what you do when you are in front of your students delivering instruction in an FTF or synchronous session. The ways in which you deliver these steps will vary based upon your course delivery mode and if you are using a CPE, PSI, or TPSR framework, but each step is a critical component in furthering student learning.

The first step in your delivery is to explain the learning outcomes to students. Frame the learning outcome as the target that they are aiming to hit by the end of the lesson. Next, you can clarify how they will know if they have hit the target—the performance criteria. The performance criteria are what will be measured to know that students have successfully met the outcome. Knowing the performance criteria in advance allows students to be able to self-monitor their performance throughout the lesson to see if they are on track to meet the outcome. Fitness education is characterized by a curricular and instructional approach that helps students develop self-management skills to maintain healthy behaviors, so teaching students how to monitor their performance toward achieving an outcome supports developing self-management skills.

In a psychomotor learning task, the performance criteria will be the skill cues for the movement. The skill cues tell the learner each of the steps of meeting the outcome of performing that movement. In an affective learning task, the performance criteria may be behaviors that students display during a cooperative-learning activity. In a cognitive learning task, the performance criteria may be their ability to summarize a health-related fitness concept in their own words without any type of assistance.

After explaining the performance criteria, you will describe the teaching strategy and learning tasks that the students will perform to accomplish the learning outcome. As described previously, the teaching strategies are the methods that you will use to engage students in the content. As students are engaged in the learning tasks, you will provide opportunities for them to receive feedback on their performance. Feedback can come from a teacher, a peer, self-evaluation, or a video recording. Feedback during the lesson helps students stay focused on the target by letting them know how close they are to meeting the outcome. The final step in the instructional delivery process is to assess the students' progress toward meeting the learning outcomes. How many students achieved the learning outcome? How many students need more practice to meet the learning outcome? The final step informs your planning for the next session. If students have not met the learning outcome for today, then what will you do tomorrow so that they will meet the outcome?

PROVIDING PERFORMANCE FEEDBACK

Feedback is one of the most powerful influences on student learning and achievement (Hattie & Timperley, 2007). It provides students with information regarding their progress toward meeting the learning outcomes. Feedback for cognitive, affective, and psychomotor outcomes will be slightly different. In general, there are two types of psychomotor performance feedback: intrinsic and augmented feedback. *Intrinsic feedback* comes from the sensory information that results from producing movements (Schmidt, Lee, Winstein, Wul, & Zelaznik, 2019). A performer can feel how her muscles tense during a movement and can watch what happens to a weight as she is lifting it as sensing the feedback from the movement. *Augmented feedback* comes from an external or supplementary source, such as a teacher, peer, or video recording that communicates performance to the student (Haywood & Getchell, 2020). The two types of augmented feedback that guide students' learning are *knowledge of results (KR)* and *knowledge of performance (KP)*. In archery, students know they

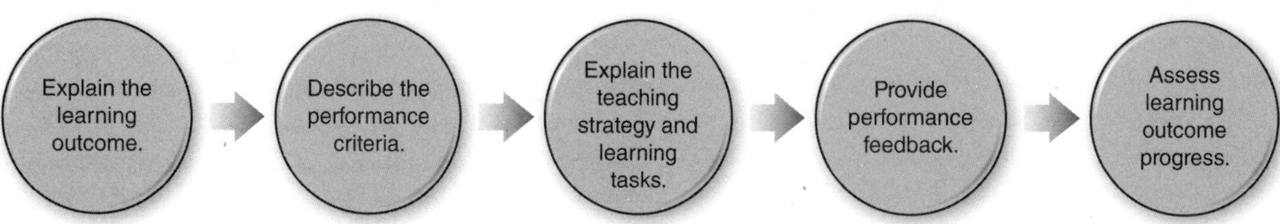

Figure 3.1 The instructional delivery process.

have hit the target when the arrow hits the bull's-eye—this is KR. They can see the outcome of their performance: whether or not they hit their goal. In fitness education, KR would include how many PACER laps, push-ups, or curl-ups that they completed during a fitness assessment. Students can then compare their fitness assessment results with the healthy fitness zone standards to know if they are on track to achieving health-enhancing fitness. The scores act as feedback that tell students if they need to improve a certain component of fitness.

Knowledge of performance (KP) is feedback about the characteristics of a specific movement pattern or skill. If students do not hit the bull's-eye, then that result indicates they need to change something, such as their stance or arm motion, which will allow them to hit the bull's-eye on their next performance. KP can come from you, a peer, or a video recording communicating to the student how his movement patterns align with the performance criteria. In fitness education, this would include providing feedback on the proper form and technique for fitness activities. When performing the push-up, an example of KP would be, "Place your hands directly under your shoulders." This feedback communicates to students the proper preparation stance. You may have noticed that the student was shifting his weight too far back and unable to keep a straight back while lowering himself. Providing the KP feedback for the proper stance may be the assistance that he needed to get his body into the right position so he could perform the push-up correctly. KP feedback is especially critical when students are struggling to achieve the learning outcome. They know they are not hitting the mark, but they may not be able to determine why they are not. KP feedback can also be referred to as *corrective feedback* since its purpose is to correct student errors in learning and performance.

KP feedback can be delivered as either prescriptive or descriptive feedback. *Prescriptive KP* tells the students specifically what the error correction is. It is a prescription for correcting the performance. *Descriptive KP* prompts the student to correct their own errors by describing a problem without providing the solution (Donnelly et al., 2017). As in the push-up example, you would say, "Your back was not in a straight line while you performed that push-up. What do you need to do so that you are able to keep your back straight?" Descriptive KP allows students the opportunity to self-diagnose their performance and demonstrate how well they know the critical elements of a skill. This is an example of a cognitive teaching strategy because you are asking the student to solve a problem by activating prior knowledge. Descriptive KP can be a motivational tool, as students can take pride in solving a problem and implementing their solution rather than you telling them what they need to do. Prescriptive KP may be necessary for beginner-level students who lack the content knowledge of the movement pattern. Selecting prescriptive or descriptive KP during an activity would be differentiating instruction for your students based upon their knowledge level and what you believe would help them improve their learning and performance the most in the moment.

CHARACTERISTICS OF EFFECTIVE FEEDBACK

Effective feedback results in the learner using the feedback to improve performance. Feedback is not effective if the learner's performance remains unchanged. Effective feedback "feeds forward" (Moss & Brookhart, 2015). This means that the learner can use the feedback to improve future performances. The following list comprises several characteristics of feedback that will feed forward in all three learning domains:

- *Effective feedback is specific and actionable.* This means that it is targeted to learners and provides a clear next step in their performance. That next step may be to either continue using their new skill or knowledge as it was performed or to correct their performance in some way to make it more accurate. Students know specifically what action they must take on their next trial that will lead to a more successful attempt. Going back to the push-up example, if you say, "You have poor form," that is not specific, and the student does not know what he needs to do to improve upon his performance. If you give him prescriptive KP such as, "Place your hands directly under your shoulders," or you lead him to that conclusion through descriptive KP, you are providing an actionable next step. That means on the next push-up he does, he will move his shoulders to be directly over his hands instead of his hands out in front of his shoulders. Feedback motivates students when they know that they can improve by implementing a correction that they understand. Students cannot act upon feedback when problems are identified without solutions. Solutions can be self, teacher, or peer generated.
- *Effective feedback is timely and ongoing.* In order for feedback to improve future performances, it must be given while the student is still learn-

ing, still has time to improve, and is provided ample opportunities to improve. That is why in the instructional delivery process "provide performance feedback" comes before "assess learning outcome progress." You do not want to reach the end of the lesson without students having had an opportunity to correct their errors. At the "assess learning outcome" step, the students should know whether or not they have met the learning outcome or what they need to do to meet it. It is possible that they may need more practice due to the complexity of the task, but they are clear about what they need to do in order to demonstrate that they met the target.

Timely and ongoing feedback is especially important when it comes to utilizing fitness assessments in fitness education. If students perform a pre-assessment with set goals to improve a fitness component but without receiving any feedback until the post-assessment, they will probably not improve. Fitness feedback needs to be ongoing in that students are consistently monitoring their progress to reach health-related fitness goals. You need to build into your instruction opportunities for students to use regular fitness feedback so that students stay on track to reach their end goal. An example of descriptive fitness assessment feedback would be, "Your PACER score has only improved by two laps in the past five weeks. Your goal was to improve by six laps at this point. Can you tell me why you think you were not able to reach your goal?"

- *Effective feedback is descriptive, not evaluative.* Feedback should not be grades focused. For students, a grade signifies the end of the learning process. When students receive a grade along with descriptive feedback comments, the grade tends to overshadow the feedback, and students do not use the feedback as formative but rather see the comments as evaluative (Brookhart, 2017). Research on the subject of grades and feedback found that grading does not appear to impact students' future performance as effectively as descriptive feedback (Schinske & Tanner, 2014). To produce greater learning gains, you want to associate feedback with learning and growth, not with rating and evaluation. For this reason, it is recommended to attach feedback to performance criteria rather than a grade (Ntuli, 2018). In fitness education, this would relate to performing fitness activities, writing fitness plans, and keeping nutrition logs. Each of these learning tasks will be ongoing tasks that students can continuously use feedback to improve, so a grade should not be attached to them until the end of the course.

Feedback is an essential instructional strategy because of its influence on student learning and performance. You will want to plan how students will receive feedback during your session to ensure that it is given in the most effective manner and that students have opportunities during class to use the feedback that they receive. Again, feedback must be timely, meaning students need an opportunity to use it immediately rather than in the next class session. Using the characteristics of specific, actionable, timely, ongoing, and descriptive feedback instead of evaluative feedback are essential to making the feedback effective, and thereby helps learners improve on future performances.

CONCLUSION

Fitness education is a curriculum model that focuses on teaching the knowledge, skills, and values that lead to a lifelong health and fitness. You must determine the best instructional approach for delivering the fitness education curriculum by analyzing the characteristics of your students, your available resources, and your instructional abilities. This chapter sought to increase your PCK so that you can more effectively deliver the fitness education curriculum to a diverse population of students. Designing an inclusive instructional approach to fitness education is important to providing students access to all aspects of the curriculum. Physical and cognitive impairments should not exclude students from participating in the learning tasks. As an educator, it is your responsibility to create learning experiences that provide flexible learning paths so that students can choose an appropriate level of challenge. By understanding how to match the learning tasks, teaching strategies, and feedback methods to your students' skills and abilities, you can improve student learning of fitness education objectives. As you continue to increase your content knowledge by reading additional chapters in this book, you will find it easier to design learning experiences that promote students achieving and maintaining a health-enhancing level of physical fitness.

Review Questions

1. Compare and contrast the PSI and the TPSR instructional approaches to fitness education. Describe when it would be more appropriate to use each of the approaches in delivering fitness education.
2. What teaching strategy would be an ineffective strategy to use in a completely online fitness education class, and why?
3. Describe three different ways that you can modify body-weight exercises to appropriately challenge and progress students' muscular fitness.
4. Explain why a UDL approach to instructional design and delivery is a key concept in delivering high-quality fitness education.
5. Describe the characteristics of effective feedback that motivate students to improve future performances.

Visit HK*Propel* for additional material related to this chapter.

CHAPTER 4

Classroom Considerations and Teaching Tips

Chapter Objective

After reading this chapter, you will understand the role that various classrooms' considerations play in impacting student performance, classroom-management constructs, and safety precautions in fitness education programs. Emphasis will be placed on three major headings: *general class and teaching considerations*; *supervision, safety, and environmental factors*; and *equity, diversity, inclusion, and social justice*. Although these could apply to any physical education class, emphasis will be placed on fitness education due to the intensity of the activities involved in the class. Physical education teachers will be provided with knowledge-based concepts as well as how to employ best teaching practices that enhance student learning and comprehension.

Key Concepts

- Class climate has a direct impact on student achievement, engagement and self-management, enjoyment, motivation, and attitudes toward physical activity.
- Communication skills serve as a conduit for class interaction between the student and teacher.
- Managerial skills promote organization, class flow, and a reduction in discipline problems and off-task behavior.
- Student safety involving facilities, equipment, and environmental conditions should be monitored at all times with an emergency plan in place.
- Equity, diversity, inclusion, and social justice are key elements to ensuring students are provided with equal opportunity and access to all parts of the curriculum and programs.
- Accommodations and modifications are recommended so that all activities and instructional materials can be adjusted and delivered to all students in the class.

INTRODUCTION

The common theme throughout this book is that *all* students enrolled in your physical education class should reap the social and emotional rewards and health benefits of participating in a fitness education curriculum. Through the implementation of developmentally appropriate activities based on the students' individual fitness plans and using the universal design for learning strategies, as discussed in chapter 3, with careful consideration, your fitness activities should easily be modified to meet the individual needs of students enrolled in your class. Although the focus is on fitness education, throughout this chapter, emphasis will be placed on *general class and teaching considerations; supervision, safety, and environmental factors*; and *equity, diversity, inclusion, and social justice*, which should be inherent in all physical education classes. By creating a class environment that respects and values diversity, student interaction will be heightened; students will feel safe, free, and confident to perform at their own levels; and your fitness education class will be motivating, engaging, supportive, and fun.

As you begin to design your curriculum and class lessons and conduct a self-evaluation insuring that the intended objectives and outcomes are met, consider some of these internal questions to ask yourself as a self-check on effectiveness:

- Were the goals and objectives of the lesson met?
- Did the students show an understanding of the fitness components involved in the exercises?
- Were all students engaged?
- Was there an easy flow of exercises for the students to perform?
- Did the workout meet the needs of all students?
- Were all exercises adaptable and easy to modify?
- Was the workout fun and challenging?
- What changes need to be made for next time?
- Will I use this lesson again?

Once you establish the direction and parameters of your course objectives and design, it's time to get teaching!

GENERAL CLASS AND TEACHING CONSIDERATIONS

In an effort to keep all students physically and emotionally safe, we as physical educators must develop a positive learning environment where all students feel physically and emotionally safe, feel free to have open and honest communication with their peers and teachers, and take responsibility for their learning and class behaviors. Once we can establish this environment, we can then begin to integrate our instructional and curricular goals and objectives with equity, diversity, inclusion, and social justice issues.

Class Climate

Through years of research on school and class climate, there is widespread belief that student learning is influenced by both the school and classroom environments in which instruction takes place. When students feel connected to their school, they are more likely to experience academic success and better health outcomes (Centers for Disease Control and Prevention, 2020). As cited by Schweig et al. (2014), these qualities of the learning environment are associated with higher student achievement (Allensworth et al., 2018; Durlak, Weissberg, Dymnicki, Taylor, & Schellinger, 2011; Shindler, Jones, Williams, Taylor, & Cardenas, 2016; Aspen Institute, 2019); effectively engaging in class lessons and self-management (Standage, Duda, & Ntoumanis, 2003); expressing enjoyment (Morgan & Carpenter, 2002; Ommundsen & Kvalo, 2007); displaying positive attitudes toward physical activity (Sproule, Wang, Morgan, McNeill, & McMorris, 2007); and becoming more physically active (Wadsworth, Robinson, Rudisill, & Gell, 2013; Ntoumanis & Biddle, 1999). Significant associations between positive climates and school engagement, motivation, and self-efficacy were also found.

When physical education and school-based physical activity were examined, results further supported that school climate played a significant role in gains for academic achievement (Rasberry, Lee, Robin, Laris, & Russell, 2011; Castelli, Glowacki, Barcelona, Calvert, & Hwang, 2015), fewer instances of bullying (Roman & Taylor, 2013), and more emotional well-being and reduced emotional problems in young people (Reid, MacCormack, Cousins, & Freeman, 2015).

The setting and surroundings of where the students are learning is just as important as the material being taught and what the students are learning. Creating a positive and motivational learning environment will play a role toward the road to success for the student, as well as the teacher. In providing for *equity, diversity, inclusion*, and *social justice*, physical education is a place of acceptance and support for everyone by everyone.

A student wants nothing more than to feel physically and emotionally safe, comfortable, and confident. Making sure that every student is an important part of the class and is evaluated as an individual is a step in the right direction. When students feel valued and comfortable in the class setting, then you as the teacher not only gain their trust but also empower them with the opportunity to be themselves and strive for higher levels of accomplishment. Knowing that the only competition is within themselves, attaining their own level of proficiency, and not being compared to their classmates just because they may be faster will speak volumes and promote hard work. This will generate more engagement and enthusiasm, increasing the work ethic allowing room to excel.

Kindness matters. It is important to practice it, promote it, and expect it. Students are faced with daily challenges, so when they arrive to your class, you want their day to become better. A simple "good morning" or "glad to see you" will make them feel welcome. A "please" and "thank you" among students needs to be encouraged. The physical education teacher further has the opportunity to create a climate of social development and relationships.

On the other hand, although competition may evolve, the lack of respect and good sporting behavior cannot, and should not, be tolerated. Allowing students to work out their differences can be done in a healthy way, and physical education class is the place where it is often challenged. Students need to abide by both the school's code of conduct, as well as the teacher's established classroom rules and policies, therefore making them aware what is acceptable and tolerated, leaving no room for violence, bullying, racism, or hate.

As the physical education teacher, especially in a fitness education class where intense effort is required of all students, your secondary role as a motivator will be in creating the eagerness, anticipation, and thrill of what is going to happen in class. High energy and high spirits will become contagious among your students. Being able to be a child's inspiration for a moment may make his entire day, so be that teacher. Remember: Your worst day may end up being your student's best.

Communication

A crucial skill that transcends all levels of educational leadership; management; and administration, teachers, and staff is the ability to effectively communicate. Within the educational system, communication occurs both internally and externally and involves many stakeholders, such as students, teachers, parents, community members, and educational policy makers. When communicating through formal or informal channels, it is important that your message is clear and concise and understood by the recipients to ensure the intended outcome is attained (Greenberg & LoBianco, 2020). Communication channels must also be sensitive to social norms and expectations, as

Positive Learning Environment

- Students feel physically and emotionally safe. They see the classroom as a place where they can be themselves and express themselves and their ideas without judgment.
- Students know that they are valued and respected, regardless of other factors such as ability, gender, sexuality, race, ethnicity, or religion.
- Students have ownership and input related to class structure and expectations. This can range from creating spaces specifically for student use to having a class discussion to establish norms and expectations.
- All students are challenged to achieve high expectations, and all students receive the support necessary to meet those expectations.
- Standards of behavior are established and are consistently and equitably enforced for all students.
- Class structure provides multiple and varied opportunities for students to experience success.
- The teacher gets to know all students and uses that knowledge to create meaningful experiences.
- There is a positive rapport (relationship) between the teacher and students and among students in the class.

Benes & Alperin (2016, p. 224).

well as cultural and language differences, to ensure that message communicated is intentional.

Whether communicating in the form of verbal, written, or electronic communication via email, text, or social media, it is essential that physical education teachers develop the skills to effectively say what they want the students to understand and do and to know what action to take based on that communication. Fundamental to teacher and student success is the teacher's ability to communicate effectively with students, parents, and colleagues. As educators, we also must acknowledge that students also have a voice, which empowers them to develop healthy relationships, learn how to resolve conflicts, and manage their own feelings and thoughts.

The ability to effectively communicate begins with three basic skills: *verbal communication*, the ability to speak; *written communication*, the ability to transmit messages in writing; and *nonverbal communication*, the ability to understand body language, facial expressions, and gestures. Effective communication skills are extremely important for a teacher in delivering classroom instruction and assignments, managing the classroom, and interacting with students in the class. To teach in accordance with the ability and capability of the individual students, a teacher further needs to adopt communication skills intended to motivate the students toward their learning process (Sng, 2012). Effective communication also involves active listening as a key skill.

Verbal communication can occur via face to face or over the phone, in-person presentations, video conferencing, Skype, FaceTime, live webinars, or other modes of technology. Communicating verbally is one of the most powerful modes of communication in that it allows you to exchange ideas and information immediately. It also provides an opportunity for the sender to provide clarification if the intent of the message is misunderstood and allows for interaction to occur naturally. Verbal communication involves the ability to speak clearly and articulate your words and thoughts so that your message is easily understood.

Whether delivering face to face or through the other types of online instructional delivery systems as discussed in chapter 3, you have the ability to maintain eye contact, observe body language, and determine levels of student engagement as the conversation progresses.

Written communication occurs in the form of emails, letters, reports, newsletters, memorandums, and other various documents. For teachers, it is the most commonly used method of communication with the purpose being to convey information through what you put on paper (hard copy) or type electronically on screen. For physical education teachers, this usually occurs in the form of *handouts* that almost all teachers prepare for their students, posters, and organizational information, which could appear on locker room bulletin boards or gymnasium walls.

Nonverbal communication, which is also commonly used but often underestimated, is characterized by using gestures, eye contact, body movements, body language, and even an individual's proximity to another person when communicating, such as when a teacher moves near a student who is exhibiting off-task or disruptive behavior. Nonverbal communication can at times be more powerful than verbal or written communication with the messages that are sent through gestures and body language. Communicating through unspoken words could send various signals and is an equally important method of communication.

Active Listening

Active listening, popularized by the work of Carl Rogers and Richard Farson in 1957, is another communication skill necessary for communication to be effective. It requires the listener to be fully focused on what the other person is saying and responding with body language, such as eye contact, so that the speaker can have some type of acknowledgment that you are listening. Asking questions and responding to what is being said by recapping the conversation also provides a confirmation that you were paying attention and listening. Active listening also involves the understanding of feelings and views that the other person has without passing judgment. Actively listening to students shows that you care about what they are saying and allows for effective teacher–student communication (Greenberg & LoBianco, 2020). Figure 4.1 shows the critical elements of active listening.

Classroom Management

Why is classroom management so important? Simply put, it sets the tone of the expectations and respect of the subject being taught along with respect for the instructor teaching it. In addition, the level of management and control within a classroom will determine the cognitive outcome of the curriculum (Rink, 2014). A well-managed classroom has a task system of protocols and routines to structure the environment and maximize time for learning (Grube, Ryan, Lowell, & Stringer, 2018). The allowance of any disruption during class time will immediately negate the teaching

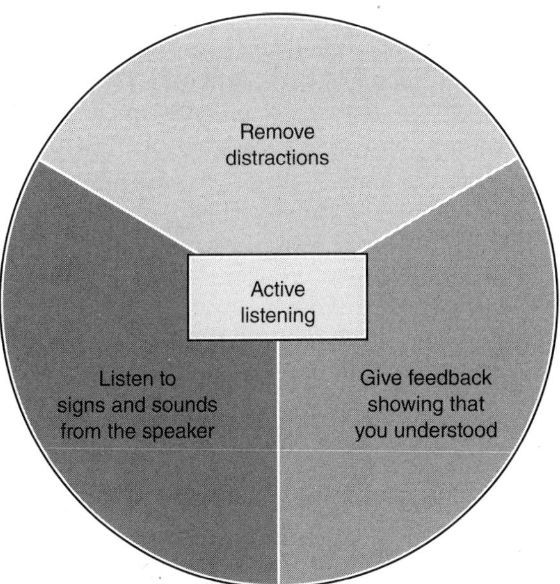

Figure 4.1 The critical elements of active listening.
Reprinted by permission from J.D. Greenberg and J.L. LoBianco, *Organization and Administration of Physical Education: Theory and Practice* (Champaign, IL: Human Kinetics, 2020).

of that day and possibly longer. There are many parts toward effective classroom management that need to be addressed and planned out, including knowing how to group students, knowing how to manage equipment distribution, and establishing locker room entrance and exit protocols. Therefore, devoting time and energy prior to the start of the school year will be a great investment toward a positive outcome.

Preparation and Practical Class Setup

From the arrival bell to dismissal, preparation and organization are major points that will allow for the class to run smoothly. Giving the students the knowledge of where to line up for attendance, which teaching stations will be used that day, and what is to be expected in advance will avoid many questions and confusion that could lead to valuable wasted minutes.

Organization is a major component in effective teaching for any educator. Having the class set up upon the students' arrival will prepare their mindset toward the lessons, activities, and goal for that class period. From excitement to disappointment, a variety of reactions will be displayed. Therefore, always taking into consideration the different levels of readiness within the class and keeping each student on task and engaged will be beneficial for everyone. Having little to no confusion as to how to complete each task is the goal, especially as the students' progress through the course and face more challenging assignments.

Although the focus of this book is on fitness education without fitness equipment, when integrating fitness education with other activities, much time is often wasted in giving out equipment in physical education classes. The physical education teacher who plans to accomplish this organizational task efficiently gains valuable activity and learning time. If the students are working on a specific fitness activity or self-assessing their progress, then providing a task for them to begin working on as soon as they have what is needed will ensure appropriate practice and activity time. If the daily lesson includes a specific circuit, then having the equipment and stations spaced around the area in the formation that the students will be working will further eliminate wasted time and increase student activity time.

As with any physical education class, students should be physically active for a *minimum* of 50 percent of actual lesson time. Through appropriate planning, fitness education instructional time and lessons can make a significant contribution to students improving and maintaining health-enhancing levels of individual fitness gains as designated in their fitness plans. Well-organized classes will further lead to greater levels of student engagement, which will foster increased participation in physical activity throughout students' life spans. Try some of these strategies to increase activity time.

Time Management

Depending on the school's daily schedule, time is always of the essence. Time management is directly related to being prepared and organized. As we all know, the failure to prepare will prepare you to fail. For that reason, the goal is to achieve the best time management possible. Considering time to be the most valuable element in teaching, we need to be sure that enough time is allotted to achieve what we set out to accomplish.

This means that everyone is on the clock. The teacher needs to make the most of the time with the students in order to be effective, and the students need to perform their due diligence in minimizing locker room time and other class managerial issues. As a result, implementing a classroom routine to allow for the unexpected obstacles, such as inclement weather for outdoor activities, will still give ample time to complete the implementation of the day's lesson and student assignments. Be cognizant that the quality of learning supersedes the quantity.

From the time students come to class until they leave at the end of the class period, they come to class ready to move and should be provided the opportunity to do so. Having the class period organized in this fashion sets a positive environment for the rest of the class lesson. For example, as the students begin to leave the locker rooms, while you are still in there performing your supervisory responsibilities, consider having music playing in the spill-out or lineup area; have student leaders begin some class exercises, dances, or other preliminary warm-up activities; or even provide a strategically placed bulletin board or informational and educational posters for students to review as they enter the gymnasium or participation area. The quicker students dress for participation and exit the locker room, the quicker the instruction and activity can begin.

Additionally, time management also refers to appropriately managing the transition between in-class activities. It is extremely important to minimize student transition and waiting times in physical education classes, not only to increase student time on task and activity times but also to eliminate any opportunities for off-task or disciplinary problems.

Physical education teacher instructions should be short and concise so that students can get moving quickly. If the teacher overloads the students with too much information, they are likely not to remember everything or simply tune themselves out. Instruction should include precise tips and demonstrations and check for learning and understanding throughout and after the lesson. Having students work with predetermined partners or cohorts will further assist in moving the instructional time along, as they can complement each other in activity time and lesson comprehension.

Although there are established and clear expectations of what is to be accomplished, sometimes things do not work out as planned. Being flexible and having the ability to deviate along the way is essential. In fact, as long as the end result and outcome is met, that deviation may even turn out to be a better plan. Sometimes we just need to go with the flow and have fun with it so that the students will as well.

Role Modeling

In the school environment, physical education teachers promote health, fitness, and wellness through modeling behaviors. Whether you realize it or not, students pay very close attention to their teachers in every way. They notice what they wear, how they speak, what they eat, and the mood that they are in that day. In many cases, we are with these students most of the day and probably more than their parents or guardians, making us their *role model* whether or not we sign up to be or realize that we are.

Although they may not hear you, they always see you. When students begin to mimic you, take it as a compliment. If they are doing it correctly, it is a sign of learning and respect. What you say and do becomes contagious, and that is the consistency that some students look for in their daily lives. Staying positive and inspirational will lead to an environment that reflects the same.

We need to be on guard and be conscious to represent how we want the students to act upon entering the classroom each day. As that relationship grows, soon the students will, too. Students will see right through to the core, so honesty and transparency in all interactions with students is a critical element to student motivation and success.

Instruction Through Interaction

Physical education teachers can assist students in appreciating the value of physical education by sharing their passion, which is imperative to creating a positive atmosphere within the class. This, in turn, will be the beginning of building relationships with the students. Physical education teachers are in a unique position for developing professional and trusting relationships with their students because, in many cases, the physical education teacher can have the same students for multiple courses or multiple years. Numerous times, that particular health and physical education instructor is the one person or staff students seem to seek out for guidance or just an ear to listen, and, more importantly, to be heard. This is especially evident when the physical education teacher may also be the athletic coach.

Knowing your students is just as critical as them getting to know you. Of course, remember to set very strong boundaries, keeping in mind that you are the teacher and they are the students. Although we know to be careful and set boundaries, we need to be there for students and be present. Remembering that being a good listener is hearing more than what is being said. Listen to anything the students want to tell you. If you do not listen to the small stuff now, they will never tell you the big stuff later!

Relationship-building does not end in the classroom. Building communication with parents is also an effective strategy in promoting effective student progress. Although most parent phone calls or emails are negative ones, it is just as important to make positive ones to inform parents that their child's behavior is improving in the right direction. This positive reinforcement will pay off in the long run. Always remember to log all of your calls with parents.

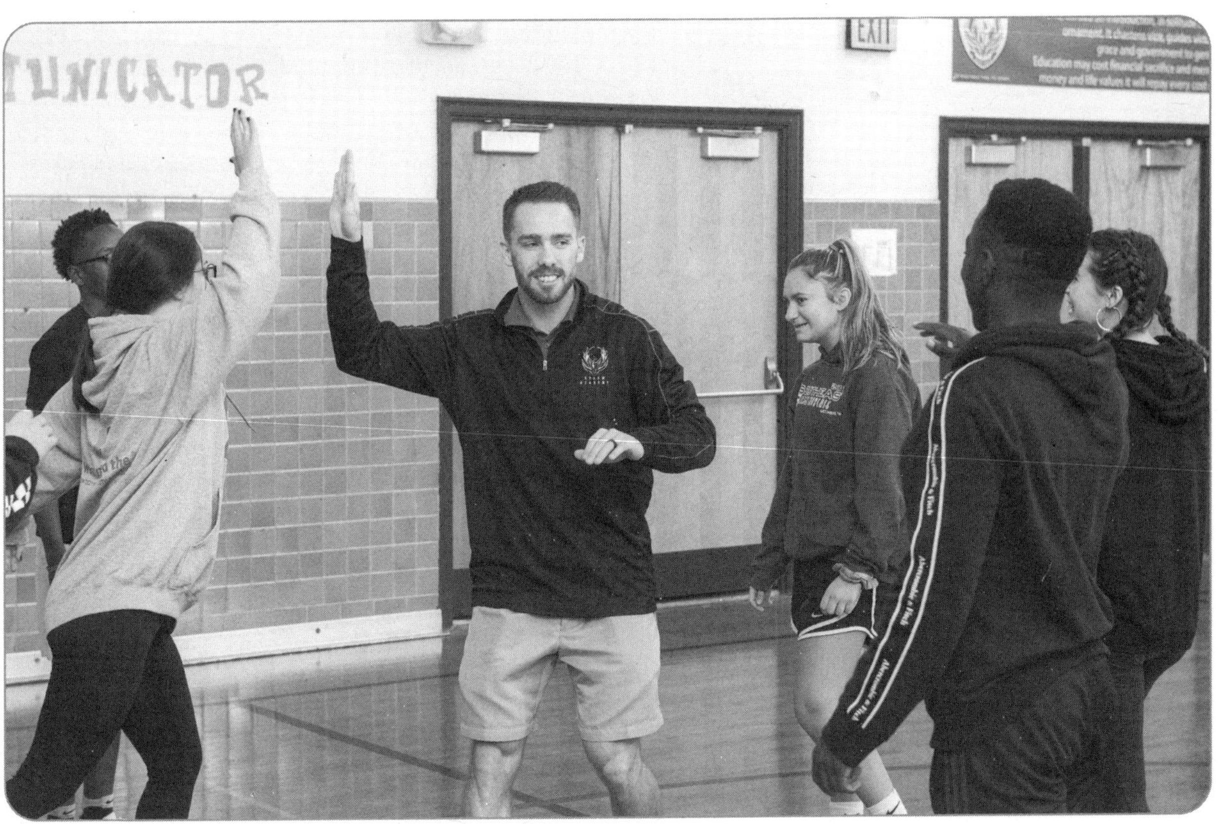

Physical education teachers are in a unique position to build positive relationships with students.

Discipline and Behavior Management

As in any other subject area, in order to have effective instruction, discipline is a vital component in the classroom. Considering the open environment where most physical education classes occur and the high number of students assigned to a class, developing and maintaining class discipline is a necessary strategy that can be used as a preventive measure and a structural component to avoid any disruptions or mishaps. Also keep in mind that, as you develop your positive learning environment as previously discussed, you will also have a positive impact on student behavior, leading to fewer disciplinary problems and a greater sense of social justice.

Consistent rules, policies, and procedures from the beginning to the end of each class and throughout the year will be most effective. Although teachers have the ability to develop their own style of discipline, certain elements should be included in order to create a safe learning environment and class atmosphere where students will feel secure and want to be.

Expectations, guidelines, and rules should be imbedded and composed in a way that the students can easily understand and follow. Along with these policies and procedures are consequences if the expectations, guidelines, or rules are undermined. It is a valuable practice to review each discipline and clearly explain what behaviors are acceptable and which are not. This approach will eliminate any misconception or variation of what is to be expected.

Prior to any disciplinary behavior being asserted, teachers should try a variety of models that include verbal cues, such as privately speaking to the pupil and offering positive alternatives, and nonverbal cues, such as maintaining physical proximity, securing eye contact, or using specific body language. The key is to be consistent and fair with all students. Always remember that, when disciplining the student, you are rejecting the behavior, not the student. As tough as it may sound, there will be times when consequences will need to be reviewed with the class. Reprimanding the entire class is not an appropriate strategy for the improper actions of one or a few students. That one student that is seeking that special attention needs to be individually addressed, but on the side as opposed to in front of the whole class. Teachers by all counts should avoid getting into public altercations with students.

SUPERVISION, SAFETY, AND ENVIRONMENTAL FACTORS

Many factors, internal and external, will affect the way you implement your class lessons to enable students to achieve greater levels of success in meeting their fitness goals. For some factors, such as supervision and safety, you will have greater control, whereas other factors, such as environmental, will be out of your control. Being prepared and always having an alternate plan will keep the students on task and your lessons successfully implemented.

Supervision

As a physical education teacher, one of your major responsibilities is to ensure that your professional responsibilities, programs, and day-to-day actions stay within the laws that govern the rights of all students enrolled in physical education and that the programs are conducted in a safe and educationally sound manner. Although several important precautions can be put into place as policies, situations may occur such that the school district or individual teachers become engaged in legal issues. This is particularly the case when students are engaged in physical activities in which there is some likelihood of accident or injury. Physical education, fitness, and sports programs place participants at relatively high risk of injury since student activities involve moving—sometimes at high speed—and possibly using implements in a confined area, which could be inherently risky. When injury does occur and the question of liability is examined, the administrator and teacher are sure to come under scrutiny. There is no guarantee that someone will not file a lawsuit for any reason or for no reason, but there are ways to limit individual liability, negligence, and liability of the school and school district. Implementing proper and intentional supervision of students at all times is paramount to student safety.

According to Spengler, Anderson, Connaughton, and Baker (2016), two of the most important issues to address with respect to supervision and the delivery of instruction involve (1) properly matching participants when choosing sides for participation and (2) teaching sport progression to ensure safety and using close and specific supervision when in specific circumstances.

It is paramount for students to engage in physical activity within an effective, age- and developmentally appropriate physical education program that is standards based and aligned to grade-level outcomes. Although it is equally important for students to be able to participate in a safe environment, accidents do and will happen. Therefore, the teacher and the administrator in the school setting must be prudent when supervising students. Physical education teachers should supervise students not only when on the playing field or in the gymnasium but also when in the locker rooms and spill-out areas waiting for class to begin or for the dismissal bell and between class periods if assigned to designated supervisory areas, such as at the entrance door to the locker room and the adjacent hallway.

Taking adequate precautions to minimize fear or intimidation is a step in the right direction. The teacher being present, visible, and approachable are all characteristics needed toward promoting the feeling of security that gives the students the opportunity to learn. A well-supervised area is required at all times.

Student Safety

Although accidents may happen and injuries could occur, it is important that students are participating in a safe and supportive environment to limit possible mishaps. In other words, it is the responsibility of the school and staff to maintain a safe environment for physical education activities. For that reason, regular inspections of facilities for damages or hazards are routine, and all problems are to be identified, addressed, and *reported*. Remembering that physical education facilities may include outdoor playing fields, tracks, tennis and basketball courts, indoor classrooms, aerobic and dance rooms, gymnasiums, weight rooms, and other activity areas, the surfaces of these areas should be clean and free of obstacles, holes, or unevenness and provide adequate traction. With this in mind, taking a daily walk-through will prevent any unexpected misfortune throughout the day.

Outdoor Areas

Outdoor areas mostly comprise a paved section, playing field, tennis and racquetball courts, baseball and softball fields, and track-and-field facilities. Many of these activity areas serve as multipurpose facilities so that a variety of activities can be performed. The most commonly used outdoor areas are the paved sections and field areas.

Paved Sections The secondary school paved section generally serves as a multipurpose facility that is used for physical education instruction and community recreation rather than for athletic competition. In general, the pavement is usual-

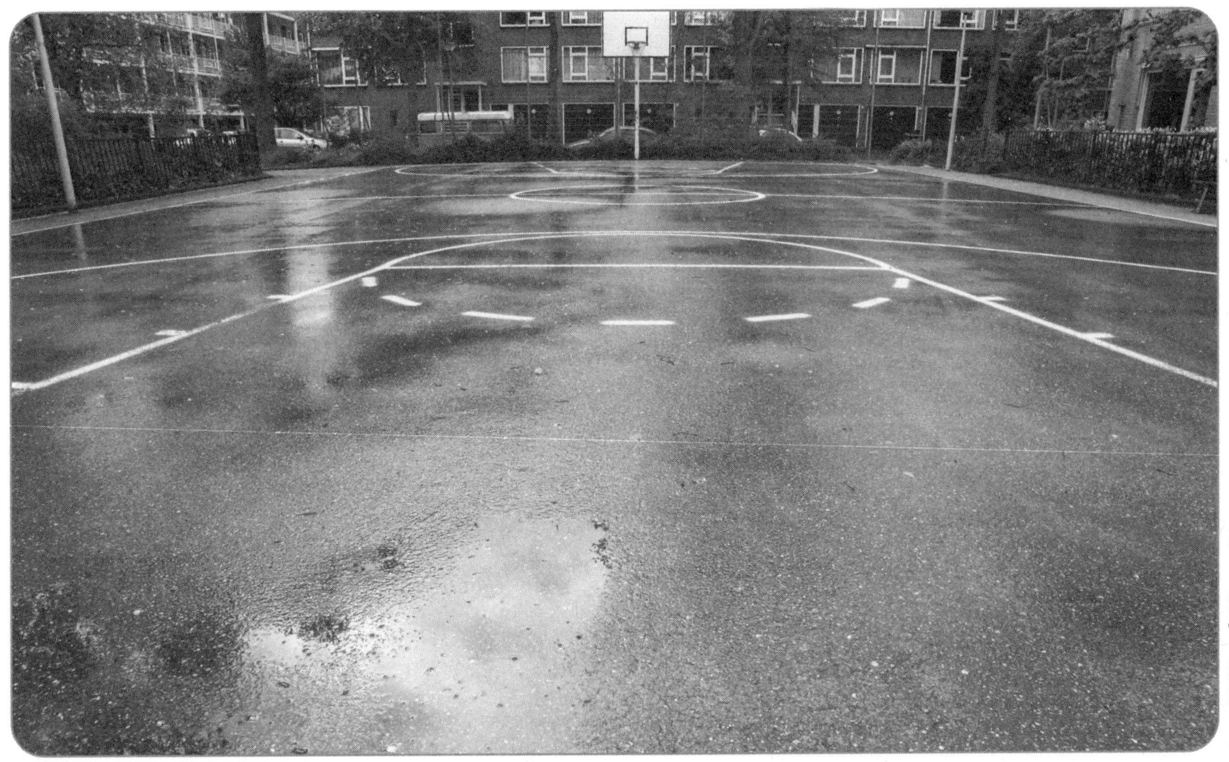
AmpH/iStock/Getty Images

Hard surfaces like pavement can be hazardous if wet, hot, or cracked.

ly marked with lines to accommodate basketball courts with goals and volleyball. Metal sleeves are often inserted into the court for removal poles, which can accommodate volleyball, badminton, and tennis, but it can also accumulate unwanted debris when not in use. Since fitness activities are often performed on hard surfaces, check for cracks in the asphalt and surface temperature prior to students sitting for roll call or performing activities such as push-ups or planks without a mat, as it may be too hot and could cause some harm to their skin.

Field Areas Prior to use, athletic fields or green play spaces should be checked daily for leftover debris from weekend activity or after-school use. The physical education teacher or custodian should immediately remove any debris found, using appropriate gloves or retrieval devices. The physical education teacher should also be aware of the placement of irrigation sprinkler heads or drainage system grates.

If working on cardiorespiratory fitness activities, the physical education teacher also needs to be aware of any divots in the grass or areas to avoid where the ground is not level. This would prevent any foot or ankle injuries if the student trips or loses balance and falls. For safety concerns, bright cones should be placed around areas of concern, such as a broken sprinkler head, or any area of the field in need of repair. All areas of concern should be immediately reported to the principal and documented. Additionally, if an installed track is being used, make sure that the surface is dry after a rainfall so that it reduces the likelihood of a student slipping on the wet surface. Accommodations should be made to ensure that students with disabilities have a safe access and egress to all playing fields and outdoor facilities used for class.

Indoor Facilities

Gymnasiums are often the largest of the indoor teaching and physical activity spaces in schools. When using the gymnasium for teaching purposes, consideration must be given to the number of teaching spaces that will be necessary to accommodate the expected enrollment of the class, the educational program, and the intended use. If multiple physical education classes will be using the facility simultaneously, then it would strongly be recommended to install movable partitions or vinyl-mesh curtains to separate instructional spaces and avoid overflow or student collisions in any given area.

All gymnasiums, as well as outdoor spaces, should also implement buffer zones, providing a 10-foot (3-m) safety zone between walls, bleachers, any obstruction, and instructional spaces. The gymnasium *floor* should be constructed of either hardwood or synthetic surfaces, and it should provide not only appropriate surface friction to allow for sliding and appropriate shock absorption for jumping but also for adequate ball bounce.

Equipment and Supplies

Although this book focuses on fitness activities that can be performed without equipment, purchasing quality equipment and supplies, using them in an appropriate manner, and making sure that they are suitable for secondary school–aged youth may prevent possible negligence or liability if involved in an injury. Common sense of examining the equipment and testing it prior to making it available to the students goes without saying. But, it does not stop there. Again, safety of our students is an ongoing activity. Equipment and supplies must be inspected, maintained, repaired, replaced, and stored throughout the year.

If your program will include use of the weight room, then it is recommended that you refer to *ACSM's Health/Fitness Facility Standards and Guidelines* or another appropriate organization's manual for assistance and guidance.

Universal Design–Built Environment

To ensure that students with disabilities have access to all activities, including indoor facilities, the Americans with Disabilities Act (ADA) provides precise requirements and guidelines pertaining to the building of public facilities. Spaces for physical education and physical activity for a school must meet the Federal Americans with Disabilities Act Accessibility Guidelines, Federal Register July 23, 2004 and Amended August 5, 2005. These guidelines can be found online and in print from the federal government.

As noted in *ACSM's Health/Fitness Facility Standards and Guidelines* (2012), several key elements must be addressed when designing and building physical education and physical activity facilities as follows:

- *Elevation changes.* This requires any change in elevation in excess of 0.05 inches (0.13 cm) must have a ramp or lift, with a slope of 12 inches (30 cm) for every inch (0.25 cm) of elevation change. A mechanical lift or elevator can be used in place of a ramp in cases of extreme changes in height.
- *Passageway width.* This requires that doors, entryways, and exits have a width of at least 36 inches (91 cm) to accommodate wheelchair access. Hallways and circulation passages need to have a width of at least 60 inches (152 cm).
- *Height of switches and fountains.* This requires that all light switches (15 to 48 inches [38 to 122 cm]); water fountains (no higher than 36 inches [91 cm] from the floor); fire extinguishers (no higher than 48 inches [122 cm] above the floor); and AED devices (no higher than 48 inches [122 cm]) must be at a height that can be reached by a person in a wheelchair.
- *Signage.* This requires facilities to provide essential signage, particularly signage on emergency exits and signage that identifies other key space locations, that can be viewed by people with visual impairments.
- *Clear floor space.* This requires that each piece of equipment have an adjacent clear floor space of at least 30 inches by 48 inches (76 cm by 122 cm).

The U.S. Access Board further provides guidance for the following:

- *Lockers.* If lockers are provided, at least 5 percent, but not less than one of each type (full, half, quarter, etc.), must be accessible. Accessible benches should be located adjacent to the accessible lockers.
- *Benches.* Accessible benches are required in dressing, fitting, and locker rooms. Benches must have a clear floor space positioned to allow persons using wheelchairs or other mobility devices to approach parallel to the short end of a bench seat. Benches must have seats that are a minimum of 20 inches (51 cm) to a maximum of 24 inches (61 cm) in depth and 42 inches (107 cm) minimum in length. The seat height should be a minimum of 17 inches (43 cm) to a maximum of 19 inches (48 cm) above the finished floor.

To ensure equitable access for all students to engage in physical education activities, other facilities that should be addressed are locker room, shower, and bathroom accessibility; accessible pathways to all indoor and outdoor facilities and courts; and indoor and outdoor bleachers. A complete list of ADA Standards for Accessible Design can be found at https://www.ada.gov (Greenberg & LoBianco, 2020).

Environmental Factors

For the following text, when we speak about environmental conditions that impact the delivery of physical education instruction, direct reference will be targeted on the weather conditions, student hydration, the importance of identifying heat illnesses, and the recommendation that every student and physical education teacher be either certified or trained in administering cardiopulmonary resuscitation (CPR).

Weather Conditions

Rain, snow, sleet, hail, or sunshine will change the playing field and may result in an interruption in that day's lesson plans. However, the notion that physical education will be cancelled due to weather should be dismissed.

Although physical education primarily takes place outdoors when feasible, weather conditions can change in an instant, and we need to be aware of the different elements of weather conditions, the danger inherent in severe weather conditions, and the appropriate course of action to take. All types of weather conditions could be detrimental to students, as well as your own safety and learning environment. From common elements of temperature, humidity, precipitation, wind, cloudiness, and rain to more severe elements of thunderstorms, tornados, hurricanes, and winter storms and blizzards, all can disrupt our teaching and learning. Whether it is the sound of an alarm or a whistle to take cover, students must be taught the proper action and protocol when this type of situation occurs. As the teacher, you will be looked upon for guidance, solutions, and calmness, as immediate action will be required. And, with preparedness, flexibility, and some adaptations, the class needs to quickly adjust and continue. The best course of action and most expedient move would simply be to take the class indoors and modify your lessons.

Hydration

Although hydration is discussed extensively in chapter 5, it's worth mentioning here, as well: Regardless of the weather, students need to hydrate as often as needed, especially since we are working with high-intensity fitness activities. Keeping the body hydrated helps the heart more easily pump blood through the blood vessels to the muscles and helps the muscles work efficiently (AHA, 2014). It further regulates your body temperature and lubricates your joints, helps transport nutrients to give you energy, and helps you perform at your highest level. Conversely, if dehydrated, students may fatigue quicker, or have muscle cramps, dizziness, or other serious symptoms, which would then require some medical attention (Bushman, 2017; Wolfram, 2018).

Whether planning for indoor or outdoor activities in hot or cold weather, students should have the opportunity to hydrate frequently, whether in physical education, recess, athletics, or before- and after-school programs. Water fountains and hydration stations should be readily available in or near locker rooms, hallways near physical education facilities, and in outdoor spaces. The American Academy of Pediatrics (2011) reminds parents and caregivers that "Water is generally the appropriate first choice for hydration before, during, and after most exercise regimens." For supervision purposes, students should be encouraged to bring their own water if no water fountain is available in the vicinity of the class. Students should never share their water bottles with other students, and physical education teachers should not withhold water breaks for students in need of hydration.

Heat Illnesses

Taking the proper precautions, especially ensuring adequate hydration, will prevent students from experiencing heat illnesses during exercise, especially when the students are participating in intense cardiorespiratory fitness activities and maintaining high levels of exertion. Heat illnesses such as *heat rash*, a mild skin irritation caused by heavy sweating; *heat cramps*, muscle cramps caused by the loss of body salts and fluid within the muscles; *heat exhaustion*, the body's reaction to losing salt and fluid through heavy sweating, during which you may experience nausea, vomiting, weakness, headache, fainting, sweating, and cold and clammy skin; or *heat stroke*, a life-threatening emergency condition when the body is no longer able to cool itself, which can occur when exercising and participating in a physical activity when temperatures and humidity are high. Your skin may be dry from lack of sweat, and you may develop confusion, irritability, headache, heart rhythm problems, dizziness, fainting, nausea, vomiting, visual problems, and fatigue. If this occurs, you need immediate medical attention to prevent brain damage, organ failure, or even death.

It is *essential* that heat illnesses and their symptoms are taught and recognized through lesson planning, emphasizing the importance of how serious and quick a situation can turn into a 911 emergency if not detected or treated. Some factors that could lead to heat illnesses are dehydration, obesity, drug use, other illnesses, or a prior history of heat-related illness. All types of heat illnesses can occur in a physical education class, so students and teachers need to know the signs and act promptly if they suspect someone is suffering from any of the types of heat illnesses. Although knowing that heat illness can cause serious problems can make the situation seem alarming, teachers need to be prepared with an emergency plan in place, stay calm, and be in control of the situation.

Many times, the teacher is not the first to realize that a student may be suffering; therefore, reviewing guidelines with your students for any circumstance is helpful. If a student observes another student in distress, students should be taught to do the following:

- Call for help immediately.
- Alert the teacher.
- Assist the student but do not try to move the student until the teacher arrives.
- Do not leave student alone.
- Stay calm.
- Keep the student alert.

Although these guidelines are for class purposes, these same situations can happen at home, in the park, at the beach, on the playground, or in other classrooms. For that reason, having informational posters that describe how to manage and treat heat illnesses around the physical activity area and in the classroom, gymnasium, and locker room would be beneficial (see figure 4.2). If students in your physical education class are outside of the building and you suspect that a student is experiencing a heat illness, call the front office for immediate assistance.

To avoid heat-related illness, it's important to watch the temperature when exercising in hot, humid climates; get acclimated to the weather; know your fitness level, which would impact your heat tolerance; drink plenty of fluids; and dress appropriately.

CPR and AED

One of the most important skills you can teach your students in any physical education class, whether for certification or for training, is cardiopulmonary resuscitation (CPR). CPR is an emergency lifesaving procedure performed when the heart stops beating. Immediate CPR can double or triple chances of survival after cardiac arrest. We hold a firm belief that all physical education teachers should hold CPR and AED certifications or training and that all students in middle and senior high school should be trained in hands-only CPR.

According to the American Heart Association, hands-only CPR is CPR without rescue breaths. If you see a teen or an adult collapse, you can perform hands-only CPR with just two easy steps:

1. Call 911.
2. Push hard and fast in the center of the chest to the beat of the Bee Gees' classic disco song "Stayin' Alive." The song is 100 beats per minute—the minimum rate you should push on the chest during hands-only CPR.

With 70 percent of all out-of-hospital cardiac arrests happening at home, if you're called on to perform hands-only CPR, you'll likely be trying to save the life of someone you know and love. Hands-only CPR carried out by a bystander has been shown to be as effective as CPR with breaths in the first few minutes during an out-of-hospital, sudden cardiac arrest for an adult victim. Remember that there is no age limit for a person experiencing a sudden cardiac arrest. Since sudden cardiac arrests occur in teens, it is also essential that secondary school students be taught how to use an automated external defibrillator (AED). The goal of an AED is to increase the rate of survival of people who have had sudden cardiac arrests.

A Final Word About Safety

Teachers are ultimately responsible for ensuring the safety of their students. The responsibility to keep our children safe and to take every precaution necessary to do so is of utmost importance. To assist teachers, the following list of safety tips should also be considered:

- Discuss and emphasize safety practices and precautions with students when introducing a new activity or reviewing an activity previously taught to the students.
- Provide proper supervision of activities at all times. There is no excuse for lack of supervision.
- Ensure an adequate warm-up to prepare students for physical activity and an adequate cool-down after the activity.
- Watch for students showing signs of fatigue and be prepared to adjust or change activities as appropriate.
- Organize activity areas so there is ample space between students, groups, and obstacles (e.g., fences, poles, walls, other equipment, etc.).
- Pay careful attention to the surface where the activity is to be performed (field conditions, hard courts, wet tracks, and other surfaces that involve students moving and changing direction quickly).
- Ensure that students are dressed appropriately for physical activity, especially footwear, which helps prevent accidents.
- Select equipment that is appropriate for students' abilities.
- Encourage students to drink water regularly to prevent dehydration.

In order to promote learning, the creation of a safe learning environment for the students is

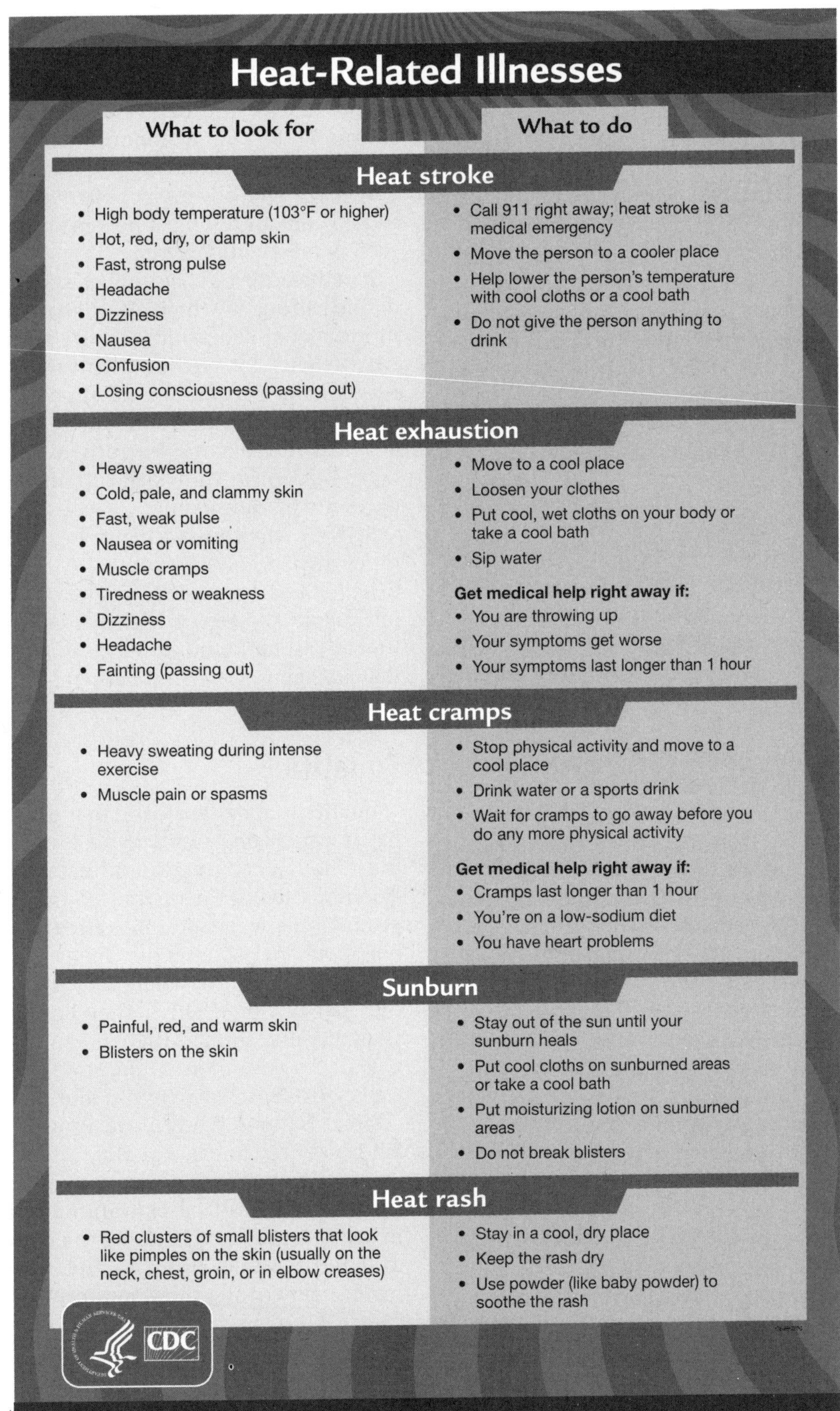

Figure 4.2 CDC heat-related illnesses chart.

Reprinted from Centers for Disease Control and Prevention, *National Disasters and Severe Weather.* https://www.cdc.gov/disasters/extremeheat/warning.html

monumental. The students need to feel safe to learn, secure to participate, protected around their peers.

EQUITY, DIVERSITY, INCLUSION, AND SOCIAL JUSTICE

A deliberate practice of focusing on equity, diversity, inclusion, and social justice should be a part of everyday modeling of physical education teachers and instructional lessons and practices for students. Our role as educators is to create a learning environment in which all students feel welcomed, respected, supported, and valued to fully participate in all physical education activities.

Equity

Before we can address issues of equity in our physical education classes, we first need to get a grasp on what equity means. Many times, we may see the words *equity* and *equality* used interchangeably when referring to educational equity. However, although they may seem similar, there are distinct meanings between the two.

Equity, by simple definition, is fairness, impartiality, or justice in the way people are treated. It's about getting what we individually need to survive or succeed, and it involves access to opportunity, resources, and supports. Social determinants also include levels of poverty, food security, and educational levels. It is further based on where we are and where we want to go. According to the American Library Association (2007) "equity recognizes that some are at a larger disadvantage than others and aims at compensating for these people's misfortunes and disabilities to ensure that everyone can attain the same type of lifestyle." Equity recognizes this uneven playing field and aims to take extra measures by giving more to those who are in need than to others who are not. Equity aims at making sure that everyone's lifestyle is equal. This leads to social justice in education, striving to ensure equitable outcomes for students.

Educational equity is a measure of achievement, fairness, and opportunity in education. "Educational equity means that every student has access to the educational resources and rigor they need at the right moment in their education across race, gender, ethnicity, language, disability, sexual orientation, family background and/or family income" (Council of Chief State School Officers, 2017, p. 3). Educational equity depends on two main factors: The first is fairness, which implies that factors specific to one's personal conditions should not interfere with the potential of academic success; and the second important factor is inclusion, which refers to a comprehensive standard that applies to everyone in a certain education system (Organization for Economic Co-Operation and Development, 2008). A fair and inclusive system that makes the advantages of education available to all is one of the most powerful levers to make society more equitable.

In education, an equitable system would be defined as one in which all students, independent of individual characteristics, are treated equally. All students are provided with the same opportunities and curriculum, taught by teachers with the same certifications and same level of expertise; are held to the same learning expectations and outcomes; and are provided with the same amount of resources and support.

SHAPE America further recognized equity in their *Appropriate Instructional Practice Guidelines, K-12*. Table 4.1 includes the appropriate practices for middle and senior high school. The full document can be found at: www.shapeamerica.org/upload/Appropriate-Instructional-Practice-Guidelines-K-12.pdf.

Equality

"Equality is about ensuring that every individual has an equal opportunity to make the most of their lives and talents" and is not treated differently or discriminated against because of the individual's personal characteristics. "It is also the belief that no one should have poorer life chances because of the way they were born, where they come from, what they believe, or whether they have a disability" (Equality and Human Rights Commission, 2018). *Equality* by definition is "the state of being equal, especially in status, rights, and opportunities" (United Nations World Food Programme, 2021). Within our schools, equality in sport is about recognizing and removing the barriers faced by the students involved or wanting to be involved in sport. It is about changing the culture of sport to one that values diversity and enables the full involvement of all groups in every aspect of sport. Figure 4.3 depicts an illustration of what reality, equality, equity, and social justice would look like in a real-world setting.

Social Justice

Social justice is a concept that is based on fair and just relations between individuals and society. It asserts the idea that all people should have equal access and distribution of wealth, health, well-be-

Table 4.1 Appropriate Practices for Middle and Senior High School: Equity

Appropriate practice: middle school	1.5 Equity	1.5.1 All students (boys and girls, high- and low-skilled) have equal opportunities to participate and interact with the teacher (e.g., leadership, playing "skilled" positions, teacher feedback). All students, regardless of developmental level and ability, are challenged at an appropriate level.	1.5.2 All students are encouraged, supported, and socialized toward successful achievement in all content taught in physical education (e.g., dance is for everyone).	1.5.3 Physical educators use gender-neutral language (e.g., "students," "person-to-person defense")
Appropriate practice: high school	1.5 Equity	1.5.1 All students (boys and girls, high- and low-skilled) have equal opportunities to participate and interact with the teacher (e.g., leadership, playing "skilled" positions, teacher feedback). All students, regardless of developmental level and ability, are challenged at an appropriate level.	1.5.2 All students are encouraged, supported, and socialized toward successful achievement in all content taught in physical education (e.g., dance is for everyone).	1.5.3 Physical educators use gender-neutral language (e.g. "students").

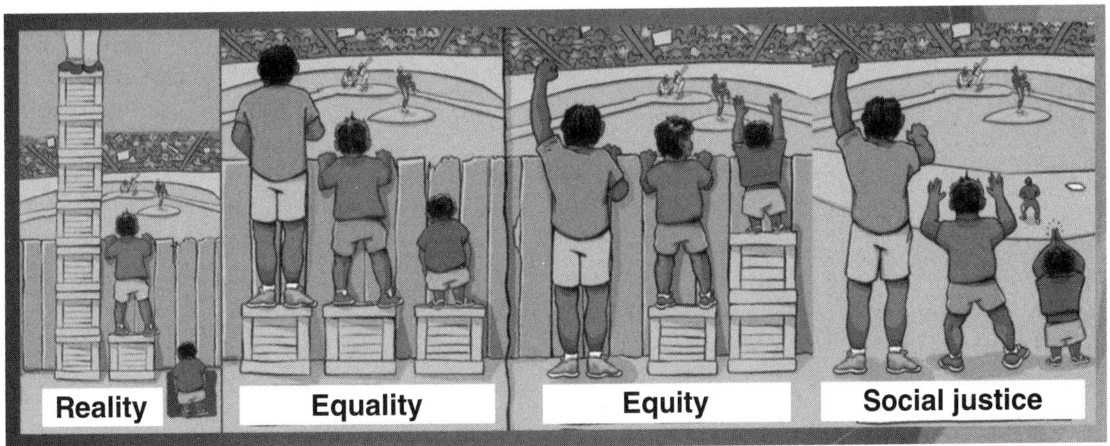

Figure 4.3 Equality Versus Equity Versus Social Justice
Equality/Equity/Liberation image collaboration between *Center for Story-based Strategy & Interactive Institute for Social Change*. Artist: Angus Maguire. Reality panel created by Andrew Weizeman. Copyright Permission Granted by Angus Maguire.

ing, justice, social privileges, and opportunity. "Social justice includes a vision of a society in which the distribution of resources is equitable and all members are physically and psychologically safe and secure" (Bell, 2013, p. 21). As individuals, our thoughts are often shaped by race, ethnicity, nationality, religion, gender, and sexuality, which contribute to our own self- and personal identity.

Through the development of a positive learning environment, where all students feel safe and respected, physical education teachers have the opportunity to address equity, diversity, inclusion, and social justice through not only curricular lessons but also the *actions* taken in the class.

Lynch, Sutherland, and Walton-Fisette (2020) assert that issues surrounding social justice in physical education have been around for several years and there are strategies that can be implemented to work toward achieving the goals and objectives. Although this list is not exhaustive, the following are some actions for immediate consideration:

- ability awareness
- being aware of your bias
- diverse forms of assessment
- gender equity
- identity
- knowledge of minority groups
- language
- policies
- standards-based practices

- values-based instruction
- xenophobia
- youth centered and empowering
- zeal

In considering the aforementioned actions, physical educators need to ask themselves some basic questions when planning for an opening of the new school year and deciding what and how to teach that will be different from previous years, which will address the eight strands of oppression represented in social justice in figure 4.4 (Lynch & Landi, 2018). Physical education teachers can engage students in open conversation, allow students to develop co-curriculum activities and experience games from different cultures.

The National Education Association (NEA) recommends the following strategies for addressing equity, diversity, and inclusion:

- *Focus on diversity.* Awareness of the diversity in communities is critical to fostering social justice.
- *Address real consequences of oppression.* When discussing social justice in lessons or staff meetings, it is important to acknowledge the real social and economic disadvantages that oppressed people face in society, not simply the psychic harm of oppression.

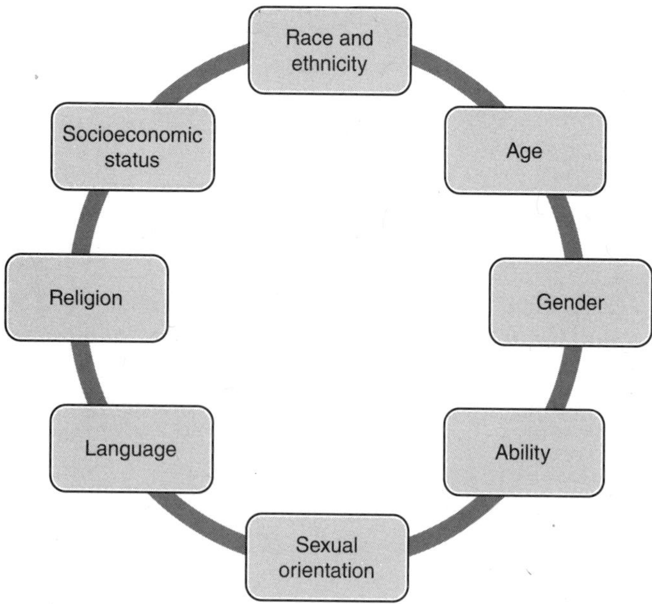

Figure 4.4 Social justice in physical education and the eight strands of oppression.

Reprinted by permission from S. Lynch and D. Landi, *Social Justice in Physical Education* (Blog). Cited in SHAPE America online, 2018). https://blog.shapeamerica.org/author/slynch/. Permission granted by author Shrehan Lynch.

- *Understand the mechanisms that perpetuate oppression.* These are attitudes and behaviors (e.g., racism, sexism, ageism, heterosexism) from a position of privilege.
- *Resist hierarchies of oppression.* Form strategies to foster justice with an inclusive mindset: Who is being left out?
- *Seek to address social justice on three levels.* The levels are (1) personal (self), (2) institutional (school), and (3) societal (community).

Play Equity

The *Healthy People 2030 Framework,* launched on August 18, 2020, by the U.S. Department of Health and Human Services, set forth as their vision of "a society in which all people can achieve their full potential for health and well-being across the lifespan," and identified the "health and well-being of all people and communities as essential in a thriving equitable society" as one of its foundational principles. Based on this new prevention agenda, we need to ask, "Do all youth have access to equitable play spaces and opportunities to be physically active in schools and the communities in which they live?"

Based on the work and research performed by the LA84 Foundation (LA84 Foundation, 2018), Play Equity means fairness. Play Equity means opportunity. Play Equity means that how much exercise kids get must not be determined by their income. Renata Simril, President & CEO of Play Equity Fund stated, "The lack of equal access for all kids to play is a crisis hiding in plain sight." Research by the Aspen Institute, Project Play (2019, 2020), LA84 Foundation (2018), and Active Living Research (2011) discovered the following inequity trends in the United States:

- Fifteen million kids are in poverty across the United States.
- Many school districts have eliminated or reduced investment in enrichment programs including sports.
- Many school districts mandate physical education for only one to two days per week and many no longer offer recess in schools.
- Black and Latinx youth are two times as likely to reside in areas with subpar park space per capita.
- Kids from households below US$25K are five times less likely to participate in sports.
- Eighty percent of young people, many poor, do not meet federal guidelines for daily physical activity.

- Kids in poor communities have an obesity rate that is nearly two times higher than kids from affluent communities.
- Deeper, negative impacts occur in communities of color: Black and Latinx youth have the highest rates of stress, anxiety, and depression.

Active Living Research (2011), further asserted that "lower-income groups and racial and ethnic minorities have limited access to well-maintained or safe parks. The presence of parks, open space and other recreational facilities is consistently linked with higher physical activity levels among children and adolescents." Inactivity also is disproportionate among children living at or below poverty level and among children living in neighborhoods that parents perceived to be unsafe.

The Equity Project by the Women's Sports Foundation defines their vision as "inspire the nation and create meaningful change so that all girls and women have equitable access to physical activity and sport, to help unlock limitless possibilities in their lives" (Women's Sports Foundation, 2021). Looking back, "nearly 50 years ago, Title IX opened the doors for sports participation. Today, women and girls still lag behind in access, leadership and coaching opportunities, pay, and media coverage" (Women's Sports Foundation, 2021).

What solutions can we set forth to provide play equity for all of our youth? We begin with empowering schools to be the hub of the community in providing more physical education, physical activity, and sports programs, as frequently addressed in the Comprehensive School Physical Activity Program, also known as CSPAP (CDC, 2019); through collective action, engaging community partnerships and forming coalitions to work toward proactive policies leading to lasting impact; collaborating with public health, law enforcement, planners, and civic groups to develop strategies that can simultaneously improve neighborhood safety and encourage physical activity; and developing joint-use agreements that allow community members to use school-owned recreational facilities. In turn, communities can offer facilities to schools, such as swimming pools, and mobilize stakeholders, such as local businesses and organizations, to become active participants in their communities.

Additionally, if we look at play equity in terms of physical education, physical activity, and sports in both the school environment as well as the community setting, and we correlate that with the health benefits of maintaining a healthy lifestyle, as documented in chapters 1 and 2, then we begin to see a relationship between physical activity, healthy behaviors, and the benefits of physical activity to academic performance in the school setting, which is well documented in the research. Figure 4.5 further supports the need for advocacy around the right to play and play equity in the schools and communities.

Diversity

Diversity recognizes that everyone is different from one another and that we each possess a unique blend of diverse qualities, skills, experiences, background, heritage, beliefs, and many other characteristics. Diversity is about celebrating and valuing how different we all are and how those differences are linked with promoting human rights and freedoms, based on principles such as dignity and respect. Diversity is about recognizing, valuing, and taking account of people's different backgrounds, knowledge, skills, and experiences, and encouraging and using those differences to create a productive society.

It is important for physical education teachers to set the norms in their classes that promote inclusion and openness while promoting equity and diversity. It will be a conscious effort teaching students how to be respectful of each other, accept each other and individual differences and identities,

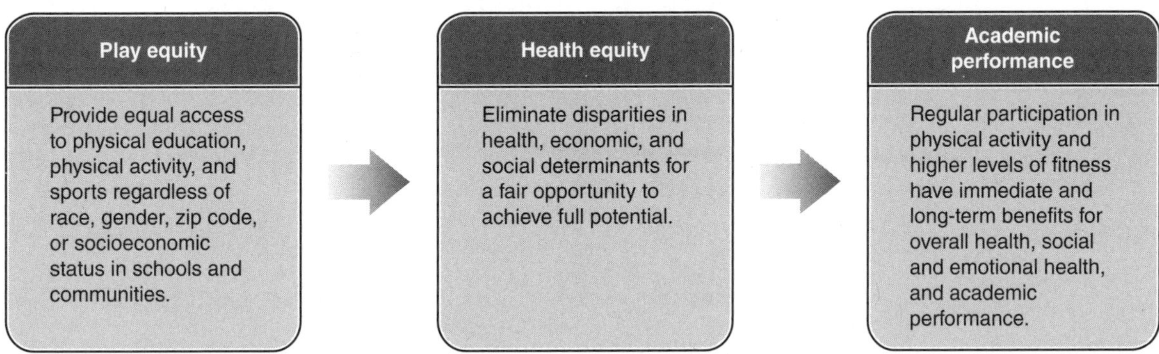

Figure 4.5 Play equity, health equity, academic performance.
Source: Concept developed by Dr. Jayne D. Greenberg

and share ideas and thoughts in open and respectful conversation. Table 4.2 provides examples of appropriate practices for teachers to consider when creating diverse educational environments in secondary school physical education classes.

There are several resources that are available to assist physical education teachers in developing lesson plans and delivering instruction in equity, diversity, inclusion, and social justice that should be explored. Some that have had overall school board approval across the United States are: *Welcoming Schools,* aligned with Common Core State Standards, by the Human Rights Campaign Foundation; *Positive Behavioral Interventions and Support (PBIS),* U.S. Department of Education, Office of Special Education; the *Second Step Program;* and the *Gay, Lesbian & Straight Education Network (GLSEN).* Additionally, the *Social Justice Standards* from Teaching Tolerance provide a road map for anti-bias education for K-12 instruction through anchor standards and age-appropriate learning outcomes. The four domains—identity, diversity, justice, and action—"represent a continuum of engagement in anti-bias, multicultural, and social justice education." Teaching Tolerance's Anchor Standards for identity (2020, p. 5) include the following:

- Students will develop positive social identities based on their membership in multiple groups in society.
- Students will develop language and historical and cultural knowledge that affirm and accurately describe their membership in multiple identity groups.
- Students will recognize that people's multiple identities interact and create unique and complex individuals.
- Students will express pride, confidence, and healthy self-esteem without denying the value and dignity of other people.
- Students will recognize traits of the dominant culture, their home culture, and other cultures and understand how they negotiate their own identity in multiple spaces.

Accompanying lesson plans, activities, and anti-bias scenarios can be found at www.tolerance.org/sites/default/files/2019-06/TT-Social-Justice-Standards-June-2019.pdf.

Teachers interested in securing additional resources are invited to visit https://www.cbhpe.org/edi-social-justice for books, resources, posters, and other educational materials.

Inclusion

Classrooms are composed of diverse learners who have different ethnicities, races, cultures, abilities, and genders. Being able to deliver quality instruction requires that you learn who your students are. Physical activity preferences can be influenced by cultural and ethnic norms. In addition, students' cognitive, physical, and communicative abilities will guide how you deliver the curriculum and choose instructional strategies. Possibly one of the most challenging aspects of instruction is to develop a positive and inclusive environment in which all students feel safe, supported, and challenged to achieve. It is considered not only appropriate instruction to develop an inclusive environment but also a legal responsibility for physical educators.

As discussed extensively in chapter 3, universal design for learning (UDL) is a concept, set of principles, and framework that supports accessibility and encourages teachers to explore new ways of delivering instruction in what would be a heterogeneous environment (Bowes & Tinning, 2015). According to Lieberman and Houston-Wilson (2018), the UDL curriculum provides students with disabilities access to the same learning outcomes as their peers without disabilities.

Table 4.2 Appropriate Practices for Middle and Senior High School: Diversity

Appropriate practice: middle school	1.4 Diversity	1.4.1 Teachers create an environment that is inclusive and supportive of all students, regardless of race, ethnic origin, gender, sexual orientation, religion, or physical ability. Such differences are acknowledged, appreciated, and respected.	1.4.2 Teachers intentionally select activities that represent a culturally diverse environment (e.g., dances and games from around the world).
Appropriate practice: high school	1.4 Diversity	1.4.1 Teachers create an environment that is inclusive and supportive of all students, regardless of race, ethnic origin, gender, sexual orientation, religion, or physical ability. Such differences are acknowledged, appreciated, and respected.	1.4.2 Teachers intentionally select activities that represent a culturally diverse environment (e.g., dances and games from around the world).

The Individuals with Disabilities Education Act (IDEA) is a federal law mandating that all children with disabilities receive physical education and that they are educated in the least restrictive environment (LRE) to meet their unique needs. The LRE is one that allows children with disabilities to interact and participate with their peers to the maximum extent possible while affording them the most success. For some students with disabilities, this may mean inclusion—integrating them into the general physical education setting. Inclusion requires providing adapted physical education strategies since students with a disability learn alongside their peers without disabilities and need modifications and or accommodations to fully participate. Adapted physical education is a *service*, not a *placement*, and provides the best opportunities for success to students with disabilities in the most appropriate environment (Lieberman & Houston-Wilson, 2018).

Options for inclusion might look like any of the following scenarios:

- Full inclusion with no adaptations or support (no IEP needed)
- Full inclusion with curriculum adaptations and modifications
- Full inclusion with trained peer tutors
- Full inclusion with para-educators
- Full inclusion with specialists
- Modified physical education (small class) with able-bodied peers

Options for part-time, self-contained and part-time, integrated placement might look like the following:

- Split placement without additional support
- Split placement with additional support

For some students, the LRE may be a segregated class; however, removal from the general classroom setting is only to be used when the nature or severity of the disability will not allow for inclusion with the use of supplementary aids or services. If participating in an inclusive class is not the best service for specific students, then alternate placements should be considered. The following list of reasons explains why students with disabilities may require an alternative environment:

- There is a probability of harm to the student with a disability or probability of harm to other participants inside the general education classroom (based upon reasonable medical judgments).
- The student with a disability is a disruptive force and detracts from other students' ability to learn.
- The student with a disability will not receive educational benefits in the general classroom, and having a separate instructional setting significantly outweighs the benefits of inclusion (French, Henderson, Kinnison, & Sherrill, 1998; Yelm, 1998).

It is possible that, in a classroom of 30 students, you may have three students with individualized education programs (IEPs)—plans that ensure students receive specialized instruction and services to reach personalized goals—because roughly 12.9 percent of the public school population receives special education services (National Center for Education Statistics, 2016). Therefore, when delivering appropriate instruction to all students, you will want to understand the students' disabilities and instructional strategies that you can use to meet their unique needs. Throughout this section, you will see that there are many ways to adapt the fitness curriculum for students with disabilities. Children's current fitness needs must be specifically modified, and the modifications should be based on valid assessments. Although many teachers may feel a bit uncomfortable, or feel that they do not have the appropriate training to accommodate students with disabilities in their classes, it is best to ask supervisors for support or solicit assistance from adapted physical education teachers in the school, school district, or state. This chapter, as well as chapter 3, provides some teaching strategies for including students with disabilities by ensuring that your curriculum is accessible and that all students have the opportunity to achieve success.

Table 4.3 presents the 13 categories of disabilities as defined by IDEA, listed in order according to the greatest number of students receiving services for that disability. Students diagnosed with any of these disabilities may require an IEP. An IEP team will examine a variety of factors and determine the appropriate placement for those students. Typical components of a physical education IEP include present level of performance, short-term goals, annual goals, evaluation procedures, assessment modifications, support services, and supplementary aids (Lieberman & Houston-Wilson, 2018). Successful inclusion occurs when physical education teachers can use the information in the IEP and adapt or adjust the regular curriculum setting to meet the needs of students. There are several strategies that physical educators can use for improving the learning outcomes of students with disabilities in an inclusive environment. Using these strategies can help students be fully included in the class as opposed to being mere spectators. Those strategies include

- implementing peer tutoring and cooperative learning strategies,
- enlisting the help of paraprofessionals and adapted physical education specialists or occupational therapists,
- collaborating with all members of the IEP team, and
- using a universal design for learning framework to plan for and structure learning experiences (Lieberman & Houston-Wilson, 2018; Grenier, Miller, & Black, 2017; Qi & Ha, 2012).

Additionally, some students in your classroom may have 504 plans as governed by another federal law known as Section 504 of the Rehabilitation Act of 1973. This law prohibits discrimination based upon disability and applies to students who have a disabling condition that is not specifically listed under IDEA but need accommodations or services (French et al., 1998). According to Section 504: "An individual with a disability means any person who: (i) has a mental or physical impairment that substantially limits one or more major life activity; (ii) has a record of such an impairment; or (iii) is regarded as having such an impairment" (U.S. Department of Education, 1995). For example, in physical education, many students with asthma or diabetes may have a 504 plan that requires teachers to modify exercise intensities to meet students' needs, but the plan does not require a specialized program.

Students without diagnosed disabilities may also bring a unique set of individual constraints (e.g., fitness levels, motor skills competency, motivation, anxiety levels) that affect learning and performing skills for which teachers will also have to make accommodations to ensure success (Gagen & Getchell, 2004). Limitations can be in the form of structural or functional characteristics related to students' fitness level, intellectual capabilities, social skills, or emotional well-being. All of these factors will affect how students interact with the

Table 4.3 IDEA Disability Categories

Federal disability term	Alternative terms and descriptions	% of students receiving special education services (12.9%)
Learning disability	Disorders related to difficulty in processing information (reading, writing, and computing)	4.5
Speech or language impairment	Communication disorder	2.7
Other health impairment	Disease, disorder, or condition that limits a child's strength, energy, or alertness; such as cancer, diabetes, or heart disease	1.6
Autism	Autism spectrum disorder	1.1
Mental retardation	Intellectual disability, cognitive impairment	0.9
Developmental delay	Nonspecific disability category for students ages 3-9 that may need special education services due to delays in physical, cognitive, communicative, social emotional, and/or adaptive development	0.8
Emotional disturbance	Behavior disorder, emotional disability	0.7
Multiple disabilities	Presence of two or more disabilities so that one cannot be identified as the primary disability	0.3
Hearing impairment	Deaf or hard of hearing	0.2
Visual impairment	Low vision, blind	0.1
Orthopedic impairment	Physical disability; impaired ability to move or perform motor activities	0.1
Traumatic brain injury	Brain injury that may affect learning, behavior, social skills, and language	0.1
Deaf-blindness	Significant hearing and vision loss	>0.1

National Center for Education Statistics. (2016): Adapted from Donnelly, Mueller, and Gallahue (2017, pg. 173).

curriculum, instruction, and environment. If you know that students have an individual limitation, you want to consider how that limitation will interact with the environment, equipment, task and game rules, or your instructional methods. Knowing students' limitations and how to adapt activities allows physical educators to create a positive, inclusive environment and deliver instruction that allows all students to be successful. As you prepare to implement your own strategies, it is recommended that you use the Lieberman-Brian Inclusion Rating Scale for Physical Education (LIRSPE) to measure the actions taken by teachers to ensure students with disabilities are offered physical education opportunities alongside their peers without disabilities. The Basic Principles for Adapting Activities sidebar includes Lieberman and Houston-Wilson's (2018) basic principles for adapting physical activities to assist physical education teachers in providing for an inclusive environment.

Lieberman and Houston-Wilson (2018) also propose several inclusion strategies that physical education teachers can incorporate into their classes to ensure that all students have the opportunity to participate in class activities. However, the following specific strategies are designed for physical education teachers to teach students how to work with and support their peers with disabilities, leading to a successful environment for all. Although it is not a comprehensive list, it does provide a few ideas to get you started.

Autism

Characteristics

- Children with autism have a difficult time relating to people.
- They may be more interested in playing with an object or watching their hand than in talking to a person.
- They may play in a corner all by themselves or run around for no apparent reason.
- They may have very limited communication or no communication, and what they do say may not make very much sense.
- They may react to touch, noise, or lights very differently. Sometimes a low noise will seem very loud to them, so much that they will cover their ears.
- They may cry from a soft touch or cover their eyes from a dim light.
- Other kids may appear deaf when there is a loud noise, may seek out deep pressure or

Basic Principles for Adapting Activities

- When possible, include students with disabilities in adaptation decisions. Some students will not mind having the activity modified to ensure success. In middle school and high school, however, many students with disabilities prefer to fit in rather than be successful, and they may not welcome an adaptation that makes them seem different. You must first consider the student's attitude toward the activity, peers, and him- or herself. Universal design for learning applies to all students, so if the modifications are for all students then students with disabilities may not feel as marginalized as if the modifications were just for them.
- Give the student as many choices as possible. The more types of equipment, teaching styles, rule modifications, and environmental options you provide, the greater the chance that the student can make a choice that will enable him or her to be successful in the activity. You can also discuss all options with the student prior to the unit and allow him or her to try out a few to make the best decisions. This way, the student can start the unit with success, and you can make further adaptations if needed (Haegele & Sutherland, 2015).
- Physical assistance is acceptable and is preferred over sitting out of an activity. Physical cues, hand-over-hand aid, and total physical assistance are appropriate to ensure participation in the activity. The amount of assistance should be decreased when possible (Grenier & Lieberman, 2018).
- If a modification is not working, change it as soon as possible to facilitate success.

Source: Lieberman, L.J. and Houston-Wilson, C. (2018). Strategies for inclusion: Physical education for everyone (3rd ed., p. 82). Champaign, IL: Human Kinetics.

textured feelings on their skin, or may look for very bright lights to stimulate themselves.

- Each person with autism is different, and you need to understand what she wants and needs in order to be able to cope with the environment.

Inclusion Ideas

- You can help classmates with autism by talking clearly and asking them only one or two things at a time.
- You can help them when they don't know what to do, redirect them when they are doing the wrong activity, and help other people understand what they are good at and what they need help with.
- You can learn what makes them mad, frustrated, and happy, and you can help convey these feelings to other classmates and the teacher.

Blindness and Visual Impairment

Characteristics

- Children who are blind or visually impaired have difficulty seeing.
- They have this disability because of a birth accident, an accident after birth, or a sickness.
- Some kids can see a little bit and walk around by themselves; some kids can see a little bit but need some help getting around; and some kids cannot see anything and need help in getting around.
- With practice and a cane or a seeing-eye dog, kids may be able to walk around school and their neighborhood by themselves.
- These kids will eat by themselves and use the "clock system" for knowing where things are. You can tell them their milk is at 12:00, which means their milk is at the very top of the plate, and their fork is at 9:00, which means their fork is just to the left of the plate.
- These students can dress themselves, and they know which clothes are which color by reading braille writing on the tag of the shirt.
- They find out what is happening in their environment, who is around them, and where they are going by having people tell them.
- Do not be afraid to use words like *see* or *look* in a sentence. Students who are blind or visually impaired will use these words, and you can, too.

Inclusion Ideas

- You can guide your classmates by allowing them to grab your elbow and walk one step behind you. This will allow them to let go if they want to.
- You can assist them in getting their food in the lunch line, and you can tell them where their food is on their plates.
- You can describe their environment to them, such as who is in the room, what the weather is like, and what equipment is located around the gym.
- You can answer their questions and make sure they are included in conversations.
- Do not ever leave a room without telling them you are leaving. They may want to talk to you and not know you are gone, and this is embarrassing.
- You can make sure they are included in games and activities in your neighborhood or on the playground by adapting the equipment, the playing area, or the rules.

Deafness and Hardness of Hearing

Characteristics

- Children who are deaf or have difficulty hearing cannot hear like you and I can.
- They hear much less than we do, and, in some cases, they cannot hear at all.
- Some kids wear hearing aids, cochlear implants, or other hearing devices to help them hear better.
- Some kids with hearing difficulty can talk clearly; you can understand them, and they can read your lips.
- Some kids communicate using hand gestures and sign language.
- Some kids with hearing difficulty are not able to talk with their voices, and they may not be able to understand everything you say.
- Some kids with hearing difficulty will prefer to talk mostly with other deaf kids; others will talk and make friends with anyone, regardless if that person can hear or is deaf.

Inclusion Ideas

- Because your classmates with hearing difficulty cannot hear, you can help them in many ways.
- If they use their voices and read lips, you can help by making sure you are looking at each other when you talk.
- You can tap them on the shoulder to get their attention if the teacher is talking, if there is a fire drill, or if someone wants to talk to them.

- You can make sure they understand the instructions when you are in class, and you can answer any questions they have.
- If your friends are completely deaf and use signs, you can learn some signs to aid in communication; if you don't know the signs, you can look at your friends when you are talking, and the interpreter will interpret what you say.
- Many kids who are deaf feel lonely and left out, so it is important to try to include them in all activities, both in and out of school.
- It is also important that you do not make students with hearing difficulty feel bad if they do not understand something; instead, you can try to increase their understanding the best that you can.
- If you want to help students who are deaf or have difficulty hearing, always remember that you can make sure they are included in games and activities in your neighborhood or on the playground. Do this by communicating the rules, talking with them, and helping other kids understand them. Students who are deaf or have difficulty hearing are just like you in many ways.

Intellectual Disability

Characteristics

- Students who have an intellectual disability may not be able to think the same way you do. This is because they had an accident before, during, or after they were born, involving their heads or the chemicals in their bodies.
- They will sometimes be able to understand parts of what you say but not everything. They may also react to what they are asked in an unusual way because of the lack of understanding.
- These classmates may also have trouble communicating with you, taking care of themselves (such as feeding themselves), or putting on their coats.
- They may walk away when you are talking to them or laugh for no reason. They may have trouble going out into the community on their own to do things, such as taking a bus or going shopping.
- Sometimes during the day, they may not know what they want to do, they may not be aware of danger in the environment, or they may need help to do classwork or recreational activities such as walking, riding a bike, or bowling.

Inclusion Ideas

- You can help these classmates by talking clearly and asking them only one or two things at a time.
- You can help them when they don't know what to do, redirect them when they are doing the wrong activity, and help other people understand what they are good at and how they can be helped.
- You can make sure they are included in groups, games, and activities by giving them clear instructions and demonstrations throughout the activity and praising them when they do something right.
- These classmates have the same feelings you have. They are hurt when other students don't want to play with them; just like you, they enjoy things like eating ice cream, watching cartoons, and being part of the game.

Physical or Orthopedic Disability

Students with physical disabilities are often characterized by having either an acquired or congenital physical or motor impairment; they may exhibit some form of paralysis, variations in muscle tone, and loss or inability to use one or more limbs and may have difficulty with select gross- or fine-motor skills. These may be associated with spinal cord injuries, TBI, cerebral palsy, amputation, multiple sclerosis, spina bifida, musculoskeletal injuries, and muscular dystrophy, to name a few. When preparing your physical education lessons, it is important to take the needs of all students into consideration.

Inclusion Ideas

- Create a physically accessible environment that is not mobility limited.
- Eliminate time limits.
- Modify the activity if needed and activity area.
- Adapt the rules if needed.
- Use a variety of teaching methods, including visual aids, verbal cues, and modeling.
- Use a variety of equipment that includes size, weight, and texture of balls and other equipment and objects that can be tossed and caught.
- Limit the number of players on a team.
- Incorporate breaks or rest periods.
- Provide for partner and peer support.
- Listen to students and allow them to tell you what their needs are.

When delivering a standards-based instructional program, physical education classes have control over many internal and external factors.

Table 4.4 Appropriate Practices for Middle and Senior High School—Inclusion

Appropriate practice: middle school	1.6 Inclusion	1.6.1 Physical educators implement the special education process for students with disabilities as outlined in the students' individualized education programs and/or the school's accommodations.	1.6.2 Lessons/activities are adapted for students at all fitness levels (e.g., distance and pace runs are made appropriate). Students are encouraged to complete appropriate levels of activity for their own improvement.	1.6.3 Physical educators provide appropriate experiences for students with temporary medical limitations (e.g., a student with a broken arm can ride an exercise bike).
Appropriate practice: high school	1.6 Inclusion	1.6.1 Physical educators implement the special education process for students with disabilities as outlined in the students' individualized education programs and/or the school's accommodations.	1.6.2 Lessons/activities are adapted for students at all fitness levels (e.g., distance and pace runs are made appropriate). Students are encouraged to complete appropriate levels of activity for their own improvement.	1.6.3 Physical educators provide appropriate experiences for students with temporary medical limitations (e.g., a student with a broken arm can ride an exercise bike).

The ability to create an inclusive environment is essential for successful teaching as well as student learning. Table 4.4 shows appropriate practices as recommended by SHAPE America.

It cannot be said enough, and often throughout this text, that as teachers, what we do in physical education classes has direct impact on the behaviors that students learn, independent of the written curriculum. We must practice the behaviors that we expect our students to adhere to and make sure that every child in the class is provided an equal opportunity to succeed, feels physically and emotionally safe, and is respected.

CONCLUSION

At the end of the day, we are all given the responsibility to keep students safe and be aware of the liability and neglect that we may face. Teachers are to be in compliance of the health and well-being of student guidelines and take every safety precaution to avoid any and all liability and negligent behavior.

Physical education classes need to be a place that children enjoy and give them the experience that will continue their motivation toward lifelong activity. For this reason, always strive to ensure that facilities and instruction are both inclusive and adaptable for all students, allowing easy modifications and making no student feel isolated. This can only happen if we, as teachers, pledge to continue to educate in an environment in which students feel mentally, emotionally and physically safe and provide quality instruction and adequate resources.

Review Questions

1. Explain the importance of class climate and describe some strategies to develop it.
2. Describe the types and roles of various modes of communication.
3. Describe some of the legal issues surrounding supervision.
4. Explain the difference between equity and equality.
5. Identify some strategies to make your class an inclusive environment.

Visit HK*Propel* for additional material related to this chapter.

CHAPTER 5

Nutrition, Wellness, and Consumer Issues

Lisa Dorfman

Chapter Objective

After reading this chapter, you will understand the role that nutrition and healthy eating habits play in overall cognitive and physical performance in secondary age students; know how to deliver, develop, and assess students' knowledge in key nutrition topics; and employ best teaching practices that enhance student learning. Key research findings will further allow for creative and innovative class discussions during the delivery of instruction.

Key Concepts

- Proper nutrition and healthy eating habits are essential to teenagers' enhanced physical activity performance, as well as everyday activities.
- Dietary challenges, such as irregular snacking, poor sleep habits, and supplement use and abuse, during the teen years affect future overall health and physical activity and sports performance.
- Lifestyle behaviors, eating disorders, social media, and an understanding of caloric input and output have an impact on weight management.
- Intake of fluids, vitamins and minerals, nutrients, supplements, and steroids and other consumer issues affect performance and health.

INTRODUCTION

Having healthy eating habits during the teenage years is essential for growth and cognitive development. Research suggests education pertaining to food, fitness, and healthful lifestyle habits can help young people to attain the knowledge and the skills that they need to make proper food choices and develop lifelong healthy eating patterns, which can impact the quality of their entire lives (Sadegholvad, Yeatman, Parrish, & Worsley, 2017).

High school and middle school educators play a pivotal role in teaching students about performance nutrition for health, sport, and life. Nutrition education can help teens to attain the knowledge and skills they need to make healthy food decisions and improve their energy levels, mood, appearance, and, most importantly, lifelong eating behaviors.

This chapter will help guide physical educators in teaching hands-on, practical information about nutrition and wellness pertinent to the teenage years. Instruction can be delivered through lectures, handouts, journaling, or group discussions. Topics in this chapter include basic nutrition requirements, exercise fuel, weight management and dieting, supplement safety, behavior, and mental health dietary-related issues such as eating disorders. In addition, this chapter addresses special dietary considerations—food allergies and intolerances—while aiming to improve students' knowledge, skills, self-efficacy, and behaviors associated with dietary guidelines.

At the end of each section, teachers will find suggested discussion topics, questions for students, and activities or journal prompts. Students can start a journal at the beginning of the semester to log introspective questions and activities into each section. References and support resources, along with additional references for further reading, can be found within and at the end of the chapter.

NUTRITIONAL NEEDS IN ADOLESCENCE

Adolescence is the period of development that begins at puberty and ends in early adulthood. It is one of the most exciting yet challenging stages in the life cycle. Most commonly, adolescence is divided into three developmental periods: early adolescence (10-14 years of age), late adolescence (15-19 years of age), and early adulthood (20-24 years of age) (Das et al., 2017).

The time between 12-21 years old is a period of tremendous physiological, psychological, and cognitive transformations from a child to an adult. The physical process of growing from a child into an adult is the only time after birth that the velocity of growth increases. Teens gain about 20 percent of their adult height and 50 percent of their adult weight during adolescence. Most of this growth is gained during an 18- to 24-month period, called the growth spurt, during the five to seven years of puberty. Everyone goes through growth spurts at different times and can continue into the early 20s (Larson et al., 2017). During this process, body composition changes too. Prior to puberty, body composition for boys and girls are about the same, but during puberty, boys gain about twice as much lean mass as girls do. The nutritional requirements for teens also vary because of the variations in growth rate and training.

Diet deficiencies during the teen years can impose short-term health risks, such as weight gain, inadequate bone mineralization, negative impact on hormone development, and poor academic performance. In the long-term, poor diets developed during this period often continue into adulthood, influencing the risk of chronic diseases including diabetes, cardiovascular disease, and certain cancers (Winpenny, Penney, Corder, White, & van Sluijs, 2017). We'll go into greater depth in this chapter about what constitutes a healthy diet.

While the physical changes during puberty to adolescence transform the child into a young adult, the social and emotional development often lags behind with some teens maturing faster than others (Larson et al., 2020). Discrepancies between the teen's body, mood, and behaviors often result in a food rebellion—a search for autonomy using food for independence, whether it means becoming vegetarian or making impulsive food and beverage decisions. These often-irrational dietary decisions can have short- and long-term effects on body image, trust, and respect for adults, including food educators and nutrition experts. Irregular meals and snacking; fast food and the media; and the influence of poor sleep, alcohol, and use or abuse of recreational drugs, steroids, and supplements are additional challenges for meeting nutrition and physical activity goals for teenagers. As a result, teens take risks with themselves, their health, and their diet. Meal patterns are often chaotic: Teens stop eating at home; they often skip breakfast and lunch; and, if a nighttime social activity is scheduled, teens may overlook dinner. According to a 2019 USDA report, more than one in four (27 percent) adolescents obtained 30 percent or more of their total daily energy from late evening eating.

Topics for discussion include teen physical changes and challenges, influences on eating, importance of diet during teen years, and consequences of poor teen diets.

Questions:

1. Why is it important to eat well during the teen years?
2. What type of physical and growth changes take place during adolescence? What changes have you seen in yourself during puberty to teenage years?
3. What are some of the consequences of nutrition deficiencies during teen years?
4. Why are the teenage years a period of nutrition transition? What impact does this period have on dietary choices?
5. What are three ways teens may change their diet during this period?

Journal Prompts:

1. Keep a three-day food diary (a template is provided in HK*Propel*). Provide the time you eat, the specific food you eat (fluids, snacks, and candy), the amount of all food consumed, and the circumstances of your food decision making (e.g., Were mealtimes at home, with friends, or in a social setting such as a party? Did you experience boredom or stress?). What do you see in the timing of your meals? Did you skip meals, leave too much time between them, or eat too little at mealtime, which causes excess eating and drinking in the evening? At any given time, were you emotional eating?
2. Based on your evaluation of your food diary, select three dietary changes that you believe can improve and enhance your health, weight, social and emotional well-being, and overall performance.
3. How does your diet affect your mood, energy levels, concentration, performance in physical education, sports, high-intensity recreational activities (e.g., hiking up mountains, long bike rides, and kayaking), and physical tasks? What would you like to improve about how you are feeling? Do you want more energy, be in a better mood, or get better sleep?
4. What is holding you back from changing your eating habits at home, at school, and within you and your beliefs?

NUTRITION EDUCATION

There is no doubt that teens can benefit and are interested in learning more about nutrition despite very little research in this area with the exception of examining active teens (Larson et al., 2017). In a recent study, general and sport nutrition knowledge, dietary habits, and attitudes toward nutrition education were collected by survey among active middle and high schoolers. Seventy-nine percent of middle school students and 92.5 percent of high school students stated feeling they could benefit from advice about nutrition (Partida, Marshall, Henry, Townsend, & Toy, 2018). In the case of adolescent athletes, the belief is that diet is important for exercise training and performance despite diets being less than adequate. Less than 40 percent of students stated their diet meets their nutritional needs (Partida et al., 2018).

Adolescent athletes have unique nutritional requirements because of daily activity, training, and competition in addition to the demands of growth and development (Desbrow et al., 2014). For teen athletes, research suggests nutrition knowledge, behaviors, and beliefs are limited (Manorel, Patton-Lopez, Meng, & Wong, 2017). Misconceptions about activity nutrition among teens also persist. For example, in one study, only 35.5 percent of questions regarding protein and exercise were answered correctly by active high school students while 28.5 percent of questions were answered correctly by active middle school students prior to a nutrition intervention (Partida et al., 2018). Both middle school and high school students stated a desire to learn more about nutrition, but most nutrition information currently received comes from non-nutrition-related professionals, such as parents and coaches.

According to a recent review of 34 studies, secondary schools are a good environment to educate students and model good health behaviors (McHugh et al., 2020). Multimedia and web-based intervention programs for adolescents have also been shown to be successful in improving diet and physical activity behaviors and promoting weight loss, especially programs that engage adolescents in the program development (Cullen, Thompson, Boushey, Konzelmann, & Chen, 2013).

In addition to the best delivery modalities for nutrition education and regardless of whether teens are sedentary, active, or competitive athletes, providing reliable sources of nutrition and nutrition information and advice is imperative. Often, teens obtain their diet and health info from the Internet, social media, coaches, friends, teammates, advertising, and impressionable testimonials by celebrities and athletes (Stang & Larson, 2020; Lapierre, Fleming-Milici, Rozendaal, McAlister, & Castonguay, 2017). Nutrition misinformation can have immediate and long-term negative consequences on food choices, eating behaviors, and long-term health. It can also result in unnecessary purchases of vitamins, minerals, and nutritional supplements that have health risks due to tainted ingredients; include caffeine and herbs, which can affect cognitive and physical health; and, in some circumstances, lead to death (Medina-Caliz et al., 2018).

Social media also have a strong influence on dieting, body image, and lifestyle behaviors in teens. Teenage vulnerability to online food marketing and digital promotions is a result of cognitive and emotional factors, peer-group influence, and high levels of exposure to advertising messages (Elliott, 2019). In a recent study, the influence of social media use on disordered eating in adolescents was reported by 51.7 percent of girls and 45 percent of boys, with strict exercise and meal skipping as the most common behaviors (Wilksch, O'Shea, Ho, Byrne, & Wade, 2020). A total of 75.4 percent of girls and 69.9 percent of boys had at least one social media account, with Instagram being the most commonly used: 68.1 percent of girls and 61.7 percent of boys (Wilksch et al., 2020).

Nutrition experts are people with undergraduate and often graduate degrees in nutrition and dietetics who have accredited onsite internship practice and have passed a national board exam to become Registered Dietitians (RDs) and licensed (LDN) in most U.S. states. These experts can give teens reliable resources. Most RDs are members of the Academy of Nutrition and Dietetics (AND), a professional organization with more than 70,000 members nationwide. The website for this group, www.eatright.org, offers valuable resources, handouts, and educational materials that are especially helpful for educators of middle and high school nutrition.

For dietitians who specialize in sports nutrition, acquiring additional internship experiences and passing a national board exam offers the Board-Certified Specialist in Sports Dietetics (CSSD) credential. Sports dietitians are members of specialty practice groups such as the Sports, Cardiovascular, and Wellness Nutrition (SCAN), a dietetic practice group of the Academy of Nutrition, or the Collegiate and Professional Sports Dietitians Association (CPSDA). Each group freely offers current topic-focused handouts, research, and activity nutrition information.

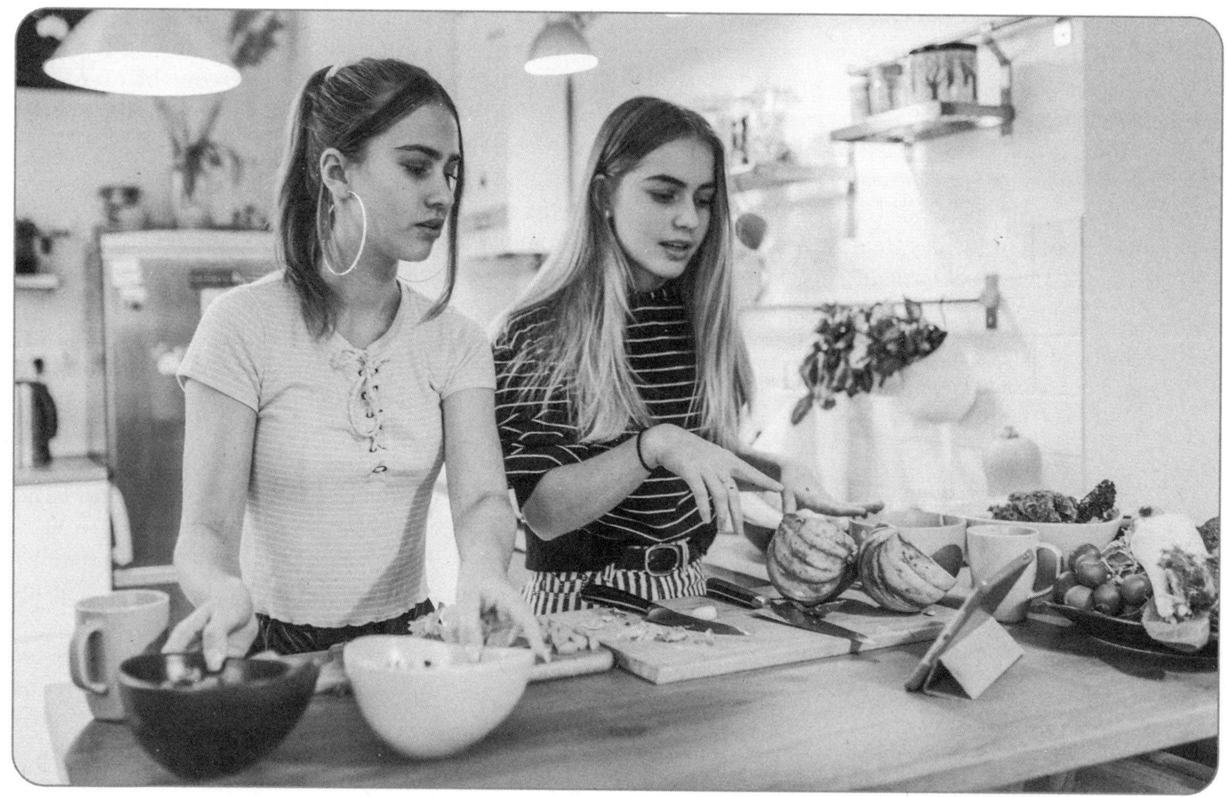

Teens using the internet and social media need to learn how to judge the reliability of information obtained there.

Topics for discussion include diet quality, nutrition knowledge, registered dietitians (RD, LDN), Certified Specialists in Sports Dietetics (CSSD), and social media and misinformation.

Questions:

1. How can teens benefit by understanding nutrition from credible resources?
2. Where do teens get their nutrition information? What are some of the consequences of getting nutrition information from non-nutrition-related professionals or educators such as the Internet and celebrities?
3. Who are the experts in nutrition and sports dietetics?
4. How has taking nutrition advice from non-expert sources affected your food choices, eating behaviors, and overall health?
5. Interview a Registered Dietitian who works with teens or athletes in your area. What does the RD do to help guide teens to optimal health and performance?

Journal Prompts:

1. Draw a picture of your present diet—breakfast, lunch, dinner, snacks, and beverages—for one day. Include the time of the meal, the specific food and preparation (e.g., fried, baked, or steamed), and the approximate amount on a plate. If possible, use colored pencils or crayons. Then, in a separate chart, draw a picture of what you think the nutritious meals and beverages for a typical day should look like.
2. Compare the two pictures. What differences did you find in the two diets?

DAILY CALORIE NEEDS FOR WEIGHT MANAGEMENT

To be healthy, the body must be continuously supplied with food energy, called calories. Recommended calorie requirements for teens are designed to help them maintain health, promote optimal growth and maturation, sustain energy for daily living, and support training needs. Teens who compromise their diet by taking in too many calories or not getting enough can negatively affect their overall adult growth and health.

The formula for calculating daily calorie needs is dependent on three factors: (1) basal metabolic rate (BMR), the minimum number of calories for basic functions that you burn while at rest; (2) energy expended for physical activity (EEPA), the energy expended during physical activity directly related to intensity, duration, and skill level; and (3) the thermic effect of food (TEF), the amount of energy you spend digesting food and extracting nutrients while eating (also known as specific dynamic action, or SDA).

To calculate daily total calories required to support everyday activities like going to class, doing homework and household chores, exercising, digesting and metabolizing food, or maintaining a weight or reaching a goal weight, you can use the *Formula for Calculating Daily Calorie Needs*. Additional guidelines for physical activity can be found in chapters 1 and 2.

Several online tools help determine how many calories you expend for a physical activity. The Calorie Control Council offers one simple tool at their website, https://caloriecontrol.org/healthy-weight-tool-kit/get-moving-calculator/, in which calories are based on moderate activities. You can find another calorie counter resource at the website of American Council on Exercise (ACE), www.acefitness.org/education-and-resources/lifestyle/tools-calculators/physical-activity-calorie-counter/.

Topics for discussion include calories, BMR, EEPA, SDA, and TEF.

Questions:

1. What three factors are used for calculating daily calorie needs?
2. What is basal metabolic rate (BMR)? Which factors affect BMR?
3. What is EEPA? How does exercise affect the number of calories you use each day when you exercise verses being sedentary?
4. How much exercise do you do in one week? Which type of exercise do you do? Do you meet the U.S. Department of Health and Human Services guidelines for exercise? If you aren't meeting the guidelines, what are the reasons? (Refer to chapters 1 and 2 for more on physical activity recommendations.)

Journal Prompts:

1. Using the formula provided, calculate the number of calories you need in one day.
2. You can use the DRI calculator, based on the Dietary Reference Index (DRI) established by the Health and Medicine Division of the National Academies of Sciences, Engineering and Medicine, to calculate how many calories you need each day.

HEALTHY WEIGHT RANGE

There are several tools to guide teens on determining their healthiest weight range. The best tool depends on how teens feel. In other words, it is not about weight; instead, it is about how people hold the weight, as in your body composition, which is the percent of body fat relative to total weight. RDs or exercise physiologists can measure people's body fat and help determine healthiest weight and percent body fat. On the National Institute of Health's (NIH) website (www.niddk.nih.gov/bwp), people 18 and over can use an easy-to-use free online tool to start planning for their best body weight.

Another tool for determining a healthy body weight range is the body mass index (BMI). The BMI is a formula: weight in kilograms divided by the square of height in meters. According to the Centers for Disease Control (CDC) BMI is age- and sex-specific for teens and is often referred to as BMI-for-age. The CDC offers a free tool for calculating BMI for children and teens at its website, www.cdc.gov/healthyweight/assessing/bmi/childrens_bmi/about_childrens_bmi.html.

Once the BMI is calculated, it is expressed as a percentile, which can be obtained from either a graph or a percentile calculator. These percentiles express the BMI relative to other teens in the United States who participated in national surveys that were conducted from 1963 to 1965 and 1988 to 1994. Because weight and height and their relation to body fat change during growth and development, an individual teen's BMI is interpreted as weight relative to others in the same age and gender group. The U.S. categories (underweight, normal weight, overweight, and obese) and their corresponding percentiles are as follows:

- Underweight: Less than the 5th percentile
- Normal or healthy weight: 5th percentile to less than the 85th percentile
- Overweight: 85th to less than the 95th percentile
- Obese: Equal to or greater than the 95th percentile

Source: www.cdc.gov/healthyweight/assessing/bmi/childrens_bmi/about_childrens_bmi.html

If a teen needs to lose or gain weight in order to get into the normal category, he will have to adjust calorie intake or expenditure gradually in order to gain or lose over a period of time.

To *lose* one pound per week, deduct 500 calories daily for an extra 3,500-calorie difference each week. A person can also expend more calories by increasing activity levels to 500 calories expenditure a day. The following list provides suggestions for reducing calories through food intake:

- Eat more fruits and vegetables.
- Limit fast food or choose fewer fried and more grilled selections.
- Drink more water; drink less soda, juice, and whole milk.
- Limit sweets; avoid simple sugars found in candy and desserts.
- Eat at least three smaller meals and three snacks daily.
- Decrease portion sizes to fist-sized meat portions and tennis ball complex carbohydrate portions.
- Increase intake of fresh or frozen vegetables and fruits to five per day.
- Cut back on the extras (condiments like mayonnaise, oils, and sauces).
- Eat portion-sized snacks instead of eating directly out of the box or bag.

To *gain* one pound of lean muscle per week, add 500 calories daily for an extra 3,500 calories a week:

- Eat five to six meals daily, including two to three snacks of shakes and bars before and after exercise.
- Add a glass of whole milk to mealtimes and snacks; whole soy, almond, or rice milk if lactose intolerance is an issue.
- Do not drink at mealtime until food has already been consumed because beverages can be filling.
- Replace low-calorie beverages such as water with juice, sports drinks, milk, and shakes.
- Add the equivalent of about three to four ounces (85 to 114 g), the size of a deck of cards, of lean protein daily.
- Double the portion sizes of complex carbs such as whole grain pasta, bread, rice, and potatoes.
- Snack between meals on healthy, high-calorie choices such as trail mix and nut butter sandwiches.
- Use higher-calorie foods for every meal, for example: granola instead of plain cereal, muffins instead of toast, pan-fried meats cooked in olive oil instead of grilled and oil free.
- Eat a bar or shake before and after training that has at least 0.1 gram of protein per pound of body weight (e.g., 13 grams for the 130-pound [59 kg] athlete), with good sources of carbohy-

drates, about one gram per pound body weight (130). Options can include a fruit smoothie with Greek yogurt, protein-fortified milk, or a whole-food sports bar (protein bars generally limit carbohydrates).

For athletes, meeting minimal daily calorie needs beyond weight and performance goals also presents challenges. If athletes are juggling training, studies, and occasional family responsibilities, it often means eating on the run. School schedules, budgets, social schedules, and appetites can compromise the quantity, quality, and timing of meals. Preparing ahead with healthy snacks and portable meals such as sandwiches and shakes can improve dietary intake of calories and nutrients. More recommendations on snacking can be found later in the chapter in tables 5.14 and 5.15.

Compromising the nutritional quality of the diet and the timing of the meals can also affect energy levels, performance, and weight by underestimating the number of calories used for BMR and training. Getting enough calories by eating the right foods more frequently throughout the day is just as important as the amount one is consuming.

Topics for discussion include weight management, BMI, weight loss, weight gain, and strategies for weight loss and weight gain.

Questions:

1. What is your BMI? How does it compare to others in your age and gender groups? Which category does your BMI indicate?
2. How do you know if you need to reduce or increase calories to attain and maintain a healthy weight?
3. What kinds of changes can you make to either reduce calories or increase calories to meet your goal weight?
4. If you are outside a healthy range of body fat, how do you think this is affecting your mood, performance, and energy levels?

Journal Prompts:

1. Are there changes you think you need to make this semester in order to lose or gain weight, have more energy, or improve performance? Provide three strategies.
2. From your three-day food diary, identify where most of the calories come from in your diet. Is it chips, soda, and sweets? Or, is it too much protein, cereals, or added fats such as oils, dressings, and sauces?
3. How can you change some of the foods you eat to improve the nutrition quality of your food options?

DIETING AND EATING DISORDERS

Attempts at weight control are common across a person's life span. Estimates suggest that one-third of adolescents and two-thirds of adults engage in dieting—using willful but not always healthy approaches to weight control and often restricting themselves to small amounts or specific foods or food groups to lose weight. Most research has examined the prevalence of these behaviors in adolescence and adulthood (Haynos et al., 2018). Dieting and unhealthy weight-control behaviors have been associated with negative outcomes such as malnutrition and obesity. According to the National Center for Health Statistics (NCHS) latest report (2017), the adolescent obesity rate in the United States has nearly doubled over the past three decades.

Currently, 20.6 percent of U.S. adolescents are obese. Recent research suggests teens' diets are reflecting excesses in calories and deficiencies in expenditure since there has been a tenfold increase in child and adolescent obesity figures globally over the last four decades (McHugh et al., 2020). According to the World Health Organization (WHO), 80 percent of the world's adolescents are not active enough, have high sugar diets, and do not consume the recommended amount of fruit and vegetables (McHugh et al., 2020).

A smaller, but still considerable, portion of adolescents engage in unhealthy and disordered forms of weight control, such as disordered eating, severely restricting intake, fasting, or purging through vomiting or laxatives (Bould, De Stavola, Lewis, & Micali, 2018). Although certain forms of weight management may be nonthreatening and often recommended, even relatively common weight-control behaviors have been associated with negative psychological consequences.

Dieting has also been shown to increase the risk of eating disorders such as anorexia nervosa, bulimia, binge eating, anorexia athletica, and muscle dysmorphia (MD), and other psychological concerns, such as depressive symptoms and substance use (Haynos et al., 2018). Eating disorders are one of the most common and serious health problems affecting teenagers in the U.S. According to the American Psychiatric Association's (APA) *Diagnostic and Statistical Manual (DSM-5)*, eating disorders affect several million people at any given time, most often women between the ages of 12 and 35 (APA, 2020). The NIH cites the lifetime prevalence of eating disorders among U.S. adolescents aged 13 to 18 years was 2.7 percent, twice as prevalent among females (3.8 percent) than males (1.5 percent). The prevalence of eating disorders among adolescents continues to increase.

Recent evidence suggests the estimated lifetime prevalence of eating disorders is approximately one in five females and one in seven males, with the initial onset concentrated during adolescence and young adulthood (Ward, Rodriguez, Wright, Austin, & Long, 2019). The Growing Up Today Study of 9,031 U.S. females ages 9 to 15 years old shows a lifetime prevalence of bulimia nervosa was 2.1 percent and 6 percent for binge-eating disorder (Glazer et al., 2019). The occurrence of anorexia nervosa, bulimia nervosa, and binge-eating disorder appear to be 0.3 percent, 0.9 percent, and 1.6 percent, respectively (Swanson, Crow, & Le Grange, 2011).

Symptoms of eating disorders have been shown to be more common in teens who are overweight or obese. Although most symptoms tended to have higher prevalence among girls than boys, boys with obesity had higher prevalence of binge eating and excessive exercise than girls with obesity (Hughes et al., 2019). The most unhealthy and extreme weight-control behaviors have also been associated with negative psychological consequences, including increased risk of suicide attempt (Nagata et al., 2018; Solmi et al., 2015; Zuromski & Witte, 2015).

The three main types of eating disorders are (1) anorexia nervosa, (2) bulimia nervosa, and (3) binge-eating disorder. Disordered eating behaviors specifically in athletes have been termed anorexia athletica (AA), where the goal is to perform at one's best as opposed to achieving thinness in and of itself. Muscle dysmorphia, also known as bigorexia or reverse anorexia, is a disorder in which people are preoccupied with their bodies not being muscular enough or big enough.

Athletes who are more vulnerable to AA are those who participate in lean-build sports, such as cross country running, swimming, gymnastics, cheerleading, dance, yoga, and wrestling. These athletes may think they need to be a certain weight or body type, often far less than what it is realistic to attain and maintain to be competitive (Dorfman, 2019). Figure 5.1 depicts the differences between men and women with a lifetime prevalence of eating disorders.

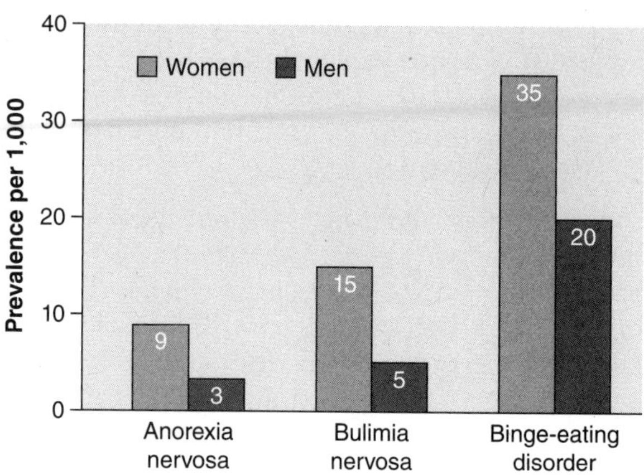

Figure 5.1 Lifetime prevalence of eating disorders.
Reprinted by permission from Mirror-Mirror. https://mirror-mirror.org/facts-staticstics/graphs-on-eating-disorders.

Anorexia Nervosa

Anorexia nervosa is diagnosed when patients weigh at least 15 percent less than the normal healthy weight expected for their height. People with anorexia nervosa do not maintain a normal weight because they refuse to eat enough, often exercise obsessively, and sometimes force themselves to vomit or use laxatives to lose weight (APA, 2020).

Signs

- Limited food intake
- Fear of being "fat"
- Problems with body image or denial of low body weight

Long-Term Consequences

- Cessation of menstrual periods
- Osteopenia or osteoporosis (thinning of the bones) through loss of calcium
- Brittle hair and nails
- Dry skin that can take on a yellowish cast
- Mild anemia
- Atrophy of muscles, including the heart muscle
- Severe constipation
- Drop in blood pressure and slowed breathing and pulse rates
- Reduced internal body temperature, causing person to feel cold all the time
- Depression and lethargy

Bulimia Nervosa

Bulimia nervosa is identified in those who binge eat frequently and may eat an astounding amount of food in a short time, often consuming thousands of calories that are high in sugars, carbohydrates, and fat. They can eat very rapidly, sometimes gulping down food without even tasting it. Compared to people with anorexia nervosa, people with bulimia nervosa typically are not underweight and can have a normal weight or be overweight or even obese.

People who binge often stop only when they are interrupted by another person, fall asleep, or their stomach hurts from being stretched beyond normal capacity. During a binge, the person feels out of control. After a binge, stomach pains and the fear of weight gain are common reasons that those with bulimia nervosa purge by throwing up or using a laxative. This cycle is usually repeated at least several times a week or, in serious cases, several times a day.

Many people do not know when a family member or friend has bulimia nervosa because people almost always hide their binges. Since people with bulimia nervosa do not become drastically thin, their behaviors may go unnoticed by those closest to them.

Signs

- Chronically inflamed and sore throat
- Swollen salivary glands in the neck and below the jaw; puffy cheeks and face, causing sufferers to develop a "chipmunk"-looking face
- Tooth decay when enamel wears off due to exposure to stomach acids
- Gastroesophageal reflux disorder due to constant vomiting
- Intestinal problems due to laxative abuse
- Kidney problems due to using diuretics (water pills)
- Severe dehydration from purging of fluids

Long-Term Consequences

- Rare but potentially fatal complications including esophageal tears, gastric rupture, and cardiac arrhythmias
- Damage to the heart, teeth, kidneys, and gastrointestinal tract
- Reduced metabolism
- Negative mental and emotional effects

Binge-Eating Disorder

People with binge-eating disorder have episodes in which they consume very large quantities of food in a brief period and feel out of control during the binge. Unlike people with bulimia nervosa, they do not try to get rid of the food by inducing vomiting or by using other unsafe practices such as fasting or laxative abuse. Binge eating is chronic and can lead to serious health complications, including particularly severe obesity, diabetes, hypertension, and cardiovascular diseases.

According to information from the National Institutes of Mental Health (NIHM, 2020), *Cognitive Behavior Therapy With Adolescents With Eating Disorders* (Grave & Calugi, 2020), and the APA (2020), binge-eating disorder involves frequent overeating during a discrete period (at least once a week for three months) combined with lack of control and is associated with three or more of the following:

- Eating more rapidly than normal
- Eating until feeling uncomfortably full
- Eating large amounts of food when not feeling physically hungry
- Eating alone because of feeling embarrassed by how much one is eating
- Feeling disgusted with oneself, depressed, or very guilty afterward
- Having significant distress

The long-term effects of binge eating include the following:

- Heart disease
- Gastrointestinal distress
- Struggles with body image and self-esteem
- Psychological distress

Eating Disorders in Teen Athletes

Although drive, perfection, and attention to detail are some of the characteristics of talented athletes, they are also some of the personality traits associated with the development of eating disorders. Disordered eating behaviors among athletes can be difficult to detect because the tendencies of athletes to maintain rigid nutritional requirements, follow intense training schedules, and push through fatigue and pain are considered normal.

This desire to be unrealistically light or lean may lead to restrictive eating, binging and purging, and excessive training far beyond what is required for their sport. Chronic dieting by female athletes can lead to the *female athlete triad (FAT)*, which consists of three interrelated health disorders: low energy availability with or without an eating disorder, osteoporosis, and amenorrhea (lack of menstruation). The prevalence of FAT for athletes participating in lean-requiring versus non-lean-requiring sports has been shown to range from 1.5 percent to 6.7 percent and from 0 percent to 2.0 percent, respectively (Gibbs, Williams, & De Souza, 2013).

The low energy intake of *athletic energy deficit (AED)*, also known as relative energy deficit in sports (RED-S), can lead to an increase in bone fractures, lifelong consequences for bone and reproductive health, and health and performance consequences including impaired judgment, decreased coordination, decreased concentration, irritability, depression, and decreased endurance performance in developing adolescent girls and even men (Ackerman et al., 2018).

Evidence suggests it is an energy availability issue that regulates reproductive function in women, not exercise or body composition, and that ensuring adequate calorie intake is imperative to the overall health of the athletic woman (Ackerman et al., 2018; De Souza et al., 2014). Low energy intake paired with amenorrhea has been associated with poor athletic performance. Dancers frequently deal with body image and eating disorder issues. One recent study showed professional dancers consume only 70 to 80 percent of the recommended dietary allowance (RDA) for total daily energy intake (Mountjoy et al., 2014).

While many studies suggest females are more susceptible to disordered eating behaviors than males, results from project EAT (Eating Among Teens) revealed that males who consider themselves in a weight-related sport are comparative to females in the same category (West et al., 2019). In fact, with the media's portrayal of the male physique being increasingly muscular and unattainable, men have become more dissatisfied with their bodies and more vulnerable to eating, exercise, and body image (EEBI) disorders.

Muscle dysmorphia (MD) is marked by symptoms that are similar and the opposite of AN signs and symptoms. Athletes with anorexia athletica and MD experience distorted perceptions of their bodies, which, in MD, often leads to maladaptive eating, exercise, and substance-use behaviors, including preoccupation with diet and excessively high protein intakes. In addition, there is often anabolic steroid, diet pill, caffeine, and over-the-counter supplement abuse, especially of those reputed for fat-burning, ergogenic, or thermogenic effects.

A behavior of the MD-impacted athlete is participating in excessive exercise, especially with weightlifting, in an attempt to increase body satisfaction and attain the "perfect" lean and muscular physique. Many studies suggest that bodybuilders display higher MD prevalence rates and more MD features than other resistance-training athletes, with prevalence rates ranging from 3.4 to 53.6 percent within this group (Cerea et al., 2018). As with other EEBI, MD can lead to social, occupational, and relationship impairments. Research suggests that this preference for a muscular physique is already evident in boys as young as six years old and may affect up to 95 percent of college-age American men who are dissatisfied with some aspect of their body (Engeln et al., 2013; Murray, 2019).

Some of the leading characteristics of the effects of body image and eating disorders, as described by Dorfman (2019) are identified in the following lists.

Anorexia Athletica

- The need to exercise beyond the requirements for good health
- Obsessive dieting
- Fear of certain foods
- Obsessive or compulsive exercising
- Refusal to eat with teammates
- Attempts at hiding dieting
- Devotion to exercise that steals time from work, school, and relationships
- A focus on the challenge that prevents any memory that physical activity can be fun
- Self-worth defined in terms of performance
- Constant dissatisfaction with athletic achievements
- A push to keep moving on to the next challenge
- Justification of excessive behavior by defining self as an athlete or insistence that the behavior is healthy
- Desire to keep losing more pounds despite already low body weight
- Mood swings or angry outbursts
- Inability to menstruate

Source: www.eatingdisordersonline.com/explain/anorexiathleticasigns.php

Muscle Dysmorphia

- A disorder that primarily affects males
- Preoccupation with getting bigger, including thinking about diet, working out, or appearance
- Self-image of looking small or "puny" despite having a typical or muscular appearance to others
- Constant concerns with body fat percentage
- The use of baggy clothing to hide a physique that is perceived as a source of shame
- Precedence of workouts over other significant events or time spent with family and friends

- Fear that missing one workout session will be a setback or stymie progress, and works out despite injuries
- Abuse of anabolic steroids to enhance appearance
- Extreme anxiety and crushing self-esteem triggered by missing a workout or eating a "forbidden" food item
- Added workout sessions, skipped meals, or punishment for diet cheating
- Frequent symptoms of depression

Source: www.eatingdisordersonline.com/lifestyle/general/recognizingmuscle-dysmorphia-bigorexia

Topics for discussion include eating disorders, disordered eating behaviors, anorexia nervosa, bulimia nervosa, muscle dysmorphia, anorexia athletica, female athletic triad (FAT), and athletic energy deficit (AED).

Questions:

1. What is an eating disorder? Name three eating disorders and provide a description for each.
2. Why are eating disorders harmful to health?
3. Give three signs and symptoms of each of the following eating disorders: anorexia nervosa, bulimia nervosa, binge-eating disorder, muscle dysmorphia, anorexia athletica, female athletic triad (FAT), and athletic energy deficit (AED).

Journal Prompts:

1. Have you or someone you know experienced an eating disorder?
2. What signs and symptoms did you or the person experience?
3. How have media, social media, your friends, family, coaches, or teammates affected the way you feel about your body, your physique, and yourself?
4. Write a letter to yourself or someone you know or believe to have an eating disorder. Share your specific concerns for that person's health and provide resources and recommendations for help. Use the resource section or online research organizations that provide help for these disorders.

DIETARY COMPOSITION

Overall good nutrition for teens is the balanced consumption of nutrients from a variety of foods to meet daily calorie (energy) needs. *Nutrients* are compounds in foods essential to health and life. Nutrients provide us with energy in the form of calories to help us to grow, repair, and provide substances required to regulate chemical processes. There are six essential nutrients that the body needs to accomplish these goals. The essential *macronutrients* that give the body calories—carbohydrates, protein, and fat—can be found in varying amounts in all foods. The essential *micronutrients* that also help the body to use energy, but do not have calories, include vitamins, minerals, and water.

While the composition (proportion) of carbohydrates, protein, and fats in a diet needs to be individualized and based on personal health and athletic and performance goals, ideal ranges for teens are recommended to fall within a range determined to be ideal for overall health. The chart for the *Nutritional Goals for Age-Gender Groups Based on Dietary Reference Intakes and Dietary Guidelines Recommendations* can be found in HK*Propel*.

The 2015-2020 Dietary Guidelines for Americans 8th Edition offers guidance on the ideal dietary composition: https://health.gov/sites/default/files/2019-09/2015-2020_Dietary_Guidelines.pdf. The Institute of Medicine (IOM) Food and Nutrition Board also established guidelines for protein, carbohydrates, and fats. It is called the Acceptable Macronutrient Distribution Range (AMDR). The AMDRs define appropriate ranges for carbohydrates, protein, and fat designed to avoid deficiencies (Manore, 2005).

The AMDR recommendations based on total calorie intake are as follows:

- 45 to 65 percent from carbohydrates
- 10 to 35 percent from protein
- 20 to 35 percent from fat

Topics for discussion include calories, macronutrients, micronutrients, dietary composition, IOM guidelines, and macronutrient percentage recommendations.

Questions:

1. What are nutrients and why are they important for the body?
2. What are the three macronutrients?
3. What are the three micronutrients?
4. What are the IOM's recommended guidelines for distribution of calories from carbohydrates, proteins, and fats?

Journal Prompts:

1. Analyze your three-day diet journal by using an online dietary analysis calculator. Use the following link for a free analysis: www.choosemyplate.gov/startsimpleapp.

2. How does your diet compare to the recommended nutrients distribution guidelines?
3. What are three changes you can make to the dietary distribution of calories in your diet?

Macronutrients

Carbohydrates, proteins, and fats are all calorie sources for meeting daily energy needs. An individual teen's age, gender, physical fitness level, and diet can all potentially affect the amount and proportion of carbohydrates, fats, and proteins needed.

Carbohydrates

Carbohydrates are the main energy fuel for the body. There are two types of carbohydrates, simple and complex. Simple carbohydrates are found in sweet foods, soft drinks, candy, cookies, and fruit. Complex carbohydrates, also known as starch, are found in pastas, breads, potatoes, rice, beans, peas, crackers, cereals, and vegetables.

When the body consumes simple or complex carbohydrates, they are digested and broken down into glucose, the simplest form of energy that every cell in the body uses. When not used for energy, glucose is stored in the muscles and liver as glycogen, which is an especially important energy source for athletes. Eating enough total daily carbs and fueling with carbs is particularly important before, during, and after exercise.

It is recommended that simple carbohydrates or sugars should not exceed more than 10 percent of total calories. Why? The reason is that simple carbohydrate–rich food such as candy, soft drinks, and desserts actually tend to rob the body of energy. They provide quick, empty fuel that is lower in vitamins, minerals, fiber, and compounds called *phytonutrients*. These compounds are the plant nutrients found naturally in vegetables, fruits, beans, and whole grains that help the body to use fuel, stay fit, recover faster, and reduce the risk for injury and illness. Complex carbohydrates, on the other hand, are slower than simple carbohydrates to metabolize because they take longer to digest. They are generally higher in vitamins, minerals, and fibers that cannot be digested because the body lacks the enzymes needed to break them down and assist in keeping your gut and digestion fit. Whole grains, fruits, and vegetables are not only rich in complex carbohydrates and fibers but also more nutritious for overall health.

Choosing complex carbohydrates will fuel the body with better nutrition—more fiber, vitamins, minerals, and protein, and less of the fat, saturated fat, and simple sugars typically found in fried foods and sweets. Selecting fewer fried high-carbohy-

Table 5.1 Carbohydrate Food Sources

Complex carbohydrates	Simple carbohydrates	Fibers
Fresh fruits and vegetables	Canned or dried fruits	Fresh, frozen, canned, or dried fruits
Canned or cooked vegetables	Cereals	Fresh, frozen, canned vegetables
Vegetable-based soups	Breakfast bars	Beans and lentils
Brown rice	Fruit tarts	Sprouts
Risotto	Honey and agave	Whole grain–based: cereals, pastas, breads, crackers
Potatoes	Snack pudding	Hot cereals: oatmeal and quinoa
Bean pastas	Barbeque sauce	
Whole grain–based: pizza crusts*, pastas, breads, crackers, cereals, bagels, pancakes*, and waffles*	Sherbet and sorbet	
English and bran muffins	Brownies	
Hot cereals: oatmeal and quinoa	Cakes*	
	Cookies*	
	Sports bars and drinks	
	Frozen yogurt	
	Energy gels and chews	

*Contains extra fats with food preparation . . . can be modified

drate foods like french fries or doughnuts will also help to prevent excessive gains in weight and body fat, poor energy levels, and upset stomachs especially when consumed prior to exercise. Table 5.1 shows some common sources of simple and complex carbohydrates and fiber.

Table 5.2 lists foods that are rich in carbohydrates. Additionally, please refer to online content in HK*Propel* to learn the formula for calculating total carbohydrate needs.

Topics for discussion include simple and complex carbohydrates, food sources, and calculation of carbohydrate needs.

Questions:

1. What is the difference between simple and complex carbohydrates?
2. What are the benefits of complex carbohydrates?
3. What are some of the drawbacks of simple carbohydrates?
4. List three food sources of both simple and complex carbohydrates.

Journal Prompts:

1. Calculate your recommended daily complex and simple carbohydrates.
2. How does your dietary intake compare with the guidelines?
3. What changes can you make to improve your intake of carbohydrates?
4. How do you think these changes will help improve the way you feel and your energy, weight, mood, and performance?

Protein

Protein is important for growth and development. It helps to build and repair muscles, contract and relax muscles, build ligaments and tendons that hold muscles and support bones altogether, and assist with exercise recovery by rebuilding muscle (anabolism) and preventing muscle breakdown

Table 5.2 Carbohydrate Amounts in Select Foods

Food	Serving size	Calories	Total carbohydrates (g)
Complex carbohydrates			
Garbanzo beans	1 cup	269	45
Navy beans	1 cup	259	28
Dates	Dried, 10	228	61
Raisins	1/2 cup	302	79
Sweet potato	1 large	118	28
Bagel	1 regular	165	31
Cereal	1 cup	110	24
Cornbread	1 square	178	28
English muffin	1	130	25
Noodles	1 cup	159	34
Pizza	Cheese, 1 slice	290	39
Pretzels	1 oz (26 mL)	106	21
Tortilla	Flour, 1	85	15
Apple	1 medium	81	21
Simple carbohydrates			
Chocolate milk	1 cup	208	26
Pudding	1/2 cup	161	30
Yogurt	Low fat, 1 cup	225	42
Applesauce	1 cup	232	60

(catabolism). Protein is also needed for building hormones such as insulin which regulates blood sugar and metabolism for the thyroid. Protein is also necessary to the immune system and for regulating digestion. While protein is not the primary fuel for athletic training, it is a crucial part of the support system.

In times of extreme need, protein also provides energy, especially when the total calorie expenditure is greater than the consumption or when the body is healing after injury. Competitive teen athletes may also need additional protein timed carefully throughout the day before and after workouts, especially when trying to build muscle mass during preseason or postseason. Failure to meet daily protein needs increases risk of weight loss and illness.

A complete protein comprises 20 amino acids, 11 of which our bodies produce. The remaining nine building blocks are referred to as essential amino acids because they make a protein whole, or complete. Animal-based food sources are complete proteins and include chicken, fish, turkey, red meat, pork, game, eggs, cheese, and milk. Very few plant-based foods are complete proteins, but they include quinoa, buckwheat, hempseed, blue-green algae, and soybeans. Other plant-based foods, such as vegetables, beans, legumes, whole grains, nuts, and the nondairy milks, cheeses, and yogurts, are incomplete sources of protein because they do not contain all of the essential amino acids found in animal-sourced foods. For vegetarians, getting enough protein and eating a variety of plant-based foods daily is critical for matching the amino acid profile of animal sources because plant-based complete proteins do not provide as much protein per serving as animal-sourced proteins. Vegetarian diets are further discussed later in the chapter. Table 5.3 lists protein-rich foods, and table 5.4, which follows, provides the amounts of protein in some foods.

The formula for calculating protein needs can be found in HK*Propel*.

Topics for discussion include proteins and their functions, essential amino acids, and ways to calculate protein needs.

Questions:

1. What are the differences between animal- and plant-based proteins?
2. List three health reasons for why you need to eat protein daily.
3. What are the most nutritious sources of protein, and why do you think some foods with protein are healthier than others?

Journal Prompts:

1. Calculate your recommended daily protein needs.
2. How does your dietary intake compare with the guidelines?
3. What kinds of changes can you make to improve your intake of protein?
4. How do you think these changes will improve the way you feel and your energy, weight, mood, performance, and risk of injury and illness?

Fats

Dietary fats are a dense energy source that fuels the body slowly and for long-duration exercises. Fats

Table 5.3 Protein-Rich Foods

Animal-based proteins	Plant-based complete proteins	Plant-based protein combinations that make complete proteins
Beef, pork	Quinoa	Beans and rice
Fish, shellfish, seafood	Buckwheat	Cereal with low-fat or soy milk
Turkey, chicken	Hempseed	Vegetable lasagna
Milk, cheese, yogurt	Blue-green algae	Tofu, vegetables, and rice
Eggs, egg whites	Soybeans	Macaroni and cheese
Sport shakes and bars		Peanut butter and jelly sandwich
		Hummus with carrots
		Mixed vegetables
		Tofu, tempeh

Table 5.4 Protein Amounts in Select Foods

Food	Serving size	Calories	Protein (g)
Ground beef, 85% lean	4 oz	243	21
Steak top round	4 oz	188	25
Skinless chicken breast	4 oz	110	26
Chicken drumsticks	4 oz	110	14
Ground turkey, 93% lean	4 oz	170	23
Canned tuna in water	4 oz	140	28
Alaskan wild salmon	3.5 oz	142	19.8
Eggs	2	140	12
Egg whites	4	69	14.4
Low-fat milk, 1%	8 oz	110	8
Peanut butter	2 tbsp	180	7
Tofu	5 oz	70	7

transport the fat-soluble vitamins A, E, D, and K essential for muscle development and immunity to red blood cells and bones. Fats also provide essential fatty acids, the omega-3s and omega-6s required for brain function, healthy skin, normal blood pressure, and blood clotting.

Fats are a concentrated energy source that provide twice as many calories (nine calories a gram) as proteins or carbohydrates (four calories per gram). In excess consumption, fats are apt to be stored as body fat faster than carbohydrates and protein, leading to extra unnecessary weight and undesirable changes in body composition. The minimal amount of fat required to perform body functions is actually only three to six grams (27 to 54 calories fat) per day; however, with energy expenditure, the daily amount recommended is higher and can be calculated in the activity for this section.

Fats are especially essential for teen athletes as a source of long-term energy use, the stored form of calories when the body runs out of carbohydrates and protein. This is especially true for leaner athletes who burn a lot more calories or in preseason when training can boost the calorie needs to double or more. The two major dietary fat groups are *unsaturated* and *saturated* fats.

Monounsaturated and polyunsaturated fats comprise the unsaturated fats group. Both types of fats are liquid at room temperature and heart healthy. The difference between these fats is a chemical one, as it is the structure of the fats—mono containing only 1 carbon bond "mono" in its molecule while polyunsaturated has more than one "poly" carbon bond in its structure.

Polyunsaturated include the essential omega-3s found in salmon, flax, soy, and walnuts and the omega-6s found in whole grains and vegetables. Both contain the same amount of fat as saturated fat, 9 calories per gram.

Saturated fats look hard at room temperature, the kind you find in marbled meat, bacon, cheese, ice cream, cakes, and pastries. These fats have been shown to increase inflammation; blood cholesterol to unhealthy levels for some individuals; and the risks for diabetes, obesity, high blood pressure, and compromised performance. *Trans fats*, those found in processed foods like some types of crackers, cookies, and margarines, are also saturated and can compromise performance and overall health. Table 5.5 shows common sources of saturated, monounsaturated, polyunsaturated, and trans fats.

The dietary recommendation for fat is 20 to 35 percent of total calories, depending on weight and calorie needs and goals and a nutritional periodization plan for athletes' performance.

The recommendation for saturated fats is less than or equal to 10 percent of total calories and less than or equal to 1 percent for trans fats for overall health. Some of the healthiest fats from food are fish such as salmon, sardines, and tuna; olives and olive oils; and nuts such as almonds, walnuts, pistachios, and peanuts. HK*Propel* provides the formula for calculating the amount of daily total fat and saturated fat needed. The menu provided at the end of the chapter highlights the healthiest fat options.

Table 5.5 Sources of Saturated, Unsaturated, and Trans Fats

Saturated fats	Monounsaturated fats	Polyunsaturated fats	Trans fats
Palm oil	Olive oil	Safflower oil	Cookies
Animal fats	Canola oil	Soybean oil	Crackers
Coconut oil	Sunflower oil	Corn oil	Chips
Lard	Peanuts, peanut oil	Sunflower oil	Fast food
Palm kernel oil	Avocados	Fish oil	Hydrogenated fats in food
Animal fats	Cashews	Almonds	Margarine
Cream	Poultry	Cottonseed oil	
Whole milk		Fish such as salmon and tuna	
Shortening		Walnuts	
Cocoa butter		Mayonnaise	
Hydrogenated oils			
Cheese			

Topics for discussion include saturated, unsaturated and trans fats, and the functions of fat.

Questions:

1. What is the difference between saturated, unsaturated, and trans fats?
2. List three health reasons for why you need to eat fat daily.
3. Which sources of fat are the most nutritious?

Journal Prompts:

1. Calculate your recommended daily fat and saturated fat needs.
2. How does your dietary intake compare with the guidelines?
3. What changes can you make to improve or limit your intake of dietary fats?
4. How do you think these changes will improve the way you feel and your energy, weight, mood, and performance?

Micronutrients: Vitamins and Minerals

Micronutrients are essential nutrients for overall health, assisting in such basic health factors as immune function, energy production, and blood clotting. They are needed in much smaller amounts than macronutrients, and they do not have calories. Both vitamins and minerals are important micronutrients.

There are about 40 vitamins and minerals that the body needs daily to perform all healthy body functions. Those most commonly seen in deficiency states are vitamins A, C, D, and the minerals potassium, magnesium, and calcium. These vitamins and minerals affect health and performance in numerous ways. While nutrition surveys of teens appear to suggest that vitamin and mineral needs can most likely be met through diet, deficiencies are consistent for most teens, especially those in high school with imbalanced diets.

Diets lacking in vitamins and minerals can negatively affect energy levels, recovery, inflammation, bone strength, and muscle contraction. Electrolyte deficiencies such as potassium, magnesium, and calcium can cause cramping and muscle spasms. The best way to meet the vitamin and mineral guidelines is eating whole foods. The sample menus at the end of the chapter provide a route to meeting the needs, but no one eats perfectly. In this case, a daily vitamin supplement or fortified shake or bar can help teens meet the daily vitamin and mineral needs. Safe supplementation guidelines are offered later in the chapter. In the meantime, selecting a wide variety of foods from all the food groups enables teens to get closer to reaching the goals. Table 5.6 shows the function of select vitamins, signs of their deficiency, and foods that are rich in each vitamin; table 5.7 shows the same information for minerals.

Table 5.6 Key Vitamins

Vitamin	Functions	Signs of deficiency	Major food sources
A (retinol)	Supports vision, skin, bone and tooth growth, immunity, wound healing, and reproduction	Night blindness, dry eyes, poor bone growth, impaired resistance to infection, skin issues	Deep yellow and green vegetables, mangoes, broccoli, butternut squash, carrots, tomato juice, sweet potatoes, pumpkin, beef liver, egg yolks
B_1 (thiamin)	Essential for growth, normal appetite, digestion, and nerves; supports energy metabolism—carbs, protein, fats	Edema (swelling), heart failure, numbness, and nerve pain	Whole grains and enriched foods, legumes, potatoes, lean pork, wheat germ
B_2 (riboflavin)	Supports energy metabolism, growth	Light sensitivity, cracks and sores around the mouth and nose	Fortified grains, breads, and cereals; dark green vegetables, legumes, egg yolks, milk, liver, oysters, clams
B_3 (niacin)	Supports energy metabolism, skin health, nervous and digestive systems	Dermatitis, depression, dementia	Egg yolks, meat, fish, poultry, enriched and whole-grain breads, fortified cereals
B_6	Amino acid and fatty acid metabolism, red blood cell production	Anemia, irritability, convulsions	Legumes, potatoes, whole-grain breads and cereals, liver, meat
Folacin (folate)	Important for heart health and cell development; prevents birth defects	Poor growth, anemia, impaired immunity	Legumes, dark green leafy vegetables, oranges, cantaloupes, enriched whole-grain breads, fortified cereals, lean beef
B_{12}	Helps body make red blood cells, works with folate and central nervous system metabolism	Anemia, neurologic deterioration	Meats, poultry, fish, shellfish, milk, eggs; fortified milk and dairy products, cereals, and whole grains
Biotin	Energy storage and protein, carbohydrate, and fat metabolism	Rare	Avocados, cauliflower, eggs, raspberries, liver, pork, salmon, whole grains
C (ascorbic acid)	Collagen synthesis, amino acid metabolism, iron absorption, immunity, antioxidant	Scurvy, hemorrhages in skin, diarrhea, bleeding gums, easy bruising	Spinach, broccoli, red bell peppers, citrus fruits such as oranges, papaya, strawberries, potatoes, cabbage
D	Promotes bone mineralization, muscle growth and strength, builds immune system	Soft bones, bowlegs, weak immune system	Self-synthesis via sunlight, fortified milk products, egg yolks, liver, fatty fish
E	Antioxidant, regulation of oxidation reactions, supports cell membranes	Anemia, retina degeneration	Egg yolks, fortified cereals, nuts and nut butters, plant oils (soybean, corn, and canola oils), dark green leafy vegetables, wheat germ, sunflower seeds
K	Synthesis of blood-clotting proteins, synthesized by intestinal bacteria	Defective blood coagulation	Dark green leafy vegetables, pork, liver, vegetable oils

Sources:
https://www.accessdata.fda.gov/scripts/InteractiveNutritionFactsLabel/assets/InteractiveNFL_Vitamins&MineralsChart_March2020.pdf
https://wicworks.fns.usda.gov/wicworks/Topics/FG/AppendixC_NutrientChart.pdf

Table 5.7 Key Minerals

Mineral	Functions	Signs of deficiency	Major food sources
Sodium	Maintains fluid and electrolyte balance, supports muscle contraction and nerve impulse transmissions	Nausea, cramps, vomiting, exhaustion, dizziness, apathy	Sodium chloride (table salt), foods with added salt, processed foods, salted snack foods like chips and fast food
Chloride	Maintains fluid and electrolyte balance, aids in digestion	Usually accompanied with sodium depletion	Sodium chloride (table salt)
Potassium	Maintains fluid and electrolyte balance, cell integrity, muscle contractions, and nerve impulse transmission; controls blood pressure	Nausea, anorexia, muscle weakness, irritability, cardiac arrhythmias	Potatoes, bananas, yogurt, milk, meat, fish, poultry, soy products, vegetables
Calcium	Formation of bones and teeth, supports blood clotting	Rickets in children; osteomalacia (soft bones), and osteoporosis in adults	Milk, yogurt, hard cheeses, fortified cereals, kale, dark green leafy vegetables, tofu (if made with calcium sulfate), sardines, salmon
Phosphorus	Helps with energy production, normal cell activity, and bone growth	Muscle weakness, decreased intestinal tone and distension, cardiac arrhythmias	Milk and dairy products, peas, meat, egg yolks, whole-grain breads, cereals, and other whole-grain products
Magnesium	Helps with heart rhythm, muscle and nerve function, bone strength	Nausea, irritability, muscle weakness, twitching, cramps, cardiac arrhythmias	Dark green leafy vegetables, nuts, dairy products, beans, potatoes, tofu, whole grains, and quinoa
Iron	Needed for red blood cells and many enzymes	Skin pallor, weakness, fatigue, headaches	Fortified cereals, beans and legumes, beef, turkey (dark meat), liver, soybeans, and dark green leafy vegetables
Zinc	A part of many enzymes, involved in production of genetic material and proteins, transports vitamin A; helps with taste perception, wound healing, sperm production, and normal development of the fetus	Slow healing of wounds, loss of taste, retarded growth	Egg yolks, oysters and other seafood, whole-grain breads and cereals, legumes
Selenium	Antioxidant that protects cells from damage and helps manage thyroid hormone	Muscle tenderness and pain, cardiac, and red blood cell issues	Whole-grain breads, cereals, other fortified products, onions, meats, seafood, and vegetables
Iodine	Helps produce thyroid hormones that help regulate growth, development, and metabolic rate	Depressed thyroid function	Iodized salt, dairy products, seaweed, seafood
Copper	Necessary for the absorption and utilization of iron, supports formation of hemoglobin and several enzymes	Slow growth, anorexia, edema	Liver, kidney, poultry, shellfish, whole grains
Choline	Brain development, cell signaling, lipid (fat) transport and metabolism, liver function, muscle movement, nerve function, normal metabolism	Rare, but can cause muscle damage, liver damage, and nonalcoholic fatty liver disease	Beans and peas, egg yolks, fish, liver, beef, chicken, milk, nuts, salmon, soy foods, broccoli, cauliflower, spinach
Fluoride	Helps with formation of bones and teeth and resistance to tooth decay	Increased dental caries	Fluoridated water

Mineral	Functions	Signs of deficiency	Major food sources
Chromium	Helps control blood sugar associated with insulin, required for the release of energy from glucose	Impaired glucose tolerance and growth, numbness in extremities	Meat, whole-grain breads, fortified grains, brewer's yeast, corn oil
Molybdenum	Produces enzymes	Unknown	Organ meats, breads, cereals, dark green leafy vegetables, legumes

Sources:

https://www.accessdata.fda.gov/scripts/InteractiveNutritionFactsLabel/assets/InteractiveNFL_Vitamins&MineralsChart_March2020.pdf

https://wicworks.fns.usda.gov/wicworks/Topics/FG/AppendixC_NutrientChart.pdf

Topics for discussion include vitamins and minerals and their functions and food sources.

Questions:

1. Why are vitamins and minerals considered essential nutrients?
2. How much of each selected vitamin and mineral is recommended daily?
3. Provide three food sources for five selected vitamins and minerals.

Journal Prompts:

1. How do you believe you are meeting or not meeting your vitamin and mineral needs each day?
2. What foods or food groups are missing from your diet that can provide these nutrients?
3. Which signs of deficiency are you experiencing that lead you to believe you are missing specific vitamins and minerals?

Water

Water is an essential nutrient. Adequate hydration from fluids is critical for health, performance, and life. Fluids help to maintain blood volume, which in turn supplies blood to the skin for body temperature regulation. Fluid needs can vary greatly due to body size, physical activity, and environmental conditions. Environmental conditions have a large effect on regulating core body temperatures. Humidity also affects the body's ability to drive away heat to an even greater extent than air temperatures alone. As humidity increases, the rate at which sweat evaporates decreases, meaning more sweat drips off the body without transferring heat from the body to the environment.

Because exercise produces heat, which must be eliminated from the body to maintain appropriate temperatures, fluids are even more essential when exercising. Imbalance between fluid intake and fluid loss during prolonged exercise may increase the risk for dehydration, which increases the risk of hyperthermia, heat exhaustion, and heat stroke. Combining the effects of a hot, humid environment with a large exercise heat load produced during exercise taxes the body to its maximum.

Ensuring proper and adequate fluid intake is key to reducing the risk of heat stress, especially in environments with high temperatures and humidity. A fluid loss of just 1 to 2 percent of total body weight can affect performance. With a 2.5-percent body-weight loss, the blood becomes thicker and loses volume, the heart works harder, and blood circulation of oxygen becomes less efficient, affecting overall health. The general fluid recommendations are 3.7 liters per day (130 ounces per day, or 16 cups of fluid per day) for males and 2.7 liters per day (95 ounces per day, or approximately 12 cups per day) for females.

Athlete Hydration

Despite the evidence that dehydration is detrimental for all teens, *especially teen athletes*, there is no general agreement on how much or which types of fluids are needed, nor the conditions under which additional fluids are needed. One study on endurance athletes suggests that mild dehydration during workouts of one hour or less does not affect performance (Perreault-Briere et al., 2019). However, other studies have shown that two percent or more weight loss either before or after hour-long exercise negatively affects performance (Casa, 2019). Three percent fluid loss in a 130-pound (59 kg) person equates to a fluid loss of four pounds at minimum.

Athletes need to rehydrate on a timed basis rather than drink to thirst because thirst perception appears to alter during exercise (Armstrong et al., 2014). When possible, fluids should be consumed at a rate that closely matches sweating rate. One way to measure sweat rate is outlined in HK*Propel*. Fluid intake should be enough to maintain pre-exercise weight. Depending on the amount, duration, and intensity, plain water may not be the best beverage to consume following exercise, as large amounts of electrolytes may have also been lost in sweat and need to be replaced. Approximately 20 percent of daily water needs can be met by water found in fruits and vegetables. The remaining 80 percent should come from beverages such as water, juice, milk and milk alternatives, soup, sports drinks, and shakes.

Fluids, Electrolytes, and Sugars

Electrolytes are minerals involved in the movement of water in and out of cells and in nerve and muscle transmission. Both electrolytes and water are lost through sweat. Electrolyte depletion during exercise can be even more serious and detrimental to performance than dehydration itself. Electrolyte depletion can cause leg cramps or painful contractions in the gut, and it can also cause the misfiring of information between the stomach and the brain and from the muscles to the kidneys. Athletes who must wear heavy gear and train two to three times a day in preseason are especially prone to electrolytes depletion.

For teen athletes who lose heavy amounts of sodium, a component of salt, during high rates of sweating, the replacement of electrolytes—primarily sodium in addition to water—is essential for complete rehydration. Rehydration with water alone potentially increases blood volume but dilutes the contents of blood while also stimulating urine output. Blood dilution lowers both sodium and the volume-dependent part of the thirst drive, removing much of the drive to drink and replace fluid losses. For training or competing in events lasting more than two hours, electrolytes (sodium and potassium) should be added to fluids to replace losses and to prevent hyponatremia, or low sodium levels in the blood. An easy way to accomplish this is to lightly salt foods at mealtime or consume sports drinks.

Active teens who live in a warm environment are reported to have daily water needs of approximately six liters, and serious athletes may even have markedly higher needs of more than 10 liters per day. Exercise hydration guidelines set by the American College of Sports Medicine (ACSM), the National Athletic Trainers Association (NATA), the American Academy of Pediatrics (AAP), Australian Institute of Sports (AIS), the Academy of Nutrition and Dietetics (AND), the Dietitians of Canada, the International Olympic Committee (IOC), International Marathon Directors Association (IMDA), the Inter-Association Task Force on External Heat Illnesses, and USA Track and Field (USA T&F) are as follows:

- Before exercise: Drink 14 to 22 ounces of water or sports drink (approximately 17 ounces) two to three hours before the start of exercise.
- During exercise: Drink 6 to 12 ounces of fluid every 15 to 20 minutes, depending on exercise intensity, environmental conditions, and tolerance. Drink about one cup (8 to 10 ounces) every 15 to 20 minutes, although individualized needs vary.
- After exercise, consume as follows:
    - Twenty-five to 50 percent more than existing weight loss to ensure hydration, four to six hours after exercise.
    - Sixteen to 24 ounces of fluid for every pound of body weight lost during exercise.
    - When participating in multiple workouts in one day, 80 percent of fluid replacement is advised prior to the next workout.

Topics for discussion include fluids, heat illness, electrolytes, and fluid recommendations for exercise.

Questions:

1. Why is water considered an essential nutrient?
2. How much water is recommended daily? What are sources of water and fluids in the diet?
3. What are electrolytes? Why are electrolytes important for staying hydrated?
4. What are the symptoms of heat illness?
5. What are fluid recommendations for before, during, and after exercise training?
6. If a teen athlete loses two pounds of fluid between pre- and post-training, how many ounces of fluid should the athlete replace for the next exercise session?

Journal Prompts:

1. Describe how you would know if you are experiencing heat illness. Describe a real (or imagined) situation in which you encountered heat illness by neglecting to drink enough water and fluids.
2. How much fluid do you lose when exercising? Use the formula provided or calculate your daily fluid loss with the Gatorade Sports Science Institute tool: https://www.gssiweb.org/toolbox/fluidLoss/calculator

3. How do you meet your daily water and fluid recommendations? What are some ways you can improve your fluid intake through healthier beverage and food choices?

SPECIAL DIET CONCERNS

In considering their nutrition choices, teens should be aware of considerations related to consumption of dairy products, foods that contain gluten, and vegetarian diets.

Dairy and Skin Health

Dairy products can provide important nutrients, but they also can potentially present challenges for some people. For teens, dairy has been associated with severity of acne, which affects more than 17 million Americans. The appearance of acne peaks during adolescence, affecting 80 to 90 percent of U.S. teens, and is moderate to severe in about 15 to 20 percent of those affected (Stang & Larson, 2020; Juhl et al., 2018). Acne can have a significantly negative impact on a teen's quality of life, potentially leading to social withdrawal, anxiety, and even depression (Ferdowsian & Levin, 2010).

Diet appears to influence and aggravate the development of acne. The role of dairy products and high-glycemic-index foods in influencing hormonal and inflammatory factors has been shown to increase acne prevalence, severity, and duration. The glycemic index (GI) is a measure of the relative potential of food to raise glucose levels in blood as compared to equal amounts of carbohydrates within the food. It gives a sense of the quality of the carbohydrates present in food by reflecting the rate of carbohydrate absorption. Glycemic load (GL) is a food's potentiality to increase blood glucose as well as insulin and accounts for the glycemic index of a food quality and the amount of food consumed (Mahmood & Bowe, 2014).

Several studies suggest young adults with moderate to severe acne compared with those with milder forms have diets containing a higher glycemic index with more added and total sugars, milk servings, and saturated and trans fats (Stang & Larson, 2020). Studies have been inconclusive regarding the association between acne and other foods. There is little evidence to suggest a correlation between the intake of chocolate or salt and acne severity.

The Western diet includes many dairy sources that contain hormones. In a meta-analysis of 78,529 children, adolescents, and young adults globally, any dairy, such as milk, yogurt, and cheese, was associated with an increased prevalence of moderate to severe acne in 13.9 percent of people ages 7 to 30 years (Juhl et al., 2018). A higher, full-fat dairy consumption of more than two glasses daily was associated with moderate to severe cases (Ulvestad, Bjertness, Dalgard, & Halvorsen, 2017). A review of 26 studies suggests cow's milk intake appeared to increase acne prevalence and severity. The relationship between milk and acne severity may be due to the presence in dairy of normal reproductive steroid hormones or the enhanced production of other hormones such as IGF-1, which can increase androgen exposure, and acne risk (Juhl et al., 2018).

Dairy Sensitivity and Allergy

According to the NIH, about 65 percent of the U.S. population is lactose intolerant. In athletes, one study reported 86.5 percent of athletes felt better after the removal of lactose in their diets (Lis et al., 2016). Lactose intolerance suggests a lactase deficiency. Lactase is the enzyme responsible for breaking down lactose, the sugar that is found in milk and dairy products. Lactose intolerance is different than a milk allergy, which is an immune response to the protein in milk. When people with lactose intolerance eat foods with lactose, they may experience gas, bloating, abdominal pain, nausea, and diarrhea. Individuals may have varying levels of intolerance. Some experience symptoms from a very small amount of dairy while others can eat a cheese pizza or frozen yogurt and avoid symptoms.

For lactose-sensitive teens, consuming 10 or fewer grams of lactose per day is recommended, ideally spread throughout the day. Table 5.8 shows the amount of lactose in select foods. If symptoms progress, a complete lactose elimination may be necessary. There are many obvious foods, milk and ice cream for example, that include lactose, but other no-so-obvious foods, such as margarine, bread, and hot dogs, can also contain small amounts of lactose.

Eliminating dairy from the diet may leave some teens challenged with meeting ample dietary protein and calcium needs, although there is an abundance of alternatives to dairy on the market, such as soy, rice, almond, oat, flax, and hemp milks, all of which can be fortified with calcium (though it's important to check the nutrition label to be sure). Lactose-intolerant teens who need extra protein should avoid milk-, whey-, and casein-based protein powders, shakes, and bars and instead, opt for whey isolate in products, which has nearly no lactose. There are also many plant-based

Table 5.8 Lactose Content of Selected Foods

Food	Portion	Lactose amount (g)
Milk	1 cup	11
Butter, margarine	1 tsp	Trace amount
American cheese	1 oz	1
Sharp cheddar cheese	1 oz	0.4-0.6
Parmesan cheese, grated	1 oz	1
Swiss cheese	1 oz	1
Mozzarella cheese	1 oz	0.8-0.9
Cream cheese	1 oz	1
Ice cream	1/2 cup	6
Sour cream	1/2 cup	4
Yogurt, low fat	1 cup	5

proteins-shake powders and ready-to-drink shakes for athletes looking for a milk-like protein boost.

For lactose-intolerant teens who want to eat dairy without experiencing gas or cramping, over-the-counter lactose digestive aids are widely available at pharmacies and grocery stores. Additionally, some milk products, such as Lactaid, already include the enzyme.

GLUTEN INTOLERANCE AND SENSITIVITY

Gluten is a protein found in wheat products, such as pasta, cereals, crackers, cookies, and cakes. It can also be found in foods with small amounts of wheat, such as marinades, cheese sauces, vitamins, and chips. Avoiding bread and products with gluten has been a growing trend over the past several years. Some people follow gluten-free diets incorrectly thinking gluten causes extra weight gain and calories. The truth of the matter is gluten does not cause extra weight gain, but it can affect people who have celiac disease.

Celiac disease is a serious autoimmune disease in which people have an immune response to the wheat protein gluten, which attacks the small intestine (Singh et al., 2018). Celiac disease affects 1.4 percent of the global population. In Europe, the United States, and Australia, prevalence estimates range from 1:80 to 1:300 children (Frühauf, Nabil El-Lababidi, & Szitányi, 2018). Non-celiac gluten sensitivity (NCGS) and non-celiac wheat sensitivity (NCWS) share similar symptoms with celiac disease, and the Celiac Disease Foundation estimates that those who are affected by gluten sensitivity prevalence is equal to or even exceeds those with celiac disease.

Hereditary factors cause celiac disease, which can be triggered by stress, surgery, or infection. According to the Celiac Disease Foundation, people with celiac disease are two times more likely to develop coronary artery disease and four times more likely to develop small bowel cancers than people without celiac disease (Celiac Disease Foundation, n.d.).

Non-celiac gluten sensitivity is diagnosed in people who do not have celiac disease or wheat allergy. People with non-celiac gluten sensitivity experience general gastrointestinal symptoms or physical symptoms after eating gluten such as bloating, gas, diarrhea, headache, lethargy, and joint pain. Removing gluten-containing foods from the diet helps prevent symptoms. Some research suggests up to 41 percent of U.S. athletes adhere to a gluten-free diet with the belief that it will and does reduce gastrointestinal discomfort experienced during exercise (Lis, 2019). Another study found that 41 percent of the 910 athletes, including 18 world and Olympic medalists, follow a gluten-free diet 50 to 100 percent of the time, despite only 13 percent choosing so for medical reasons. Fifty-seven percent of these athletes self-diagnosed their gluten sensitivity (Lis et al., 2015).

Teens who have symptoms of bloating after eating meals containing gluten can learn more about foods, food products, and other edibles, such as supplements and medications that may contain gluten or are at risk for cross-contamination with gluten. Information can be found at The Gluten Intolerance Group, www.gluten.org/category/getting-started/.

VEGETARIAN DIETS

Eating a plant-based diet has become a growing trend, especially among teens with health, ethical, moral, and religious reasons. Vegetarian diets emphasizing plant foods have been shown to have a positive impact on long-term health, weight, body composition, and risk factors for chronic disease. Being a vegetarian means following a diet rich in non-animal-based foods such as vegetables, fruits, grains, nuts, and seeds. Vegetarianism involves a wide spectrum of people, from vegans who refrain from all animal products to flexitarians, who eat fish, chicken, and meat on occasion. Table 5.9 describes types of vegetarian diets, from most restrictive (fruitarian) to most inclusive (flexitarian), along with potential concerns related to each.

Vegetarian teens eating a well-balanced diet can be assured of getting generous amounts of vitamins, minerals, phytonutrients, healthy fats, and protein. However, like any diet, animal based or not, those who eat poorly are at risk for deficiencies in iron, calcium, zinc, vitamins D and B_{12}, essential fats, and amino acids and excesses of compounds such as fiber, which can bind essential nutrients and decrease absorption.

While vegetarian diets can provide enough calories to meet daily needs, for teens, it can be challenging getting enough variety for optimal growth and health due to plant-based foods often being lower in calories and higher in fiber. Another concern are the unhealthy but often popular options among teens that are considered vegetarian—french fries, chips, soda, and the like. One way to overcome either challenge is by including nutrient-dense vegetarian foods whenever possible.

Nutrient-dense vegetarian meals and snacks include

- nuts, nut butters, seeds, and oils;
- soy-based meat alternatives (tofu and tempeh);
- almond, hemp, and soy milks;
- textured vegetable proteins;
- fruit juices and smoothies;
- salad toppings such as avocados, soy cheese, and nutritional yeast; and
- bean and hummus dips with baked tortilla chips.

Another strategy for meeting calorie needs is to prepare multiple small meals instead of the more traditional three larger meals. To make planning vegetarian diets higher in protein easier, some companies offer vegetarian protein alternatives now more commonly found in grocery stores, such as plant-based "meats:" vegetarian burgers, meatballs, chicken strips, cheeses, milks, yogurts, and toppings for salads or snacks. The downside to many of these alternatives, however, is they are highly processed foods, reducing their nutritional value compared to other less-processed vegetarian and whole foods. A sample of a vegetarian menu can be found at the end of the chapter.

As previously mentioned, plant-based diets can present vegetarians with challenges for getting enough of certain vitamins and minerals. The following section identifies those vitamins and minerals.

- *Iron.* The daily recommended amount of iron for vegetarians can be up to 1.8 times the RDAs because of low bioavailability. While iron can be found in both meat- and plant-based foods,

Table 5.9 Types of Vegetarian Diets

Type	Food specifics	Potential nutrition deficiencies
Fruitarian	Most restrictive: raw and dried fruits, seeds, honey, and oil only	A wide range of vitamins, minerals, protein, and essential fatty acids
Vegan	Very restrictive: excludes all products derived from animal sources, including dairy and eggs (exclusively plant-based)	Vitamins B_{12} and D, zinc, calcium, omega-3s, and essential amino acids
Lacto-vegetarian	Restrictive: includes milk and other dairy products derived from animal sources	Omega-3s, protein, and iron
Lacto-ovo-vegetarian	Less restrictive: includes dairy products and eggs derived from animal sources	Omega-3s and iron
Pesco-vegetarian	Inclusive: includes fish	Typically meets nutrient needs with a well-balanced diet
Flexitarian	Most inclusive: typically excludes red meat but on occasion includes other animal products	Typically meets nutrient needs with a well-balanced diet

the form found in plants, called non-heme iron, has lower absorption rates than heme iron from animal sources. Vegans usually get more iron than lacto-based vegetarians since dairy is a poor iron source. Some compounds, such as phytates, that are found in soy and tea can inhibit the absorption of iron, while consuming fruits and vegetables rich in vitamin C with iron can enhance absorption. Vegetarians can get enough iron through their diet by including beans, fortified cereals, greens, and dried fruits on a regular basis.

- *Zinc.* This mineral has been shown to be lower in vegetarian athletes since about 50 to 70 percent of zinc typically comes from meat and dairy products. Zinc is essential for protein synthesis, immune function, and blood formation. The recommended daily amount is 11 milligrams. Zinc bioavailability is an additional challenge for vegetarians because high amounts of phytate, a plant compound, may act as an inhibitor to absorption. Plant-based sources of zinc include beans, grains, and seeds. Soaking dried beans, grains, and seeds in water before cooking can help increase the bioavailability of zinc, as will eating zinc-rich meals with foods rich in vitamin C such as citrus fruits and bell peppers.
- *Calcium.* Some research suggests that vegetarians may have lower calcium needs than those eating a diet high in animal protein and sodium because vegetarians excrete less calcium; however, this isn't entirely clear (Rogerson, 2017). For vegetarians and vegans, calcium can be found in fortified dairy alternatives like soy, rice, and almond milks, cheeses, and yogurts; tofu; some fortified juices and shakes; and greens. Compounds such as oxalates in spinach and phytates found in grains might hinder calcium absorption.
- *B_{12}.* Strict vegans may be at greater risk than other vegetarian types for B_{12} deficiency. Vitamin B_{12} is naturally found only in animal products, but there are also some foods fortified with it. B_{12} is an important coenzyme required for the normal metabolism of protein, carbohydrates, and fats. The daily requirement is 2.4 micrograms (mcg). For vegans, vitamin B_{12} can be found in fortified cereals, bars and shakes, rice and soymilk beverages, and nutritional yeast.

Table 5.10 shows good vegetarian sources of select vitamins and minerals.

Topics for discussion include acne, lactose intolerance, gluten and celiac diseases, and vegetarian diets.

Questions:

1. What are some of the foods that may cause acne? Which food substitutions can you select to improve your skin?
2. What is lactose intolerance? How might you suspect if you are lactose intolerant? Which foods should be limited with lactose intolerance?
3. What is gluten intolerance? How might you suspect if you are gluten intolerant? Which foods should be limited with gluten intolerance?
4. What is a vegetarian diet? What are the types of vegetarian diets? What are the benefits or drawbacks of a vegetarian diet?

Journal Prompts:

1. Do you or someone you know have acne? Lactose or gluten intolerance?
2. For each condition, outline three recommendations you can make to possibly help people to improve or manage their condition.

Table 5.10 Vegetarian Sources of Select Vitamins and Minerals

Vitamin or mineral	Sources
Zinc	Legumes, whole grains, nuts, seeds, soy, dairy, and fortified shakes and bars
Iron	Legumes, fortified grains, beans, soy, nuts, dried fruits, dark green leafy vegetables, and fortified shakes and bars
Vitamin B_{12}	Dairy; eggs; and fortified soy, grains, sports bars, and drinks
Vitamin D	Dairy; eggs; and fortified soy, grains, sports bars, and drinks
Riboflavin (vitamin B_2)	Dairy; fortified soy milk, yogurt, and cheese; fortified grains; and texturized vegetable protein
Calcium	Dairy; fortified soy milk, tofu, and yogurt; cereal; low oxalate vegetables such as broccoli, bok choy, and kale; tahini; almonds; calcium-fortified orange juice; blackstrap molasses; and texturized vegetable protein

3. If you or someone you know were thinking about becoming a vegetarian, summarize the benefits and concerns and provide a one day recommended menu example of a nutritious vegetarian diet.

SUPPLEMENTS AND STEROIDS

The best way to meet dietary needs for vitamins and minerals is by eating whole foods, which, in most cases, eliminates the need for additional supplements, such as vitamins, minerals, enzymes, and many other ingredients that would need to be added to the diet. According to the Academy of Nutrition and Dietetics (AND) Position Paper-Nutrient Supplementation, 2009,

> The best nutrition-based strategy for promoting optimal health and the risk of chronic disease is to choose a variety of nutrient-rich foods. Additional nutrients from supplements can help some people meet their nutritional needs as specified by science-based standards such as the Dietary Reference Intakes (DRIs). (Marra & Bailey, 2018)

The United States Department of Agriculture (USDA) Food and Nutrition Information Center has a free interactive tool to calculate daily nutrient recommendations for dietary planning based on the DRIs. According to the website, the tool is based on the most current scientific knowledge on nutrient needs, developed by the National Academy of Science's Institute of Medicine, although, depending on personal health, activity, and dietary factors, individual requirements may be higher or lower than the DRIs. The link to this interactive tool is www.nal.usda.gov/fnic/dri-calculator/.

After visiting the site to determine your daily needs, you can track your dietary intake and determine the amounts of vitamins and minerals you get through your diet before considering supplementation. To track intake, keep a dietary log and have a nutrition expert perform a dietary analysis to determine how much you are getting and how much is missing through the food you eat. You can also analyze it for free online. If you do come up short on one or more of the vitamins and minerals, check tables 5.6 and 5.7 to see if you are experiencing symptoms associated with deficiency in that vitamin, mineral, or nutrient. Making an informed decision about taking supplements can save you money. It can also help you avoid the potential risks of consuming products with either too little or too much, or products tainted with ingredients like amphetamines, steroids, or toxic metals like lead that may be harmful to health.

Teens who may benefit from a supplement due to risk for dietary deficiencies include the following situations:

- Teens with medical issues such as iron or vitamin D deficiencies
- Vegetarians, vegans, or athletes who are on restrictive diets with allergies, food sensitivities, or personal aversions where whole food groups are eliminated or avoided, such as dairy, whole grains, and vegetables
- Teens with eating disorders or who are undernourished due to low-calorie dieting or those trying to make weight for sport (e.g., jockeys, wrestlers, rowers, and boxers and athletes who take prescription medications or have spinal cord injury)

The Taylor Hooton Foundation (n.d.) estimates that 7 percent of U.S. high school students, or roughly 1.5 million teens, take steroids. Of the 1.4 percent of NCAA athletes who admit to using, about 42 percent say they started in high school, while 15 percent report using in middle school or before. This is probably due to the pressure of growing larger and faster, without having to train hard or eat well and wait for the body to go through the natural puberty growth cycle. Teenage girls are the fastest growing users, with 62 percent reporting they do it to improve their looks.

Originally designed for clinical use for healing from injury, nontherapeutic usage is increasing among adolescents. Anabolic effects include increases in muscle mass, bone mineral density, and blood cell production and a decrease in body fat. These effects may sound appealing to adolescents, but there is a price to be paid for such quick development that goes beyond a positive drug test: Increased heart, liver, and kidney sizes; vocal cord changes; and psychiatric symptoms including aggression, violence, mania, psychosis, and suicide also come with the package. Additional side effects are as follows:

- *Skin.* Acne and cysts, oily scalp
- *Hormonal.* Disturbance in endocrine and immune function
- *Physical.* Short stature, tendon rupture
- *Children.* Premature closing of growth plates
- *Males.* Increased sex drive, acne, enlarged breasts, testicular hypotrophy, infertility
- *Females.* Male-type body hair (mustache, beard), male baldness pattern, deepened voice,

breast shrinkage, abnormal menstrual cycles, enlarged clitoris

- *Metabolic.* Changes in hemostatic system and urogenital tract, altered glucose metabolism, immune system suppression, low thyroid hormone levels
- *Heart.* Increased blood pressure, reduction of the "good" cholesterol called HDLs
- *Liver system.* Cancer, peliosis (purpura), hepatitis, increased liver enzymes, jaundice
- *Mental health.* Increase in aggressive behavior, mood disturbances (e.g., depression, hypomania, psychosis, homicidal rage, mania, delusions)
- *Infection.* HIV-AIDS, hepatitis from injectable
- Source: Taylor Hooton Foundation at https://taylorhooton.org/anabolic-steroids/

Topics for discussion include supplements and the pros and cons of supplementation, dietary deficiencies and requirements, and the risks associated with steroid usage.

Questions:

1. What are some ways to determine if you need a dietary supplement?
2. Who might be at risk for dietary deficiency and may benefit from supplements?
3. What are the health risks of taking steroids?
4. What steps can you take to assess your dietary needs for vitamins and minerals and determine which foods you need to include to eliminate deficiencies in your diet?

Journal Prompts:

1. What leads you to believe you need to take a supplement?
2. What information did you use to determine whether you need a dietary supplement?
3. Which vitamin and mineral deficiencies do you believe you have on a regular basis? Which factors are sabotaging your efforts to include the foods you need with the nutrients you are missing? Preference? Allergies? Medical conditions?
4. What can you eat or drink to obtain the missing vitamins and minerals in your diet before investing in dietary supplements?
5. Do you or someone you know take steroids? What changes in looks and attitude have occurred? What concerns would you share about taking steroids?

ADOLESCENT STRESS

In 1904, G. Stanley Hall proposed that adolescence is inherently a time of storm and stress. Researchers agree that not much has changed since adolescence is a period in life that is difficult, and conflict resides within each child transforming to adulthood, including mood disruption, conflict with parents and adult authority, and risk behaviors (Arnett, 1999). Along with the physical changes, emotional and intellectual changes take place, enabling teens to mature into accomplished adults. Cognitive development allows teens to have insight into their nutritional needs, although, more often than not, the motivation is for appearance.

Psychological and emotional changes that might hold teens back from reaching their goals include being influenced by peers and mistrustful toward adults and becoming more independent in thinking. As a result, teens take risks with themselves, their health, and their diet. Meal patterns of teens are often chaotic. Teens stop eating at home, breakfast and lunch are often skipped, and, if a nighttime social activity is scheduled, dinner can be overlooked as well.

In addition, teen diets and eating behaviors are also complicated by numerous internal and external factors, including food availability, preferences, cost, and convenience; personal and cultural beliefs; parental modeling; peer pressure; mass media; and body image (Das et al., 2017). Challenges for meeting nutritional goals for teenagers include irregular meals and snacking; fast foods; the media; and the influences of poor sleep, caffeine, alcohol, and use and abuse of recreational drugs and supplements.

SLEEP

The natural sleep and wake patterns, school and practice schedules, mealtimes, and social calendars of most teens shift during adolescence, making earlier bedtimes and wake times more difficult. The result is a chronic sleep deficit, poor concentration, stunted growth, mood swings, and a greater occurrence of overtraining syndrome. Issues related to weight management and eating and diminished cognitive and physical performance have also been reported (Tarokh, Saletin, & Carskadon, 2016).

A study published in the *Journal of Adolescent Health* reported that 10 percent of teens sleep only five hours, while 23 percent sleep only six hours on an average school night. High school seniors suffer about 20 percent more than freshman with sleep deficits, and African Americans and Whites have more deficits than Hispanics have. Although no formal sleep guidelines exist, the National Sleep Foundation recommends nine hours per night as optimal for adolescents, eight hours as borderline, and anything under eight as not enough. Of the four stages of sleep (see table 5.11), stage 4 (REM, or rapid eye movement, sleep) is the most important for growth, and especially so for building muscle mass.

It is important for teens to find a way to get enough rest, but even more importantly, to get a good, deep rest every night. Studies have shown that sleep deprivation lowers levels of testosterone, the anabolic hormone that enhances growth and immune and hormonal functions and increases muscle protein synthesis and strength, size, and performance for athletes (Pujalte & Benjamin, 2018). Other typical lifestyle factors in teens include alcohol and recreational and steroid drug use. The effect of these chemicals on nutritional status depends on the amount, duration used, and health of the individual teen. More information about sleep health is available at www.sleepfoundation.org/sleep-topics/children-teens-sleep.

ALCOHOL

Alcohol is a central nervous system depressant. Alcohol consumption affects perceptual motor performance, gross motor skills, balance, and coordination, thereby having an impact on daily activity and sports performance. Testosterone and growth hormone levels also decrease in just one acute alcohol drinking session, which can have an impact on teens' ability to build muscle mass (Martinsen & Sundgot-Borgen, 2014).

Pure alcohol supplies seven calories per gram, almost the same amount as fat. It is either metabolized as fat or to a compound that limits the body's ability to use fat as an energy source during training. Beer drinkers have been shown to eat 30 percent more than those who don't drink, typically high-fat calorie snacks and meals that can affect body composition.

For alcohol to be used by muscle, it must first be metabolized in the liver. Over time, alcohol clogs the arteries to the liver, which causes liver disease. Alcohol also reduces glycogen release from the liver, which leads to low blood-sugar levels, called hypoglycemia, and early fatigue during training.

For obvious reasons, alcohol consumption immediately before or during exercise has a detrimental effect on performance. For some teen athletes, drinking or taking a recreational drug before workouts or competition may reduce feelings of insecurity, tension, and discomfort; however, it gives teen athletes an unrealistic perception of their abilities and can lead to injury. Some athletes incorrectly believe that they can load up on beer to improve their performance because alcohol contains carbohydrates (Lisha & Sussman, 2010).

Alcohol after workouts is also detrimental to restoring hydration, which is critical to a teen's performance and overall health. Alcohol acts as

Table 5.11 Sleep Stages

Stages	Percent of total sleep time	Description
1	5%-10%	• Floating or drifting sensation • Insomniacs have longer stage 1 than others and more difficulty falling into a deeper sleep
2	50%	• Rolling eye movements • Easily awakened during this stage in those sensitive to noise
3	5%-20%	• Deep sleep • Hard to arouse • Sleepwalking • Talking in sleep • Night terrors • Bed-wetting occurs in this stage
4	20%-25%	• REM, active, paradoxical, dream types of sleep occur during this stage • Voluntary muscles relaxed • Brain waves quicken • This stage important for psychological health, learning, and memory • Alcohol prevents this stage of sleep

Adapted from Dorfman (2010).

a diuretic, having an impact on blood-sugar and glycogen recovery. Chronic alcohol use causes the loss of many nutrients important for performance and health, including vitamin A, which helps to make testosterone, vitamins B_1 and B_6, and the minerals calcium, magnesium, and zinc, all of which can affect skin, the immune system, bones, and overall health. Alcohol can also be a contributing factor to hypothermia, the inability to maintain body temperature in cold weather (https://www.drinkaware.co.uk/alcohol-facts/health-effects-of-alcohol/lifestyle/can-alcohol-affect-sports-performance-and-fitness-levels/). Additional information about alcohol and drug use and their impact on sports performance can be found at https://blog.insidetracker.com/how-does-alcohol-affect-your-athletic-performance.

BREAKFAST AND SNACKS FOR OPTIMAL HEALTH AND PERFORMANCE

Breakfast is one of the most important meals of the day and a great way to get the day started on the right foot. The problem is fewer than half of U.S. teens wake up early enough or stop for breakfast at school.

Breakfast is a wake-up call for pure physical energy. A morning meal helps to replenish blood sugar, an immediate energy source for a morning workout, training, or daily responsibilities such as doing household chores or staying sharp in school. The morning meal breaks the physiological fast that the body has endured overnight—that is what makes "break-fast" just that. It helps recoup energy, also know as the calories expended during sleep, and raise the blood sugar to a healthy level to enable longer-term energy in the form of glycogen stored in muscle and the liver for morning classes.

Research suggests that breakfast can make the difference between being at normal weight or overweight, being alert or having a poor attention span, fighting infection, or succumbing to diseases like colds and the flu. Some recent studies imply that skipping breakfast may be associated with a susceptibility to gaining weight and increased prevalence of obesity, especially when eating breakfast away from home or by including heavy meats, super-stack pancake specials, or whole-egg omelets with whole-fat cheese on croissants or buttered biscuits.

The morning meal can be the easiest strategy for meeting one-third of the required daily needs for carbohydrates, proteins and fats, vitamins, minerals, fiber, and phytochemicals. Breakfast may be the best, most convenient, and consistent opportunity to incorporate a nutritious daily meal.

Eating something first thing in the morning is not easy for many teens. That is why fast food choices such as smoothies, shakes, breakfast bars, or even a glass of fortified juice can make it easier to get the day started. As long as some form of complex carbohydrates, such as a whole-grain bagel, piece of fresh fruit, or a few vegetables in an omelet, is included along with a low-fat, protein or calcium source such as yogurt or an egg-white omelet, breakfast can keep the body energized through mid-morning snack and even lunchtime.

Research shows that adding a high-quality protein source (such as egg whites or whey in dairy) and citrus to the diet may help expend additional calories throughout the day compared to high-carbohydrate, high-fat meals.

However, not all breakfasts are healthy. Starting the day with empty calorie choices such as high-sugar cereals, pop tarts, or soda and chips can be as bad as not starting it at all. Fast food choices are often excessive in calories, fat, and sodium and low in vitamins and minerals.

Although snacking can be a concern when poor choices are made, for teens, it can actually be an opportunity to get substantial calories and nutrition. Because teens tend to skip meals, nutritious snacks can provide essential calories and nutrients in these smaller meals. When teens wake up or stay up late, they can include a snack of fortified breakfast bar and milk as a valuable source of complex carbohydrates and protein. If they skip lunch, teens can include a fruit smoothie, nut butter sandwich, or trail mix. These snacks and many others can help meet vitamin and mineral needs, too. For instance, one cup of yogurt can help meet 25 percent of calcium needs, a handful of nuts and dried fruits provides 100 percent of biotin and 22 percent magnesium, and 10 baby carrots provide more than 100 percent of vitamin A. Following are some healthy snack options to consider:

High-Carbohydrate Snacks

- Fresh fruit (orange slices, bananas, grapes)
- Fresh vegetables (celery with dip or carrots with hummus)
- Baked potato or tortilla chips, pretzels, rice cakes with nut butter
- Dry whole grain cereals
- Breakfast bars

- Saltine crackers, whole-wheat crackers, rice crackers
- Air-popped popcorn
- Baked potato with broccoli and low-fat cheese or salsa
- Whole-grain bagels, English muffins with nut butter
- Canned or plastic pack fruit in its own juice
- Applesauce, no added sugar
- Fruit or vegetable "pouches"
- Fresh fruit smoothies
- Fruit bars or whole-fruit frozen pops
- Vegetables with low-fat dressing or hummus
- Low-fat, low-sugar, or frozen yogurt

High-Protein Snacks

- Greek or Icelandic yogurt smoothie, nut butter shakes, whole-food sports bars
- Beef, turkey, or vegan jerky
- Hard-boiled eggs
- Lean, organic, or low-fat sliced turkey, chicken, beef, or ham
- String cheese, Babybel cheese, Laughing Cow wedges
- Cottage cheese
- Dried edamame, dried chickpeas

High-Fat Healthy Snacks

- Trail mix
- Pistachios, almonds, walnuts
- Nut butter on crackers
- Fruit smoothie with whole milk
- Granola or muesli cereal
- Whole-fat chocolate milk
- Whole-fat yogurt
- Whole-fat ice cream shake

Portable Snacks

- Almonds, walnuts, pistachios, trail mix
- Breakfast cereal bars
- Single portion whole-grain cereal boxes
- Baby food fruit and vegetable pouches
- Fresh fruit (apples, bananas, pears)
- Fruit leathers or dried fruits
- Meat or veggie jerky
- Whey- or plant-based sports bars or shakes

Selecting Healthy Breakfast and Sports Bars

The goal of a breakfast or sports bar is to boost energy and endurance and maintain stamina before or after sports, in between classes, or in the afternoon as a snack. While there are no specific guidelines for selecting a healthy bar, the following section identifies ingredients to look for and others to avoid.

Wholesomeness. Look for bars without unnecessary additives: coloring and flavoring agents, preservatives, hydrogenated or trans fats, and industrial oils of the corn and soy varieties. Bars with flax, nuts, or seed fats offer a healthier fat profile and vitamins and minerals, which can help to meet daily nutritional requirements.

Total calories. This is dependent on the individual teen's calorie needs, activity level, and fitness or physique goals. Teens with high-calorie needs should eat a nutritious, wholesome bar with 200 to 250 calories for an after-school, pre-training, or practice snack. For lighter and younger teens, or female teens with lower total calorie needs, a bar with 100 to 150 calories or half of a 200-calorie bar may suffice as a pre-workout snack.

Sugar. For long-term energy, consume bars containing sugar in the form of complex carbohydrates, such as maltodextrin, waxy maize, or glucose polymers. For quick energy, bars with more natural sources of sugar, such as dried fruits, brown rice syrup, molasses, or honey, are recommended.

Protein. If immediate energy fueling is important, then bars with five or fewer grams of protein are sufficient and allow for a higher carbohydrate composition to fuel exercise. If building muscle or recovering from a training session is the goal, then a bar with 15 to 25 grams is sufficient to meet post exercise recovery needs. Bars that exceed 40 grams of protein are unnecessary and not advised.

Fiber. Bars with 1 to 3 grams of fiber are sufficient. Some bars have much higher amounts of fiber and are not encouraged before physical activity due to the possibility of stomach distress, gas, and pain.

Topics for discussion include breakfast, snacking, and breakfast bars.

Questions:

1. What makes breakfast the most important meal of the day?
2. How can snacking be healthy for you? Unhealthy?
3. Compare three healthy and three less-healthy snacks. Describe the reasons why one is more nutritious than another, e.g., less fat, less sugar, more protein, and more calcium.

Journal Prompts:

1. How are you going to change your breakfast and snacking habits based on the information you have learned?
2. Look at your food diary. At what times during the day can snacks provide a good source of nutrition and energy in your diet?

BECOMING A SMART CONSUMER

Just as fitness education courses are designed with the ultimate goal of teaching teens how to live physically active lives as adults, nutrition education should prepare teens to make healthy eating choices as adults.

Teens should be encouraged to develop skills that enable them to minimize eating out. Several health organizations recommend eating at home, which appears to improve the nutritional density (nutrition per calorie ratio), versus dining out. Eating out has been associated with a higher intake of total energy, sugar-sweetened beverages, and fat, and a lower intake of healthful foods and key nutrients, linking it to increased risks for obesity, insulin resistance, and metabolic syndrome (Larson, Neumark-Sztainer, Laska, & Story, 2011). Home-cooked meals have been shown to be more healthful, less costly, and higher in many of the nutrients of concern in a teen's diet, including fiber; calcium; folate; iron; and vitamins B_6, B_{12}, C, and E (Fulkerson et al., 2011; Larson et al., 2011). More frequent family dinners were also associated with higher-quality dietary intake. In one study of 2,728 14- to 24-year-old females (1,559) and males (1,169), more frequent family dinners were associated with higher intakes of fruits and vegetables and lower intake of sugar-sweetened beverages for males (Walton et al., 2018). Research by the Food Marketing Institute (n.d.) also suggests that with each additional family meal shared each week, adolescents are less likely to show symptoms of violence, depression, and suicide and less likely to use or abuse drugs, run away, and engage in risky behavior or delinquent acts.

Teens also should learn about the surprising impact that watching television has on their nutrition. Television watching has been shown to negatively affect the quality of food choices. In a recent meta-analysis, 13 studies of 61,674 English-speaking children ages 1 to 18 years old showed a positive association between TV viewing and consumption of pizza, fried foods, sweets, and snacks and a negative association with fruit and vegetable consumption (Avery, Anderson, & McCullough, 2017). The influence of watching television while eating is associated with a less nutritious diet among children, including more frequent consumption of sugar-sweetened beverages; high-fat, high-sugar foods; and fewer fruits and vegetables (Avery et al., 2017).

Grocery shopping as a family might have a positive effect on nutrition choices. In a recent study of 2,008 Canadians ages 16 to 24, 37 percent who engaged in shopping at least once weekly had increased only their vegetable and fruit consumption, while the 84 percent who helped with dinner preparation not only increased their vegetable and fruit consumption but had more frequent breakfast consumption and fewer meals that were prepared away from home (Vanderlee, Hobin, White, & Hammond, 2018).

Preparing healthful meals at home starts with well-planned grocery shopping. According to the book, *Shopping on a Budget for Athletes*, planning is the first step. Planning meals saves money and time, as well as preventing food waste. It also helps you to consume balanced meals with more variety. Surveying one's household and writing a list of the groceries needed helps avoid "mindless" shopping (Turpin, 2014). Other strategies for budget-conscious shopping include eating before shopping to avoid "hunger" purchases; carving out time to avoid rushing; looking throughout store shelves for bargains on nutritious items; buying in bulk and portioning foods into baggies or BPA-free plastic containers; looking through weekly coupon flyers; or searching websites such as www.coupons.com and www.Valpak.com. Buying fruits and vegetables in season can also be a money-saver and build nutritious meals. One suggested guide to buying in-season produce is available free online at www.fruitsandveggiesmorematters.org/what-fruits-and-vegetables-are-in-season.

Ultimately, it's important as an adult to consistently make good choices about which foods to consume. Table 5.12 shows an overall guide to choosing foods that are more nutritious.

Table 5.12 Nutrient-Dense Food Recommendations

Instead of this	Choose this	Nutrition benefits
White, processed grains and baked goods such as cookies, cakes, croissants, and muffins	100% whole grains, such as cereals, brown rice, bread, crackers, pasta	More B vitamins, iron, magnesium, and zinc; less fat, saturated fat, trans fat, sodium
Powdered juice or ready-to-drink juice drink, soda, energy drinks, sweet tea	Water, natural sparkling water, 100% fresh juice, unsweetened green tea	Less added sugar and caffeine; more vitamins and minerals in fruit juice
Canned or frozen fruit with syrup, dyes, artificial colors and flavors; fruit-flavored frozen pops, candy, or treats	Fresh, frozen, or canned unsweetened fruit	Less added sugar; more vitamins, fiber, minerals
Canned or frozen vegetables that have sauce or cheese or are in cream sauces and creamed soups	Fresh, frozen, canned low-sodium vegetables	Less sodium, saturated fat, cholesterol
High-fat flavored yogurts, milk, or cheese	Low- or nonfat milk, yogurt, cheese	Less fat, saturated fat, cholesterol
Processed luncheon meats such as bologna, salami, frankfurters, bacon, sausage	Lean protein without skin and limited fat such as chicken, turkey, eggs, lean beef, turkey or veggie burgers, tofu	Higher-quality protein; less fat, saturated fat, trans fat, cholesterol
Butter, vegetable shortening, cashews, palm oil, margarine	Healthy fats such as olive or canola oil, almonds, walnuts, pistachios, peanut butter, avocados	More essential omega-3s and omega-6s; less saturated fat, trans fat, cholesterol

For more information, follow this link:
www.fmi.org/family-meals-movement/make-meals-happen/view/nfmm-news-page/2020/04/17/recipes-practical-easy-and-delicious

Topics for discussion include planning affordable meals, eating in versus eating out, and making wise food choices.

Questions:

1. What are three benefits of eating at home instead of dining out?
2. Name three wise food choices you can make instead of fast food options.
3. How do media influence people's eating habits?

Activities:

1. What is your favorite fast food recipe? How can you take the same dish and make it lower in fat, sugar, or sodium and higher in vitamins, minerals, and fiber?
2. Create a 15-minute PowerPoint presentation of your favorite dish recipe conversion describing which ingredients you substituted to make it more nutritious and why you chose the new ingredients.
3. Have a competition. Challenge students or classes to convert their favorite traditional recipe to a healthier dish. Take a one-pot dish like chili (see recipe, Dorfman, 2010, p. 243), pizza, or macaroni and cheese and have students create healthier options for these traditionally high-fat, high-calorie, popular meals.
4. Create a class cookbook. Include recipe modifications, recipe nutritional analysis, and tips for other students in finding cost-effective ingredients. The class cookbook should include all the recipes submitted by students and can be used as the basis for an end-of-semester potluck celebration meal or fundraiser for a cause that supports feeding homeless, hungry, or other children.
5. Play nutritional Jeopardy. Seek the support of a local grocer or restaurant to provide store coupons or gift certificates for the winner. Students can also be tested on their nutrition knowledge and skills by changing at least three ingredients in a traditional dish, such as pizza, paella, or even chili con carne, to create a vegetarian option.

SAMPLE MENUS

Table 5.13 shows sample menus for 1,800 calories and 3,500 calories. Each menu also features examples of pre- and post-workout meals. Table 5.14 shows a sample vegan menu.

Table 5.13 Sample Menus

	1,800-calorie menu	3,500-calorie menu
Breakfast	• 2-egg omelet with veggie toppings and low-fat cheese • 1 mini whole-grain bagel with 1 tsp almond butter • 6 oz low-fat yogurt • 1/2 cup strawberries	• 1 cup 100% orange juice • 1 bowl whole-grain cereal • 1 cup low-fat milk or milk alternative • 1/2 cup strawberries • 1 banana
Morning snack	• 1 oz string cheese • 1 apple	• 1 string cheese • 6 whole-grain crackers • 1 apple
Lunch	• 1 cup tomato soup • Sandwich on whole-grain bread with 4 oz lean meat, veggie toppings, and 1 tsp olive oil–based dressing • 1 cup mixed tropical fruit salad with diced kiwi and citrus sections	• 1 green salad with carrots and tomatoes • 1 oz olive oil–based salad dressing • Sandwich on whole-grain bread with 6 oz lean meat, variety of veggies, and lite cheese • 1 bag baked chips • 12 oz low-fat milk or milk alternative • 1 orange
Pre-workout snack	1 lite natural sports drink and 1 banana	1 whole-grain breakfast bar or sports bar
During workout	Water and sports drink, as needed	Water and sports drink, as needed
Post-workout snack	Recovery smoothie with fresh fruits and Greek yogurt	Recovery smoothie with fresh fruits and Greek yogurt
Dinner	• Green salad with shredded carrots, tomatoes, beans, mushrooms, grilled corn, and low-fat feta cheese crumbles • 5 oz grilled lean meat or veggie burger on a whole-grain bun • Baked sweet potato fries • Stir-fried mixed vegetables	• 1 cup vegetable soup • 1 whole-grain roll with 1 tsp butter • 8 oz grilled fish • 1 cup brown rice and beans • 1 cup peas and corn • 1 cup steamed broccoli with parmesan cheese • 1 cup mixed berries with whipped cream
Evening snack	Frozen fruit pop or 1 cup frozen yogurt	1 cup frozen yogurt or low-fat ice cream with 1 whole grain muffin

CONCLUSION

Adolescence is one of the most exciting yet challenging stages in the life cycle. Healthy eating habits during the teenage years are essential for growth and cognitive development. As secondary school physical educators, you have empowered yourselves with information for educating, engaging, and assessing nutritional knowledge from the basics of nutrition and calculating nutritional needs—vitamin, mineral, and fluid requirements—for teaching this course. You are armed with tools, activities, and resources for teaching more sensitive topics, such as eating disorders, skin health, and supplement and steroid use.

Teachers play the most important role outside of caregivers in shaping a child's life, especially during the transitional period of adolescence. Your lessons in nutrition will help teens to attain the knowledge and skills they need to make healthy food decisions and improve energy levels, mood, appearance, and, most importantly, lifelong eating behaviors.

There are no easy answers in understanding or generalizing the teen years. The impact of the psychological and hormonal changes that take place in your students during a school year may influence you to make changes in the content, organization, and delivery of the material provided. Additionally, there is neither a best way nor only one way for sharing, shaping, and guiding teens with the information you have acquired. To help you develop your lesson plans and class format, there are valuable resources and references for you in HK*Propel*.

Table 5.14 Sample Vegan Menu

Breakfast	• Whole-grain blueberry waffles • Tofu egg scrambler • 1 cup mixed fresh fruit • 12 oz plant-based milk	
Morning snack	• Nut butter and jam sandwich • Cashew yogurt • 100% fruit juice	
Lunch	• Black bean soup with multigrain crackers • Veggie wrap with whole-grain tortilla and grilled tempeh • Fruit salad • Almond yogurt	
Afternoon snack	Fresh fruit smoothie with almond yogurt and vegan protein scoop	
Pre-workout snack	1 lite natural sports drink and 1 banana	1 whole-grain breakfast bar or sports bar
During workout	Water and sports drink, as needed	
Post-workout snack	Recovery smoothie with fresh fruits and plant based yogurt	
Dinner	• Vegetarian chili with whole-grain crackers • 3 cups whole-grain or bean-based pasta with veggie meatballs, red sauce, and mixed vegetables • Vegan parmesan cheese • 2 whole-grain rolls with vegetable-based butter • Green salad with mixed vegetables and olive oil • Almond milk	
Evening snack	Dairy-free frozen dessert	

Visit HK*Propel* for additional material related to this chapter.

CHAPTER 6

Social and Emotional Learning

Chapter Objective

After reading this chapter, you will understand how and why to create a positive and motivational learning environment by incorporating social and emotional learning into the fitness education curriculum and instruction, be able to describe how you can use social and emotional skills to support culturally diverse students and students affected by trauma, know how to influence students' motivation levels in a fitness education setting, and understand how students can maintain a physically active lifestyle using self-management strategies.

Key Concepts

- Creating a positive fitness education experience that motivates students to continue engaging in physical activity outside of the classroom requires developing a positive, motivational class climate.
- Students need to feel physically safe from violence or injury and emotionally safe from embarrassment, threats, abusive language, and bullying so that stress and anxiety do not interfere with their ability to engage in the fitness education learning experiences.
- Using the social and emotional competencies of self-management, self-awareness, and relationship skills in health and fitness education have all been shown to increase physical activity, improve nutritional habits, and reduce body fat percentage in the adolescent population.
- Goal setting is one of the most effective strategies for increasing adolescent physical activity behavior and improving health-related fitness.

INTRODUCTION

When adolescents enjoy physical activity, they develop positive attitudes toward it and choose to engage in it more frequently, creating regular physical activity patterns that lead into adulthood (Graham, Sirard, & Neumark-Sztainer, 2011). Recent research on adults' memories of their K-12 physical education experience shows that people who had positive memories, such as enjoyment of class activities and experiences of feeling physical competence, developed positive attitudes toward physical activity, engaged in less sedentary behavior, and had intentions to remain physically active as adults (Ladwig, Vazou, & Ekkekakis, 2018). Those who had negative memories, such as being embarrassed, being bullied, or experiencing a lack of enjoyment in activities, were more likely to be sedentary, had negative attitudes toward physical activity, and had fewer intentions of being physically active as an adult (Ladwig et al., 2018). Several studies have shown that students' experiences in physical education class affect their attitude toward physical activity and their adoption of a physically active lifestyle, so helping them to have a positive experience in physical education is crucial to accomplishing the goal of lifetime physical activity (Castillo, Molina-García, Estevan, Queralt, & Álvarez, 2020; Ladwig et al., 2018; Trudeau & Shephard, 2008).

CREATING A POSITIVE AND MOTIVATIONAL LEARNING ENVIRONMENT

Creating a positive fitness education experience that motivates students to continue engaging in physical activity outside of the classroom requires developing a positive and motivational class climate. As mentioned in chapter 4, the learning environment is just as important as the content that is taught because of its impact on student learning and achievement. The motivational climate is the psychological environment that you create by how you structure learning tasks, interact with students, deliver feedback, and set expectations for peer interactions. It is the prevailing mood and attitudes that students feel during class. Depending on the class climate, they may either feel welcomed, respected, safe, motivated, and supported or excluded, guarded, and unwilling to participate. The motivational climate is how well you can support students' social and emotional well-being in your class so that they feel safe and want to engage in the learning experiences.

Feeling safe is a prerequisite for learning. Feeling safe and secure is a basic human need according to Maslow's hierarchy of needs, a motivational theory that suggests our behavior is motivated by our attempts to fulfill various needs classified as basic, psychological, and self-fulfillment (see figure 6.1). People are more likely to reach their fullest potential, or self-actualization, when their basic physiological and psychological needs are met. Your students need to feel physically safe from violence or injury and emotionally safe from embarrassment, threats, abusive language, and bullying so that stress and anxiety do not interfere with their ability to learn to their fullest potential. Students experiencing stress can have impaired memory retrieval and difficulty encoding new information to memory, which negatively affects academic achievement (Vogel & Schwabe, 2016).

Bullying is a common reason that students feel unsafe at school. One in every five students ages 12 to 18 report being bullied at school, and the reasons for being bullied most often reported include physical appearance, race or ethnicity, gender, disability, religion, and sexual orientation (National Center for Educational Statistics, 2019). Students may be more vulnerable to bullying and victimization in a physical education class because their physical capabilities are on display. It is difficult to hide low levels of fitness or poor motor-skill competency in a physical education class without sitting out of the activities. Bullying can have several negative outcomes for youth who bully others, youth who are bullied, and even those who have observed but not participated in bullying behavior (Centers for Disease Control and Prevention, 2014). Potential negative outcomes associated with bullying behavior include feelings of helplessness, social isolation, depression, anxiety, poor academic performance, poor attendance, substance abuse, and involvement in interpersonal violence (Center for Disease Control and Prevention, 2014). Roughly 20 percent of the students in your class may not be able to reach their learning potential as a result of bullying if you do not proactively and relentlessly work to establish an emotionally safe environment. In addition, there are factors other than how their peers treat them that can negatively affect a student's ability to feel emotionally safe. Such factors include experiencing childhood trauma, not being understood due to a language barrier, being misunderstood because of cultural differences, or lacking the social skills and confidence to ask for help (Souers & Hall, 2019).

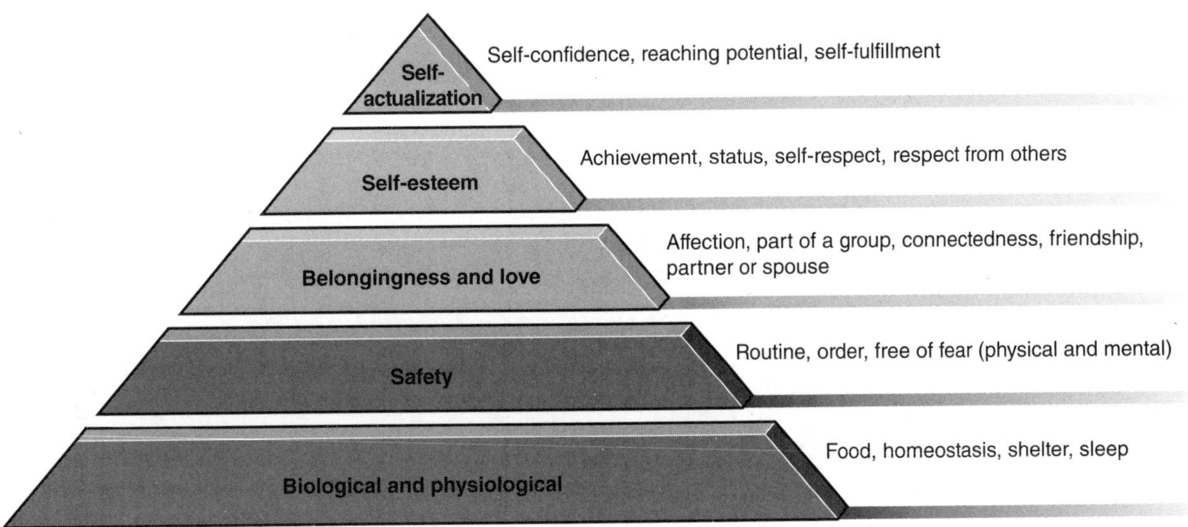

Figure 6.1 Maslow's hierarchy of needs
Reprinted by permission from S. Benes and H. Alperin, *The Essentials of Teaching Health Education* (Champaign, IL: Human Kinetics, 2016), 41.

TRAUMA-INFORMED TEACHING

According to the Substance Abuse and Mental Health Services Administration (SAMHSA), individual trauma results from an event, series of events, or set of circumstances experienced by a person as physically or emotionally harmful or life-threatening with lasting adverse effects on the person's functioning and mental, physical, social, emotional, or spiritual well-being.

SAMHSA (2020) estimates that more than two-thirds of children will experience at least one traumatic event by the age of 16. Examples of traumatic events include the following:

- Physical, emotional, or sexual abuse
- National disasters such as fires, hurricanes, or floods that affect their living situation
- Military family related stressor (e.g., deployment, loss of a parent, injured parent)
- Physical or emotional neglect
- Witnessing or experiencing school, domestic, or community violence
- Refugee or war experiences
- Life-threatening illness or serious accident
- Sudden loss of a loved one (SAMHSA, 2020)

When students enter our classrooms, as teachers, we have a tendency to see their immediate behaviors, but what we don't necessarily see is what lies beneath the surface. Figure 6.2 provides an illustration of what a student experiencing trauma could be dealing with internally.

Traumatized students may have difficulty trusting their environments, tend to struggle in forming relationships, and are prone to extreme behaviors that range from complete withdrawal to excessive, disruptive, acting-out behavior (Terrasi & de Galarce, 2017). Teachers who do not understand why traumatized students display aggression, are defiant, isolate themselves, and inappropriately express emotions can feel such behaviors as antagonistic (Minahan, 2019). Students who have two or more traumatic events, referred to as adverse childhood experiences (ACEs), have increased absenteeism, lower rates of engagement, difficulty focusing, and increased behavioral issues (Ellison, Walton-Fisette, & Eckert, 2019). For students affected by trauma, the basic need of emotional safety must first be met before any meaningful learning can take place. Otherwise, they may be in a constant state of survival mode that stimulates an overreactive stress response leading to numerous negative physical and emotional health consequences (Ellison et al., 2019).

As teachers learn to understand how the behaviors of traumatized students interfere with the teaching and learning process, they realize that student responses are not directed toward them and can employ thoughtful interactions, build trusting relationships, and provide supportive feedback instead of negative thinking (Minahan, 2019). According to the Council of Chief State School Officers (CCSSO, 2017), once teachers can change their mindset and understand the behaviors of traumatized students, their approach and language begins to provide a supportive and safe

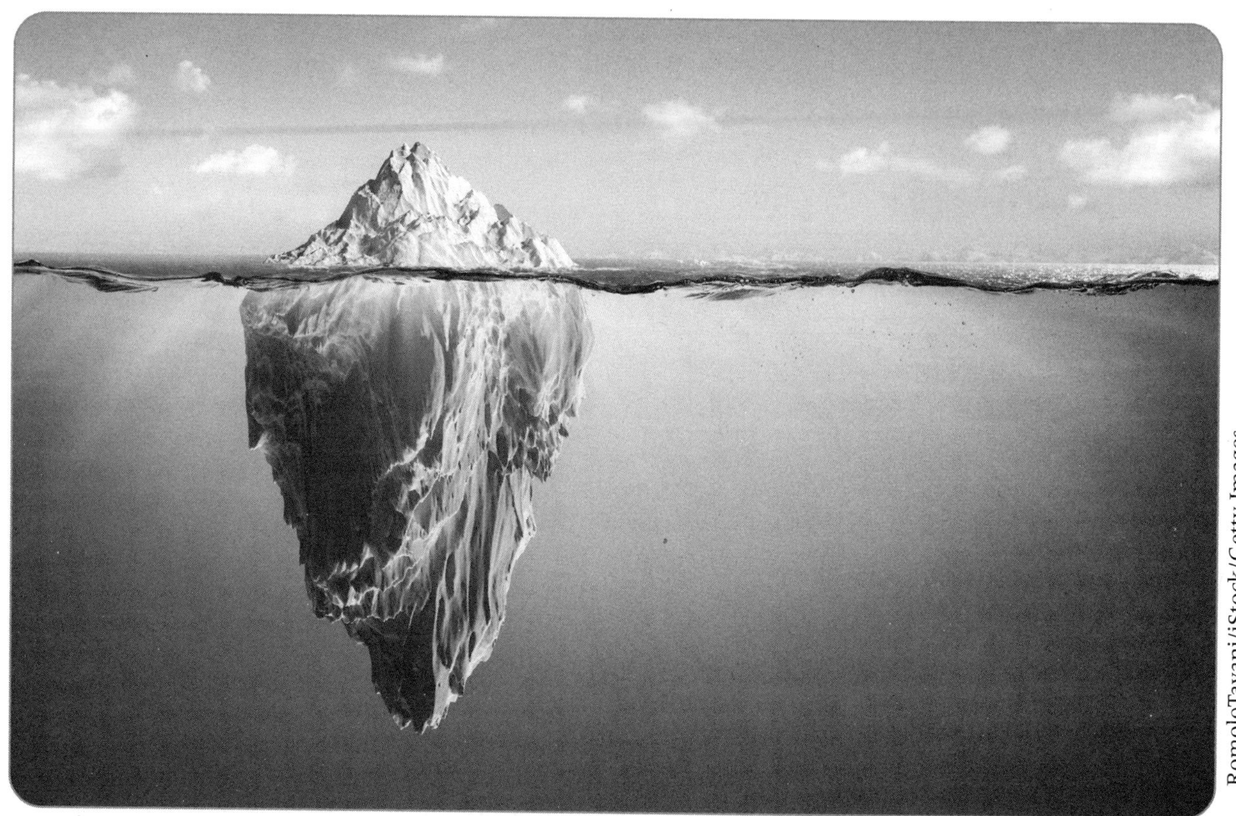

RomoloTavani/iStock/Getty Images

Figure 6.2 Just as only the small top of an iceberg is visible to others, teachers can see only a small part of a student's internal workings from observing classroom behavior. Most of what a student is dealing with is invisible to outsiders.

environment through transformative social and emotional learning.

People who are not trauma informed may wonder "what's wrong" with a person who has experienced trauma when they see the symptoms. Figure 6.3 exemplifies a process for teachers, which begins by showing how incorrect judgments and conclusions can be misconstrued if teachers are not looking at a person through a trauma-informed lens.

Some people will say that, in order to act in a trauma-informed way, you should shift your thinking in all your interactions to ask and wonder, "What happened to you?" when you see a person exhibiting symptoms of trauma. As teachers, though, it is usually not our place to ask such questions of students. It could be a huge overstep of their personal privacy. Remember, you don't need to know exactly what caused the trauma to be able to help.

It is recommended that teachers move toward this third question, "What's right with you?" It fits much better with our focus as educators. It brings a holistic, strengths-based approach to all our interactions with students. The single, solid circle represents that strong, strengths-based approach, with the focus on the positive attributes of students.

DEVELOPING SOCIAL AND EMOTIONAL LEARNING

Socially and emotionally competent behaviors are essential in creating a safe and supportive learning environment that facilitates positive experiences and enjoyment for every student. Social and emotional competence is the ability to positively interact with others, regulate one's own behavior and emotions, and communicate effectively (Center for the Study of Social Policy, 2015). The Collaborative for Academic, Social, and Emotional Learning (CASEL, 2020) has identified five core competencies—self-awareness, social awareness, relationship skills, self-management, and responsible decision making—as shown in figure 6.4, that contribute to healthy social and emotional development and positive social behaviors (e.g., kindness, empathy, cooperation) in the classroom. Social-awareness and relationship skills represent *interpersonal* competencies, responsible decision making represents *cognitive* competencies, and self-awareness and self-management represent *intrapersonal* competencies.

"What's wrong with you?"
"What happened to you?"
"What's right with you?"

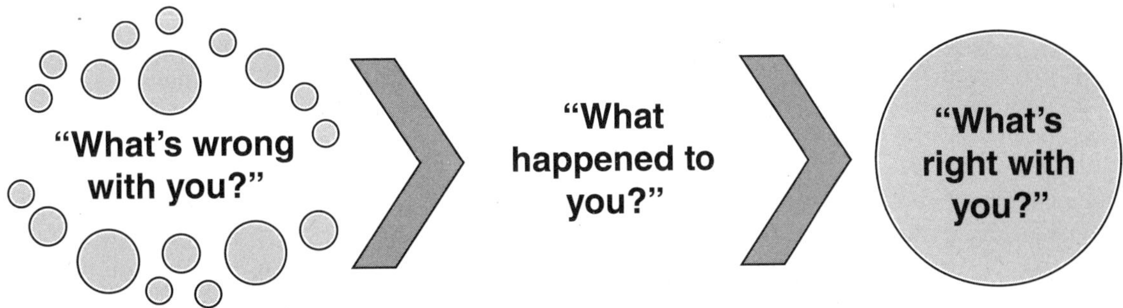

Figure 6.3 Changing our mindset changes our approach.
Introduction to Trauma Informed Care in Adaptive Sports, www.cotipusa.com, Copyright 2020 by Christine Cowart.

Implementing social and emotional learning (SEL) in the classroom can develop these competencies. SEL is an educational process that facilitates students learning and applying the knowledge, attitudes, and skills necessary to manage emotions, set and achieve positive goals, feel and show empathy for others, establish and maintain positive relationships, and make responsible decisions (CASEL, 2020). Having social and emotional skills makes students more capable of managing their feelings, building healthy relationships, controlling their impulses, solving problems, and supporting others.

Incorporating SEL into the curriculum and instruction is vital to delivering quality fitness education because of the need to establish a safe, inclusive, and motivational learning environment. Explicitly teaching students the SEL competencies and holding them accountable for demonstrating responsible and respectful behaviors are necessary for physical and emotional safety. Responsible behaviors are key to safety in fitness education, and not abiding safety protocols can lead to bodily harm. Respectful and inclusive behaviors promote emotional safety so that when students are performing fitness activities in

Social and Emotional Learning (SEL) Competencies

Self-awareness

The ability to accurately recognize one's own emotions, thoughts, and values and how they influence behavior. The ability to accurately assess one's strengths and limitations, with a well-grounded sense of confidence, optimism, and a "growth mindset."

- Identifying emotions
- Accurate self-perception
- Recognizing strengths
- Self-confidence
- Self-efficacy

Social awareness

The ability to take the perspective of and empathize with others, including those from diverse backgrounds and cultures. The ability to understand social and ethical norms and behavior and to recognize family, school, and community resources and supports.

- Perspective-taking
- Empathy
- Appreciating diversity
- Respect for others

Responsible decision-making

The ability to make constructive choices about personal behavior and social interactions based on ethical standards, safety concerns, and social norms. The realistic evaluation of consequences of various actions, and a consideration of the well-being of oneself and others.

- Identifying problems
- Analyzing situations
- Solving problems
- Evaluating
- Reflections
- Ethical responsibility

Self-management

The ability to successfully regulate one's emotions, thoughts, and behaviors in different situations – effectively managing stress, controlling impulses, and motivating oneself. The ability to set and work toward personal and academic goals.

- Impulse control
- Stress management
- Self-discipline
- Self-motivation
- Goal setting
- Organizational skills

Relationship skills

The ability to establish and maintain healthy and rewarding relationships with diverse individuals and groups. The ability to communicate clearly, listen well, cooperate with others, resist inappropriate social pressure, negotiate conflict constructively, and seek and offer help when needed.

- Communication
- Social engagement
- Relationship building
- Teamwork

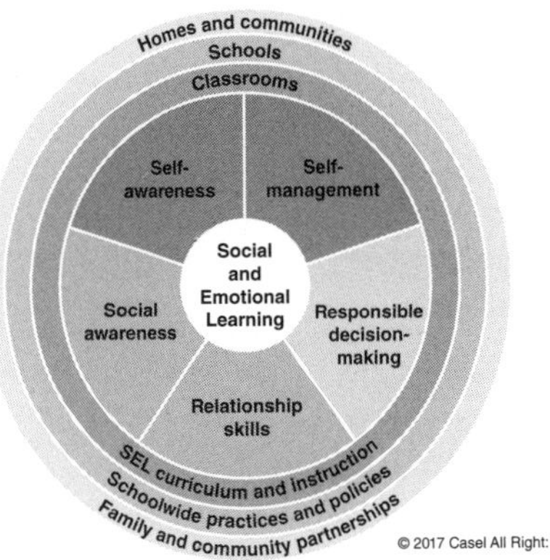

Figure 6.4 CASEL: The five core SEL competencies.
7 Steps for Choosing and Using SEL Assessments. Source: ©2020 CASEL. All Rights Reserved.

front of their peers, they feel comfortable enough to fully engage in the activities without fear of being judged, embarrassed, or put down.

It may feel overwhelming to think about teaching something else in your fitness education course. You already have numerous cognitive and psychomotor objectives that you want students to master, and adding SEL to your program may not seem possible. Fortunately, SEL is not just another add-on to fitness education. The SEL competencies are the affective objectives of fitness education that sometimes get neglected in a program due to a concern over lack of time to teach fitness concepts and activities. The self-management and responsible decision-making competencies directly align with a distinguishing feature of fitness education curriculum and instruction that was described in chapter 1: "helps students develop self-management skills to maintain healthy behaviors" (SHAPE America, 2012). Therefore, SEL is, in fact, necessary to accomplish the goals of fitness education.

In the long run, greater social and emotional competence can increase the likelihood that students will have better mental health outcomes; benefit from healthy relationships; and achieve goals such as graduating high school, attending college, and acquiring a successful career (Weissberg, Durlack, Domitrovich, & Gullotta, 2015). In addition, students with greater social and emotional competence will be more likely to attain and maintain a health-enhancing level of physical fitness using self-management (e.g., goal setting, self-monitoring strategies), enhancing self-awareness (e.g., improving self-efficacy), and using relationship skills (e.g., social engagement, social support), which have all been shown to increase physical activity, improve nutritional habits, and reduce body fat percentage in the adolescent population (de Bruin et al., 2012; Hortz & Petosa, 2008; Shimon & Petlichkoff, 2009; Thomason, Lukkahatai, Kawi, Connelly, & Inouye, 2016; Laird, Fawkner, Kelly, McNamee, & Niven, 2016). Greater social and emotional competence can be acquired in a similar fashion to proficient motor-skill competence by practicing the skills to refine them so that they can be used in a variety of situations. Effective approaches to SEL typically incorporate four elements represented by the acronym SAFE (CASEL, 2020):

- *Sequenced.* Connect and coordinate activities so that they are integrated into the instruction rather than taught in isolation. In addition, progressively sequence the development of the skills. Scaffold the learning experiences to match your students' social and emotional competence developmental levels. Students may not be able to perform self-directed skills without first engaging in teacher-directed skills. They may need to be prompted, encouraged, and specifically directed to demonstrate positive social behaviors. Table 6.1 shows an example of how students can demonstrate greater levels of personal and social responsibility in their social engagement. The key here is that you will have to provide opportunities for students to demonstrate these levels and refrain from instructing them to assist peers once you believe they have the ability to self-direct. Design activities that encourage cooperation and allow students to demonstrate an ability to self-direct with you, gradually decreasing behavior prompts.
- *Active.* Students must be given opportunities to practice the skills through active learning. This means that they are not simply told about SEL competencies; rather, they have opportunities to engage with peers in practicing the SEL competencies in an authentic environment.
- *Focused.* Some component of the lesson or unit emphasizes developing personal and social skills. This means that you have created space within your instructional framework to deliver SEL. In the teaching personal and social responsibility (TPSR) model, for example, this would be done in the awareness talk lesson component because that framework intentionally teaches a personal and social responsibility theme in each lesson. You can create an SEL-focused component in your daily lessons with any instructional framework.
- *Explicitly.* The targeted social and emotional skill is clearly identified and taught with intention. Teachers do not use vague references to social and emotional behaviors. If the SEL competency is "Social awareness: Respecting others" and the identified standard is S4.H2.L1: "Exhibits proper etiquette, respect for others and teamwork while engaging in physical activity and/or social dance" (SHAPE America, 2013), then teachers will provide examples of what proper etiquette is in that situation and describe criteria for what respect looks like. In addition, students are assessed and receive feedback on their social and emotional skills similar to how they receive feedback on their psychomotor skills.

To create a safe, positive, and motivational environment, you must demonstrate social and emotional competency and also teach students how to demonstrate social and emotional competence so that you and the class are working together to create a climate that motivates every student to engage. Your competency allows you to model positive social behaviors, coach students through inappropriate

Table 6.1 Levels of Personal and Social Responsibility for Social Engagement

Level 1	Students assist peers when directed to.	Teacher-directed: Teachers design learning experiences where peers have to assist each other, explicitly explain how to assist a peer, and model the expectations of assistance.
Level 2	Students assist peers when asked for help.	Peer-directed: Teachers design learning experiences where peers have to assist each other, explain that peers can ask for help to accomplish the task, and model how to ask classmates for help
Level 3	Students recognize when peers need assistance and assist them.	Self-directed: Teachers design learning experiences where peers may need to assist each other, provide no direct instruction on assisting students, and observe if students engage in supporting each other when appropriate.

behaviors, and develop relationships with students that promote positive interactions. In addition, your social and emotional competence equips you to design lessons that will foster greater SEL for your students. The next section describes how you can provide opportunities for students to develop each of the social and emotional competencies through SEL experiences, as well as how you can use your social and emotional competence to create the best learning environment for your students in a fitness education class. It should be noted that many of these behaviors are embedded in physical education standards, GLOs, and, most importantly, in the behaviors of both students and teachers. The full document can be found at http://www.shapeamerica.org/standards/guidelines/sel-crosswalk.aspx.

INTERPERSONAL COMPETENCIES: SOCIAL AWARENESS

> The ability to take the perspective of and empathize with others, including those from diverse backgrounds and cultures. The ability to understand social and ethical norms for behavior and to recognize family, school, and community resources and supports; standards and outcomes. (CASEL, 2020)

Table 6.2 shows fitness education learning outcomes that promote the interpersonal competency of social awareness. As schools become increasingly diverse with students of many religions, languages, ethnicities, economic groups, and other cultural groups represented in each classroom, more and more teachers face the challenge of having the ability to understand the impact of our culturally diverse student body. Students' cultural patterns of behavior, which include communication, beliefs, customs, values, and relationships, may interfere with the learning process if teachers lack the cultural sensitivity and competency to engage students.

While you are teaching to a classroom of students, it is important to remember that all students in your class have their own perspective and beliefs specific to their experiences. To create an inclusive environment for a culturally diverse classroom, you must understand that students from varying cultural backgrounds have diverse perspectives and differing social norms. When you are socially aware and cognizant of diverse perspectives, you can respectfully respond to students' unique ways of interacting with their environment.

Table 6.2 Fitness Education Learning Outcomes That Promote Social Awareness

SHAPE America standard categories and SEL components	Middle school (grades 6-8) SHAPE America grade-level outcomes	High school (grades 9-12) SHAPE America grade-level outcomes
Working with others (appreciating diversity) Working with others and rules and etiquette (respect for others)	Accepts differences among classmates in physical development, maturation, and varying skill levels by providing encouragement and positive feedback. (S4.M4.6) Responds appropriately to participants' ethical and unethical behavior during physical activity by using rules and guidelines for resolving conflicts. (S4. M4.8)	Accepts others' ideas, cultural diversity, and body types by engaging in cooperative and collaborative movement projects. (S4.H4.L2) Exhibits proper etiquette, respect for others and teamwork while engaging in physical activity and/or social dance. (S4.H2.L1)

Modified from "Crosswalk for SHAPE America National Standards & Grade-Level Outcomes for K-12 Physical Education and CASEL Social and Emotional Learning Core Competencies."

Cultural Competence

According to the National Association of Social Workers (2015, p. 13), being socially aware means that you are culturally competent, which can be defined as follows:

> Cultural competence refers to the process by which individuals and systems respond respectfully and effectively to people of all cultures, languages, classes, races, ethnic backgrounds, religions, spiritual traditions, immigration status, and other diversity factors in a manner that recognizes, affirms, and values the worth of individuals, families, and communities and protects and preserves the dignity of each.

We want our students to develop social awareness competencies so that they are able to appreciate diversity; exhibit empathy; understand social and ethical norms for behavior; and recognize family, school, and community supports. Social awareness can reduce the negative impacts of bullying in your classroom as well as potential communication problems. For example, empathetic students are more likely to intervene in a bullying situation and support students who are different than the social norm (Swearer & Cary, 2007). You can help develop empathy in your students by having them engage in perspective-taking learning experiences. Perspective-taking is when you consider a situation from someone else's point of view by putting yourself in that position and imagining what you would feel, think, or do to help you determine an empathetic response. For example, you could present this scenario to students:

"Imagine if you were running on the track and you tripped and fell. How would you want your classmates to respond?" Have students think, and then solicit responses. Use their responses to formulate a class norm for how to respond empathetically in a similar situation, such as:

"Now if this happens in class, please respond in an empathetic way by not laughing, pointing, or name-calling but rather by assisting them and asking if they are okay."

Students of various cultures may communicate quite differently than you based on their past experiences and upbringing. Teachers lacking cultural competence may subsequently interpret students' responses as disrespectful and evoke unjustified disciplinary actions. When communicating with students from different countries, it is important to recognize that their social norms or communication styles may vastly differ from yours. For example, you may request that Tran, a Vietnamese student, look you in the eyes when you are addressing an inappropriate classroom behavior. When she refuses to make eye contact, you consider that to be a sign of disrespect and proceed to write a referral for her lack of compliance. However, Tran has been taught that direct eye contact is aggressive, confrontational, and rude, so she believes she is being respectful by listening and not making direct eye contact (Hansen, 2014).

Culture determines a person's behavioral characteristics. Learning about your students' culture, what they value, what their beliefs are, and how they communicate will help you to better understand why they behave in certain ways. Giri (2006) and Pratt-Johnson (2006) provide several examples of how a person's culture can affect ways of communicating (see table 6.3). This table can be used for self-reflection and personal improvement in developing social awareness for interacting with culturally diverse students. The more that you can learn about your students' culture and how it influences their learning experience, the more capable you will become in supporting them to achieve their learning potential.

Stokes and Schultz (2007) assert that teachers must do a self-evaluation to determine their own thoughts, language, behaviors, and attitudes regarding other cultures before they can interact with their students to bring about an understanding of cultural diversity. Some strategies and teaching tips might include the following:

- Get students to interact with each other as individuals, not as people in a particular ethnic group.
- Confront remarks made by students by telling students that you find these comments out of taste. You must send a message in the classroom that you will not tolerate words or actions that degrade anyone for any reason.
- Structure noncompetitive games or activities. Use cooperative games, trust-building activities, and teamwork.
- Provide cross-cultural experiences such as guest speakers and field trips.
- Include information about the contributions of people from different cultures, including games and sports.
- Display people from diverse cultures on bulletin boards.
- Encourage students to get to know each other better. Assign partners and have them intro-

Table 6.3 Cultural Differences in Communication

Communication type	Description	Examples
Verbal versus nonverbal and directive versus nondirective cues	How do people interact with each other?	Nondirective communicators are attentive and relaxed, acknowledge others, and follow others' leads. Directive communicators are dramatic and animated, talk frequently, and take control.
Contact	What are the frequency of touch, close interaction distances, rates of gaze, and gestural animation?	Contact cultures prefer frequent use of touch, have higher rates of gaze, and use more gestural animation. Noncontact cultures prefer the opposite of contact cultures: less touching or no touching, very little or no eye contact, and less gestural animation.
Silence	How is silence interrupted in a conversation?	Some cultures prefer to express feelings and emotions verbally and think of silence as a cue for being disengaged, so they interrupt it. Other cultures use silence to express acceptance and agreement and it is not viewed as avoidance or lack of interest.
Conflict resolution	How are conflicts resolved?	Some cultures prefer face-to-face encounters to solve conflict with the belief that dealing with it openly is a positive way to solve the problem. Other cultures do not prefer open conflict and regard it as demeaning and embarrassing. Conflicts must be worked out quietly, without making a scene.

Adapted from Giri (2006); Pratt-Johnson (2006).

duce each other by telling one unique quality about their partner.

When teachers fail to consider cultural issues in their instructional design and delivery, many students feel disengaged, bored, alienated, and, at times, fearful of being embarrassed (Spencer-Cavaliere & Rintoul, 2012). A culturally relevant and sensitive learning experience helps all students to find value in the content, feel as if they belong, and experience interactions with you and their classmates as emotionally safe. Table 6.4 provides examples of how to incorporate social-awareness skills into fitness education lessons.

Table 6.4 Examples of Developing Social-Awareness Skills in Fitness Education

Social-awareness skill	Fitness education examples
Perspective-taking	• Incorporate ParaSport activities into the curriculum, such as goalball or sitting volleyball. • Have students do fitness activities with a blindfold or seated in a chair to get perspective on how people with disabilities engage in exercise.
Empathy	• Create an exercise buddy system for running and circuit-training activities. • Before exercising, have buddies discuss barriers to achieving health-related fitness and encourage them to create a strategy for success in the exercise activity. • Students should engage in active listening to support each other's struggles for obtaining health-enhancing fitness. • Have students reflect on their strategy after the session and then plan for exercise outside of the classroom.
Appreciating diversity	• Incorporate culturally diverse physical activities into the curriculum and explain the how and why of the activities in relationship to their cultural background. • For example, learn a cultural dance or have students teach a playground game that originated from another country.
Respect for others	• Have the class create a set of class norms for how students want to be treated and how they will treat each other. • Have students identify types of communication that show respect and types that show disrespect and then have them sign a commitment to use only respectful communication in the classroom.

INTERPERSONAL COMPETENCIES: RELATIONSHIP SKILLS

The ability to establish and maintain healthy and rewarding relationships with diverse individuals and groups. The ability to communicate clearly, listen well, cooperate with others, resist inappropriate social pressure, negotiate conflict constructively, and seek and offer help when needed (CASEL, 2020).

Table 6.5 shows fitness education learning outcomes that promote the interpersonal competency of relationship skills. Teaching SEL can help you create an inclusive and supportive environment by incorporating relationship-building activities. Building relationships is key to establishing an emotionally safe environment in fitness education. Trust needs to be built between you and your students and also between students so that they feel safe enough taking risks when challenging themselves to improve and comfortable asking for help. Building relationships starts with actions as simple as greeting students by name and creating opportunities for students to get to know you and for you to get to know them within appropriate boundaries. You may need to implement more complex and intentional relationship-building strategies for students who have been affected by trauma.

A recommended strategy for building relationships with struggling students is the 2 by 10 conversation strategy. With this strategy, you aim to have brief, two-minute conversations about anything other than school with a student for 10 consecutive days. The hope is that these conversations provide the opportunity for a relationship to develop and students see that you genuinely care for them as people before you address any academic or behavioral concerns (Fisher & Frey, 2016). Chances are that students affected by trauma will not respond to behavioral interventions unless you have established a rapport with them and they believe they can trust you. The Example Questions for the 2 by 10 Conversation Strategy sidebar shows examples of relationship-builder questions and academic- and behavioral-concern questions to use in the 2 by 10 conversation strategy. You can start with the relationship-builder questions for 10 consecutive days before moving to questions related to students' performance in school.

You are directly supporting the goal of adopting a physically active lifestyle when you help students learn the skills to build relationships. When students have diverse friendship groups they are more likely to engage in physical activity (Jago, Brockman, Fox, Cartwrith, Page, & Thompson, 2009). Access to diverse groups means that when one friend cannot go for a walk, then another friend might be available to play soccer. Students create more options for physical activity engagement when they have more friendship groups. Adolescents are more likely to engage in physical activity when their friends participate with them (Zook, Saksvig, Wu, & Young, 2014). By teaching students the SEL skill of how to build relationships, you are teaching them how to develop friendships that can support a physically active lifestyle.

Building relationships is just as important, if not more so, in the online learning environment because there are fewer face-to-face interactions. Social isolation can be a negative aspect of the remote learning experience if students are unable to interact with their classmates or teacher. As

Table 6.5 Fitness Education Learning Outcomes That Promote Relationship Skills

SHAPE America standard categories and SEL components	Middle school (grades 6-8) SHAPE America grade-level outcomes	High school (grades 9-12) SHAPE America grade-level outcomes
Accepting feedback and working with others (communication and social engagement)	• Provides corrective feedback to a peer using teacher-generated guidelines and incorporating appropriate tone and other communication skills. (S4.M3.7) • Problem-solves with a small group of classmates during adventure activities, small-group initiatives, or game play. (S4.M5.7)	• Uses communication skills and strategies that promote team or group dynamics. (S4.H3.L1) • Assumes a leadership role (e.g., task or group leader, referee, coach) in a physical activity setting. (S4.H3.L2)
Social interaction (relationship building)	• Demonstrates respect for self by asking for help and helping others in various physical activities. (S5.M6.8)	• Evaluates the opportunity for social interaction and social support in a self-selected physical activity or dance. (S5.H4.L2)

Modified from "Crosswalk for SHAPE America National Standards & Grade-Level Outcomes for K-12 Physical Education and CASEL Social and Emotional Learning Core Competencies."

Example Questions for the 2 by 10 Conversation Strategy

Relationship-Builder Questions

- What are your plans for this weekend?
- What is your all-time favorite movie or TV show?
- What physical activity do you do the most?
- Do you have any songs that get you pumped up when you work out?
- How do you spend your time outside of school?
- Who do you most admire? Why?

Academic- and Behavioral-Concern Questions

- What are we doing in class that is helping you reach your goals?
- What assumptions do teachers make about you that are not true?
- What obstacle is holding you back from being successful in this class?
- I want to help you make a plan for where you want to be. If we start with what is most important to you in this class, what would that be?
- How can we communicate respect to each other? (Smith, Fisher, & Frey, 2015)

mentioned previously, according to Maslow's hierarchy, belonging, connection, and relationships are psychological needs that help to promote self-actualization. Humans have an innate desire to create meaningful connections with one another. Social isolation can lead to loneliness, and there is a clear association between loneliness and mental health problems in adolescents (Loades et al., 2020). Establishing social support and creating meaningful connections are protective factors that can prevent students from disengaging from the course and developing mental health problems such as depression or anxiety.

To avoid students experiencing social isolation in your class, it is important that you provide opportunities for them to connect with you and other students in the class. You can start your online sessions with a nonacademic question of the day and have every student type into the chat box a response to the question. When using discussion strategies, you can have students answer a relationship-builder question before responding to the academic content question. You can also help students in the class get to know each other by using the strategy of "student mentions." Student mentions are when you intentionally and relevantly mention facts about your students during direct instruction of the lesson. For example, if you know that your student Alan is an excellent swimmer, when you discuss how swimming can be a great cardiorespiratory fitness activity, mention Alan by name: "Speaking of swimming, Alan, I heard that you won the 50-meter freestyle event last weekend. Congratulations! That is a fantastic accomplishment. Can you tell us what the different swimming events are and show us how the strokes are different?"

In either online or face-to-face classes, you can have students answer several getting-to-know-you questions on a survey so that you can use that information as topics to include in class instruction. The goal is to mention every student in the class at some point during the course. With this strategy, you show students that you care about their interests, while also helping other students know how to possibly start a conversation with their classmates. Now, you have just provided students in your class with a way to engage Alan in a conversation: They can talk to him about swimming and ask him how he is doing at his swimming competitions. Through student mentions, you model to students how to show interest in each other's lives and how to have engaging, relationship-building conversations. Table 6.6 provides examples of how to incorporate relationship skills into a fitness education lesson.

COGNITIVE COMPETENCIES: RESPONSIBLE DECISION MAKING

The ability to make constructive choices about personal behavior and social interactions based on ethical standards, safety concerns, and social norms. The realistic evaluation of consequences of various actions and a consideration of the well-being of oneself and others (CASEL, 2020).

Table 6.6 Examples of Developing Relationship Skills in Fitness Education

Relationship skills	Fitness education examples
Communication	• Use the reciprocal coaching teaching strategy for students to provide feedback to each other on a fitness activity. • Model to students how to use appropriate communication skills to deliver corrective feedback in a positive and constructive manner.
Social engagement	• Use the jigsaw cooperative learning strategy to have students teach each other new information, such as which sources of calcium are good for students who are lactose intolerant or new skills such as eight different ways to do planks in small groups. Give students the choice to teach something that they want to become experts at and that they would like to engage in conversations with others about.
Relationship building	• Using the strategy of student mentions in your direct instruction. • Use the think-pair-share strategy when checking for understanding during the direct instruction portion of your lesson and instruct students to answer a relationship-builder question before the content question. • Survey students to find out their fitness goals and then create exercise groups by interest and common goals (e.g., improving athletic performance, flexibility, or body composition). Have students work in these exercise groups for a few weeks before changing groups. The goal is for students to find someone that they could be active with outside of the school day.
Teamwork	• Have students set individual goals for fitness improvement and then create equal exercise teams according to pretest fitness assessments. Have the team set a goal for how many collective push-ups they will do on a fitness assessment and how many collective PACER laps they will run. Have the teams train for several weeks together (e.g., circuit-training and aerobic-training activities). Teach them how to encourage and hold each other accountable for giving their best effort to support the team at the final fitness assessment.

Table 6.7 demonstrates the fitness education learning outcomes that promote responsible decision-making. Students with responsible decision-making skills can solve problems effectively, exhibit responsible behaviors in various contexts (e.g., school, community, basketball court), realistically evaluate the potential consequences of their actions, and apply ethical standards to personal and social behavior. Decision-making skills can be developed in fitness education by giving students choice in a variety of contexts and promoting self-evaluation of those decisions. The emphasis is on proactive decision making, where students evaluate decisions before they are made to avoid the negative consequences and promote personal and social well-being. The Example Self-Evaluation Questions for Decision-Making Skills sidebar presents several questions that you can use with students to foster proactive, health-related decision-making skills, whereas table 6.8 provides examples of how to incorporate those skills into the fitness education lesson.

Table 6.7 Fitness Education Learning Outcomes That Promote Responsible Decision Making

SHAPE America standard categories and SEL components	Middle school (grades 6-8) SHAPE America grade-level outcomes	High school (grades 9-12) SHAPE America grade-level outcomes
Safety (analyzing situations)	Independently uses physical activity and fitness equipment appropriately, and identifies specific safety concerns associated with the activity. (S4.M7.8)	Applies best practices for participating safely in physical activity, exercise, dance (e.g., injury prevention, proper alignment, hydration, use of equipment, implementation of rules, sun protection). (S4.H5.L1)
Physical activity knowledge (solving problems & reflecting)	Identifies barriers related to maintaining a physically active lifestyle and seeks solutions for eliminating those barriers. (S3.M1.7)	Analyzes the impact of life choices, economics, motivation and accessibility on exercise adherence and participation in physical activity in college or career settings. (S3.H5.L2)

Table 6.8 Examples of Developing Responsible Decision-Making Skills in Fitness Education

Responsible decision-making skills	Fitness education examples
Identifying problems	• Have students engage in writing prompts or having in-class discussions about the problems that adolescents face in maintaining a physically active lifestyle. • Give students case studies that have a person's health profile: height, weight, blood pressure, mile time or PACER score, push-up score, and curl-up score. Ask students to identify potential health-related fitness red flags based upon the person's current health status.
Analyzing situations	• After students have identified the problem(s) in the health-case study, direct them to analyze the person's health by describing how they think those fitness scores were attained and what decisions the person most likely made that resulted in that health profile.
Solving problems	• You can give students an inquiry-guided question, such as "Emilio wants to improve his muscular strength over the summer. However, he does not have access to any resistance-training equipment. Which eight body-weight exercises would you recommend to Emilio that would be the best ones he could use to improve his upper- and lower-body muscular strength?" • Tell students to be prepared to defend their answer.
Evaluating	• Present a current event from the fitness and health field and discuss the decision that was made in that event. Have students evaluate the impact of the decision on the person and the community as well as the quality of the decision. Guide students to discuss an alternative solution to the problem.
Reflecting	• Have students complete a self-reflection sheet that asks them to evaluate their decision making in the class over the past week. The reflection questions can address if the students acted in a safe manner, if they exerted maximal effort on fitness activities, and if they demonstrated respect to their peers. In the reflection, students can describe the consequences of those decisions and how they may change their decisions for the next week.
Ethical responsibility	• Give direct instruction on what ethical responsibility is and the process of ethical decision making. Have students brainstorm which ethical decisions may arise in the fitness and health field. Using the student-generated scenarios, organize students into discussion groups and have them discuss how they would respond to the ethical decision.

Example Self-Evaluation Questions for Decision-Making Skills

- Safety: Does this choice put others or me at risk for physical harm?
- Ethical standards: Does this choice violate my personal values or the norms of the classroom?
- Well-being of others: Does this choice have an impact on others' emotional, mental, or social well-being?
- My present and future well-being: Will this choice have an impact on my present or my future well-being?
- Empathy: Will my actions represent how I want to be treated in this situation?

INTRAPERSONAL COMPETENCIES: SELF-AWARENESS

The ability to accurately recognize one's own emotions, thoughts, and values and how they influence behavior. The ability to accurately assess one's strengths and limitations, with a well-grounded sense of confidence, optimism, and a 'growth mindset' (CASEL, 2020).

Students with self-awareness skills can identify emotions, recognize their strengths, maintain an accurate and positive self-concept, and experience a sense of self-efficacy. Having self-awareness is the foundation for physical activity behavior change and behavior maintenance. As stated in chapter 1, an estimated 80 percent of adolescents do not participate in the recommended 60 minutes of daily physical activity levels, so there are significant barriers and motivational issues that students must be able to overcome to develop the habit of regular physical activity. Table 6.9 shows fitness education outcomes that promote the interpersonal competency of self-awareness, and table 6.10 provides examples of how self-awareness skills can be integrated throughout fitness education lessons.

Students who are self-aware recognize if they need to make behavioral changes to achieve health-enhancing fitness and have the mindset to be able to overcome challenges to changing their behavior. Students with a growth mindset view challenges as tasks to overcome rather than feeling

Table 6.9 Fitness Education Learning Outcomes That Promote Self-Awareness

SHAPE America standard categories and SEL components	Middle school (grades 6-8) SHAPE America grade-level outcomes	High school (grades 9-12) SHAPE America grade-level outcomes
Challenge (accurate self-perception and recognizing strengths)	Recognizes individual challenges and copes in a positive way, such as extending effort, asking for help or feedback, or modifying tasks. (S5. M3.6) Develops a plan of action and makes appropriate decisions based on that plan when faced with an individual challenge. (S5.M3.8)	Chooses an appropriate level of challenge to experience success and desire to participate in a self-selected physical activity. (S5.H2.L2)
Self-expression and enjoyment (identifying emotions)	Identifies and participates in an enjoyable activity that prompts individual self-expression. (S5.M5.8)	Selects and participates in physical activities or dance that meet the need for self-expression and enjoyment. (S5.H3.L1)

Table 6.10 Examples of Developing Self-Awareness Skills in Fitness Education

Self-awareness skill	Fitness education examples
Accurate self-perception	• Have students engage in self-assessments of health-related and skill-related physical fitness. • Have students engage in regular journal writing activities. This could be a thought journal where students track self-talk to determine if they use more negative or positive self-talk in certain situations. • Have students ask for feedback on different tasks (e.g., exercise technique and written assignments).
Identifying emotions	• Either through discussion strategies or writing prompts, have students reflect on emotions during and after the activity to determine the following: – Which emotions are they experiencing and what is triggering those emotions (e.g., enjoyment, frustration, boredom)? – What can they change to experience more positive emotions? For example, if they are not enjoying the activity, how can they make it more enjoyable? Or how can changing some aspect of the activity make it less frustrating?
Recognizing strengths	• Students can use self-assessments of health-related and skill-related physical fitness to identify personal strengths and where improvement is needed. • Have students engage in cooperative activities that allow students to select a role in completing a task.
Self-confidence	• Provide positive reinforcement during which you and student peers give students sincere compliments on their performances during learning tasks.
Self-efficacy	• Use developmentally appropriate fitness activities that allow students to choose the appropriate level of challenge that will lead to success. • Have students watch demonstrations of peers succeeding in the assigned task to build confidence in the ability that it can be done.

discouraged or defeated by something they do not get right away. A growth mindset will influence students' motivation to learn and improve. If they believe that they can learn and improve through effort and perseverance, then they are more motivated to engage in behaviors that lead to the desired change. In addition, students with a growth mindset use constructive feedback, while students with a fixed mindset typically ignore constructive feedback, which can hinder their ability to improve (Dweck, 2007; Saunders, 2013). Table 6.11 exhibits the differences between the two mindsets.

In addition to having a growth mindset, students will enhance their effort and ability to persevere in achieving goals by having high self-efficacy. *Self-efficacy* is a main principle in social cognitive theory (SCT), one of the most frequently applied theories of health behavior to understand how to regulate behavior that can be maintained over time (LaMorte, 2019). Self-efficacy is people's belief in their capacity to perform the behaviors necessary to achieve a specific goal (Bandura, 1997). Self-efficacy is task-specific, meaning that people's belief in their ability is specific to a given behavior. Your students may have self-efficacy in their ability to perform cardiorespiratory-fitness workouts, but that does not translate to a high self-efficacy to perform resistance-training workouts. Their confidence or self-efficacy in cardiorespiratory-fitness workouts is most likely affected by how successful they have been in the past and how they have witnessed their peers also being successful in their ability to do aerobic fitness training. Many students may not have self-efficacy when it comes to activities such as push-ups because they have not been able to perform push-ups correctly. In addition, they may not see very many of their peers be able to improve their push-ups. Thus, they have low confidence in their ability to actually improve their push-up performance. A student who has repeatedly failed to perform one correct standard push-up may develop the belief that she cannot perform a push-up and give up trying.

Push-ups, like all other fitness activities, will require applying the principles of overload and progression for the physiological changes to occur so that students are strong enough to perform a standard push-up. Many physical education teachers may not use or know how to use developmentally appropriate progressions to help their students perform fitness activities like a standard push-up, leaving it up to students to figure out how to get strong enough to do one. Unfortunately, repeated failure may lead to self-doubt and a decrease in self-confidence, so students do not even attempt to improve their push-ups. If you want your students to persevere until they can perform a standard push-up, then you need to provide them with tasks that they can successfully perform to develop the self-efficacy to continue exercising until they achieve the goal. Table 6.12 shows an example of how to help students who cannot do one correct

Table 6.11 Fixed Versus Growth Mindset Fitness Education Examples

Fixed mindset	Growth mindset
• Achieving healthy physical fitness is for athletes. I am not an athlete. • My physical fitness level will not change. I do not have the right genetics or body type to become fit. • I can either do it or I can't do it. If I can't do the exercises at first, then I will just stick with what I know I can do.	• Achieving healthy physical fitness is for everyone. Physical fitness is not exclusive to athletes or fit people. • Everyone can improve their physical fitness if they increase their effort. No matter what my fitness level is, I can always improve by engaging in training. • Challenging exercises help me to improve my physical fitness. I want to put in the effort to see what I can achieve.

Table 6.12 Mastery Experience Example: Progress to a Push-Up Checklist

Challenge levels	Challenge task to master	Workout routine
Level 1	High plank: hold for 60 sec	3 sets per day, holding for as many minutes as you can, with 2-min rest breaks between each set, performed 3 times per week on nonconsecutive days until you can accomplish this level
Level 2	High-plank shoulder taps: perform for 45 sec without stopping	
Level 3	Low plank: hold for 60 sec	
Level 4	Alternating plank-up push-ups: perform for 45 sec without stopping	
Level 5	Knee push-ups: perform 10 consecutively with perfect form	
Level 6	Incline push-ups: perform 10 consecutively with perfect form	
Mastery task: Perform a standard push-up with perfect form.		

standard push-up. Using challenge levels and matching an appropriate workout to that challenge level gives students a sense of control over how they can achieve their goal. As they move up the challenge levels, they develop higher levels of self-efficacy as they see that they are getting closer to achieving the goal. If they have success in level 1, that will provide the confidence and motivation to move to level 2, and that continues with success at each level until students reach the mastery task. After that mastery task is completed, then a new set of challenge levels and challenge tasks can be created to master a more difficult task.

Self-efficacy is one of the strongest and most consistent predictors of *exercise adherence* (Sherwood & Jeffery, 2000). Therefore, if you want your students to engage in physical activity for life, the most likely and effective way is by having them increase their self-efficacy for doing physical activity. Self-efficacy is developed through observational learning, which involves observing others successfully performing the behavior and by past experiences. Success in a past experience increases self-efficacy, while failure in a past experience decreases self-efficacy. When you design learning experiences, it is critical that you consider how each student in your class can achieve success. This is an example of the UDL approach described in chapter 3—proactively determining modifications that students may need to experience success.

Growth Mindset for Teachers

In addition to students needing to develop a growth mindset, teachers need to continue to expand their mindset as well. Over 30 years ago, Dr. Carol Dweck coined the terms *fixed mindset* and *growth mindset* (Dweck, 2007). The idea of mindset is related to our understanding of where ability comes from. Educators have recently begun using it as a tool to explore our knowledge of student achievement and its improvement. Fixed mindset can be described as the belief that your abilities, and consequently your successes and failures, are innate. A growth mindset can be characterized as the belief that success is based on learning, persistence, and hard work. People with fixed mindsets dread failure. They feel that it reflects badly upon themselves as individuals, while people with growth mindsets instead embrace failure as an opportunity to learn and improve their abilities. However, it is possible and desirable to shift from a fixed mindset to a growth mindset.

While most mindset studies related to education have been conducted with students, the implication for teachers is obvious. If we help teachers shift to a growth mindset, they can model this for students, and everyone benefits. The school setting provides multiple opportunities for teachers to try new things and make mistakes. This can seem difficult for teachers, but it is essential for developing a growth mindset. A key principle of growth mindset is the willingness to try new approaches (Gerstein, 2014). As part of creating this opportunity, it is important to ask, "What will teachers and the school learn as part of the process?" It is the process that reflects the learning, not whether there was success or failure. Teachers should be given time to reflect on this, and administrators should urge them to take chances.

INTRAPERSONAL COMPETENCIES: SELF-MANAGEMENT SKILLS

The ability to regulate one's emotions, thoughts, and behaviors effectively in different situations. This includes managing stress, controlling impulses, motivating oneself, and setting and working toward achieving personal and academic goals (CASEL, 2020).

Students with self-management skills can regulate emotions; manage stress; set effective goals; and utilize self-motivation, self-discipline, and organizational skills to achieve them. Self-management skills provide students with the ability to change their behavior so that they are thinking, feeling, and acting in ways that support their health and the health of others. The primary goal of fitness education is exercise adherence, or maintaining physical activity behavior for life, to acquire the benefits of disease prevention and health promotion. Therefore, self-management skills are an essential component of the fitness education curriculum and instruction. Learning outcomes that promote self-management are shown in table 6.13, and table 6.14 provides examples of developing self-management skills in fitness education. Without teaching students self-management skills, the likelihood that they will change sedentary behavior habits and maintain a physically active lifestyle is very low. Some students may get fit during class, but then fail to maintain that behavior over time and relapse back into their old patterns of sedentary behavior once the class has ended. You must be able to apply motivational strategies that help students not only engage in fitness activities during class but also maintain the motivation to continue using self-management skills to remain active after the class has ended.

Table 6.13 Fitness Education Learning Outcomes That Promote Self-Management

SHAPE America standard categories and SEL components	Middle school (grades 6-8) SHAPE America grade-level outcomes	High school (grades 9-12) SHAPE America grade-level outcomes
Personal responsibility (self-discipline)	Uses effective self-monitoring skills to incorporate opportunities for physical activity in and outside of school. (S4.M2.8)	Employs effective self-management skills to analyze barriers and modify physical activity patterns appropriately as needed. (S4.H1.L1)
Stress management	Identifies positive and negative results of stress and appropriate ways of dealing with each. (S3.M18.6)	Applies stress-management strategies (e.g., mental imagery, relaxation techniques, deep breathing, aerobic exercise, meditation) to reduce stress. (S3.H14.L2)
Engages in physical activity (self-motivation)	Participates in self-selected activity outside of physical education class. (S3.M2.6)	Participates several times a week in a self-selected lifetime activity, dance, or fitness activity outside of the school day. (S3.H6.L1)
Goal setting	Sets and monitors a self-selected physical-activity goal for aerobic and/or muscle- and bone-strengthening activity based on current fitness level. (S3.M8.6)	Develops and maintains a fitness portfolio (e.g., assessment scores, goals for improvement, plan of activities for improvement, log of activities being done to reach goals, time line for improvement). (S3.H11.L2)

Modified from "Crosswalk for SHAPE America National Standards & Grade-Level Outcomes for K-12 Physical Education and CASEL Social and Emotional Learning Core Competencies."

Table 6.14 Examples of Developing Self-Management Skills in Fitness Education

Self-management skills	Fitness education examples
Impulse control	• Teach students positive self-talk strategies to use when stressful situations become overwhelming. • Assign "control buddies" to students who may have impulse-control issues. Control buddies can monitor their buddy for signs of being triggered and proactively intervene with strategies to reduce frustration, anger, or tension.
Stress management	• Teach a cognitive lesson on the mental and emotional benefits of exercise. Discuss how different types of exercise have different effects on a person's emotional health. For example, aerobic exercise can be used for muscular meditation because it uses large muscle groups in a rhythmic, repetitive fashion. Exercise reduces levels of stress hormones in the body. • Have students keep a journal that tracks their levels of stress and how much exercise they get on each day for several weeks. After a few weeks, have students analyze if there are any associations between types of physical activity they do or how much and their stress level changes.
Self-discipline	• Have students self-monitor their SMART goal progress over several weeks by completing weekly reflections on if they are meeting their short-term goals. Have them identify barriers to accomplishing their short-term goals and discuss strategies for overcoming those barriers in the next week.
Self-motivation	• Get to know students' physical activity interests and design learning experiences around those interest areas. • Allow for students to choose their level of challenge that will build self-efficacy.
Goal setting	• Use the process in table 6.19 to help students set effective SMART goals for improving their health-related fitness.
Organizational skills	• Have students develop a weekly plan for all of their required activities. Then, have the students organize their schedule to include the recommended physical activity minutes. The objective is for them to prioritize getting the recommended amount of physical activity by organizing their schedules.

Types of Motivation

Motivation is the starting point for developing a physically active lifestyle. Students must first be willing to initiate changing their sedentary behavior before they will start doing any physical activity. *Social determination theory (SDT)* is a theory of motivation that suggests a person's motivation to engage in certain behaviors is influenced by the degree to which their behavior is self determined. People want to perform behaviors out of their own self-determination rather than feeling controlled by an external source (e.g., reward, praise, recognition) to perform. When people feel that what they do will have an effect on the outcome, they are more motivated to take action. *Intrinsic motivation* describes the most self-determined form of motivation. When individuals are intrinsically motivated, they perform activities simply for the enjoyment, interest, or satisfaction of engaging in the activity. *Extrinsic motivation*, however, is just the opposite—it is not self-determined. When individuals are extrinsically motivated, they feel more controlled by external sources to succeed than in control and determined to succeed for their own satisfaction. Extrinsic motivation is a drive to achieve something as a means to an alternative end. The Examples of Extrinsic and Intrinsic Motivation sidebar shows examples that differentiate extrinsic from intrinsic motivation.

Students in your class may be motivated to engage in physical activities to earn a good grade. Unfortunately, engaging in physical activity out of fear of receiving a poor grade will not be a factor that motivates a student to continue with physical activity once the class is over. Grades are a form of extrinsic motivation that control or motivate students' short-term behavior, but externally driven motivators typically do not lead to sustained behavior change (Teixeira, Carraça, Markland, Silva, & Ryan, 2012). Those who regularly adhere to physical activity report that enjoyment is their primary reason for continuing to engage in physical activity (Edmunds, Ntoumanis, & Duda, 2006). Therefore, to meet the goals of a lifetime of physical activity, we want students to develop an intrinsic motivation to exercise—they choose to do it because they enjoy it.

How, then, do you influence students' self-determined motivation? According to SDT, motivation is influenced by the psychological needs of autonomy, competence, and relatedness. When these three needs are met in the fitness education environment, students will yield more self-determined motivation to engage in physical activity behavior and learning experiences. Fitness education can promote exercise adherence when you intentionally create a motivational climate that meets these three needs featured in table 6.15. Examples of how those needs can be met or potentially undermined in a fitness education class are also shown in the table.

Examples of Extrinsic and Intrinsic Motivation

- *Extrinsic.* I don't feel like studying for my exam, but I don't want to fail it and then possibly fail the class. I feel controlled to have to study because the teacher will not let me pass this class if I don't pass the exam. My behavior is driven by a desire to receive a passing grade.
- *Intrinsic.* I choose to study the materials for the exam because I want to learn about the topic and I enjoy becoming more knowledgeable about the information. I don't feel controlled by the consequence of the exam because I like learning about the topics and want to be able to use the information to better myself. My behavior is inspired by my pleasure of learning and becoming competent in the content.
- *Extrinsic.* I choose to exercise because I feel like I should so that I don't gain weight. I hate running, but I know that is the best way to burn calories. I run so that I burn more calories. My behavior is driven by the guilt of gaining weight and the hope that running, despite my dislike of it, is the best thing I can do to avoid the guilt.
- *Intrinsic.* I choose to exercise because I enjoy being active. I like doing workouts with my friends because we have a good time challenging each other to get better. My behavior is driven by how much I enjoy being active with my friends.

Table 6.15 Self-Determination Theory: The Psychological Needs of Motivation

Needs	Supported by	Hindered by
Relatedness: social connections to others reflected by feelings of acceptance and belonging	• Inclusive environment • Respect • Empathy • Trust	• Competition • Cliques • Criticism • Social hierarchy
Competence: sense of success and being effective in one's environment	• Credible and corrective feedback • Appropriate level of challenge	• Inappropriate level of challenge (e.g., too difficult) • Minimal and/or ineffective feedback
Autonomy: feelings of personal choice or control	• Choice • Rationale for activities • Confidence in abilities	• Self-doubt • Assigned goals • Too many teacher-directed activities

Adapted by permission from M. Standage, T. Curran, and P.C. Rouse, "Self-Determination-Based Theories of Sport, Exercise, and Physical Activity Motivation, in *Advances in Sport and Exercise Psychology*, 4th ed., edited by T.S. Horn and A.L. Smith (Champaign, IL: Human Kinetics, 2019), 302.

Lack of motivation is a significant student-related barrier in fitness education. Motivation directly affects the level of effort students put into the learning tasks and performing the fitness activities. When students are motivated, they eliminate distractions, focus on completing the task well, choose behaviors that lead to goal attainment, and sustain those behaviors despite adversity to achieve goals (Burton & Raedeke, 2008). Higher motivation will equal greater gains in learning and in health-related fitness outcomes, and those gains lead to greater competence and confidence. The next section discusses how it is possible to create a classroom climate that increases students' motivation levels.

Develop a Mastery-Oriented Environment

In general, there are two types of motivational climates that teachers can create: a *mastery-oriented climate*, also referred to as a *task-oriented climate*, or an *ego-oriented climate*, also referred to as a *performance-oriented climate*. Motivational climates are influenced by different factors such as how success is defined, which behaviors the teacher has reinforced, and how errors in performance are addressed. Studies consistently indicate that a mastery-oriented climate promotes feelings of enjoyment, commitment, confidence, and perceived competence more than an ego-oriented climate (Alesi, Gómez-López, Chicau Borrego, Monteiro, & Granero-Gallegos, 2019; Harwood, Keegan, Smith, & Raine, 2015). An ego-oriented climate can create feelings of boredom, frustration, worry, anxiety, and apathy because of the fear of failure and the potential display of demonstrating poorly in front of others (Bortoli, Bertollo, Comani, & Robazza, 2011; García-González, Sevil-Serrano, Abós, Aelterman, & Haerens, 2019). Table 6.16 lists the characteristics of each type of motivational climate and can be used to conduct a self-evaluation of the type of motivational climate that you may be creating by how you structure your class and deliver instruction. Table 6.17 provides specific examples of teacher behaviors that can contribute to developing either a mastery- or ego-oriented climate in fitness education.

It can be visibly apparent what type of motivational climate a teacher has created by the number of students sitting on the sidelines. Fitness education is inclusive and designed for all students to participate and improve their health-related fitness. Your responsibility is to establish a motivational climate in which students never want to sit out of activities, and if they do have a limitation, you are there to provide them with a modification to keep them engaged. In order for students to have a positive experience in fitness education that translates into positive attitudes toward fitness and adopting a physically active lifestyle, teachers must create a mastery-oriented motivational climate.

You can promote a mastery motivational climate that emphasizes effort, learning, accomplishment, and enjoyment of fitness by using the TARGET structure in your instructional design and delivery. As shown in table 6.18, the decisions that you make in task structure, student choice, delivering feedback, grouping students, evaluating progress, and time management will impact your students' intrinsic motivation to engage in the learning experiences. Think of these principles as your way to target students' self-determined motivation to

Table 6.16 Characteristics of Mastery- and Ego-Oriented Motivational Climates

Climate factors	Mastery-oriented climate	Ego-oriented climate
Definition of success	Individual progress and improvement	Winning or outperforming others
How to set goals	Self referenced (compare only to your own performance)	Norm referenced (compare to others' performance)
What is valued by the teacher	Giving maximal effort to the learning process and activities	Achieving results and demonstrating high ability
Reasons for student satisfaction	Hard work, challenging self to improve, overcoming obstacles	Outperforming others, being the best
View of competition	Compete with yourself	Compete with your peers
View of cooperation	Help others learn, be a good teammate	Take care of yourself first
View of mistakes	Part of the learning process, opportunity for growth	Mistakes are punished, there are consequences for poor performance
Reasons for effort	Skill development, learning new knowledge, and self-improvement	Recognition of ability and social status
Feedback	All students receive positive reinforcement when they work hard and demonstrate improvement	High-ability students receive the most attention and recognition
Evaluation criteria	Self-comparison of skill improvement, progress toward mastery of the learning outcomes	Normative comparisons—how skill compares to others' performances
Focus of attention	Learning process "How can I do better?"	Performance outcomes "How did I do?"

Adapted by permission from C. Ames and J. Archer, Achievement Goals in the Classroom: Students' Learning Strategies and Motivation Processes," *Journal of Educational Psychology* 80 (1988): 260-267.

Table 6.17 Examples of Fitness Education Teacher Behaviors in Mastery- and Ego-Oriented Climates

Mastery-oriented climate	Ego-oriented climate
• If many students in the class performed poorly on the PACER exam, the teacher would individually speak to students to determine the cause of the poor performance and help them to set goals for improvement. • To increase intensity of an activity, the teacher may use competitive-type activities in which rules are designed so that all students must participate. Winning is not the focus; instead, teamwork and putting forth full effort are emphasized. • Students are encouraged and expected to congratulate each other on high-quality performances and their demonstration of teamwork and putting forth exceptional effort. • All students receive feedback on their performance and are praised when they improve upon their performance in some way. • Students are encouraged to set personal fitness goals that they want to achieve and are realistic for them.	• If many students in the class performed poorly on the PACER exam, the teacher would have students run the PACER every class session for two weeks as punishment for poor performance. • The teacher frequently uses competitive activities, such as relays, to determine a winner, and students who have low fitness levels are allowed to sit out of activities to help their team win. • The teacher posts students' fitness testing scores and encourages students to try and beat their classmates on the next fitness test. • Students who cannot perform exercises properly are not given feedback unless they ask for it. • Praise is most often given to students who excel on the fitness tests or the cognitive exams. • Students are encouraged to "max out" on fitness performances, such as the push-up test, and poor form is often overlooked so that students can achieve a high score. • Students with high fitness levels get special privileges that students with low fitness levels do not get.

perform their best in the fitness education environment.

The teacher's role in creating and regulating the climate is important to establishing a sense of security for students to learn and perform in fitness education. You develop an emotionally safe environment for all students when you establish the expectations of a positive, mastery-oriented motivational climate and then hold students accountable to behaviors that support that type

Table 6.18 TARGET Principles for Developing a Mastery-Oriented Climate

TARGET principles	Psychological need addressed by principle	Strategies for a mastery-oriented climate
Task: the design of the learning task, how students engage with the content, what they will learn	Competence: tasks are designed for learning; students are provided with the resources they need to be successful in the task	• Have students set self-referenced goals for improvement • Differentiate tasks to match appropriate level of challenge
Authority: the kind and frequency of participation in the decision-making process for the class and the learning experiences	Autonomy: students feel as if they have choices and that they can exert personal responsibility in the class	• Involve students in decision making, such as allowing them to select activities • Give students leadership roles • Allow for student choice in a variety of tasks
Recognition: how students are motivated and recognized for their progress and achievement	Relatedness: students feel cared for by the teacher when the teacher acknowledges their progress and perseverance	• Give individualized recognition of improvement and effort • Emphasize learning from mistakes
Grouping: the ways in which students are grouped or interact with each other during class	Relatedness: students have the opportunity to develop friendships and connections through cooperative activities and social interaction	• Create mixed-ability groups that encourage inclusion and cooperation to avoid creating cliques • Design small, flexible groups that can be regrouped to meet different purposes and help students get to know more classmates
Evaluation: how assessment of learning is conducted, the standards that are used to evaluate performance	Competence: students have criteria that they can compare their progress to and they can track improvement in a meaningful way Autonomy: students are able to choose ways to assess progress based upon their needs (not a one-size-fits-all approach)	• Base your evaluation criteria on effort, improvement, persistence, and progress toward individual goals • Vary the assessment methods • Design assessments that will show individual progress toward mastery of the outcomes
Time: how time is controlled in the learning process: pacing, deadlines, schedules	Autonomy: when students are demonstrating effort and commitment, allow them to have flexible time lines for learning that don't create unnecessary pressure to perform	• Create flexible task completion deadlines to accommodate students' needs • Ask students to schedule improvement time lines to meet the learning outcomes that avoid overwhelming performance anxiety

Adapted by permission from J. Liukkonen et al., *Psychology for Physical Educators: Student in Focus*, 2nd ed. (Champaign, IL: Human Kinetics, 2007), 5.

of environment. In the fitness education setting, some students may be ego-oriented and want to show how dominant they are in fitness activities. These students may expect to receive special treatment based upon their athleticism and may make remarks about other students' lack of fitness or motor-skill competency because that is how they acted in previous situations. Other students may be experiencing toxic stress due to trauma, which may lead to hyperactivity (the inability to contain anxious energy), or hypoactivity (the inability to engage due to lack of energy). Students impacted by trauma may find it difficult to focus, solve problems, or work with others and can be prone to emotional outbursts if something triggers them (Keels, 2018).

You must be attentive to what students are saying, how they are behaving, and how they are responding to instruction to know if your strategies are supporting all students. Security is created by predictability, and you create predictability through consistent behaviors such as treating all students with respect, providing equitable learning opportunities, confronting disrespect, and holding all students accountable to the behavioral expectations. Students will be more inclined to learn more and perform better when they can trust you to consistently operate with their best interests in mind.

Self-Management Strategies: Goal Setting

A mastery-oriented motivational climate sets the stage for students to develop the intrinsic motivation to improve their health-related fitness by regularly engaging in physical activity. Motivated students who apply self-management strategies can create a pattern of sustained physical activity. Motivation leads to participation, participation leads to competence, competence leads to self-efficacy, and self-efficacy fosters greater motivation to continue being active (Jefferies, Ungar, Aubertin, & Kriellaars, 2019). Competence and self-efficacy are more likely to be established when students experience success from their participation. Success in physical activity participation relies specifically on effective goal setting and self-monitoring. Goal setting has been found to be one of the most successful strategies in increasing adolescent physical activity behavior and improving their health-related fitness (Calkins, 2015; Matthew & Moran, 2011; Rose et al., 2017).

Goal-Setting Strategies in Fitness Education

Goal setting is a specific, observable self-management skill that you can teach and assess. Goals are a major component of the fitness education curriculum because they influence students' decision-making, keeping them dedicated and committed to completing learning tasks (Morisano, 2013). While research clearly shows that goal setting can improve learning as well as health and fitness outcomes, not all types of goals are equally effective in bringing about results. Goal setting is a skill that students must learn to do, which means you must teach them how to set effective goals. Steps to teaching the goal-setting process that will help your students be able to create effective goals can be seen in table 6.19.

Types of Goals

A major characteristic of developing a mastery-oriented motivational climate is to have students set self-referenced goals. The reason that self-referenced goals will promote a more positive climate is that students only have control over their own effort; they do not have control over anyone else's performance. Outcome goals are problematic in that (1) students could achieve the goal without it even being a challenge, depending on the performance of others, and (2) even students' absolute best effort may not be enough to achieve the goal. To increase motivation, instruct students to set goals that they have control over so that only their efforts will be the deciding factor in goal attainment.

As seen in table 6.20, process and performance goals are both self-referenced goals. Performance goals focus more on the product of performance, so it can be used to track improvement of health-related fitness components. Process goals focus more on behaviors that will lead to better performance.

Table 6.19 How to Teach Goal Setting in Fitness Education

Step order	Step component	Description of the component
Step 1	Conduct a self-assessment	• Provide information about what may need improvement—the "what" of the goal. • Examples include fitness tests, 3-day nutrition tracking, and 5-day hydration tracking.
Step 2	Teach components of goal setting	• List types of goals (e.g., process, performance, outcome). • Use the SMART framework.
Step 3	Introduce the goal-setting learning task	Elements of an effective goal-setting learning task include being • developmentally appropriate for students' level of maturity and content knowledge and • relevant to course outcomes and student interest.
Step 4	Engage in goal-directed learning experiences	• Provide opportunities in class for students to engage in learning experiences that support their goal. • Refer to students' goals regularly so they do not forget about them.
Step 5	Monitor goal progress	• Have students track their progress with a self-monitoring strategy. • Provide feedback on students' progress and help them determine if they need to make changes to their behavior to attain the goal.
Step 6	Evaluate goal-attainment process	Have students complete a reflection process that asks them if they attained their goal. If they answer "yes," ask the following questions: • What strategy was most beneficial to attaining your goal? What advice would you give to others who have the same goal? If they answer "no," ask this question instead: • What obstacle interfered with you reaching your goal and what changes will you make to your plan so you are successful the next time?

Table 6.20 Types of Goals in Fitness Education

Goal type	Goal description	Fitness education example
Process	Use self-referenced goals that focus on a process rather than a product or goals that focus on performing behaviors that contribute to outcomes.	Setting a goal for physical activity behavior: I am going to participate in 30 minutes of moderate to vigorous physical activity for 5 days this week. Or Setting a goal for technique: I will keep my knees behind my toes and my heels on the ground when I perform a body-weight squat.
Performance	Use self-referenced goals that focus on improvements relative to one's own past. These goals are normally based upon numerical critiera that can be measured.	I will increase my current push-up score by 4 push-ups after training for 5 weeks.
Outcome	Use norm-referenced goals that describe one's performance relative to the performance of others. There is social comparison of performances.	I will perform more PACER laps than any other student in the class.

These types of goals would be used in developing physical activity habits and in achieving proper form for various fitness activities.

The SMART Framework

An effective goal is like a map: It gives you the directions for how to get to where you want to be. The specific, measurable, achievable, realistic, and time-bound (SMART) framework (see table 6.21) is a template you can use to fill in the directions for your destination. Goals work as a motivational factor in fitness education if students can reach their goals and experience the satisfaction of accomplishment. Efforts to set and track goals deteriorate when students believe that goals are unattainable and their effort is a waste of time.

Introducing the Goal-Setting Learning Task

When you design a goal-setting learning task, you want to consider if it is developmentally appropriate for your students' cognitive capacity and their level of content knowledge. Students may lack the content knowledge to understand how to set a realistic fitness goal if they have not learned any of the fitness-training principles and the training adaptations that happen as a result of applying those principles. They most likely could not write an appropriate fitness goal if they don't know how to use FITT in achieving health-related fitness. Middle school students may lack the cognitive capacity to understand the cause and effect of goal setting because it may be too abstract (DeMink-Carthew,

Table 6.21 The SMART Goal Framework

Specific	Target a specific area of improvement. Make sure the goal is something that you can measure and you can say "yes" or "no" to achieving it. Avoid general goals, such as "to get in shape," that include multiple components and aren't specific enough to know what to measure.
Measurable	The goal must have some way that it can be quantified. How will you measure it? What self-monitoring strategies (e.g., apps, journals, planner) will you use to track your progress?
Achievable	The goal is achievable through a defined plan that uses the necessary steps to accomplish the goal.
Realistic	The goal is realistic and reasonable given the resources available. It should be challenging so that you have to exert considerable effort but remain possible. Keep in mind that for goals related to improving health-related fitness, it can take time for training adaptations to occur, so it may not be realistic to improve your cardiorespiratory fitness by 25% in 2 weeks, but 10% may be a more realistic goal in that time frame.
Time-bound	The goal needs a deadline so that you can work backward to plan what you need to do each day, week, month, etc., to achieve the goal. Each long-term goal should be accompanied by short-term goals or progress checkpoints. If your goal is to lose four pounds in one month, translate that goal into a short-term goal of losing one pound each week. Then, create another short-term goal for what you must do each day to accomplish the weekly goal of losing one pound.

Olofson, LeGeros, Netcoh, & Hennessey, 2017). As they develop higher-level thinking skills, students start understanding how their current behavior may cause a future outcome. For these reasons, you may choose to utilize more teacher-directed goal-setting learning tasks with students. Teachers determine *teacher-directed goal-setting learning tasks,* the content and structure of the goal-setting task. *Student-centered goal-setting learning tasks* are the content and structure of the goal-setting task that students primarily control. Figure 6.5 shows how different types of goal-setting learning tasks can be more teacher directed or more student directed along a continuum. On one side of the continuum are self-set goals, which students have complete control over; on the other side are assigned goals, which teachers have complete control over. Tables 6.22 and 6.23 provide the details to help you know how to select an appropriate goal-setting learning task.

Keep in mind that the purpose of fitness education goal setting is to motivate students to direct their efforts toward accomplishing learning tasks or fitness activities that improve their health-related fitness knowledge. Part of that motivational process is determining which type of goal-setting learning

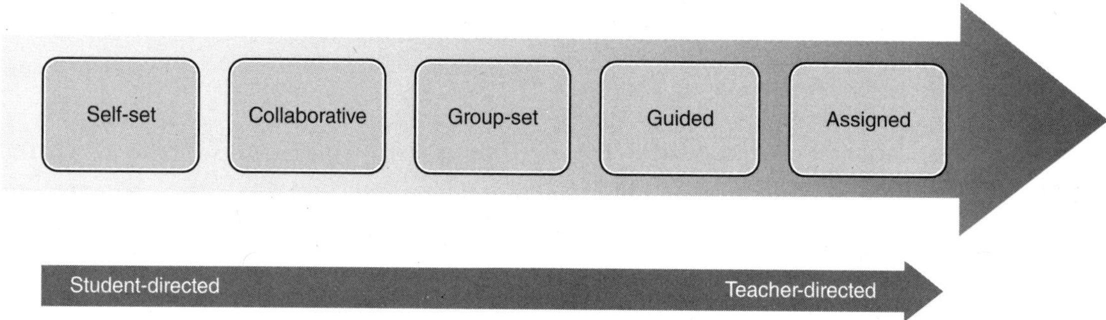

Figure 6.5 The continuum of student-centered and teacher-centered goal-setting learning tasks.

Table 6.22 Student-Centered and Teacher-Centered Goal-Setting Learning Tasks

Type	Description	Fitness education example
Self-set	Goals are chosen and designed by the student.	"Set a goal to improve some aspect of your physical health."
Collaborative	Goals are chosen and designed jointly by the teacher and the student.	The student must set a goal to improve some aspect of health-related fitness; the teacher works with the student to select the most appropriate goal.
Group-set	The class and the teacher decided upon a goal that everyone in the class will work to achieve, or small groups of students work together on a small-group goal. Each member of the group will have to report progress toward the goal.	"Everyone in class, including me, will participate in 30 minutes of moderate to vigorous physical activity for five days this week."
Guided	The teacher designs multiple goal choices, and the student selects a goal.	The teacher designs several goal-setting sheets that provide a framework for achivieng the goal. For example: Hydration goal: Drink eight glasses of water each day for two weeks. Nutrition goal: Eat one serving of vegetables at lunch each day this week. Physical activity goal: Walk for 20 minutes five days a week for two weeks. Students select which goal they want to work toward and follow the directions for monitoring that goal.
Assigned	Goals are chosen and designed by the teacher without the student's input.	"Set a goal to improve your muscular-endurance fitness test score (for example, a push-up score)."

Adapted by permission from M.K. Shilts, M. Horowitz, and M.S. Townsend, "Goal Setting as a Strategy for Dietary and Physical Activity Behavior Change: A Review of the Literature," *American Journal of Health Promotion* 19, no. 2 (2004): 8-93.

Table 6.23 How to Select an Appropriate Goal-Setting Learning Task

Type	Recommended for students who	Not recommended for students who
Self-set	• have been taught effective goal-setting guidelines such as the SMART framework and who understand how to analyze their current level of physical fitness or health with appropriate assessments and • are self-motivated and have a high level of personal responsibility.	• have minimal content knowledge on effective goal setting or do not know how to assess their current fitness and health status and • lack the maturity to recognize their own strengths and needs for improvement.
Collaborative	• have been taught effective goal-setting guidelines such as the SMART framework and • may need help in analyzing their current level of physical fitness or need teacher-guided direction to determine appropriate strategies for goal attainment.	• have minimal content knowledge on effective goal setting and • lack the maturity to have a conversation with the teacher about their progress.
Group-set	• will act personally and socially responsible in trying to achieve the group goals, • are comfortable working in group settings, and • can demonstrate several SEL competencies.	• may refuse to participate due to their lack of trust (e.g., the first few weeks of a course, students do not yet feel safe in the classroom environment or do not yet know others in the class) and • are unable to demonstrate several SEL competencies.
Guided	• are beginning to learn effective goal-setting guidelines and • need practice designing effective goals.	• have had a lot of goal-setting instruction and practice, are self-motivated, and have a high level of personal responsibility.
Assigned	• have disabilities that limit their ability to provide input on their goals. Note: IEP team members may work together to create an appropriate prescribed goal for their students' performance.	• like the autonomy to choose what and how they improve their health and fitness and • may feel controlled to perform certain behaviors by teacher-imposed goals.

task students will experience the most success with. Depending on your students and context, you may start your fitness education course with teacher-directed goal-setting learning tasks, and then, as the course progresses, have students set different goals with more student-directed goal-setting learning tasks. Teacher-directed goal-setting learning tasks eliminate the possibility of students setting inappropriate goals that are unattainable or too general to be measured. However, because assigning goals decreases students' self-determination, you will want to provide students with some type of choice that supports their ability to be autonomous. Figure 6.6 provides an example of a guided goal for improving cardiorespiratory fitness. This is a guided goal because the teacher has provided the structure and the content for setting the goal. One option has students choose from the PACER or the mile test to set a goal; the other option has the teacher provide similar frameworks for muscular fitness and flexibility and then allow students to select one of the health-related fitness components to write a goal for.

With the SMART goal structure, you can teach students how to set realistic goals based on the time frame and what is physiologically possible. The improvement rates used in this framework are only intended to be a starting point to help students understand that fitness improvement takes time and is based on current fitness status. In general, students may see between a 5 to 10 percent improvement in their cardiorespiratory fitness each week if they are increasing their training duration or intensity by 5 to 10 percent above what they normally do in a week (Reuter & Dawes, 2016). However, fitness improvement is confounded by the principle of diminishing returns. This principle suggests that the rate of fitness improvement diminishes over time as your fitness approaches its ultimate genetic potential. For example, it is much more difficult for someone who runs a mile in five minutes to improve than a person who runs a mile in 12 minutes. To give an idea of the room for improvement, the current record-time for the mile-run is 3:43.13 minutes (World Athletics, 2020). As students become fitter, the room for improvement lessens to the point that a 1 percent improvement rate over several weeks may be all that is possible.

When designing your fitness education course, you will want to provide opportunities for students to engage in goal-directed learning experiences. This means that you don't want to simply have students set a goal, expect them to work on it outside of class, and then only talk about that goal again

Time-bound	I have ____ weeks to train before the next fitness test. My current mile time is ____ or My current PACER score is ____.
Realistic	This is the realistic amount of improvement that I can expect if I give 100% effort on my pretest, follow the principles of training, and commit to engaging in the recommended FITT prescription for cardiorespiratory fitness. **For the mile**: If over 9 minutes, I can decrease time by 10 seconds for every week. If 7 to 9 minutes, I can decrease time by 5 seconds for every week of training. If under 7 minutes, I can decrease time by 5 seconds for every 2 weeks of training. **For the PACER**: I can increase by 2 lines for every week of training. If over 75 lines, I can increase by 1 line for every week of training.
Achievable	This goal is achievable if I commit to following the principles of training and the FITT principle. I will participate in cardiorespiratory training at least ____ times per week for ____ minutes and I will work out in my target heart rate zone which is ____.
Measurable	I will track my improvement by recording my FITT process goals. My improvement is measurable by how many seconds I can decrease my mile time or how many more PACER laps I can complete.
Specific	I am going to run a ____-minute mile on the next fitness test in ____ weeks. OR I am going to complete ____ PACER laps on the next fitness test in ____ weeks.

Figure 6.6 A guided SMART goal for improving cardiorespiratory fitness.

at the end of the course. To be effective, goals must be regularly monitored for progress, and providing time in class for students to participate in activities related to their goal makes achieving it much more likely. At the conclusion of any goal-setting learning task, you will want students to evaluate their goal-setting process. Since goal setting is a skill that you want students to master, it is valuable to have them reflect on what did or didn't work. As students move on to create their next goal, the hope is that they learned a strategy that would help them to be more successful or just as successful the next time.

CONCLUSION

Students who have a positive learning experience in physical education are more likely to engage in physical activity in adulthood. You will want to use every strategy possible to provide students with a positive learning experience that translates into adopting a physically active lifestyle. Strategies for creating a positive learning experience include incorporating SEL competencies into the curriculum and instruction, creating a mastery-oriented motivational climate, structuring lesson design and delivery to meet students' psychological needs, and being sensitive to the needs of trauma-affected students and students from culturally diverse backgrounds. The goal of engaging in lifelong physical activity relies on using the social and emotional competencies of self-management, self-awareness, and relationship skills. When students can consistently, autonomously, and effectively use these skills, they greatly increase their ability to achieve and maintain a health-enhancing level of physical fitness. You can teach students how to use these skills in the fitness education setting to promote overall health and wellness.

Review Questions

1. What are the five core SEL competencies and how do they support the goal of fitness education?
2. Describe three learning experiences that you can use for developing self-awareness in the fitness education setting.
3. What are two strategies that you can use to build relationships with students so that they feel safe and supported in the fitness education setting?
4. Explain how the TARGET principles can be used to enhance students' intrinsic motivation.
5. Contrast the major characteristics of the mastery-oriented and ego-oriented motivational climates.

Visit HK*Propel* for additional material related to this chapter.

CHAPTER 7

Standards, Grade-Level Outcomes, and Assessment

Chapter Objective

After reading this chapter, you will understand the role that fitness assessment plays in the delivery of a standards-based instructional program; the manner in which fitness education is aligned with specific grade-level outcomes and instructional frameworks; ways to develop cognitive fitness assessments; the role that technology plays in fitness assessments; the method for administering fitness assessments; and strategies for grading students in a fitness education course. Physical education teachers will be provided with knowledge-based concepts as well as details for how to employ best teaching practices that enhance student learning and comprehension.

Key Concepts

- Fitness education and assessments are aligned with physical education national standards and grade-level outcomes.
- Fitness education affects all learning domains, cognitive, affective, and psychomotor, and student assessments should measure student learning.
- Alternative assessments are recommended to address student learning in authentic settings.
- Accommodations and modifications are recommended so that all activities, assessments, and instructional materials can be adjusted and delivered to all students in the class.

INTRODUCTION

Assessment is an essential component of the curriculum and instructional process because it demonstrates student progress in achieving the outcomes and meeting standards. Student assessments enable instructors to measure the effectiveness of their teaching by linking student performance to specific learning objectives (Fisher, 2020). It is the "proof" of progress and achievement. In designing assessments, teachers must ask, "What will students do to demonstrate proficiency in the outcomes?" The primary purpose of assessment in physical education is to provide stakeholders with evidence of students' learning as well as their attainment of the national standards and grade-level outcomes (Chepko, Holt/Hale, Doan, & MacDonald, 2019). In the curriculum development process, it is important to identify common assessments so that you know if students are learning what you intend for them to learn and achieve. In physical education, assessment measures and validates student learning in a variety of skill-related activities and health-related fitness. Feedback from assessment factors into increasing student motivation and engagement, which, in turn, helps create a positive learning environment, as previously discussed in chapter 4.

Summative and formative assessments are the two forms of student assessment most frequently used in determining teaching and learning. *Summative assessments* evaluate student learning outcomes at the completion of an instructional unit by using an identified standard of performance. Rubrics, checklists, portfolios, written exams, and skills tests are all tools that you can use to assess learning in physical education. These assessments help communicate the expectations to both students and teachers. Students understand that they must demonstrate a certain level of learning or performance in order to succeed in the class, and teachers can design learning experiences that will prepare students to master the assessments. *Formative assessments* involve the evaluation of learning throughout the course at various points. Teachers should employ a wide variety of formative assessment methods or tools to determine student readiness, skill acquisition, and learning progress toward common assessment achievement. Formative assessment allows students to receive immediate, corrective feedback and provides teachers with information to guide future instruction. This type of assessment is informal and can use peer-, self-, or teacher-led tools to determine progress. Using formative assessments helps students remain focused on the process of learning and the purpose of activities within the class. You can help students develop the skills and knowledge that they need for lifelong physical activity by consistently providing feedback on their performance related to the objectives.

Selecting and administrating assessment techniques that are appropriate for the goals of instruction as well as the developmental level of students are crucial components of effective assessment for learning. Physical education teachers need to know the characteristics of a wide variety of assessment techniques and how these techniques can be adapted for various fitness education content and skills and student characteristics. Teachers also should understand the roles that reliability, valid-

Characteristics of Student Assessment

- Student assessment is aligned with national and/or state physical education standards and established grade-level outcomes and is included in the written physical education curriculum along with administration protocols.
- Student assessment includes evidence-based practices that measure student achievement in all areas of instruction, including physical fitness.
- Grading is related directly to the student learning objectives identified in the written physical education curriculum.
- The physical education teacher follows school district and school protocols for reporting and communicating student progress to students and parents.

ity, and the absence of bias should play in choosing and using assessment techniques.

According to Aschbacher and Winters (1992), when deciding on the type of assessment to deliver, the following questions should be asked in choosing and designing effective assessments:

- Does the assessment match the specific instructional objectives and targeted learning domains?
- Does the assessment enable students to demonstrate their progress and proficiency level?
- Does the assessment use authentic, relevant tasks?
- Can the assessment be structured to measure several objectives?
- Does the assessment provide students with feedback they can use to improve future performance?
- Is the assessment time efficient and realistic for my context?

Keep in mind that continuously evaluating student learning to determine your effectiveness is a key element in delivering appropriate instruction. Embedding assessment into the curriculum and instruction will not only greatly benefit students but also allow you to adapt instruction to your students' needs in order for students to progress. Assessment data may show that you need to reteach a concept or that you can provide more challenging tasks for students.

Additionally, fitness education classes need to be inclusive, safe, and respectful of diversity in order for *all* students to thrive. Teachers can offer content that is culturally relevant and responsive to individual students' needs and allow for choices in assessment practices. Through appropriate assessment, students will further display knowledge of the benefits of engaging in physical activity and fitness education as well as the consequences of physical inactivity through a fitness education perspective and the *Instructional Framework for Fitness Education in Physical Education* (IFFEPE) as exhibited in table 7.1.

As we progress throughout this chapter, you will begin to see how fitness education aligns with the National Standards for Physical Education and specific Grade-Level Outcomes (GLOs) and is identified in the Instructional Framework for Fitness Education in Physical Education (IFFEPE). Tables referencing GLOs and the IFFEPE are strategically placed throughout this chapter as examples of how a fitness education curriculum and materials can be developed and implemented. We highly recommend that physical education teachers familiarize themselves with SHAPE America's complete documents, which can be found at https://www.shapeamerica.org/.

FITNESS EDUCATION ASSESSMENT STRATEGIES

Chapters 1 and 2 clearly define what fitness education is and why it is an essential component of physical education programs for all students in understanding the importance of being physically active throughout their life span. This chapter will explain the how of fitness education and fitness assessment.

Table 7.1 IFFEPE Benchmarks for Knowledge of PA Benefits and Dangers of Inactivity

Descriptor	Grades 6-8 benchmark	Grades 9-12 benchmark
Knowledge: Demonstrates understanding of fitness concepts, principles, strategies and individual differences needed to participate and maintain a health-enhancing level of physical fitness.		
Benefits of physical activity/dangers of physical inactivity	• Analyze the empowering consequences of being physically fit (e.g., improved cognition, stamina, confidence). • Recognize physical activity as a positive opportunity for stress reduction and social interaction. • Identify positive mental and emotional aspects of participating in a variety of physical activities.	• Compare and contrast the health-related benefits of various physical activities (e.g., improved cognition, increased strength and flexibility, cardiovascular endurance, social interaction). • Explain the interrelationship of physical activity to physiological responses and physical, mental/intellectual, emotional, and social benefits. • Analyze the benefits of a healthy lifestyle and the consequences of poor nutrition and inactivity.

Developing Written Cognitive Assessments

For many physical education teachers, administrating fitness assessments as well as physical activity and sport skills assessments has become second nature. But all too often it becomes a bit more challenging to develop cognitive assessments. Using an example from SHAPE America's National Physical Education Standard 3, Grade-Level Outcome for grades 6 through 12 as shown in tables 7.2 and 7.3, the following section provides guidance on how to appropriately develop physical education written tests that will allow you to develop your own test bank for both formative and summative assessments. EduMeasure Inc. provides guidance and walks you through a step-by-step process, enabling you to develop the same types of questions used on standardized assessments in all subject areas.

Developing Multiple-Choice Items

Effective multiple-choice items should assess significant information and be aligned with the standards and grade-level outcomes. The first step in developing a cognitive assessment is to understand the terminology used in developing a multiple-choice item, or test question. A *stimulus* is the reading material or graphic information that precedes the question posed and provides information pertinent to answering the question. Multiple-choice items may include stimuli. An individual or a discrete item may require a stimulus to provide students with enough context to answer the question. A group of items, commonly called a cluster or a set, may be based on a passage or graphic, and thus each item may not require an additional stimulus. Every multiple-choice item comprises the following specific element: the stem, options, key, and distractors.

The *stem* is the statement that poses the problem to be solved or the question that must be answered. Every multiple-choice item must include a closed stem, meaning the question posed is a complete sentence punctuated with a question mark.

Options are the choices provided from which students must select an answer. Every multiple-choice item must include options, but the number of options can vary. Most assessments use three- and four-option multiple-choice items. All the options should be approximately the same length and ordered according to length (shortest to longest or vice versa) or alpha or numeric order. The options should not contain the words *all, always, only,* or *never,* but they may use limiting words like *usually* or *sometimes*.

Table 7.2 Fitness Knowledge: Grade-Level Outcomes for Middle School

Standard 3	Grade 6	Grade 7	Grade 8
The physically literate individual demonstrates the knowledge and skills to achieve and maintain a health-enhancing level of physical activity and fitness.			
S3.M13 Fitness knowledge	Defines resting heart rate and describes its relationship to aerobic fitness and the Borg rating of perceived exertion (RPE) scale. (S3.M13.6)	Defines how the RPE scale can be used to determine the perception of the work effort or intensity of exercise. (S3.M13.7)	Defines how the RPE scale can be used to adjust workout intensity during physical activity. (S3.M13.8)

Table 7.3 Fitness Knowledge: Grade-Level Outcomes for High School

Standard 3	Level 1	Level 2
The physically literate individual demonstrates the knowledge and skills to achieve a health-enhancing level of physical activity and fitness.		
S3.H10 Fitness knowledge	Calculates target heart rate and applies that information to personal fitness plan. (S3.H10.L1)	Adjusts pacing to keep heart rate in the target zone, using available technology (e.g., heart rate monitor), to self-monitor aerobic intensity. (S3.H10.L2)

The *key* is the correct answer choice, which should answer the question in the stem. Every multiple-choice item must include only one key. The key must be correct and defensible as the one and only correct answer. In addition, it should not contain significant language from the stem.

Lastly, *distractors* are the incorrect answer choices. The distractors should be attractive and make sense. They should look like possible answers to the question posed in the stem and not be so far removed from the question that they are ludicrous or throw-away choices. However, they must be incorrect and should avoid using opposing statements. Most importantly, distractors should not use the choices *all of the above* or *none of the above*. Figure 7.1 provides an example of the components involved in developing a multiple-choice question.

The following guidelines should be considered when writing and reviewing effective multiple-choice items. The item content should be correct, accurate, realistic, and succinct. The facts, dates, documents, people, and events presented in an item should be verified as correct. Dates, spelling of people's names and place names, titles of documents, and so on should be confirmed as accurate. Data and graphical information provided in an item should be realistic and not contain values that could not be found in the real world. Items should not have a negative stem, which is a sentence or question that asks students to find the incorrect answer (key) among the correct answers (distractors). Negative words such as *not, never, except,* and *none* should be avoided, and the options should not contain repeated information. Items should have a closed stem; in a closed stem, the question posed is a complete sentence and punctuated with a question mark. Items should be *aligned to the standard and grade-level outcome* and fair and free from racial, ethnic, gender, and socio-economic bias. When developing assessment items, teachers should use the following language accessibility, bias, and sensitivity (LABS) protocols and become familiar with the sensitivity inherent in unintentional bias:

- Stereotyping
- Sensitive or controversial subjects
- Advice
- Dangerous activities
- Population diversity and ethnocentrism
- Differential familiarity
- Language accessibility

Additionally, items should be written in the active voice because most of us have more difficulty processing text written in the passive voice. Here is an example of a sentence written in the passive voice:

A game of tennis was played by John and Mary.

Here is the same sentence written in the active voice:

John and Mary played a game of tennis.

Developing Constructed-Response Items

Constructed-response items assess how students apply their knowledge, skills, and critical-thinking skills to real-world problems. Constructed-response items are generally referred to as prompts because they may appear in the form of written questions or as photos, data tables or graphs, or interactive computer stimuli. These items can include a large variety of end products from all domains of education and are standards driven. Items should be aligned to the standard or grade-level outcome being assessed, can range from low to high

Stimulus

Student name	Heart rate		
	Day 1	Day 2	Day 3
Tiffany	115	125	130
Maria	120	135	125
Sandy	115	115	120

Stem — Look at the chart above. Which is the correct explanation of the heart rate readings?

Options

a. Sandy had the lowest mean heart rate.* — **Key**

b. Maria had a median heart rate of 135.

c. Tiffany had the lowest mean heart rate.

d. Maria and Tiffany had the same mean heart rate.

(b–d: **Distractors**)

Figure 7.1 Sample multiple-choice question.

complexity, and should require a more complex response than the stem of a multiple-choice item. Prompts should have enough information to focus attention on the task that must be accomplished. The most common way of scoring constructed-response items is through the use of rubrics. Rubrics should be aligned with the prompt, allow for multiple-response solutions or for multiple ways to achieve a correct response, and clearly delineate what a student must do to achieve each score point within the score-point descriptors.

Often called open-ended questions, constructed-response items require students to construct and develop their own answer without the help of other suggestions or choices. Because of this, there are ways to correctly answer constructed-response questions. Constructed-response items measure students' ability to apply, analyze, and synthesize information into their own words (Tankersley, 2007). Student responses can be a written response, a performance, or a product. Through the use of short-answer responses and essay items on an assessment, which require more elaborate answers and explanations of reasoning, students are able to show their knowledge and exemplify their understanding of a set of academic skills.

As with developing multiple-choice items, constructed-response items should include the *stimulus* or a *prompt*, and a scoring *rubric*. The stimulus can take many forms, such as written questions, photographs, data tables, graphs, or interactive computer stimuli of various types. The prompt is a written statement of the question students must answer. The scoring rubric is a description of how to score student responses. Figure 7.2 shows an example of a constructed-response item.

When physical education is presented online or in a hybrid model, other means of cognitive assessment should be implemented. Ensuring that students understand concepts related to physical education is very important. Assessing students' ability to understand the subject matter in an

Prompt: Identify two activities that a person should do before running in order to exercise safely.

Sample response: One activity that a person should do before he or she runs is engage in a short cardiovascular warm-up. After this, the person should engage in some gentle stretching.

Rubric	
2 points	The student correctly identifies two activities that a person should do before running in order to exercise safely. Activities include, but are not limited to: • Various cardiovascular warm-up activities: - Jumping rope - Jumping jacks • Various stretches - Quad stretches - Hamstring stretches - High knees - Wall stretch - Lunges
1 point	The student correctly identifies one activity that a person should do before running in order to exercise safely.
0 points	The response indicates inadequate or no understanding of the concept needed to answer the item. The student may have written on a different topic or written "I don't know."

Reprinted by permission from American Institutes for Research, *Florida Physical Education Test Item Bank Specifications.*

Figure 7.2 Sample constructed-response item.

online setting can be done a few different ways. Scheduling a one-on-one video conference with students allows you to discuss the physical education subject matter with them and check for understanding. If one-on-one video conferencing is not an option, teachers can have students submit written, audio, or video answers to questions related to cognitive objectives.

Developing Performance Tasks or Psychomotor Assessments

Performance tasks require students to demonstrate knowledge of the content. They can be asked to perform an action, provide a verbal response to a standard set of questions, or be given a standard set of materials with which to show an understanding of a concept. Performance tasks can assess one or more GLO and range from medium to high complexity. A performance task takes approximately 5 to 10 minutes of testing time to answer, and each item is worth one to four score points (American Institutes of Research, 2016).

Performance task terminology includes all of the specifications as identified in constructed-response items, including the task—directions provided to students prior to students beginning the task—and the rubric—the scoring guidelines to assess the student responses. Table 7.4 provides an example of how a standard and grade-level outcomes are used to develop a performance task in determining what a student should know, and be able to do, as a result of quality physical education instruction.

A sample performance task in a psychomotor format is presented as another form of assessment that should be administered in physical education classes. The following are definitions of the specific terms used for the parts of a performance task along with a sample task with each term identified (see figure 7.3).

- Materials: the materials that must be provided to students
- Setup: the setup for the presentation of the task
- Prompt: the directions that are stated prior to students beginning the task
- Rubric: the scoring guidelines for student responses
- Score points: the points that can be awarded for a response
- Score point description: the student response that will earn each of the score points

A performance task can also be administered in a written format where students are asked to describe a skill, such as the step-by-step instructions on how to correctly perform a push-up, and are scored with a rubric.

Since assessments should include a spectrum of difficulty levels ranging from low to high, physical education teachers need to become familiar with Webb's Depth of Knowledge (DOK) levels, a framework used to identify the level of rigor for an assessment. Webb (1997) developed the DOK framework to categorize activities according to the level of complexity in thinking. The creation of the DOK stemmed from the alignment of standards to assessments. Figure 7.4 identifies the four levels of DOK: Level 1, Recall; Level 2, Skill/concept; Level 3, Strategic thinking; and Level 4, Extended thinking.

Developing Affective Assessments

Teaching students to value physical education is crucial to their participation later in life. The affective domain encompasses student perceptions, values, interests, emotions, attitudes, and feelings toward particular physical education or fitness components, or even physical education as a whole. In order to effectively assess behaviors in the affective domain, the behavior must first be defined, and you must identify the acceptable indicators of students meeting those expectations (Lund & Veal, 2013). Table 7.5 provides a sample GLO for standard 4, and table 7.6 provides a sample GLO for standard 5.

Table 7.4 Standard 3: Grade-Level Outcomes for Middle School

Standard 3	Grade 6	Grade 7	Grade 8
The physically literate individual demonstrates the knowledge and skills to achieve and maintain a health-enhancing level of physical activity and fitness.			
S3.M9 Fitness knowledge	Employs correct techniques and methods of stretching. (S3.M9.6)	Describes and demonstrates the difference between dynamic and static stretches. (S3.M9.7)	Employs a variety of appropriate static stretching techniques for all major muscle groups. (S3.M9.8)

Materials: 4 cones; gym, track, basketball court, or open space for running and stretching

Setup: Place the four cones in a square, with each cone 60 feet (18 m) apart.

Prompt: Move around the cones in a way that is meant to improve cardiorespiratory endurance. Complete one lap around the cones. Then, perform one stretch designed to improve leg flexibility.

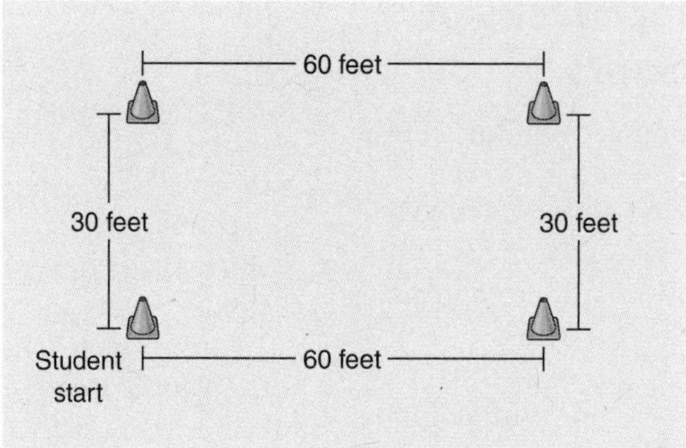

Rubric	
2 points	The student successfully travels one lap around the cones while performing a movement that is meant to improve cardiorespiratory endurance, including but not limited to: • Jogging • Running • Skipping • Sliding AND the student successfully performs one stretch designed to improve leg flexibility.
1 point	The student successfully travels one lap around the cones while performing a movement that is meant to improve cardiorespiratory endurance OR The student performs one stretch designed to improve leg flexibility.
0 points	The student is unable to perform the task, does not understand how to complete the task, or unsuccessfully completes the task.

Figure 7.3 Sample psychomotor performance tasks.

Affective domain assessments can measure constructs such as acceptable social and personal behaviors when engaged in physical activities or students' behaviors toward other classmates. Additional affective behaviors can be observed and assessed through students' effort in participation; acts of fair play (usually demonstrated through fair play); and willingness to cooperate and be scored by rubrics, journaling, or portfolios (Mitchell & Walton-Fisette, 2016).

For students taking physical education online or in a hybrid model, determining how they value physical education while attending an online course can seem complicated. Examples of how to measure and assess students' value of physical education include having them participate in a

Depth of knowledge level	Cognitive expectation	What students will do at this level	Fitness education examples
Level 1: **Recall and reproduction**	Focus is on the acquisition of knowledge and recalling of previously taught content such as facts, definitions, and procedures. • Working with facts, terms, definitions, procedures • Student knows it or does not know it. A clearly defined answer.	Demonstrate their understanding of information from specified topics through learning activities that have them: *List, identify, recognize, define, recite, label, restate*	• Identify two resistance training exercises that target the hamstrings. • Label the major muscle groups on a given diagram. • Define social awareness.
Level 2: **Skills and concepts**	Focus is on applying knowledge and explaining how or why information can be used to achieve an outcome. • Applying skills, explaining how or why • Compares and contrasts	Use knowledge to answer questions and accomplish tasks through learning activities that have them: *Predict, compare, distinguish, summarize, classify, modify, describe*	• Describe how you could modify the push-up exercise to make it both less and more challenging for individuals of varying fitness levels. • Compare the two nutritional plans and predict the amount of weight loss or gain that each person would experience in a month based upon their physical activity level. • Explain how and why good sport behavior impacts sport and physical activity outcomes.
Level 3: **Strategic thinking**	Focus is on knowledge analysis and how to think and examine concepts, procedures, or topics to find and explain answers. • Analysis and evaluation to solve problems, combining knowledge and skill from multiple subject areas to reach a solution • Drawing conclusions from observations or data	Use knowledge to investigate issues, solve problems, determine cause and effect, and support answers or results in learning activities that have them: *Analyze, explain, support with evidence, generalize, create*	• Design a survey to gather information on student opinions of the health benefits of being fit and design activities based on an analysis of responses. • Develop an individual fitness plan based on actual fitness assessment data that utilizes the principles of training.
Level 4: **Extended thinking**	Focus is on knowledge transfer and thinking how knowledge can be extended for use in different situations and in contexts beyond the classroom. • Conducting investigations with unpredictable outcomes that require multiple steps over a period of time to solve the problem • Multiple answers and multiple approaches with varied results	Use knowledge in tasks that require multiple steps over a period of time to solve a problem, through learning activities that have them: *Create, synthesize, design, reflect, conduct, develop, prove*	• Conduct an experiment to determine which fitness training program will produce the most improvement in a high school students' mile time. • Create a full inclusion fitness circuit, based on scientific principles and research, to address the components of fitness education as a group project. • Develop a relationship building manual that explains how students use communication skills and strategies to demonstrate respect for self and others in the fitness education setting.

Figure 7.4 Depth of Knowledge (DoK) Levels
Based on *Webb's Depth of Knowledge Guide* (2009). www.aps.edu/sapr/documents/resources/Webbs_DOK_Guide.pdf

Table 7.5 Standard 4: Grade-Level Outcomes for High School

Standard 4	Level 1	Level 2
The physically literate individual exhibits responsible personal and social behavior that respects self and others.		
S4.H1 Personal responsibility	Employs effective self-management skills to analyze barriers and modify physical activity patterns appropriately, as needed. (S4.H1.L1)	Accepts differences between personal characteristics and the idealized body images and elite performance levels portrayed in various media. (S4.H1.L2)
S4.H2 Rules and etiquette	Exhibits proper etiquette, respect for others and team-work while engaging in physical activity and/or social dance. (S4.H2.L1)	Examines moral and ethical conduct in specific competitive situations (e.g., intentional fouls, performance-enhancing substances, gambling, current events in sport). (S4.H2.L2)
S4.H3 Working with others	Uses communication skills and strategies that promote team or group dynamics. (S4.H3.L1)	Assumes a leadership role (e.g., task or group leader, referee, coach) in a physical activity setting. (S4.H3.L2)
S4.H4 Working with others	Solves problems and thinks critically in physical activity and/or dance settings, both as an individual and in groups. (S4.H4.L1)	Accepts others' ideas, cultural diversity and body types by engaging in cooperative and collaborative movement projects. (S4.H4.L2)

Table 7.6 Standard 5: Grade-Level Outcomes for Middle School Students

Standard 5	Grade 6	Grade 7	Grade 8
The physically literate individual recognizes the value of physical activity for health, enjoyment, challenge, self-expression and/or social interaction.			
S5.M4 Self-expression and enjoyment	Describes how moving competently in a physical activity setting creates enjoyment. (S5.M4.6)	Identifies why self-selected physical activities create enjoyment. (S5.M4.7)	Discusses how enjoyment could be increased in self-selected physical activities. (S5.M4.8)
S5.M5 Self-expression and enjoyment	Identifies how self-expression and physical activity are related. (S5.M5.6)	Explains the relationship between self-expression and lifelong enjoyment through physical activity. (S5.M5.7)	Identifies and participates in an enjoyable activity that prompts individual self-expression. (S5.M5.8)
S5.M6 Social interaction	Demonstrates respect for self and others in activities and games by following the rules, encouraging others and playing in the spirit of the game or activity. (S5.M6.6)	Demonstrates the importance of social interaction by helping and encouraging others, avoiding trash talk and providing support to classmates. (S5.M6.7)	Demonstrates respect for self by asking for help and helping others in various physical activities. (S5.M6.8)

guided reflection journal or digital portfolio or reflect on their participation in physical education and physical activity while at home. This provides students and teachers the opportunity to evaluate their value and importance of being physically active. This guided reflection could be done through writing or brief audio and video reflections. The feedback from this reflection helps instructors understand the value-driven concepts students derived from the online course.

RUBRICS

According to Heidi Goodrich Andrade (2014), authentic assessments tend to use rubrics to describe student achievement and are powerful tools for both teaching and assessment. Rubrics describe varying levels of student performance and provide clear criteria for observation (Mitchell & Walton-Fisette, 2016). Rubrics clearly define academic expectations and should be provided and explained to students before they begin the assignment or assessment. Rubrics can improve student performance, as well as monitor it, and they can be used to guide self- and peer assessments. When students use rubrics regularly to judge their own work, they begin to accept more responsibility for the end product and their own learning gains.

A rubric, in essence, is a scoring guide used in both formative and summative assessments for evaluating student performance, a product, or a project. It consists of three major parts: (1) the performance criteria, (2) the rating scale, and (3) the indicators, or descriptions for each performance level. For both you and your students, the rubric defines what is expected and what will be assessed.

In determining the *performance criteria*, teachers must first determine which evidence of learning should occur, which learning outcomes should be listed in the rubric, which skills are essential, and which level of competence or proficiency is required. Before developing the *rating scale*, generally a range from 1 to 5, with the highest number being the highest score, teachers must first create indicators that are present at all performance levels. The *indicators* should reflect equal steps along the scale and clearly display the characteristics of each performance level.

For physical education teachers new to assessment, *PE Metrics* (3rd edition) should become part of your professional library. *PE Metrics* is the standards-based, cognitive- and motor-skills assessment package, which offers 130 of SHAPE America's K-12 assessments.

SOFIT OBSERVATION ASSESSMENT

Getting the 60 or more minutes of moderate-to-vigorous physical activity (MVPA) daily that the *Physical Activity Guidelines for Americans* (2nd edition) recommends is one of the most important actions that youth can take to develop the foundation for lifelong health. This amount of physical activity improves cognitive functions; develops higher levels of fitness; prevents chronic disease; and activates executive function, processing speed, and attention, which leads to stronger academic performance (U.S Department of Health and Human Services, 2018). However, we know that although students spend most of their waking hours in the school setting, many are not provided with the opportunity to be physically active for 30 minutes. One way to monitor and assess the amount of time that students spend in physical activity at the school site is to use the System for Observing Fitness Instruction Time (SOFIT) tool.

Developed by Thomas McKenzie, the valid and reliable SOFIT is a comprehensive tool for assessing physical education classes by providing a simultaneous collection of data on student activity levels, the lesson context, and teacher behavior. Physical activity engagement is one of the main health-related goals of physical education, and it is needed in order for students to become both physically fit and skilled. Participation in MVPA during class is highly dependent on how physical education subject matter is being delivered (i.e., lesson context) and the behavior of the instructor delivering it (McKenzie, 2009; 2012).

The availability of instructional videos and web-based training also allows for consistency in training observers in both structured settings, such as physical education, and unstructured settings, such as recess and free play (McKenzie & van der Mars, 2015; McKenzie, 2016). Additionally, as technological advances have provided for the use of on-site data collection, iSOFIT can be downloaded as an app to facilitate entering, storing, summarizing, and exporting data.

ALTERNATIVE ASSESSMENTS

Aside from the administration of written or performance assessments, alternative, or authentic, assessment has become a valuable tool, which measures applied proficiency, in the teaching and learning process. Authentic assessment reflects on student learning, achievement, motivation, and attitudes on relevant class activities. In physical education, authentic assessment can include portfolios, journals, student and class projects, and fitness logs to name just a few.

Portfolios

The student portfolio is a purposeful collection of student work that is organized to show learning progress and provides students the opportunity to reflect on their own growth over a period of time. The content in the portfolio must be linked to the learning objectives and outcomes of the class and should represent a subset of students' work. The opportunity to select their own portfolio content makes students view the material as more motivating and feel a sense of pride and accomplishment. According to Mueller (2018), portfolios are usually created for one of three purposes: to show growth, to showcase work, or to evaluate a student's work and progress. Portfolios further encourage individualized learning, as well as document student learning, promote student responsibility, provide for continuous evaluation, encourage student self-reflection, and showcase the overall physical education program and student achievement.

Portfolios, although a form of assessment, may or may not be graded, but when used for evaluation, they usually are graded with a rubric explained to students in advance. Portfolios can be shared with parents or guardians and community members for showcasing purposes and can contain sample assignments, video clips, pictures, and fitness logs. Portfolios can either be kept in physical, hard-copy folders or set up digitally. For successful implementation of an online physical education course, a digital portfolio is a must. Standard 3, level 2 shows the use of authentic assessment by portfolio in table 7.7.

Journals

Journal writing in physical education allows students to reflect on and take charge of their learning experiences, feelings, thoughts, and emotions. Individualized journal writing allows students to organize and express their thoughts in a less-restrained manner, enhancing critical thinking and affording students self-reflection on both positive and negative feelings. By keeping journals, students become increasingly motivated by the tracking of their own goals and develop self-awareness through writing about their own thoughts and patterns of behavior in response to varying situations.

In a class setting, physical education teachers can give students the choice to either free-write in their journals without prompts or respond to a series of reflective questions. As students progress through their education, they must practice, enhance, and habitually use their reflection skills. As students develop a trust in their teachers when sharing their journals, teachers can glean the ways in which students think about how and what they are learning. If teachers decide the journals will be graded, then they should first discuss writing strategies with students.

Student and Class Projects

Implementing student and class projects is another way to engage students in real-world learning opportunities. For students in grades 6 through 12, this offers a wide range of research possibilities from issues relating to fitness, or sports in general (the Olympics, NFL, NBA, WNBA, MLS, NWSL), to equity, diversity, inclusion, and social justice issues mentioned in chapter 4 relating to sport and physical education. For example, students could present an argument for or against equal pay for men and women who are designing a fitness facility. Through selecting their own projects and developing the end product, students drive their own learning by studying a topic that was interesting and engaging for them. Encouraging students to use a variety of multimedia resources to present their projects to the class will further allow for innovation and creativity.

By working in groups, students also learn the importance of cooperation and collaboration through teamwork, group skills, problem-solving skills, time management, and the same level of shared responsibility in completing projects so that grades are fair and equitable. Group work allows teachers to learn more about students, providing teachers a path for communicating in a more progressive and meaningful way as they employ various assessments.

Opportunities for collaboration should still occur whether an online version or a hybrid model of a physical education class. Group meetings can be held through a variety of online platforms, such as Zoom, Microsoft Teams, Skype, or other agreed-upon and available platforms. With teacher and parental input and support, students who live in the same geographic location could arrange to meet in person to work on the class project. Online education does not mean that students work in iso-

Table 7.7 Standard 3: Grade-Level Outcomes for High School

Standard 3	Level 1	Level 2
The physically literate individual demonstrates the knowledge and skills to achieve and maintain a health-enhancing level of physical activity and fitness.		
S3.H11 Assessment and program planning	Creates and implements a behavior-modification plan that enhances a healthy, active lifestyle in college or career settings. (S3.H11.L1)	Develops and maintains a fitness portfolio (e.g., assessment scores, goals for improvement, plan of activities for improvement, log of activities being done to reach goals, timeline for improvement). (S3.H11.L2)

lation, therefore the social interaction is beneficial on many levels.

Fitness and Activity Logs

Having students develop and maintain fitness and activity logs is another way to validate that students are physically active and working toward reaching their individual goals. Activity logs assist students in measuring progress, helping them to develop a sense of satisfaction in working toward a goal, which, in turn, boosts their confidence in knowing that their goal is attainable and within sight. Students' self-selected goals could either reflect their overall physical activity levels in achieving the 60 minutes a day of MVPA or be specific fitness goals based on pretest results of a health- or skill-related fitness assessment.

Student activity logs can be used as part of the student portfolios or as a stand-alone assignment. Activity logs should not only record progress but also provide an opportunity for students to self-assess whether they are making adequate progress and whether changes should be implemented in subsequent weeks.

USE OF TECHNOLOGY IN STUDENT LEARNING AND ASSESSMENT

The use of technology is exciting and engaging for teachers and students in the implementation of a fitness education program. Physical education teachers should implement the use of technology when delivering instruction or assessing student knowledge and fitness performance. Technology has become an essential tool for both teachers and students within a physical education learning environment. Technology should never be used as a substitute for sound teaching practices or as a tool to just keep students busy. The use of technology in a physical education class requires teachers to shift their teaching practices as well as change their classroom habits.

As many school districts are exploring hybrid and online delivery systems, this will further require a learning shift in both teachers and students as they engage in online collaboration tools. There are several online options, including Google Drive, a cloud-based storage system; Edmodo, Schoology, and Canvas, learning management systems; Discovery's educational video content; and Gizmos, which offer interactive subject area content that teachers can integrate into their textbook series. Seeking professional development, if your district offers it, is always encouraged. While online software tools, resources, and programs may be easy to use, professional development offers effective strategies to successfully implement such resources so that your class has richer experiences with the course content.

Wearable Technology

Wearable technology devices are an effective accountability and feedback tool for both students and physical education teachers. Wearable technology includes, but is not limited to, heart rate monitors, watches, accelerometers, and pedometers. Students have the opportunity to get immediate feedback about their performance in a physical education and activity setting. Wearable technology has become increasingly more common among people who monitor their physical activity and exercise habits on a regular basis, to the extent that many students now own their own device. The ability to track students' participation in physical activity through wearable technologies has become a significant assessment asset in a physical education setting, as shown in table 7.8 for standard 3, grade 8. Depending on the wearable device, feedback can be obtained privately online or in print form. This feedback can be used to help improve teaching practices as well as student physical activity performance. Sharing information with parents or guardians and administration alike is a beneficial form of data collection and advocacy (Greenberg & LoBianco, 2020).

As technology has progressed, these measures may include step and mile (or kilometer) counts, participation in MVPA, heart rate, and other biometric measures. These devices help track students' participation in physical activity not only during physical education class but also at other times outside of the school setting. For hybrid or online-only learning environments, the data provide physical education teachers with important assessment information, as well as accountability of student performance because wearable technology allows students to submit their daily physical activity to their instructors. Exposing students to wearable technologies increases the likelihood of daily physical activity becoming a sustainable practice across students' life span.

Additionally, using multiple mobile devices in a physical education setting allows opportunities for quick and easy assessments, including formative and summative assessments, especially when developing quizzes on cloud-based platforms, such as Plickers; video-based movement analysis for

Table 7.8 Middle School Grade-Level Outcomes for Self-Monitoring Physical Activity

Standard 3	Grade 6	Grade 7	Grade 8
The physically literate individual demonstrates the knowledge and skills to achieve and maintain a health-enhancing level of physical activity and fitness.			
S3.M8 Fitness knowledge	Sets and monitors a self-selected physical activity goal for aerobic and/or muscle- and bone-strengthening activity based on current fitness level. (S3.M8.6)	Adjusts physical activity based on quantity of exercise needed for a minimal health standard and/or optimal functioning based on current fitness level. (S3.M8.7)	Uses available technology to self-monitor quantity of exercise needed for a minimal health standard and/or optimal functioning based on current fitness level. (S3.M8.8)

psychomotor assessments; and heart rate monitor classroom systems, which allow teachers to assess the whole classroom within seconds. Simply put, technology affords endless opportunities.

FITNESS EDUCATION GRADING

As stated throughout this chapter, there are many beneficial reasons to grade students in physical education and many ways of assessing and grading students, but grading students on fitness assessments is *not* one of them. Although engagement in specific types of physical activity can increase students' physical fitness, factors beyond the control of students and physical education teachers need to be considered. Heredity and genetics, caloric consumption, environmental limitation and opportunities to be physically active within and beyond the school day, and underlying health issues are just a few reasons why grading students on their fitness assessment would be unfair to students who exert high levels of effort but don't reach the criterion referenced measurement.

According to the Presidential Youth Fitness Program (PYFP, 2017, p. 16),

> because students differ in terms of interests and ability, teachers should not use student scores to evaluate individual students within K-12 physical education. Grading students on fitness might constitute holding them accountable for results that are beyond their control. Standards-based grading should reflect students' knowledge of activities and concepts related to fitness education, including their understanding of fitness concepts, their ability to plan a fitness program by using appropriate

Appropriate and Inappropriate Uses of Fitness Assessments

While assessments of student fitness levels are necessary for physical education classes, fitness results should be private; publicly posting them is unnecessary and inappropriate. Both physical education teachers and students share a responsibility in ensuring that the results of any fitness assessment are used appropriately. Additionally, fitness assessment scores should *not* be used for high-stakes accountability, and physical education teachers should not be evaluated based on their students' fitness assessment measurements.

Incorporating fitness assessment into the course further provides that health-related fitness activities are incorporated into the curriculum and instructional strategies; students gain knowledge and skills regarding fitness education concepts, programs, and opportunities; students are prepared to participate in appropriate fitness assessment activities; teachers individualize fitness assessments to meet the needs of each student and use the Brockport Physical Fitness Test (BPFT) for students with disabilities; and teachers work with students in developing and assessing their individualized personal fitness plan. For further reading, see SHAPE America's position on *Appropriate and Inappropriate Practices Related to Fitness Testing* at www.shapeamerica.org/advocacy/positionstatements/pe/upload/Appropriate-and-Inappropriate-Uses-of-Fitness-Testing-FINAL-3-6-17.pdf.

activities, their maintaining a physical activity or nutrition log, and their developing personal portfolios related to fitness.

The Appropriate and Inappropriate Uses of Fitness Assessments sidebar provides more details on this subject.

HEALTH-RELATED FITNESS ASSESSMENTS

Health-related fitness comprises five identified components of fitness: cardiorespiratory endurance (aerobic capacity), body composition, muscular strength, muscular endurance, and flexibility. It has long been one of the staples in physical education. Physical fitness testing is a highly visible and important part of physical education and fitness education programs. Several well-established and recommended health-related fitness assessments exist for use in school settings, such as the YMCA fitness assessment and the JROTC Cadet Challenge. However, Cooper Institute's FitnessGram, designed in 1982, is the most popular and widely used health-related fitness assessment in the United States.

SHAPE America (2012, p.1) defines fitness education as "the instructional and learning process of acquiring knowledge, skills and values; experiencing regular participation in physical activity; and promoting healthy nutrition choices to attain life-enhancing, health-related fitness." The use of health-related fitness assessments in physical education programs is well documented in the literature and is an essential and integral component of the overall physical education program. Linking fitness assessment to the established curriculum and encouraging students to assume responsibility for their own health and wellness is a major goal of fitness education programs. The use of health-related fitness assessment further supports the National Standards for Physical Education, predominantly Standard 3, and the corresponding Grade-Level Outcomes, as documented in this chapter and throughout the text. SHAPE America (2009) further develops these appropriate instructional practice guidelines and support for health-related fitness assessment:

Inclusion

- 1.6.2 Lessons/activities are adapted for overweight students (e.g., distance and pace runs are made more appropriate). Students are encouraged to undertake appropriate levels of activity for their own improvement.

Developing Health-Related Fitness

- 3.4.1 Health-related components provide the focus for fitness activities. Skill-related components of fitness are emphasized in their relation to skill development.
- 3.4.2 The physical educator helps students interpret and use assessment data to set goals and to develop a lifelong fitness plan.

Fitness Testing

- 4.3.1 Physical educators use fitness assessment as part of the ongoing process of helping students understand, enjoy, improve and/or maintain their physical fitness and well-being (e.g., students set goals for improvement that are revisited during the school year), not for grading.
- 4.3.2 As part of an ongoing physical education program, students are prepared physically in each fitness component so that they can complete the assessments safely.

Fitness Procedures

- 4.4.1 Physical educators make every effort to create testing situations that are private, nonthreatening, educational and encouraging.
- 4.4.2 Physical educators encourage students to avoid comparisons with others and, instead, use the results as a catalyst for personal improvement.

Reporting Student Progress

- 4.5.1 Test results are shared privately with students and their parents/guardians as a tool for developing personal goals and strategies.

To read the full document for *Appropriate Instructional Practice Guidelines, K-12: A Side-by-Side Comparison*, go to www.shapeamerica.org/upload/Appropriate-Instructional-Practice-Guidelines-K-12.pdf.

FITNESSGRAM

Assessing students in physical education is about more than giving a grade; it's a tool to use in designing the overall curriculum and instructional program. Assessments are what link student performance to specific learning objectives. The same holds for fitness assessment, as shown in figure 7.5. FitnessGram is as much an educational program as it is a battery of fitness assessments with items scored according to criterion-referenced standards that are age- and sex-specific and established according to how fit children need to be for the purpose of good health. Based on individual student assessment results, scores fall into one of

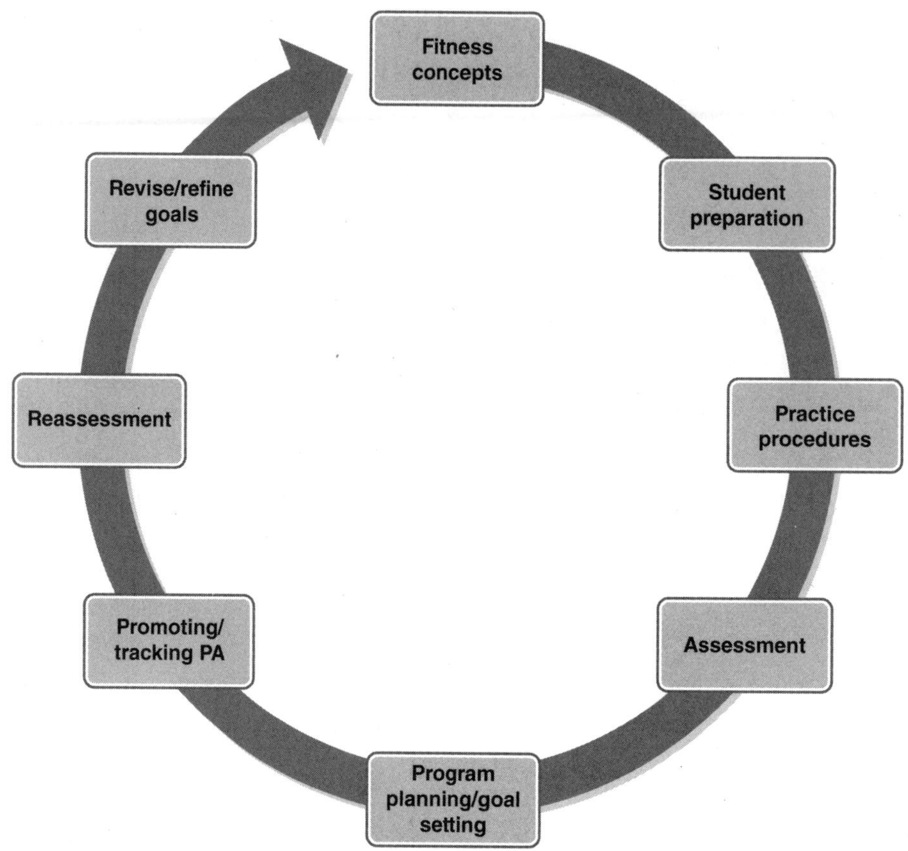

Figure 7.5 FitnessGram's instructional learning cycle: the eight steps of physical fitness programming.

three categories: the healthy fitness zone, needs improvement, or needs improvement—health risk. The FitnessGram program's specific goals are to "promote enjoyable, regular physical activity and to provide comprehensive physical fitness and activity assessments and reporting programs for children and youth." (Cooper, 2017, p. 3). Therefore, assessment-based information should be used as the foundation for designing personal programs of fitness development.

With FitnessGram being the fitness assessment most commonly administered in schools, as well as an anchor in the Presidential Youth Fitness Program, the next section focuses on the five components of health-related fitness and basic teaching tips and steps to administer FitnessGram assessment.

According to Pate and Oria (2012), to plan and conduct fitness testing in schools effectively and appropriately, test administrators should first consider the following four factors:

- Test items should be selected with consideration of contextual variables, such as access to high-quality equipment; space; cost; privacy; availability of volunteers; and cultural, racial, and ethnic factors.
- When administering tests, consideration should be given to the safety of participants, the presence of preexisting conditions, the effects of body composition and other modifiers on test results, and the confidentiality of results.
- School-based professional development that is applicable to the daily routine of teachers and includes instruction for how to integrate fitness testing into the curriculum should be provided.
- Professional development should include training in the administration of protocols and interpretation and communication of test results, with emphasis on educating participants about the importance of fitness, supporting the achievement of fitness goals, and developing healthy living habits. Those interpreting and communicating test results should ensure confidentiality, consider each student's demographic characteristics, provide for the involvement of parents or guardians, and offer positive feedback and recommendations to students and their parents or guardians.

The following section will focus on the five components of FitnessGram and the Brockport Fitness Assessment.

Cardiorespiratory Endurance

Cardiorespiratory endurance is the ability of the heart, lungs, and blood vessels to work together to provide the needed oxygen and fuel to the body during sustained workloads. Although cardiorespiratory endurance is covered extensively in chapters 2 and 8, it is important to note again that children with healthy cardiorespiratory fitness are more likely to live longer and healthier as adults and have improved academic achievement, clearer thinking, better mental health, and a higher sense of self-worth and life satisfaction (American Heart Association, 2020). Aerobic capacity, which depends on how well the respiratory system can bring oxygen into the body and how fast the heart can pump oxygenated blood to the rest of the body, is one of the most important aspects of any fitness program. Tables 7.9, 7.10, and 7.11 align cardiorespiratory endurance assessment with GLOs and the IFFEPE benchmarks. The three cardiovascular endurance assessments discussed here are the PACER and the one-mile (1.6 km) run and walk tests. When administering the tests, teachers often either have preference or are limited by space; maintaining accuracy without a track is difficult, and therefore the PACER is easier to do in a gymnasium.

PACER Test

The PACER is a maximal aerobic fitness test that requires participants to run 20-meter shuttles at increasing speeds. A 15-meter PACER test can be

Table 7.9 Middle School Grade-Level Outcomes for Cardiorespiratory Endurance Assessment

Standard 3	Grade 6	Grade 7	Grade 8
The physically literate individual demonstrates the knowledge and skills to achieve and maintain a health-enhancing level of physical activity and fitness.			
S3.M13 Fitness knowledge	Defines resting heart rate and describes its relationship to aerobic fitness and the Borg rating of perceived exertion (RPE) scale. (S3.M13.6)	Defines how the RPE scale can be used to determine the perception of the work effort or intensity of exercise. (S3.M13.7)	Defines how the RPE scale can be used to adjust workout intensity during physical activity. (S3.M13.8)

Table 7.10 High School Grade-Level Outcomes for Cardiorespiratory Endurance Assessment

Standard 3	Level 1	Level 2
The physically literate individual demonstrates the knowledge and skills to achieve and maintain a health-enhancing level of physical activity and fitness.		
S3.H12 Assessment and program planning	Designs a fitness program, including all components of health-related fitness, for a college student and an employee in the learner's chosen field of work. (S3.H12.L1)	Analyzes the components of skill-related fitness in relation to life and career goals, and designs an appropriate fitness program for those goals. (S3.H12.L2)

Table 7.11 IFFEPE Benchmarks for Assessment of Cardiorespiratory Endurance

Descriptor	Grades 6-8 benchmark	Grades 9-12 benchmark
Demonstrates competency in techniques needed to perform a variety of moderate-to-vigorous physical activities		
Technique in improving cardiovascular fitness	• Apply the appropriate form, speed and generation of force during cardiovascular activities. • Adjust pacing to keep HR in the target zone.	• Apply rates of perceived exertion (RPE) and pacing. • Adjust pacing to keep HR in the target zone for extended periods of time.

used when space is limited. Full test administration details can be found in the *FITTNESSGRAM Administration Manual* (5th ed.).

- Objective: Run as long as possible with continuous movement back and forth across a 20-meter space at a specified pace that gets faster with each passing minute.
- Equipment and facilities: flat, non-slip surface at least 20 meters long; marking cones, a 20-meter measuring tape; a computer, laptop, or handheld music device; PACER test audio; recording sheets
- Instructions:
  1. Select and download the PACER cadence; allow students to listen to the cadence a day in advance.
  2. Make copies of the PACER score sheet; mark the course to indicate lanes and end points; have students select a partner.
  3. Students being tested should run across the full marked distance and cross the line with both feet by the time the next tone sounds. At the sound of the tone, each student turns around and runs back to the other end. If students get to the line before the tone, they must wait for the tone before running in the other direction. Students continue in this manner until they fail twice to reach the line before the tone.
  4. The first time that students do not reach the line before the tone sounds, they stop where they are and reverse direction immediately, attempting to get back on pace. This lap constitutes a form break, but it is counted as a complete lap. The test is considered complete as of the next time (i.e., the second time) students fail to reach the line before the tone sounds. The two misses do not have to be consecutive; the test is over after two total misses. Upon completing the test, students should continue to walk and then stretch in the designated cool-down area.
- Scoring:
  - A lap consists of one 20-meter or 15-meter segment, which is the distance from one end of the course to the other. In other words, do not use a down-and-back count for the test.
  - The scorer records lap numbers (crossing off each lap number as it is completed) on a PACER individual score sheet (20-meter or 15-meter).
  - Failing to cross the line before the tone occurs constitutes a form break. As with many other FitnessGram test items, the first form break is counted as a completion. Therefore, the PACER score consists of the number of laps completed prior to the second time students do not get to the line before the tone.
  - The number of laps completed by students is used with their age to estimate aerobic capacity.
- Suggestions for test administration:
  - During the first minute, the 20-meter version allows 9 seconds to run the distance, whereas the 15-meter version allows 6.75 seconds. The lap time decreases by about 0.5 seconds at each successive level. Before administering the test, allow students to practice it and help them understand that the speed increases with each minute.
  - A tone indicates the end of a lap (one 20- or 15-meter distance). Students run from one end to the other between each set of tones. Caution students not to begin too fast; in fact, the beginning speed is very slow.
  - Groups of students may be tested at the same time. With this method, adult volunteers can be asked to help record scores; students can also record scores for each other.

One-Mile (1.6 km) Run Test

- Objective: Run one mile as fast as possible. If students get tired, it is okay to walk for a brief amount of time, and they should be encouraged to maintain at least a slow jog throughout the assessment.
- Equipment and facilities: a stopwatch, a pencil, score sheets; course can consist of a track or any other measured area
- Instructions:
  5. Describe the course to students and remind them to complete the distance in the shortest time possible.
  6. Remind students to listen for their time once they cross the finish line at the one-mile mark.
  7. Remind students to use appropriate pacing in order to get an accurate assessment.
  8. Provide a signal to students to initiate the assessment, such as "Ready . . . start."
  9. As students cross the finish line, call out their times and record them.
- Scoring: Scoring is based on the total time of the one-mile run.

- Suggestions for test administration:
  - Call out times as runners pass the start–stop line for each lap to help them pace themselves.
  - Test preparation should include instruction and practice pacing.
  - Students should always warm up prior to the test and cool down after the test by continuing to walk for several minutes.
  - The test should not be administered in unusually high temperatures or humidity or when the wind is strong. These elements can cause invalid estimates of aerobic capacity as well as create an environment that may be unsafe.

The One-Mile (1.6 km) Walk Test

- Objective: Walk one mile as quickly as possible while maintaining a constant pace for the entire distance.
- Equipment and facilities: a stopwatch, a pencil, score sheets; course can consist of a track or any other measured area
- Instructions:
  1. Describe the course to students and instruct them to complete the full distance at a steady and brisk walking pace that they can maintain for the entire distance.
  2. Up to 30 students can be tested at a time by dividing the group.
  3. Students select a partner; one is the walker and the other the scorer.
  4. As walkers cross the finish line, call out the elapsed time.
  5. At the conclusion of the walk, each student should take a 60-second heart-rate count.
- Scoring: The walk test is based on the relative heart rate when walking a mile at a specific speed.
- Suggestions for test administration:
  - Test preparation should include instruction and practice in pacing and in techniques for monitoring heart rate.
  - Results are better if students maintain a constant pace during most of the test.
  - Students should always warm up prior to the test and cool down after the test by continuing to walk for several minutes.
  - The test should not be administered in unusually high temperatures or humidity or when the wind is strong. These elements can cause invalid estimates of aerobic capacity as well as create an environment that may be unsafe.

Body Composition

Body composition describes the percentage of fat mass versus nonfat mass (e.g., muscle mass, body water, bone mass) in the body. The measurement of body fat tells what percentage of the body's total weight is fat.

Body Mass Index (BMI) Test

- Equipment: stadiometer and digital scale to accurately measure height and weight
- Instructions:
  1. Measure students with their shoes off.
  2. In measuring height and weight, enter fractions of an inch (2.5 cm) up to two decimal places. Do not round height and weight; fractions of an inch or a pound (0.5 kg) can make a difference in the calculated BMI.
- Scoring:
  - Age- and sex-specific values of BMI are used to access weight status for youth.
  - Scorer that fall into the Needs Improvement Zone generally indicate children weigh too much for their height.

Bioelectrical Impedance Analysis Test

- Equipment: Bioelectrical impedance analysis (BIA) devices, which estimate body composition by measuring the body's resistance to the flow or current (see figure 7.6 for an example)

A body with more muscle has more total water and therefore lower resistance to current flow. A body with more fat has less total water and therefore has a greater resistance to flow or current.

- Instructions: Follow the instructions for each individual device.
- Scoring: The output from the BIA device is the score.

Skinfold Measurement Test

- Equipment: a skinfold caliper
- Instructions: The FitnessGram protocol involves measures from the triceps and calf.
- Triceps:
  1. Measure on the back of the right arm above the triceps muscle, midway between the elbow and the acromion process of the scapula (see figure 7.7*a*).

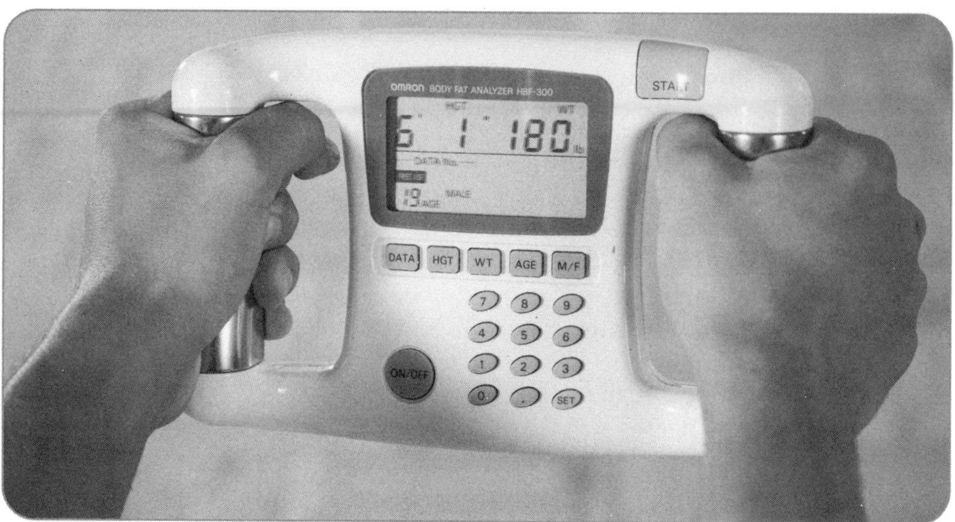

Figure 7.6 Bioelectrical impedance analysis device.

2. Pinch the skinfold slightly above the midpoint to ensure the fold is measured exactly on the midpoint.

- Calf:

1. Measure the inside of the right leg at the level of maximal calf girth.
2. Place the right foot on a flat, elevated surface with the knee flexed at a 90-degree angle.
3. Grasp the skinfold just above the level of maximal girth, and take the measurement below the grasp (see figure 7.7*b*).

- Scoring: The skinfold procedure requires accurate estimates of skinfold thickness. Each measurement should be taken three times, and the recorded score should be the median (middle) value of the three scores.

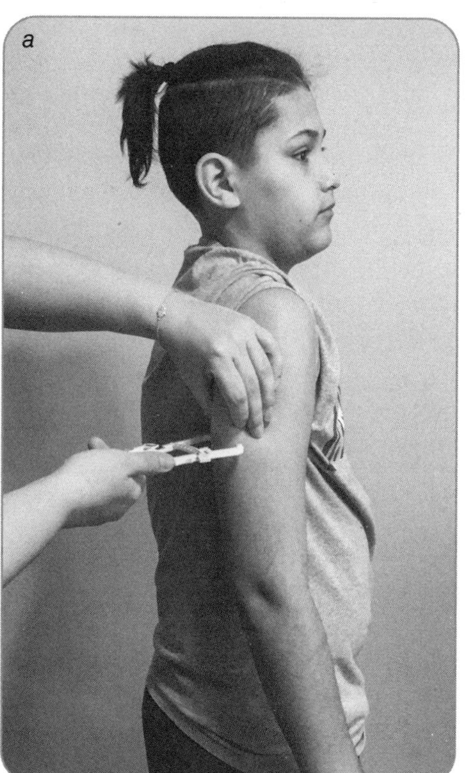

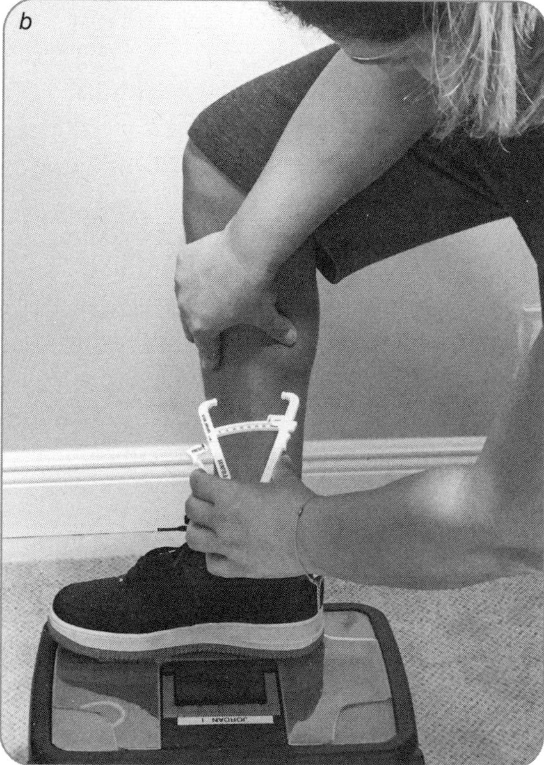

Figure 7.7 Skinfold measurement tests at the triceps (*a*) and calf (*b*).

- Suggestions for test administration:
  - Body composition testing should be conducted in a setting that provides each student with privacy.
  - Whenever possible, have the same tester conduct all measurements for the entire class of students to maximize consistency.
  - The tester should practice taking measurements prior to conducting the test.

Muscular Strength and Endurance

Muscular fitness defines your ability to use your muscles to perform work against a resistance. There are three separate yet interrelated components of muscular fitness: muscular strength, muscular endurance, and power. Muscular strength is the ability to exert maximum force in order to overcome a resistance in a single effort. Abdominal muscle strength and endurance are important in promoting good posture and correct pelvic alignment. A test of trunk extensor strength and flexibility is related to lower back health and vertebral alignment. Upper-body muscle strength and endurance help maintain functional health and promote good posture as well. Tables 7.12 and 7.13 align muscular strength and endurance assessment with the GLOs and IFFEPE (see table 7.14).

Abdominal Strength and Endurance Curl-Up Test

- Objective: Complete as many curl-ups as possible (up to 75) at a specified pace.
- Equipment and facilities: a gym mat marked with the curl-up strips, a piece of paper, the cadence from the accompanying online learning content in HK*Propel*, a device to play the cadence (laptop or other digital music player with a speaker)
- Instructions:
  1. Allow students to partner in groups of two. Partner A does the curl-ups as Partner B counts and watches for errors.
  2. Partner A lies spine on the mat, with knees bent at 140 degrees, feet flat on the floor, legs slightly apart, and arms straight and parallel to the trunk. Partner A's palms should be resting on the mat, with fingers stretched out, and head in contact with the mat.

Table 7.12 Middle School Grade-Level Outcomes for Muscular Strength and Endurance Assessment

Standard 3	Grade 6	Grade 7	Grade 8
The physically literate individual demonstrates the knowledge and skills to achieve and maintain a health-enhancing level of physical activity and fitness.			
S3.M14 Fitness knowledge	Identifies major muscles used in selected physical activities. (S3.M14.6)	Describes how muscles pull on bones to create movement in pairs by relaxing and contracting. (S3.M14.7)	Explains how body systems interact with one another (e.g., blood transports nutrients from the digestive system, oxygen from the respiratory system) during physical activity. (S3.M14.8)

Table 7.13 High School Grade-Level Outcomes for Muscular Strength and Endurance Assessment

Standard 3	Level 1	Level 2
The physically literate individual demonstrates the knowledge and skills to achieve and maintain a health-enhancing level of physical activity and fitness.		
S3.H9 Fitness knowledge	Identifies types of strength exercises (isometric, concentric, eccentric) and stretching exercises (static, proprioceptive neuromuscular facilitation [PNF], dynamic) for personal fitness development (e.g., strength, endurance, range of motion). (S3.H9.L1)	Identifies the structure of skeletal muscle and fiber types as they relate to muscle development. (S3.H9.L2)

Table 7.14 IFFEPE Benchmarks for Muscular Strength and Endurance Assessment

Descriptor	Grades 6-8 benchmark	Grades 9-12 benchmark
Demonstrates competency in techniques needed to perform a variety of moderate to vigorous physical activities		
Technique in improving muscular strength and endurance	• Analyze and differentiate basic musculoskeletal techniques (e.g., alignment, knee not in front of foot) necessary to participate safely in selected movement forms (e.g., correct musculoskeletal errors while performing stretching, yoga, modified weightlifting, etc.). • Demonstrate appropriate technique in resistance training machines and free weights (e.g., sand bells, bars, bands, homemade jug weights.	• Apply basic musculoskeletal techniques necessary to participate in strength and endurance activities. • Demonstrate proper machine adjustment and techniques on resistance training machines, and compare machines to free weight lifting.

3. After Partner A is in position, Partner B ensures that the fingertips rest on the nearest edge of the curl-up distance to the measuring strip under Partner A's legs.
4. Partner B kneels down at Partner A's head to count curl-ups and watch for breaks.
5. The test begins with feet flat on the floor, but only heels must remain in contact with the mat during the test.
6. Partner A curls up slowly, sliding fingers across the measuring strip (see figure 7.8), and then curls back down until head touches a piece of paper. Movement should be slow with the cadence of about 20 curl-ups per minute, or one every 3 seconds.
7. Partner A continues without pausing until Partner A is no longer able to continue, 75 curl-ups are completed, or the second form of correction is made.

- Scoring: The score is the number of curl-ups performed.
- Suggestions for test administration:
  - Student should be repositioned if their body moves, their head does not contact the mat at the appropriate spot, or if the measuring strip is out of position.
  - Movement should start with a flattening of the lower back, followed by a low curling of the upper spine.
  - Students hands should slide across the measuring strip until their fingertips reach the opposite side.
  - Using the cadence encourages steady, continuous movement done with the correct form.
  - Students should not reach forcibly with their arms or hands.

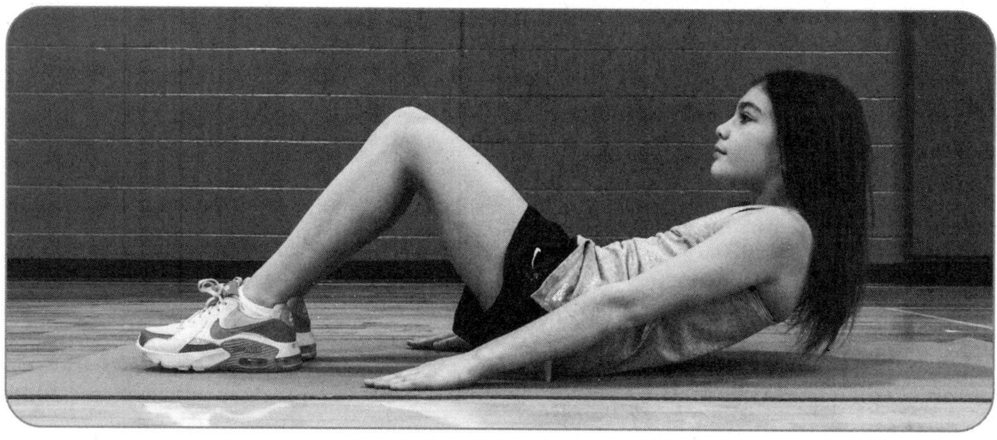

Figure 7.8 A student performing the curl-up test.

Trunk Extensor Strength and Flexibility: Trunk Lift Test

- Objective: Lift the upper body off of the floor by using the back muscles and then hold the position to allow for the measurement.
- Equipment and facilities: gym mats and a measuring device, preferably a yardstick

If using a 12-inch (30 cm) ruler, do not place it under students' chins because doing so could pose a hazard.

- Instructions:
  1. Students lie facedown on the mat with toes pointed and hands under thighs. The chin should be in a neutral position, causing the face to look directly at the mat.
  2. Place a coin or other marker on the floor in line with students' eyes. During the movement, students' face should not look forward, and their eyes should stay on the coin.
  3. Students lift the upper body off the floor in a controlled manner to a maximum height of 12 inches (30 cm; see figure 7.9).
  4. Once the measurement is made, students return to the starting position in a controlled manner.
  5. Conduct two trials and record the highest score.
- Scoring: The score is recorded in inches or centimeters; distances beyond 12 inches (30 cm) should be recorded as 12 inches (30 cm).
- Suggestions for test administration:
  - Do not allow students to do ballistic, bouncing movements.
  - Do not encourage students to lift the chin more than 12 inches (30 cm).
  - Maintaining focus on the marker on the floor helps performers keep their head in a neutral position.
  - Partner B makes the reading at eye level and therefore assumes a squatting or lying position.

Upper-Body Strength and Endurance: 90-Degree Push-Up Test

- Objective: Complete as many 90-degree push-ups as possible at a rhythmic pace (up to a maximum of 75 push-ups).
- Equipment and facilities: a mat, score sheets, 90-degree push-up cadence from HK*Propel*, a device to play the cadence
- Instructions:
  1. Pair students and have one partner perform the 90-degree push-up while the other watches to see that the performer bends the elbows at 90 degrees, with the upper arms parallel to the floor.
  2. Performers begin in a facedown position, with hands slightly wider than the shoulders, fingers stretched out, legs straight and slightly apart, and toes tucked under (see figure 7.10).
  3. Performers push up off the mat with the arms until arms are straight, keeping the legs and back straight. The back should be in a straight line from head to toes throughout the test.
  4. Performers then lower the body until the elbows bend at a 90-degree angle and the upper arms are parallel to the floor.
  5. Performers should repeat the movement as many times as possible, and their rhythm should be approximately 20 push-ups per minute, or 1 every 3 seconds.

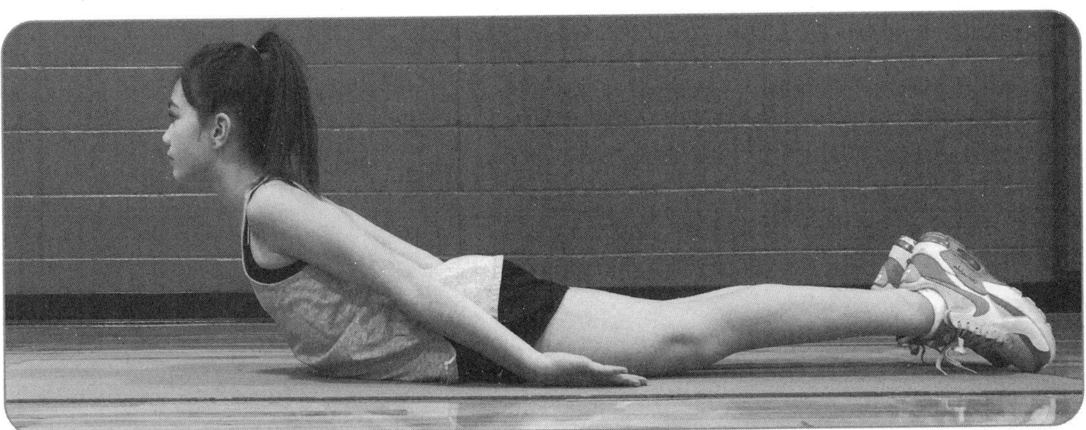

Figure 7.9 A student performing the trunk lift test.

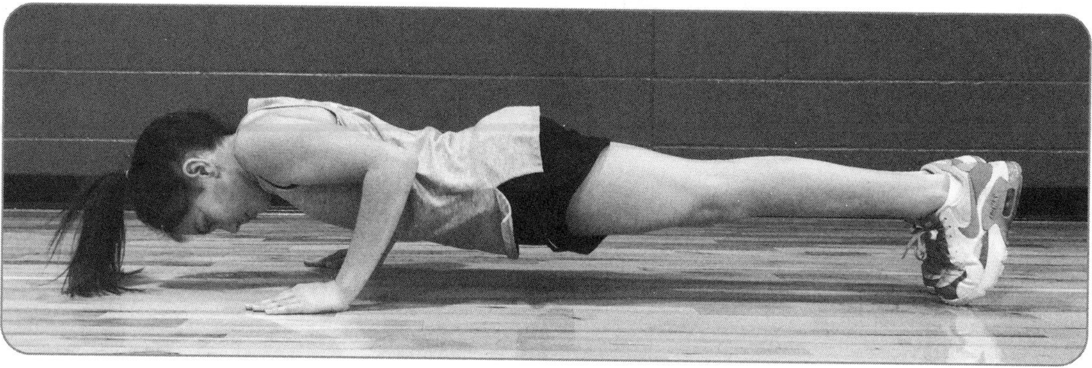

Figure 7.10 A student performing the 90-degree push-up test.

6. Partners stop performers once performers make the second mistake.

- Scoring: The score is the number of 90-degree push-ups performed.
- Suggestions for test administration:
  - The test should be stopped if students are in extreme pain or discomfort.
  - The cadence should be played from HK*Propel*.
  - Males and females follow the same protocol.
  - Use a piece of pliable equipment, such as a foam ball, that can be placed under students' chest. Students must lower to the equipment in order for the 90-degree push-up to count. The appropriate height of the equipment depends on the sizes of your students.

Flexibility

Maintaining adequate joint flexibility is important to functional health. Flexibility may be linked to various health outcomes in youth, such as prevention of back pain, injury, and posture-related problems. Tables 7.15, 7.16, and 7.17 align flexibility assessment with the GLOs and the IFFEPE.

Back-Saver Sit-and-Reach Test

- Objective: Reach the specified distance on the right and left sides of the body. The distance required to achieve the healthy fitness zone is adjusted for age and sex.
- Equipment and facilities: a sit-and-reach box, or specifications for building your own
- Instructions:

1. Students remove shoes and sit down at the test apparatus; one leg is fully extended with the foot flat at the face of the box. The other knee is bent with the sole of the foot flat on the floor, with the instep placed in line 2 to 3 inches (5-8 cm) to the side of the straight knee. The arms are extended forward over the measuring scale with the hands placed one on top of the other (see figure 7.11).
2. Students reach forward along the scale with both hands down four times, keeping the back straight and the head up, and hold the position of the fourth stretch for at least 1 second.
3. After one side is measured, students switch the position of their legs and repeat the process. Measurement must be taken for both sides.

- Scoring: Record the distance reached on each side to the nearest 0.05 inch (0.13 cm), up to a maximum of 12 inches (30 cm). To be in the healthy fitness zone, students should meet the standard on both the right and left sides.
- Suggestions for test administration:
  - The bent knee can move side to side to allow the body to move past it, but the sole of the same foot must remain on the floor.

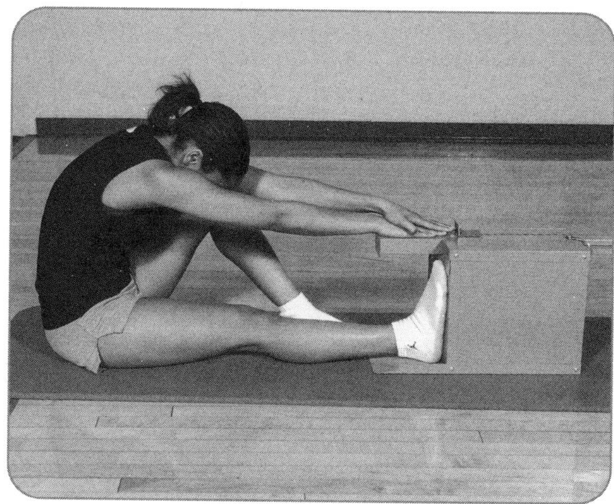

Figure 7.11 A student performing the back-saver sit-and-reach test.

- The back should remain straight and the head up during the forward flexion movement.
- The knee of the extended leg should remain straight. Testers may place one hand above performers' knee as a reminder.
- The trial should be repeated if the hands reach unevenly or the straight knee bends.
- The hips must remain square to the box.

Shoulder Stretch Test

- Objective: Touch the fingertips together behind the back by reaching over the shoulder and under the elbow.
- Equipment and facilities: score sheets only
- Instructions:
  1. Allow students to select a partner who will judge whether the stretch is complete.
  2. To test the right shoulder, students reach with the right hand over the right shoulder and down the back (see figure 7.12). Students place the left hand behind the back and reach up, trying to touch the fingers of the right hand.
  3. To test the left shoulder, students repeat the process on the other side.
  4. Partners observe on both sides whether the fingers touch.
- Scoring: If students touch their fingers on the right side, record a Y (yes) or N (no); do the same for the left side. To achieve the healthy fitness zone, a Y must be recorded on both the right and left sides.

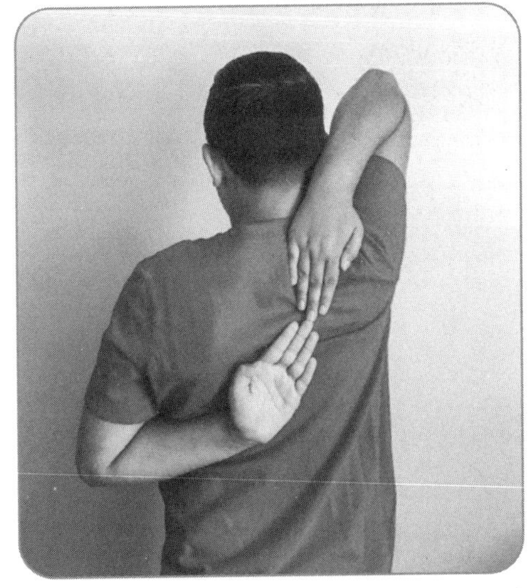

Figure 7.12 A student performing the shoulder stretch test.

Table 7.15 Middle School Grade-Level Outcomes for Flexibility Assessment

Standard 3	Grade 6	Grade 7	Grade 8
The physically literate individual demonstrates the knowledge and skills to achieve and maintain a health-enhancing level of physical activity and fitness.			
S3.M9 Fitness knowledge	Employs correct techniques and methods of stretching. (S3.M9.6)	Describes and demonstrates the difference between dynamic and static stretches. (S3.M9.7)	Employs a variety of appropriate static-stretching techniques for all major muscle groups. (S3.M9.8)

Table 7.16 High School Grade-Level Outcomes for Flexibility Assessment

Standard 3	Level 1	Level 2
The physically literate individual demonstrates the knowledge and skills to achieve and maintain a health-enhancing level of physical activity and fitness.		
S3.H9 Fitness knowledge	Identifies types of strength exercises (isometric, concentric, eccentric) and stretching exercises (static, proprioceptive neuromuscular facilitation [PNF], dynamic) for personal fitness development (e.g., strength, endurance, range of motion). (S3.H9.L1)	Identifies the structure of skeletal muscle and fiber types as they relate to muscle development. (S3.H9.L2)

Table 7.17 IFFEPE Benchmarks for Flexibility Assessment

Descriptor	Grades 6-8 benchmark	Grades 9-12 benchmark
Demonstrates competency in techniques needed to perform a variety of moderate to vigorous physical activities		
Technique in improving flexibility	• Demonstrates correct techniques and methods of stretching (e.g., alignment, no hyperextension). • Demonstrates the difference between dynamic flexibility and static flexibility and when to target each in a workout.	• Demonstrates proper alignment while stretching. • Demonstrates variety of appropriate stretching techniques (static, PNF, active, isolated, and passive).

BROCKPORT PHYSICAL FITNESS TEST

All students enrolled in physical education should have access and the opportunity to be engaged in fitness education programs and fitness assessment. The BPFT protocols and adapted fitness zone standards is a criterion-referenced, health-related test. It is specifically designed to assess the fitness of youth (ages 10 to 17) with disabilities that include intellectual disabilities, visual impairments, spinal cord injuries, cerebral palsy, congenital anomalies, and amputations. The BPFT provides assessment using three fitness components: aerobic functioning, body composition, and musculoskeletal functioning. For students who need accommodations or modifications for fitness assessment, they can use the full Brockport test battery or a combination of FitnessGram and Brockport (Winnick & Short, 2014).

The physical fitness test battery can be customized for any student, and there are several tests to choose from for each fitness component. The test items by BPFT fitness component include the following:

- Aerobic functioning
  - PACER (20-meter and 15-meter)
  - One-mile (1.6 km) run and walk
  - Target aerobic movement test (TAMT)
- Body composition
  - Percentage of body fat: skinfolds
  - Percentage of body fat: bioelectrical impedance analysis
  - BMI
- Musculoskeletal functioning
  - Reverse curl
  - Seated push-up
  - 40-meter push and walk
  - Wheelchair ramp test
  - Push-up
  - Isometric push-up
  - Pull-up
  - Modified pull-up (see figure 7.13)
  - Bench press
  - Dumbbell press
  - Dominant grip strength
  - Back-saver sit-and-reach
  - Flexed-arm hang
  - Extended-arm hang
  - Trunk lift
  - Curl-up
  - Modified curl-up
  - Target stretch test (TST)
  - Modified Apley test
  - Shoulder stretch
  - Modified Thomas test

The full *Brockport Physical Fitness Test Manual* (2nd edition) provides examples of ways to administer and score each test item, the standards, and fitness zones. It is highly recommended that physical education teachers secure a copy of this manual and become familiar with the assessments. The following list provides links to several chapters of the manual on the Presidential Youth Fitness Program website:

- Chapter 1, Introduction to the Brockport Physical Fitness Test: www.pyfp.org/storage/app/media/documents/brockport/brockport-ch1.pdf
- Chapter 4, Profiles, Test Selection Guides, Standards, and Fitness Zones: www.pyfp.org/storage/app/media/documents/brockport/brockport-ch4.pdf

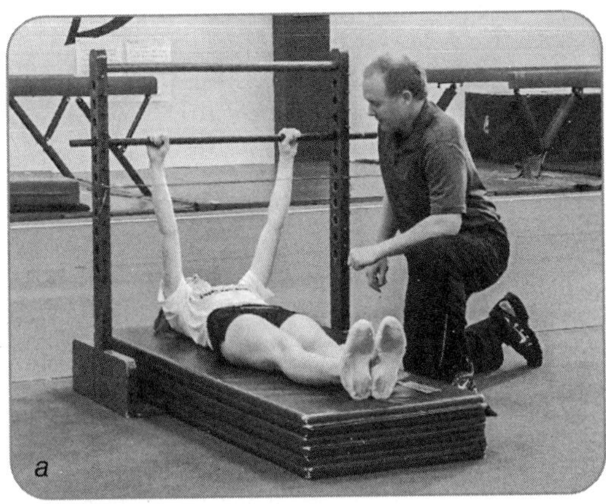

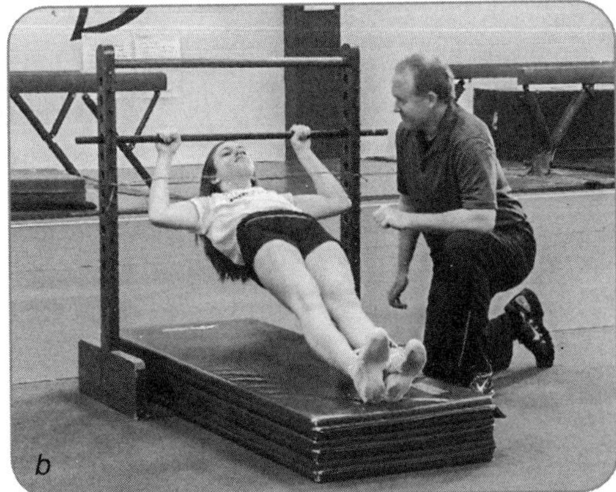

Figure 7.13 Modified pull-up: starting position (*a*) and raised position (*b*).
Reprinted by permission from J.P Winnick and F.X. Short, *Brockport Physical Fitness Test Manual*, 2nd ed. (Champaign, IL: Human Kinetics, 2014), 79.

- Chapter 5, The Test Administration and Test Items: www.pyfp.org/storage/app/media/documents/brockport/brockport-ch5.pdf
- Chapter 6, Testing Youngsters with Severe Disability: www.pyfp.org/storage/app/media/documents/brockport/brockport-ch6.pdf

A copy of the General Brockport Physical Fitness Test Form can be found at: www.pyfp.org/storage/app/media/documents/brockport/brockport-test-form.pdf.

LAB FITNESS ASSESSMENTS AND CAREER OPPORTUNITIES

Since the IFFEPE further identifies the need for fitness careers and occupational fitness needs in the benchmarks for grades 6 to 8 and 9 to 12, it is important to provide information on more advanced fitness assessment procedures, which go beyond the secondary school curriculum. Cardiorespiratory endurance assessments usually fall into two categories: maximal and submaximal tests. Maximal tests are designed to push a person to exhaustion, require specialized equipment that measures the amounts of oxygen used and carbon dioxide exhaled during the monitoring of heart rate and blood pressure, and are usually administered by a trained professional. Submaximal tests are designed to require a person to work below maximum effort, and data is extrapolated to estimate maximum capacity.

Students may choose to follow one of two tracks to earn their BS degree in sports medicine or exercise science as fitness-related careers: (1) health and human performance, the more popular track in which the following multiple certifications are an option upon graduation: personal trainer, corrective exercise specialist, and youth exercise specialist; and (2) group fitness director certification is designed to develop skills and knowledge necessary to provide safe and effective group fitness instruction using a variety of exercise modalities. The coursework includes knowledge and application of training principles and exercise techniques to develop cardiorespiratory fitness, muscular strength, muscular endurance, and muscular flexibility. The following fitness assessments, listed by fitness component, are often a component of college and university sports medicine and fitness technology programs:

- Body composition:
  - BMI
  - Hydrostatic weighing
  - Percentage of body fat: skinfolds (calipers)
  - Bioelectrical impedance
  - Waist circumference
  - Girth measurements
- Cardiorespiratory:
  - Astrand-Rhyming (lab)
  - YMCA $\dot{V}O_2$submax test (lab)
  - Field tests
  - 1-mile (1.6 km) walk
  - 1.5-mile (2.4 km) run
  - 12-minute swim test
  - Step test

Note: Use either the Karvonen or heart rate reserve (HRR) formula as seen in chapter 2 to determine the intensity of exercise in the cardiorespiratory training zone, along with the rating of perceived exertion (RPE) scale.

- Muscular strength:
  - Hand grip test: dynamometer
  - 1-RM bench press and leg press
- Muscular endurance:
  - Bench-jump
  - Modified dip
  - Push-ups
  - Abdominal crunches
- Flexibility:
  - Sit-and-reach test
  - Total body rotation test
  - Shoulder rotation test

According to Hoeger and Hoeger (2018), in addition to health-related fitness assessments, a personal trainer should also be proficient in the following skill-related assessments:

- Agility: Southeast Missouri (SEMO) agility test
- Balance: one-foot stand test
- Coordination: soda test
- Power: standing long-jump test
- Reaction time: yardstick test

Due to the decrease of physical education programs and the increase of childhood and adult obesity, some personal trainers also become certified as corrective exercise specialists (CESs). CESs prescribe specific exercises to correct any muscular imbalances that may lead to injuries during physical activities. Clark and Sutton (2014) identify the following assessments that are used for determining muscular imbalances:

- Static assessment: looking at kinetic checkpoints from the lateral, anterior, and posterior view as a person is standing
- Transitional assessments:
  - Overhead squat
  - Single-leg squat
  - Push-ups
  - Pulling: standing row
  - Pressing: standing overhead dumbbell press
  - Star Excursion Balance Test (SEBT)
- Dynamic postural assessments:
  - Gait: treadmill walking
  - Landing Error Scoring System (LESS) test
  - Tuck jump
  - Closed Kinetic Chain Upper Extremity Stability (CKCUEST) test
  - ROM tests using a goniometer

The first national certification test students must take is the personal training certification. However, to be eligible to take the corrective exercise specialist (CES) through National Academy of Sports Medicine (NASM), students must have a bachelor's degree and the personal training certification. Group fitness director certification is through the American College of Sports Medicine (ACSM).

DEVELOPING AN INDIVIDUAL FITNESS PLAN

A key element of any fitness education class or course should be the development of student individual fitness plans that are based on valid assessment data. Such plans should include goals that are short-term, intermediate, and long-term for improving or maintaining fitness levels along with selected health-related activities to improve each component. Fitness assessments facilitate the process of students developing their own individual fitness plans as they learn how to evaluate their own personal levels of fitness through formal and self-assessment (see tables 7.18 and 7.19). By setting goals, students make a commitment and take responsibility for their own behavior. Personal goals they have set should motivate them toward meeting them, be written down, and must state precisely what they wish to accomplish. Since these are personal plans, students can always modify them if unforeseen obstacles become evident. Sample personalized fitness plans can be found in HK*Propel*.

Physical education teachers should play a vital role in assisting students in creating their personal fitness plan to ensure that the plans are challenging yet achievable. Students can keep progress of their fitness gains and target goals through personal fitness logs, portfolios, journals, or self-assessment throughout the course.

As discussed in chapters 1 and 6, to assist students in developing their individual fitness plans, it is recommended that teachers follow the SMART framework for developing objectives. SMART goals and objectives should be written in simplistic terms and clearly define expectations. The type of objectives you write is contingent on whether the goal is a short- or long-term one. As a reminder, these are the principles for writing SMART goals:

Table 7.18 Middle School Grade Level Outcomes for Self-Evaluation of Fitness Levels

Standard 3	Grade 6	Grade 7	Grade 8
The physically literate individual demonstrates the knowledge and skills to achieve and maintain a health-enhancing level of physical activity and fitness.			
S3.M15 Assessment and program planning	Designs and implements a program of remediation for an area of weakness based on the results of health-related fitness assessment. (S3.M15.6)	Designs and implements a program of remediation for 2 areas of weakness based on the results of health-related fitness assessment. (S3.M15.7)	Designs and implements a program of remediation for 3 areas of weakness based on the results of health-related fitness assessment. (S3.M15.8)
S3.M15 Assessment and program planning	Maintains a physical activity log for at least 2 weeks, and reflects on activity levels as documented in the log. (S3.M16.6)	Maintains a physical activity and nutrition log for at least 2 weeks, and reflects on activity levels and nutrition as documented in the log. (S3.M16.7)	Designs and implements a program to improve levels of health-related fitness and nutrition. (S3.M16.8)

Table 7.19 High School Grade Level Outcomes for Self-Evaluation of Fitness Levels

Standard 3	Level 1	Level 2
The physically literate individual demonstrates the knowledge and skills to achieve and maintain a health-enhancing level of physical activity and fitness.		
S3.H12 Assessment and program planning	Designs a fitness program, including all components of health-related fitness, for a college student and an employee in the learner's chosen field of work. (S3.H12.L1)	Analyzes the components of skill-related fitness in relation to life and career goals, and designs an appropriate fitness program for those goals. (S3.H12.L2)

S–Specific: Goals should be attainable and clearly defined and stated and answer the questions *who, what, where, when,* and *why.*

M–Measurable: Goals should be stated in quantitative terms and be measurable.

A–Achievable: Goals should be set in challenging yet achievable and realistic terms.

R–Relevant: Goals must be relevant to the purpose and to the needs of the student or project.

T–Time-bound: Goals must have time lines to determine progress toward meeting the desired outcomes.

By setting SMART goals and objectives, teachers provide students an outline that helps them get closer to achieving their overall fitness goals. With SMART goals being set, students get immediate feedback as they progress through class and adhere to their fitness plans. The achievement of the goals and objectives will further motivate students to be physically active through their school year, and, more importantly, through their life span.

CONCLUSION

Throughout this chapter, we emphasized the role that fitness assessment plays in a fitness education course and how assessments align with the National Standards for Physical Education and Grade-Level Outcomes. Although we as physical educators have a tendency to focus on the actual health-related fitness assessments in physical education classes, we presented many other assessment strategies to offer alternative means for students to express content knowledge and learning gains including written and performance assessments, portfolios, journals, student logs, individual and class projects, and the use of wearable technology. Additionally, we provided strategies for administering the FitnessGram assessment and Brockport Physical Fitness Test to ensure that students with disabilities have the opportunity to participate in all assessment and class instruction. Lastly, when students take responsibility for improving and maintaining their fitness goals with the use of individual fitness plans, they are much better equipped to adhere to those plans and reach the goals and objectives that they developed in collaboration with their physical education teachers.

Review Questions

1. Describe the role that the National Standards in Physical Education and the Grade-Level Outcomes play in the development of a fitness education program.
2. Explain how a fitness education program can meet the objectives of the affective domain.
3. Identify an alternative form of assessment in physical education and explain how it relates to fitness education.
4. Select one component of fitness and describe the FitnessGram assessment that you would use to measure your level and which accompanying Brockport Physical Fitness Test item you would use for a student with disabilities in your class.
5. Describe how you would set up your own individual fitness plan based on your fitness assessment measures.

Visit HK*Propel* for additional material related to this chapter.

Part II

Fitness Elements and Lesson Plans

CHAPTER 8

Cardiorespiratory Fitness

Chapter Objective

After reading this chapter, you will understand how to incorporate cardiorespiratory fitness activities and concepts into a fitness education program during individual class sessions; identify the different types of cardiorespiratory fitness training programs; design age- and developmentally appropriate activities for student participation; and employ best teaching practices that enhance student learning and comprehension.

Key Concepts

- Cardiorespiratory fitness is a key predictor of health indicators in youth.
- Developing and improving cardiorespiratory fitness can be achieved without equipment.
- Various types of training methods should be offered throughout the course.
- Principles of training including specificity, individuality, overload, progression, variation, and regularity should be taught for students to comprehend components of a fitness education–training program.
- The FITT framework and HIIT activities should be utilized in applying the basic fitness education program for conceptual understanding and activity progression.
- Accommodations and modifications should be implemented to ensure all students can safely participate in the course.

INTRODUCTION

Cardiorespiratory endurance, another component of health-related fitness, is the ability of the heart, lungs, and blood vessels to work together to provide the needed oxygen and fuel to the body during sustained workloads. Although cardiorespiratory endurance is covered extensively in chapter 2, it is important for your students to develop an understanding of *why* engaging in cardiorespiratory activities is important, *what* are the benefits of developing a strong cardiorespiratory system, and *how* to safely participate in cardiorespiratory activities.

According to the American Heart Association (Raghuveer et al., 2020), "nearly 60% of American children do not have healthy cardiorespiratory fitness (CRF), which is a key measure of physical fitness and overall health," and that high levels of cardiorespiratory fitness are associated with healthy cardiovascular and metabolic profiles among children and youth (Ruiz, et al., 2007). Globally, approximately 80 percent of youth lack recommended levels of physical activity, which has a negative impact on cardiorespiratory fitness (World Health Organization, 2019). Research has further shown that children with healthy cardiorespiratory fitness are more likely to live longer and healthier as adults and have improved academic achievement, clearer thinking, better mental health, and a higher sense of self-worth and life satisfaction (Raghuveer et al., 2020).

This leads to the question of what role does physical education play in the development of increasing CRF. As explained through the conceptual physical education (CPE) model in chapter 1 (table 1.7), the curriculum designed and the delivery of instructional content plays a critical role in the delivery of fitness education concepts. Additionally, the relationship between physical activity, exercise, and physical education as identified in figure 1.1 further emphasizes how fitness levels can be enhanced through a variety of activities. According to Hildebrand and Ekelund (2017) and the World Health Organization (2019), to understand the relationship between physical activity and CRF, we first need to differentiate between habitual physical activity and exercise training. *Habitual physical activity* has been defined as "the usual physical activity carried out in normal daily life in every domain and any dimension" (Hildebrand & Ekelund, 2017). *Exercise training* consists of a planned, structured exercise program that is sustained for an adequate length of time, with sufficient intensity and frequency to induce changes in components of physical fitness, as outlined in the FITT principle.

With a deliberate emphasis on cardiorespiratory fitness, Armstrong and McManus (2011) found that appropriate training increases youth peak oxygen uptake, irrespective of sex, age, or maturity status. Collectively, the data show that either three 20-minute sessions per week of continuous intensity training at approximately 85 to 90 percent of maximum heart rate or high-intensity interval training at around 95 percent of maximum heart rate interspersed with short recovery periods will induce on average an 8 to 9 percent increase in youth peak oxygen uptake in 10 to 12 weeks. Based on this research, one semester of a fitness education program in physical education would effectively have a positive impact on students' overall CRF with deliberate instruction and opportunity to participate.

Therefore, cardiorespiratory endurance is about both the importance of fitness education and the numerous benefits of incorporating the cardiorespiratory component into the program. CRF is an essential component of any workout or fitness program. Both aerobic exercise (any form of exercise that uses oxygen to fuel your muscles) and anaerobic exercise (which does not use oxygen to fuel your muscles) are beneficial depending on your fitness instructional goals, as well as the goals that your students wish to accomplish.

Every physical education teacher will be challenged as to how to safely apply these health-related components on a daily basis while incorporating all the fitness information covered in the previous chapters. Keep in mind that each class will consist of a very diverse population of students with varying mindsets as to why they are in this particular physical education class. Several kinds of fitness methods and activities are available to accommodate all fitness levels that allow all students to feel comfortable while participating in workouts and activities. Ensuring that accommodations and modifications are included in every daily lesson plan is critical for providing an inclusive learning environment.

Chapter 2 focused on the basic principles of training—principles of specificity, individuality, overload, progression, variation, and regularity; adaptations; the FITT principle; and measuring heart rate, breathing rate, and the rate of perceived exertion. It is important to review these principles again and apply them when implementing a CRF program. Enabling students to develop their individual cardiorespiratory fitness plans based on their fitness assessments as discussed in chapter 7 should also be taken into consideration. Additionally, chapter 16 focuses on preparing students to participate in community-based events.

BENEFITS OF CARDIORESPIRATORY FITNESS

As previously discussed in chapter 2, participating in daily physical activity and developing cardiorespiratory endurance and cardiorespiratory fitness have many benefits. When done on a regular basis, moderate- to vigorous-intensity physical activity (MVPA) strengthens the heart muscle. This improves the heart's ability to pump blood to the lungs and throughout the body as more blood flows to the muscles, and oxygen levels in the blood rise. As a result, more oxygen is delivered to the body as waste products are carried away.

In particular, according to research published by the NIH (n.d.), The Lancet Global Health (2020), The MAYO Clinic (2019), the WHO (2019), ACSM (2019), Harvard School of Medicine (2016), and the *Journal of Preventative Medicine and Public Health* (2013), the many benefits of cardiorespiratory fitness include the following:

- Reduces the risk of heart disease, lung cancer, type 2 diabetes, stroke, and other diseases
- Improves cardiorespiratory functioning
- Lowers blood pressure
- Is potentially a stronger predictor of mortality than other established risk factors such as smoking, hypertension, high cholesterol, and type 2 diabetes
- Enables the heart, lungs, and cardiorespiratory system to work more efficiently in delivering oxygenated blood to the muscles
- Improves immune function
- Produces better bone health through increased bone density
- Reduces the chance of metabolic syndrome
- Promotes weight loss
- Improves brain functioning, cognitive performance, and memory function
- Improves psychological and emotional well-being
- Decreases rates of depression and anxiety

In addition, McKinney et al. (2016, p. 131) found that

> the benefits of physical activity exhibit a dose-response relationship; the higher the amount of physical activity, the greater the health benefits. However, the most unfit individuals have the potential for the greatest

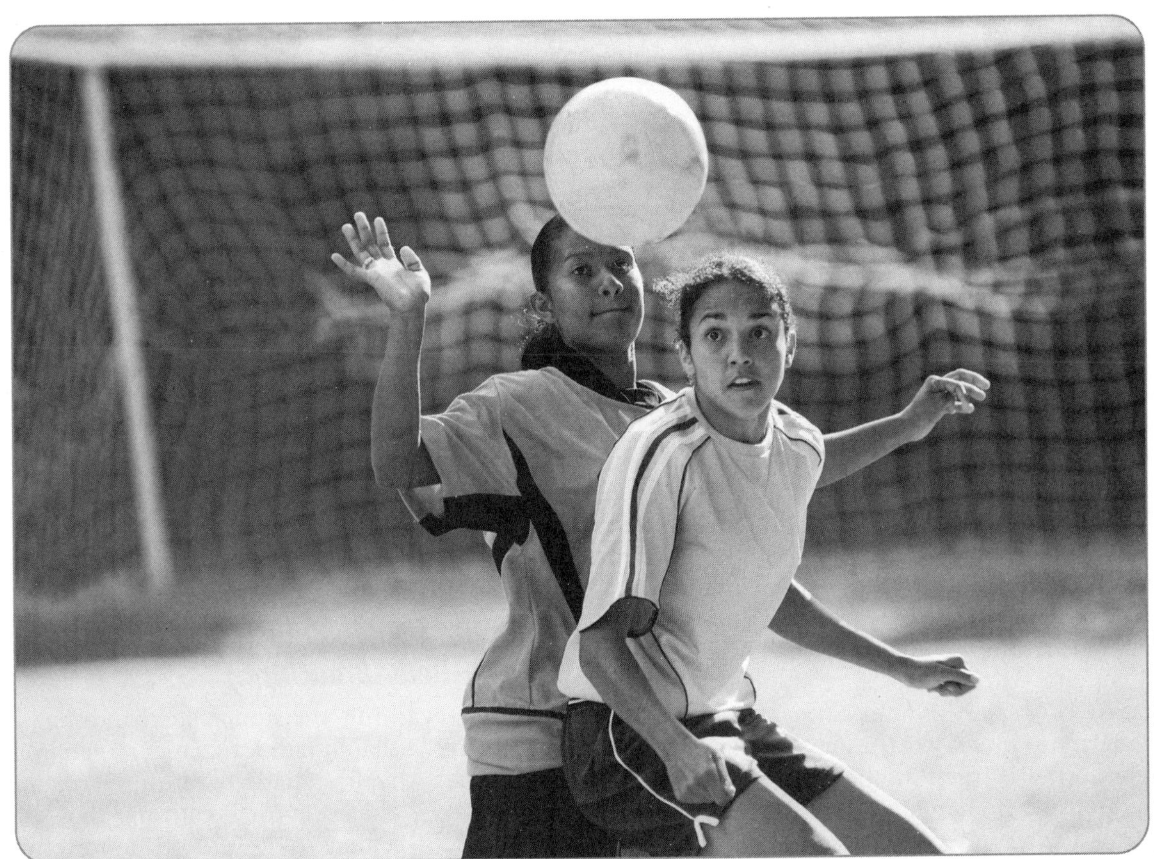

iStockphoto/Alberto Pomares

Regular MVPA strengthens the heart muscle, among many other health benefits.

reduction in risk, even with small increases in physical activity. Given the significant health benefits afforded by physical activity, considerable efforts should be made to promote this vital agent of health.

Therefore, regardless of where students are initially in their health-related fitness status and gains, including incremental gains, physical activity throughout the course of a fitness education program will have a great impact on students' immediate health. It is always important to modify all movements and exercises in order to meet the individual needs of all students so everyone can engage in full participation. As previously discussed, bringing a UDL approach to your program ensures that all students can reach their full potential. Review chapters 3 and 4 for general recommendations that should be followed for all activities.

STARTING POINTS FOR A FITNESS EDUCATION COURSE

Since CRF training and activities are this chapter's focus, we begin by providing instructional strategies on how to teach breathing while engaging in brisk walking, jogging, running, aerobic dance, stair climbing, or other rapidly paced movements during physical education class. Incorporating proper breathing techniques for physically intense exercises and activities will help students participate for longer periods of time.

Breathing Techniques

Although we often take breathing for granted, to implement an effective CRF education program, students should be taught proper breathing techniques for ease and efficiency in reaching their full potential. Since strenuous activities cause the muscles and respiratory system to work harder, the body requires more oxygen while expelling carbon dioxide. As previously discussed, more oxygen use means longer performance before fatigue sets in. Maximal oxygen uptake ($\dot{V}O_2max$), also termed aerobic capacity, is the maximal rate of oxygen that can be used during intense exercise.

Poor breathing techniques during intense physical activity will further cause students who are starting a cardiorespiratory fitness program to fatigue more quickly, gasp for air, and feel that uncomfortable "stitch" in their side, causing them to stop in the middle of the activity and give up. The quality of your breathing technique will allow for increased lung capacity and oxygen uptake.

The first question that many students will pose once you start talking about how to breathe during running is, "Do I breathe through my nose or through my mouth?" Although nasal breathing will accommodate brisk walking or slowly jogging, it may not be the best technique for more intense workouts. Beginners can also choose to inhale through their nose and exhale through their mouth. Although the research is extremely limited, many experts and professionals profess that, during more intense exercise, breathing through the mouth is more efficient because it allows more oxygen to enter the body, thus delivering more oxygen to the muscles and diaphragm, in particular. Others recommend that breathing through both the nose and mouth assists in breathing steady and engages the diaphragm for maximum oxygen uptake. However, it has been determined that elevated HR with nasal breathing indicates increased cardiovascular stress associated with this mode (Recinto, Efthemeou, Boffelli, & Navalta, 2017; LaComb, Tandy, Lee, Young, & Navalta, 2017). Breathing mode does not affect power output or performance measures during completion of a high-intensity anaerobic test, so the participant's preference should be the determining factor when a choice is available. Although nasal breathing filters large particles from the surrounding environment and may help to deliver air with fewer contaminants to the respiratory system (Carlisle & Sharp, 2001), mouth breathing further assists in relaxing the jaw muscles and reducing facial tension.

In differentiating between chest breathing and diaphragm breathing, physical education teachers should explain to students the importance of diaphragm breathing as opposed to chest breathing. Chest breathing, while shallow in nature, prohibits the lungs from receiving maximal oxygen thus impacting the lungs to fully expel carbon dioxide quicker since the air stays in the lungs for a short period of time, which inhibits a complete exchange of air. Conversely, diaphragm breathing is a more efficient technique because it uses the entire capacity of the lungs, increasing oxygen uptake by creating more space in the chest cavity (American Lung Association, 2016).

Diaphragmatic Breathing (Deep-Belly Breathing)

During breathing, the stomach expands and contracts as the diaphragm forces air into and out of the lungs. Diaphragmatic breathing strengthens the muscles that support breathing, thus allowing increased air intake during intense physical activities. It also engages the core muscles needed for body stabilization during the time of impact of the foot striking the ground. (See chapter 13 for core-strengthening exercises.) Diaphragmatic breathing should also be used during daily life because it can potentially reduce tension and provide for a more relaxed state. The following is a list of steps physical education teachers can use while teaching diaphragmatic breathing:

1. Begin by lying on the floor on your back, placing one hand on your belly and the other hand on your chest.
2. Breathe through your nose, filling your body with air and paying attention to which area rises first.
3. As your stomach expands, push your diaphragm down and out.
4. Focus on trying to exhale all of the air out of your lungs.
5. Lengthen your exhales so they are longer than your inhales.

Let your students know that this may feel a little awkward at first, explaining that the more they practice, the easier it becomes. They will eventually reach a comfort level, and diaphragmatic breathing will become second nature while engaging in cardiorespiratory activities.

Rhythmic Breathing

Now that you have taught your students the proper way to breathe more efficiently while participating in cardiorespiratory activities, the next phase should be on how to incorporate these breathing techniques into a more comfortable pace and develop rhythmic patterns. Rhythmic breathing simply describes the number of steps, or foot strikes, taken on inhale and exhale. As they begin their running, jogging, aerobic dance, or brisk walking program, it is best to have your students concentrate on a comfortable jogging pace and set realistic goals before increasing their intensity.

Determining the rhythmic patterns varies by practitioners. Some recommend a 2:2 breathing-pattern ratio of inhaling for two counts and then exhaling for two counts to ensure that you are easing into the activity and keeping a steady flow of oxygen to the muscles. Others recommend a 3:3 or 4:4 on easy runs, or a 2:1 on faster runs. Yet, for better distribution of impact across both sides of the body, a 3:2 or a 4:3 might be recommended. However, as you have your students try these various ratios, let them decide what feels most comfortable to them when getting started.

The American Lung Association (2016) further asserts that to practice rhythmic breathing, belly breathing and a five-step pattern should be used: three steps on inhale and two steps on exhale (i.e., as you step: inhale left, right, left; exhale right, left; inhale right, left, right; exhale left, right). Breathing will naturally shift so that it does not overwhelm the same foot on the inhale over and over again, reducing the pressure on the diaphragm and body during the course of the run. As the pace quickens, the body needs more oxygen to fuel the muscles, but this balance can still be maintained by shifting to a three-step pattern: two steps on inhale and one step on exhale (see figure 8.1). The five-step and three-step patterns may be hard to visualize, but, when you start to use the pattern, you can almost sense when the breathing becomes more comfortable.

To further enhance their breathing efficiency during cardiorespiratory activities, students should always focus on their posture by keeping their head in alignment with their spine, relaxing their shoulders, and avoiding slouching forward.

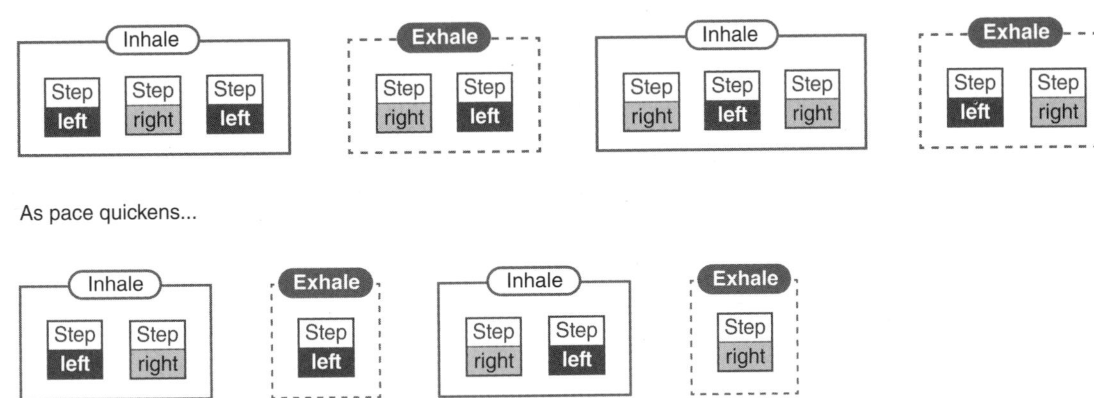

Figure 8.1 As the pace quickens, the body needs more oxygen to fuel the muscles. Shifting from a five-step pattern to a three-step pattern can help maintain this balance.

Warm-Up and Cool-Down Exercises

As with any exercise or activity, performing a series of warm-up activities prior to exercising and cool-down exercises afterward should be a part of every session, and CRF activities are no exception (see figure 8.2). In general terms, appropriate warm-up and cool-down exercises reduce the risk of injury and muscle soreness, thereby creating greater ROM; they also mentally prepare participants for the activity and improve their CRF or sports performance.

Warm-Up

According to the ACSM (2017), warm-up activities should last between 5 to 10 minutes and consist of structured low to moderately-low levels of intensity. The purpose of warming up is to prepare the body for aerobic activity and gradually activate the cardiovascular system by raising body temperature and increasing blood flow to muscles. Warm-up activities may include calisthenics that exercise large muscle groups, or lower-level activities similar to what you will be doing during the activity phase. For example, in preparation for the mile run or PACER assessment, a slow jog around the instructional area would be appropriate. Adding a variety of warm-up activities, such as grapevines or rope jumping, prior to CRF activities will also keep students motivated. If performing class sports activities, such as volleyball, then appropriate stretching activities that are sport specific should be used (see chapters 9 through 11). The point is to gradually increase the intensity from resting levels to the intensity of the next phase.

Cool-Down

Just as in the warm-up phase of the activity, the cool-down phase should also be conducted for 5 to 10 minutes, allowing the body to adjust back to resting levels. After a strenuous cardiorespiratory activity, students should understand that the purpose of the cool-down is to allow their cardiovascular system to gradually slow down so that their heart rate reaches a steady state to prevent blood from pooling in the muscles they have engaged. Throughout the cool-down phase as the muscles contract, the blood is circulated back to the heart for distribution. Similar to the warm-up phase, a slow jog or brisk walk should be performed after a strenuous CRF activity. If strenuous exercise is abruptly stopped and blood pools in the muscles used, this could result in a drop in blood pressure and students may feel dizzy or faint, which could lead to other medical issues. Keep in mind that, regardless of how fatigued students are after the activity phase of the class, they should not lie down upon completion of the activity. Additionally, continuous blood flow will assist in removing lactic acid from the muscles. Stretching exercises should also be performed during the cool-down phase.

At the beginning of a fitness education course, the initial cardiorespiratory activities that students will engage in are walking and jogging programs. These beginning activities will assist students in feeling more comfortable as they continue to reach their cardiorespiratory fitness goals and progress to more intense levels of exercises.

Beginning Walking Workout

The first thing that the physical education teacher needs to remind students of is that, before beginning any physical activity, they should have the proper clothing, which, in most cases, is their physical education uniform, and a good pair of athletic or running shoes. Students should be

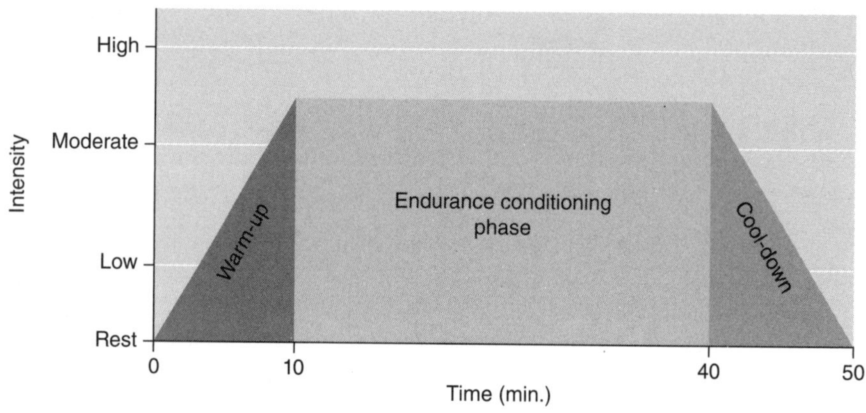

Figure 8.2 The ACSM aerobic workout overview.
Adapted from B. Bushman and J.C. Young, *Action Plan for Menopause* (Champaign, IL: Human Kinetics, 2005), 35.

reminded to maintain good posture, with the head and neck aligned with the spine, shoulders back and relaxed, chest pulled up, and abdomen pulled in; warm up and cool down appropriately; and hydrate before and after the activity, especially if the activity is taking place in extremes of hot or cold weather climates.

For students who have not engaged in cardiorespiratory exercises, either through lack of motivation, safety issues, or just sedentary behavior during those lazy summer months, they should not be expected to jump right into an intense CRF program. The best thing that you as a physical education teacher can do is start out by having them walk around the track or field to begin to get moving again. You may want to start by either time or distance; walking for 15 minutes at a target heart rate of 40 percent training level will be a good place to begin. Then you could advance to walking for 15 to 20 minutes at a moderate intensity, at a target heart rate of 64 to 76 percent of their MHR, which would be the next phase. Some students may need to start at a slower pace, but this is acceptable since fitness programs are individualized. Students should pair up with a classmate so they can provide support and motivate each other to keep moving. Remind students that walking also involves maintaining a good posture while swinging their arms comfortably at their sides when getting started. After the second week, students can begin with a brisk walk.

According to Thygerson and Thygerson (2019), students can count their steps per minute to determine their speed:

- Slow = 80 steps per minute
- Moderate to brisk = 100 steps per minute
- Fast = 120 steps per minute
- Race walking = more than 120 steps per minute

You can get additional information on walking programs from the CDC's "Step It Up! The Surgeon General's Call to Action to Promote Walking and Walkable Communities" or from the American Heart Association.

Beginning Jogging Workout

Since many students, especially at the beginning of the semester, may have not been involved in aerobic activities, it's important to inform students that they should not go all out at first and get winded before they even run half a lap around the track. Students may feel more at ease when starting a jogging or running program with a partner in their physical education class. And while the program focuses on running, teachers want students to focus on moving at their best pace, even if that pace is a brisk walk. As long as they can reach their target heart rate and maintain that pace, students are benefiting.

Week 1

- Day 1: Jog or run 100 meters (1/16 mile), walk 300 meters; repeat 3 times (track equivalent: run 1/4 of a lap, walk 3/4 of a lap)
- Day 2: Rest or cross-train
- Day 3: Jog or run 100 meters, walk 300 meters; repeat 3 times
- Day 4: Rest—other class activities
- Day 5: Jog or run 100 meters, walk 300 meters; repeat 3 times

Week 2

- Day 1: Jog or run 200 meters, walk 200 meters; repeat 3 times (track equivalent: run 1/2 of a lap, walk 1/2 of a lap)
- Day 2: Rest or cross-train
- Day 3: Jog or run 200 meters, walk 200 meters; repeat 3 times
- Day 4: Rest—other class activities
- Day 5: Jog or run 200 meters, walk 200 meters; repeat 3 times

Week 3

- Day 1: Jog or run 300 meters, walk 100 meters; repeat 3 times (track equivalent: run 3/4 of a lap, walk 1/4 of a lap)
- Day 2: Rest or cross-train
- Day 3: Jog or run 300 meters, walk 100 meters; repeat 3 times
- Day 4: Rest—other class activities
- Day 5: Jog or run 300 meters, walk 100 meters; repeat 3 times

Week 4

- Day 1: Jog or run 800 meters (1/2 mile; track equivalent: 2 laps)
- Day 2: Rest or cross-train
- Day 3: Jog or run 1,200 meters (3/4 mile; track equivalent: 3 laps)
- Day 4: Rest—other class activities
- Day 5: Jog or run 1,600 meters (1 mile; track equivalent: 4 laps)

Once students develop a comfortable pace and feel that they are progressing with this initial jogging or running program, they can begin to work on monitoring their heart rate to ensure that they are achieving their full fitness benefit in working toward CRF.

CARDIORESPIRATORY ENDURANCE, AEROBIC AND ANAEROBIC ACTIVITIES, AND MVPA

When looking at types of activity and dosage to improve cardiorespiratory fitness or aerobic capacity and the maximum rate that the respiratory, cardiovascular, and muscular systems can take in, transport, and use oxygen during exercise (Cooper Institute), most professional organizations—the Centers for Disease Control and Prevention (CDC), SHAPE America, the World Health Organization (WHO), the American College of Sports Medicine (ACSM), the National Physical Activity Plan (NPAP), and the Physical Activity Alliance (PAA)—refer to the U.S. Department of Health and Human Services *Physical Activity Guidelines for Americans* (2nd ed.) for their recommendations for school-aged youth (6 through 17 years) of 60 minutes or more of moderate-to-vigorous physical activity daily:

- It is important to provide young people opportunities and encouragement to participate in a variety of age-appropriate physical activities that are enjoyable.
- Aerobic: Most of the 60 or more minutes should be either moderate- or vigorous-intensity aerobic physical activity and should include vigorous-intensity physical activity on at least three days a week.
- Muscle strengthening: Daily physical activity should include muscle-strengthening physical activity on at least three days a week.
- Bone strengthening: Daily physical activity should include bone-strengthening physical activity on at least three days a week.

Additionally, school-aged youth (ages 6 through 17 years) can achieve substantial health benefits by doing moderate- and vigorous-intensity physical activity for periods of time that add up to 60 minutes or more each day. These activities should include aerobic activities as well as age-appropriate muscle- and bone-strengthening activities. The key to enhancing overall aerobic capacity is to provide opportunities for your students to participate in aerobic activities in which they rhythmically move their large muscles for a sustained period of time (Faigenbaum, Lloyd, & Oliver, 2020). Anaerobic activities involve quick bursts of energy and are performed at maximum capacity for a short time. Since anaerobic physical activities and select activities in sports are more intense and require specialized training, such as interval and HIIT, as a physical education teacher, it is recommended that this type of training be incorporated for students who have already achieved a good level of cardiorespiratory fitness and are ready for more vigorous activities.

As you continue to design your fitness education program, remind your students of the importance

Heart Rate Reserve (HRR) Method for Finding Target Heart Rate Zone

- Step 1: Determine resting heart rate (RHR).
- Step 2: Calculate your maximum heart rate (MHR). 220 – your age = MHR
- Step 3: Subtract your RHR from your MHR and then multiply it by the recommended THRZs for your intensity.

Recommended zones: Moderate = 40%-59% HRR, Vigorous = 60%-89% HRR

(MHR – RHR) × 0.40 + RHR = Low end of THRZ

(MHR – RHR) × 0.59 + RHR = High end of THRZ

The following example shows how to determine a moderate intensity THRZ for an 18-year-old student with an RHR of 73 bpm:

220 – 18 = 202

[(202 – 73) × 0.40] + 73= 124 Low end of THRZ

[(202 – 73) × 0.59] + 73 = 149 High end of THRZ

This THRZ would be between 124 and 149 bpm during aerobic exercise.

Note: One way to determine if you are in your THRZ if you do not have a heart rate monitor is by counting your pulse immediately after performing the activity. A recommended way to check pulse is to count for 10 seconds and then multiply by 6.

of knowing their target heart rate zone (THRZ) so that, as they participate in your class activities, they can self-assess to ensure that they are working hard enough to reach the goals of their fitness plan. See figure 2.1 and the Heart Rate Reserve (HRR) Method for Finding Target Heart Rate Zone sidebar to help determine THRZ.

This is also where the FITT principle is applied, as discussed in chapter 2. It is of greatest importance for students to understand how knowledge of intensity in meeting the MVPA recommendations is applied. The *Physical Activity Guidelines for Americans* (2nd ed.) further distinguishes between absolute intensity and relative intensity as applied to assessing the intensity of aerobic physical activity in relation to METs, or metabolic equivalents. For example, one **MET** is defined as the energy used while resting or sitting still. An activity that has a value of four **METs** means four times the energy is exerted as opposed to when resting or sitting still. See the Two Methods of Assessing Aerobic Intensity sidebar to learn more.

Students can perform light-, moderate-, and vigorous-intensity levels throughout the course, beginning with light-intensity activities as they get acclimated to more-vigorous activities as their level of CRF improves. Always remind the students that, even if they start with light-intensity activities, they are making positive gains and that some level of activity is better than none at all. Table 8.1 shows some examples of MVPA options organized by age group.

INCLUSION

Physical education teachers need to be cognizant that the *Physical Activity Guidelines for Americans* (2nd ed.) and recommendations also pertain to youth with disabilities. Students with disabilities gain the same health benefits from being physically active as their peers without disabilities. Although it would be advised to check each student's individualized education plan (IEP) to determine which activities would be appropriate, all students should be physically active in all components of health-related fitness activities. Knowing that all students in your class start at different levels of readiness, students with disabilities should engage in the amount and type of fitness activity that is right for them and start slowly based on their ability and fitness level, slowly increasing their time and intensity. Physical

Two Methods of Assessing Aerobic Intensity

Absolute Intensity

Absolute aerobic intensity is defined in terms of METs:

- Light-intensity activities are defined as waking non-sedentary behaviors of less than 3.0 METs. Walking at 2.0 miles per hour requires 2.5 METs of energy expenditure and is therefore considered a light-intensity activity.
- Moderate-intensity activities are defined as 3.0 to 5.9 METs. Walking at 3.0 miles per hour requires 3.5 METs of energy expenditure and is therefore considered a moderate-intensity activity.
- Vigorous-intensity activities are defined as 6.0 METs or more. Running a mile in 10 minutes (6.0 mph) is a 10 MET activity and is therefore classified as a vigorous-intensity activity.

Relative Intensity

Intensity can also be defined relative to fitness, with the intensity expressed in terms of a percent of a person's maximal heart rate, heart rate reserve, or aerobic capacity reserve. For example, relative moderate intensity is defined as 40 percent to 59 percent of aerobic capacity reserve (where 0 percent of reserve is resting and 100 percent of reserve is maximal effort). Relative vigorous-intensity activity is 60 percent to 84 percent of reserve.

To better communicate the concept of relative intensity (or relative level of effort), a simpler definition is useful:

- Relatively moderate-intensity activity is a level of effort of 5 or 6 on a scale of 0 to 10, where 0 is the level of effort of sitting, and 10 is maximal effort.
- Relatively vigorous-intensity activity begins at a 7 or 8 on this scale.

Source: U.S. Department of Health and Human Services (2018) *Physical Activity Guidelines for Americans, 2nd edition*, Appendix 1. Washington, DC: U.S. Department of Health and Human Services.

Table 8.1 Examples of Aerobic Physical Activities for Children and Adolescents

Type of physical activity	Preschool-aged children	School-aged children	Adolescents
Moderate-intensity aerobic	• Games such as tag or follow the leader • Playing on a playground • Tricycle or bicycle riding • Walking, running, skipping, jumping, dancing • Swimming • Playing games that require catching, throwing, and kicking • Gymnastics or tumbling	• Brisk walking • Bicycle riding • Active recreation, such as hiking, riding a scooter without a motor, swimming • Playing games that require catching and throwing, such as baseball and softball	• Brisk walking • Bicycle riding • Active recreation, such as kayaking, hiking, swimming • Playing games that require catching and throwing, such as baseball and softball • House and yard work, such as sweeping or pushing a lawn mower • Some video games that include continuous movement
Vigorous-intensity aerobic	• Games such as tag or follow the leader • Playing on a playground • Tricycle or bicycle riding • Walking, running, skipping, jumping, dancing • Swimming • Playing games that require catching, throwing, and kicking • Gymnastics or tumbling	• Running • Bicycle riding • Active games involving running and chasing, such as tag or flag football • Jumping rope • Cross-country skiing • Sports such as soccer, basketball, swimming, tennis • Martial arts • Vigorous dancing	• Running • Bicycle riding • Active games involving running and chasing, such as flag football • Jumping rope • Cross-country skiing • Sports such as soccer, basketball, swimming, tennis • Martial arts • Vigorous dancing

Reprinted from U.S. Department of Health and Human Services, *Physical Activity Guidelines for Americans,* 2nd ed. (Washington, DC: U.S. Department of Health and Human Services, 2018).

education teachers should modify the activities to ensure student engagement and success. Often, when we speak of cardiorespiratory fitness, we initially think of running the track, but consideration for modifications and accommodations for aerobic activities should also be given to the following examples: brisk walking; wheeling oneself in a wheelchair; swimming; hand-crank bicycling; and participating in water aerobics, seated volleyball, wheelchair basketball, tennis, football, softball, and in circuit-training activities.

For students with visual impairments or blindness, Williams, Ball, Lieberman, and Pierce (2020) recommend the following running techniques:

- Guided running: The runner holds the elbow of the guide runner.
- Tether running: The tether has two knots, one on each end of the rope. Both runners put the knots between their fingers to maintain contact.
- Circular running: The runner holds a rope (20 to 30 feet) attached to a stake and runs in a circle around the stake. The runner should change direction midway through the runs.
- Guide wire running: With the guide wire at elbow height of the runner, using a carabiner looped around the taught wire, or rope, the runner runs along the guide wire. A sound device should be approximately three feet from the end of the anchor to signal the runner that the end is near.
- Running to a sound source: Near the finish line, provide a sound source such as music, someone clapping, a bell, or other verbal cues to alert the runner.
- Treadmill running: Where available, the runner should work with a coach or peer using tactile modeling to learn the running technique or rhythm. Handrails should be used.

There are many strategies and techniques that could be used to engage students with disabilities in your cardiorespiratory activities. Physical education teachers should become familiar with the students' IEPs, consult with their physical education supervisors and the special education teachers at their school, or request assistance from adapted physical education teachers in their school or district if assistance is needed.

METHODS OF CARDIORESPIRATORY TRAINING

As previously discussed, several activities, whether aerobic or anaerobic, should be introduced to adolescents because the more targeted the training is, the more they improve on both measures of aerobic and anaerobic metabolism (Faigenbaum, Lloyd, & Oliver, 2020). They further assert that aerobic and anaerobic training can be developed simultaneously because common principles apply, though we often look at aerobic and anaerobic training as separate. It should be noted that implementing a fitness education class session with circuits and sample lesson plans can be found in chapter 15.

Interval training is a type of physical training that alternates short, high-intensity bursts of activity (approximately 30 seconds) with longer intervals (about one to two minutes) of less activity, with periods of rest and recovery in between. Interval training uses the body's two energy-producing systems: the aerobic and the anaerobic. The benefits of interval training are increases in cardiorespiratory endurance and fitness; more efficient workouts; more calories burned; improved aerobic capacity; and varied workouts to keep workouts fun and motivating. To assist in developing interval-training workouts, four variables should be considered:

- Duration (distance and time), or work interval
- Duration of rest, or recovery interval
- Intensity (speed) of work interval
- Number of repetitions of each interval

Since interval training is intense and demanding on the heart, lungs, and muscles, it is recommended that this type of activity be implemented one day per week for beginners, and then up to two days per week, but never on consecutive days. Additionally, for beginning level students or at the beginning of the semester, it would be recommended to begin with shorter work intervals, possibly one to two minutes of high-intensity exercises followed by longer recovery intervals, possibly five minutes of lower-intensity exercises.

As students increase their CRF, you can begin to add high-intensity interval training (HIIT) to your class. As described in chapter 2, HIIT is characterized by brief, repeated bursts of intense exercise followed by periods of rest or low-intensity exercise, in which the anaerobic interval workouts should bring the heart rate to 85 percent or more of your maximum heart rate. It has been shown to be one of the most effective ways to improve cardiorespiratory endurance, metabolic functioning, and physical performance in sports. The main goal of the HIIT protocol is to repeatedly exercise close to one's $\dot{V}O_2$max to elicit the cardiovascular training adaptations. A sample of a HIIT session might look like this:

- Run or jog for a brisk pace of about 30 seconds.
- Jog or walk at a slower pace for three minutes.
- After a rest period, run or jog for another 30 seconds.
- Continue for four bouts of exercise/rest.

Faigenbaum, Lloyd, and Oliver further professed that a *mixed-intermittent* approach for adolescents would be recommended since "it ensures exercise of sufficient intensity to stimulate positive adaptations while also providing a medium for valuable training that reflects that youth are naturally active in an intermittent manner" (2020, p. 231). Both aerobic and anaerobic training can be achieved through this approach. A mixed-intermittent approach can be achieved through activities such as traditional exercises, conditioning, small-sided games, and circuit training (see figure 8.3). These types of intense-training protocols use the entire body, so physical education teachers need to ensure that students perform proper warm-up and cool-down exercises in each session.

Continuous training, performing the same activity over an extended period of time, void of rest periods, is another approach that is beneficial for school-aged youth. Continuous training can be performed

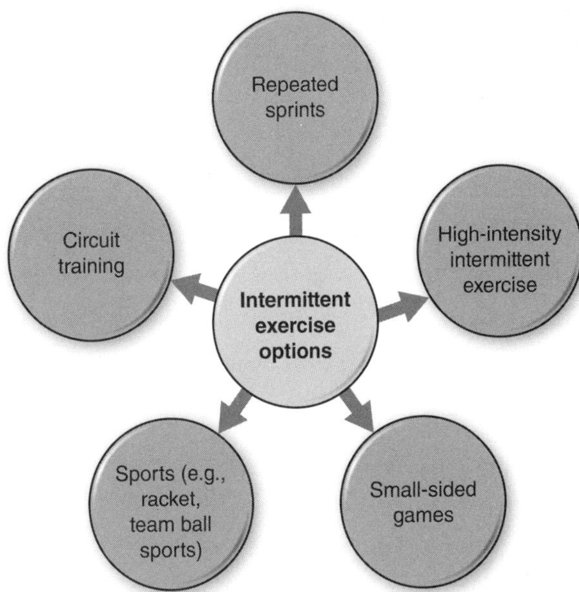

Figure 8.3 Various forms of intermittent exercise.
Reprinted by permission from A. Faigenbaum, R. Lloyd, R. Oliver, and ACSM, *Essentials of Youth Fitness* (Champaign, IL: Human Kinetics, 2020), 232.

at low, moderate, or high exercise intensities and is often contrasted with interval training or HIIT. When continuous exercises are performed in a high-intensity activity, such as a soccer match, the prolonged workload can yield about 85 percent of HR max. When used in the form of students walking to school, it can assist in meeting the daily recommendations of 60 or more minutes of physical activity for health and wellness, but it would not produce gains in aerobic or anaerobic fitness.

Fartlek training, derived from the Swedish term that means "speed play," is a form of interval training that is often used to improve running speed and endurance. Since you vary your pace while running, you can alternate the training session between fast segments and slow jogs, followed by repeated alternating periods of short sprints and slow jogs. This is motivating for students because it gives them an opportunity to experiment with pace and endurance without the activity being solely directed by the physical education teacher. Fartlek training can be done on a school track in groups of students or on various terrains.

Circuit training, another type of interval training, can be performed either outdoors, using a large space, or indoors, such as a gymnasium, with a more efficient use of space servicing many students at the same time. This type of training can combine a series of exercises that can involve muscular strength and endurance as well as aerobic exercises. The difference is that there is very little rest time between exercise stations, minimizing sedentary time often with rapid movement between stations. Once activities are learned, this is a great activity for middle school or senior high school students to develop circuit-training activities for class participation. When participating in circuit-training activities, the class can be designed for students to move through the circuit at their own pace or in groups. Students should be continuously active and, for safety and equal distribution at each station, if in large classes, students should stay with their same group until it's time to move to the next station. For students with disabilities, circuit training can be a preferred form of cardiorespiratory activity as opposed to long bouts of aerobic training such as running or wheeling on the track. National Center on Health, Physical Activity and Disability (NCHPAD) provides free inclusive fitness station posters that can be adhered to cones so that students with disabilities can participate alongside their classmates in modified activities. These can be found at www.nchpad.org/fppics/NCHPAD_PE Stations_complete.pdf. Peer tutors can also be involved to offer assistance. Figure 8.4 shows a sample circuit training that can be used in an indoor or outdoor setting. Additional examples of circuit training activities can be found in chapter 15 and in HK*Propel.*

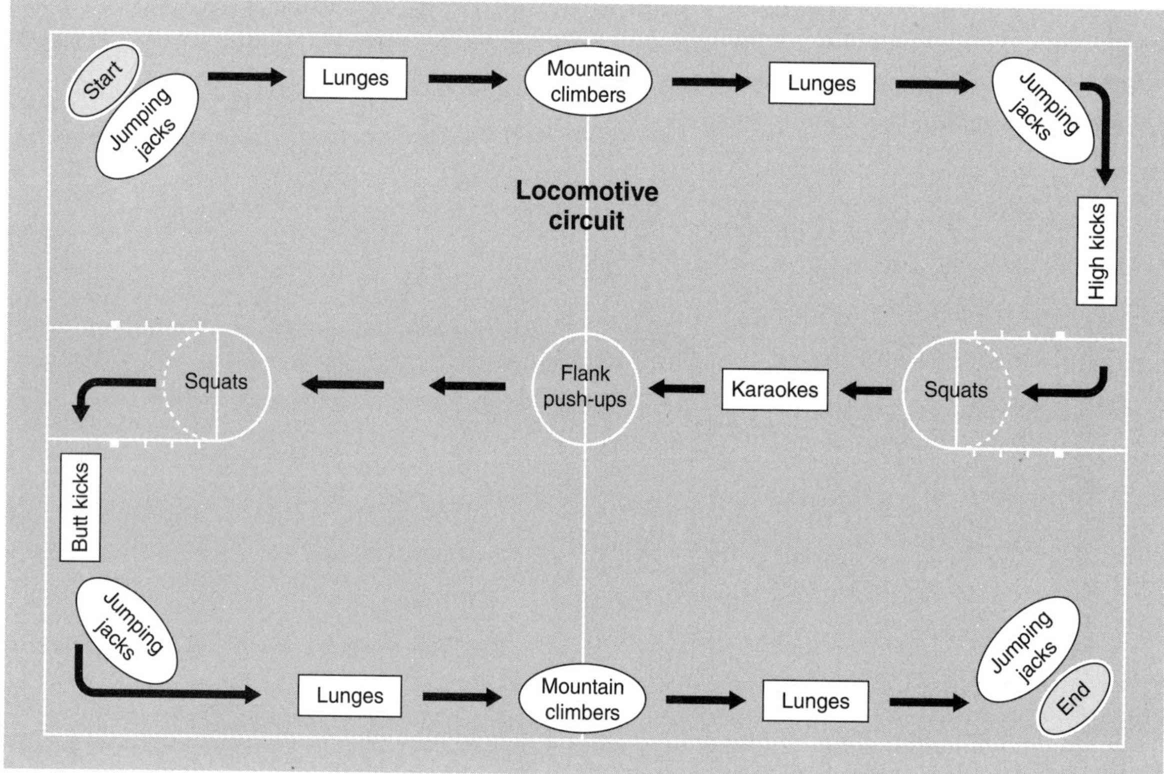

Figure 8.4 Sample circuit for indoor or outdoor activities: locomotive circuit.

SAFETY GUIDELINES

As discussed in chapter 4, safety of students should be the first and foremost when implementing any instructional program in physical education. In general, physical education teachers need to ensure the following:

- Students feel both physically and emotionally safe during physical education.
- Students are dressed appropriately for the activity. This would include physical education uniforms, or for hygiene purposes, clothing other than what students wear to school.
- Appropriate footwear is worn to prevent injuries.
- Students perform warm-up activities before participating in activities and cool-down exercises after participation.
- Teachers should select activities that are appropriate when exercising in extreme weather conditions, especially during hot and humid climates.
- Students are provided the opportunity to hydrate before and after class, as well as during class time if needed, especially when participating in high-intensity activities.
- Students should be encouraged to bring water bottles to class to limit the time students leave the supervised area to get water, but they should not share their water bottles with other students. Guidelines for hydration can be found in chapter 5.
- Teachers should supervise students at all times.

During a fitness education class, physical education teachers should do the following:

- Be knowledgeable of the physiological functions and changes that occur during fitness education activities.
- Have students begin gradually and build up to more-intense activities.
- Let students know that, if they experience pain or feel shortness of breath, they should notify the teacher immediately and stop the activity. Do not overdo it!
- Deliver appropriate instruction on all exercises and activities.
- Acknowledge that all students start at different places and that activities should be performed in alignment with their individual fitness plans based on valid assessment.
- Provide opportunities for students to self-assess and monitor their activities to ensure progress in meeting individual fitness goals.
- Be made aware of any student's medical problems.
- Make a pre-activity check of the facilities that will be used during the school day, including the gymnasium, activity rooms, hard courts, and green space playing fields.
- Modify activities according to students' age and ability level. Accommodations and modifications should be made when necessary.

Physical education teachers have a responsibility to ensure the safety of all students participating in their fitness education program or class. The safety precautions listed are not exhaustive, but both teachers and students have a shared responsibility in maintaining a safe exercise environment and program.

MONITORING AND ASSESSMENT

Both formal and informal assessments are a necessary part of a fitness education program to ensure that students are making adequate progress toward reaching their individualized fitness goals. The role of formal assessment strategies and how to use those assessment results are explained extensively in chapter 7. However, self-assessment plays a vital role in students taking responsibility for their improvements in attaining their fitness goals and monitoring their own efforts in meeting those goals. The following self-assessments can provide immediate feedback to students and should be incorporated into any fitness education program. However, since this book is developed with the understanding that no specialized equipment will be needed to implement a fitness education program, let's begin with the easiest form of self-assessing: heart rate after bouts of physical activity.

Measuring Pulse

Your pulse is the rate at which your heart beats, and it measures the number of times your heart beats per minute. As your heart pumps blood through your body, you can feel a pulsing in some of the blood vessels close to the skin's surface, such as in your wrist, neck, or upper arm. Counting your pulse rate is a simple way to find out how fast your heart is beating. You check your pulse rate by counting the beats in a set period of time (at least 15 to 20 seconds) and multiplying that number to get the number of beats per minute. Your pulse changes from minute to minute, and will be faster when you exercise (Healthwise Staff, 2018). There are two places you can easily check your pulse. The first is on the inside of your wrist below the thumb (see figure 8.5*a*). The second is on your neck, on either side of your windpipe, just below your jawbone (see figure 8.5*b*).

- Gently place two fingers, index and middle fingers, of your other hand on the artery below the base of your thumb.
- Do not use your thumb because it has its own pulse that you may feel.
- Count the beats for 15 seconds and then multiply the result by four to get the number of beats per minute.

Talk Test

The *talk test* is another low-tech method for individuals to measure their level of intensity. Developed in 1939 by Dr. John Grayson at Oxford University, it was originally used to advise mountaineers to "climb no faster than you can talk." Throughout the years, although not highly respected, it did provide some validity on determining the ventilatory threshold "since breathing frequency increases rapidly at the point of the ventilatory threshold, and the one thing you have to do to be able to talk comfortably is to control the frequency of your breathing" (Foster & Porcari, n.d.). As a result, what has been accepted as a measure of intensity is that your intensity is appropriate if you can talk but not sing. If you are too out of breath to talk, then your intensity is too high. And if you can sing, then your intensity is too low (SHAPE America, 2020).

Pedometers

Pedometers have been around for many years and have often been used as a low-cost measure in schools to determine if students are receiving their age-appropriate recommended steps per day. The original pedometers, often worn on the waistband, work by detecting movement through a spring-loaded, counter-balanced mechanism that records vertical acceleration of the hip (Pangrazi, Beighle, & Sidman, 2009). Although there are benefits to using these type of pedometers in the school setting for counting steps, along with some models that provide information on distance covered and time spent during walking, the greatest limitations on the basic models is that they cannot measure frequency or intensity of physical activity. Smartphone apps can track steps as well.

The question remains: How many steps should we ask our secondary school students to attain in working toward improving their cardiorespiratory

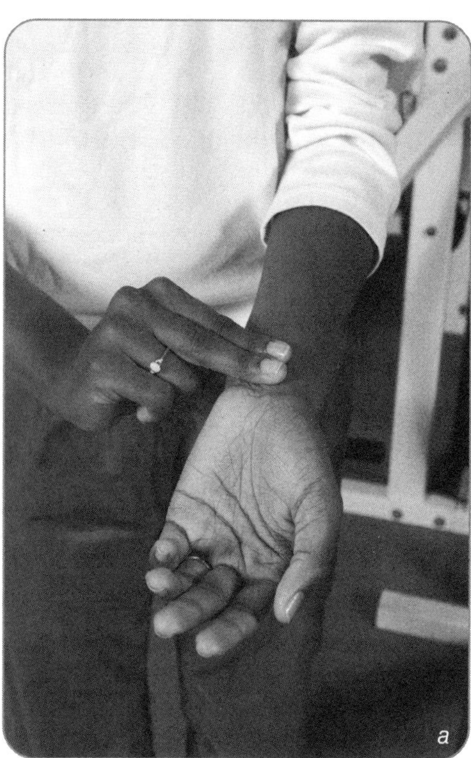

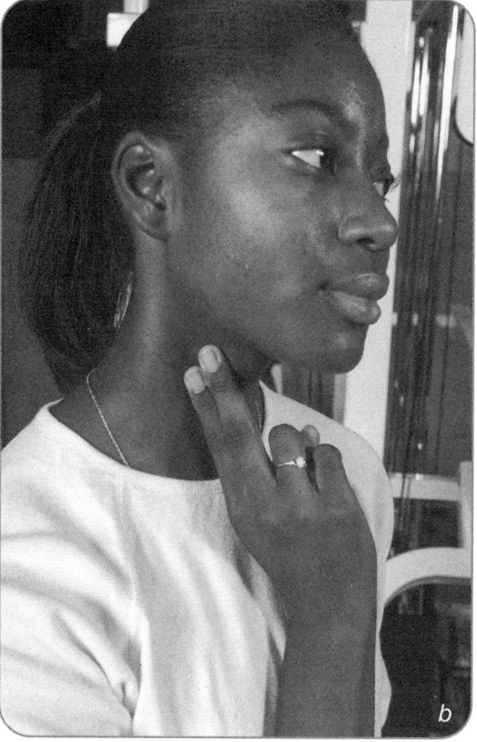

Figure 8.5 Taking the pulse at the wrist (*a*) and neck (*b*).

fitness? We typically use the 10,000 steps per day for adults to achieve fitness gains. However, Tudor-Locke et al. (2011) found that children average approximately 12,500 steps a day, boys between 13,000 and 15,000 steps per day and girls between 11,000 and 12,000 steps per day. Adolescents average between 10,000 and 11,700 steps per day. Therefore, to meet the national recommended guidelines of 60 or more minutes per day, most teens would require 12,000 steps per day (Corbin & LeMasurier, 2014). This would be a valid goal for students to put on their fitness logs to reach their cardiorespiratory fitness goals.

Fitness and Activity Trackers

A more advanced type of fitness monitor that is worn on the wrist is the fitness or activity tracker. These trackers, which include pedometers and have built-in *accelerometers*, are now available on smartwatches or can be installed as a pedometer app in which your cell phone can check its fitness-related metrics data with a variety of built-in health functions. However, it only counts steps if you are carrying your cell phone with you.

For more data collection, fitness bands usually interact via Bluetooth with an app on a mobile device that configures the device and downloads the wearer's activity data. Aside from the step count, some of the functions of fitness trackers include: distance estimate, calories burned estimate, ability to time and track specific workouts, memory to review past days, clock, stopwatch and exercise timer, alarm clock, speed or pace estimate, goal setting and progress toward daily goal, ability to upload to computer or cell phone app, pulse monitor, sitting time and inactivity tracking, sleep monitoring, and diet logging to balance calories in with calories burned. Fitness or activity trackers can assist individuals in self-monitoring their activities for fitness and overall health.

Heart Rate Monitors

Heart rate monitors (HRMs), produced by several fitness companies, have come a long way, from individual devices monitoring individual heart rates to a valid instructional tool that motivates, inspires, and assesses students and class, connecting the online environment to real class instruction. HRMs can assist schools in developing activity metrics that can be measured and assessed. Through an electronic platform, whether students are in a face-to-face classroom or participating in online instruction, student data can be stored through a mobile app on the cloud, and teachers can access that data through the class portal. In a classroom setting, student data can also be projected on a wall, enabling physical education teachers to observe individual student effort and intensity—real time data—and provide immediate feedback. This provides a level of accountability that students are performing the activities and that they can monitor their individual progress through their fitness goals.

Other Technology

In a more advanced technological application to fitness trackers, many devices now have built-in Global Positioning Systems (GPS). The advantage of having GPS on your fitness device is that it not only uses satellite systems to track your whereabouts but also can perform many functions that other devices cannot, such as using an SpO_2 sensor for blood oxygen and monitoring $\dot{V}O_2$max and even resting heart rate on more advanced models. These types of fitness trackers also include more accurate distance tracking, monitor activity on different terrains, monitor altitude, and are used in a variety of sport activities including cycling, cross-country skiing, and swimming. As technology continues to evolve, so will the ability of fitness tracking devices to provide more accurate information for reaching physical activity goals.

Tracking Student and Class Progress

Regardless of whether students are receiving face-to-face instruction or online instruction or are participating in a hybrid model, it is important for students and teachers to track their progress to show improvement over time, as well as accountability to determine if the fitness education program being implemented is accomplishing its goals. Through the utilization of several tracking devices previously mentioned, teachers and students can also use commercial apps, or teacher-developed Excel spreadsheets to assist with this record keeping. Figure 8.6 was developed using the STRAVA free app and is one example of how student data can be tracked, allowing the teacher to collect the individual and class data. The interactive STRAVA data sheets can be found in HK*Propel*.

Directions:

- Download the table and save.
- Input time with a decimal point (e.g., 8:15 should be typed as 8.15).
- Input date into the shaded cells only.

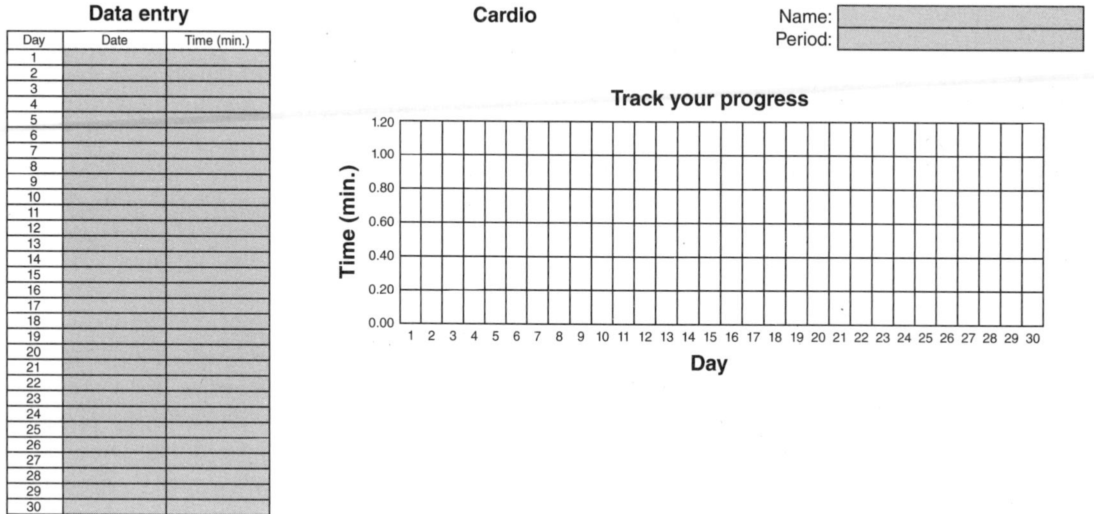

Figure 8.6 STRAVA data charts for cardio and THR.

TEACHING TIPS

As with all other health-related fitness components, it is important that every physical education teacher acknowledges the fact that students come to class with different skill sets and different motivations. As a physical education teacher, your continuous support and encouragement will empower students to reach their full potential as well as be motivated to be fit for life.

This could be especially challenging when it comes to implementing cardiorespiratory fitness activities, but throughout these chapters, the recurring theme is to meet students where they are, provide them with the knowledge and skills necessary to reach their individual goals on their fitness plans, push them to constantly improve, and always have students leave class each day feeling positive about themselves and what they accomplished. When developing your lesson plans, keep in mind that all of the principles of fitness training should be incorporated, especially progression when developing cardiorespiratory fitness to minimize unnecessary fatigue or soreness. Once students feel more comfortable in the class, they can begin to take charge and assist in designing their own circuit activities, continue to self-assess their fitness levels, and provide support to their class partners as well as other students who would benefit from their peer mentorship. Keeping activities fun and motivating should be a part of every lesson design.

Physical education teachers should also be cognizant of the fact that accommodations and modifications may be needed for some students because it is important for all movements and exercises to be modified to meet the individual needs of every student in order for all students to engage in full participation. Implementing universal design for learning (UDL) will assist the teachers in ensuring that all students can reach their full potential.

CONCLUSION

Cardiorespiratory fitness in adolescence is a key predictor of future health, but it can only happen when targeted instruction and opportunities for student participation are present. In developing the fitness education course, the physical education teacher should provide fitness-related activities that enable students to progress toward appropriate levels of intensity to develop and maintain increased levels of CRF as well as provide students with the knowledge necessary for them to understand why maintaining adequate levels of CRF is important now and throughout their lives. Understanding the principles of training would be inadequate if students did not gain the skills of how to implement those principles into developing their individual fitness education plan to reach their fitness goals.

Additionally, the physical education teacher should continue to reinforce the importance in students self-assessing throughout the course so that they can informally monitor their progress on an ongoing basis and provide positive feedback, even with incremental gains. Knowledge of target heart rate zones, exercise intensity, and types of training protocols should be included in the instructional program. Lastly, because students will be exercising at intensities beyond any other physical education class, safety considerations should be in place and practiced daily.

As you progress through the course, it is always important for the physical education teacher to remember that students start at different points in their levels of fitness and should be allowed to progress through their own individual goals with your guidance without comparing them to other students. Students with disabilities should be provided with accommodations and modifications to participate in all health-related fitness activities. Students should also be taught the intrinsic value of maintaining a healthy and fit lifestyle and be motivated to work toward improvement while having fun at the same time.

Review Questions

1. Describe cardiorespiratory activities that can be done without equipment.
2. Explain how the principles of training can be applied to cardiorespiratory fitness activities.
3. What recommendations would you make for a student who has been sedentary with low cardiorespiratory fitness levels?
4. Describe the physiological benefits of cooling down after an intense cardiorespiratory activity.
5. Explain the role that target heart rate zones (THRZ) play in improving cardiorespiratory gains.

Visit HK*Propel* for additional material related to this chapter.

CHAPTER 9

Upper-Body Stretching Exercises

Chapter Objective

After reading this chapter, you will understand how proper stretching technique enhances flexibility and improves range of motion (ROM) in the upper body. Better ROM can improve performance during activities, increase blood flow to the muscles, reduce the risk of injuries, and assist in the cool-down after exercise. You will also know how to develop lessons that teach these concepts to secondary school students; be able to effectively demonstrate a series of exercises and exercise routines designed to stretch the upper-body muscles, tendons, ligaments, and joints; and employ best teaching practices that enhance student learning.

Key Concepts

- Stretching the upper-body muscles is essential to enhanced physical activity performance as well as everyday activities for increasing the range of motion.
- The exercises presented will help you teach students to identify the muscles, tendons, ligaments, and joints involved in stretching exercises that increase flexibility.
- Warm-up and cool-down stretches should be performed before and after upper-body exercises.
- Accommodations and modifications are recommended so that all activities can be modified and performed by all students in the class.

INTRODUCTION

As a physical education teacher, you know that providing instruction in all components of fitness enables students to perform a variety of activities in a safe and healthy manner. Throughout this chapter, as well as chapters 10 and 11, we explore the importance of stretching before and after every activity. It is crucial that you explain this importance to your students and teach them to be aware of the muscles, tendons, ligaments, and joints engaged in stretching exercises and grasp the overall benefits of stretching. When you first introduce the lessons on stretching, be prepared for the usual response from students: Why is stretching important? or Why is it beneficial? Students need to understand that, although we stretch prior to exercise, it should not be mistaken for *just* being a part of the warm-up. Incorporating a stretching routine is just as essential as an exercise workout and could be 5 to 20 minutes long. Students should also be aware that levels of flexibility are individualized and that several factors, including the type of joint, age, and fitness level, have an impact on them. Lastly, students should be informed that, through stretching, they can achieve increasing degrees of flexibility.

As discussed in chapter 2, flexibility, a health-related component of fitness, along with cardiorespiratory endurance and muscular strength and endurance, are integral to any fitness education program and remain a constant part of our health and wellness. By definition, "Flexibility is the ability of a joint and surrounding muscle to move through a full or optimal range of motion" (Bushman, 2017, p. 147). Adhering to the *principle of specificity*, or stretching a specific group of muscles specific to an activity, will elongate those muscles directly associated with that activity, allowing for more fluidity of movement. The benefits of stretching are further known to improve performance during activities, increase blood flow to the muscles, reduce the risk of injuries, improve muscle extensibility, decrease muscle soreness, and assist in the post exercise cool-down.

Since there are several different types of stretches, students should become familiar with each while acknowledging the overall importance of stretching, since each type of stretch serves a different purpose. The types are as follows:

- *Static stretch.* Active or passive stretching by slowly moving a joint until you feel tension and then holding it for 10 to 30 seconds (ACSM, 2017)
- *Dynamic stretch.* Gradually increasing the ROM as the movement is repeated several times
- *Proprioceptive neuromuscular facilitation (PNF).* Contracting the muscle before you stretch it to help the muscle relax (Corbin & LeMasurier, 2014), followed by static stretching that uses a combination of active and passive stretching (Thygerson & Thygerson, 2019)
- *Ballistic stretch.* Using slow, bouncing and repetitive movements to stretch the muscle beyond its normal ROM

Stretches are just as important as the workout itself. Students should continuously be reminded that, when beginning a stretching routine, it is important to listen to your body and be cautious not to overstretch the ligaments and capsules that surround the joints, which could cause damage to tissues. Stretching should be performed with slow, continuous, and controlled movements.

It is also important for teachers to remind students that warming up prior to stretching is an essential component of the process. Warm-up routines can begin with a slow jog, rope jumping, or other cardiorespiratory activity that will increase the blood flow to the muscles, increase the heart rate, and gradually increase the core muscle temperature, enabling muscles to be stretched further while avoiding injuries.

We explore flexibility in this chapter as well as the next two, with each of the three chapters focusing on the upper body (chapter 9), core (chapter 10), or lower body (chapter 11). In this chapter, we start by examining the major muscle-tendon groups of the upper body, which include the neck, shoulders, back, chest, and arms. In all of these groups, having full ROM to perform a movement is crucial. We need to slowly acquaint students with the concepts and make students aware of the importance of each movement. If we could fast-track a kinesiology, anatomy, and physiology lesson, it would behoove us to know and understand the mechanics, the structure, and the functions of each movement in order to provide students with the proper and appropriate exercises.

The body is made up of many *joints*, defined as the union of two or more bones, of several different types. For example, the hinge joint of the elbow allows flexion and extension of the forearm, giving limited movement (see figure 9.1). The *condyloid* joint of the wrist allows flexion, extension, adduction, and abduction. The ball-and-socket joint of the shoulder is one of the largest and most complex types, allowing the greatest ROM (see figure 9.2). Each specific joint type limits and affords different movements. Therefore, we need to prepare that muscle tendon, defined as a strong, fibrous tissue attaching a muscle to a bone, within that joint to be used.

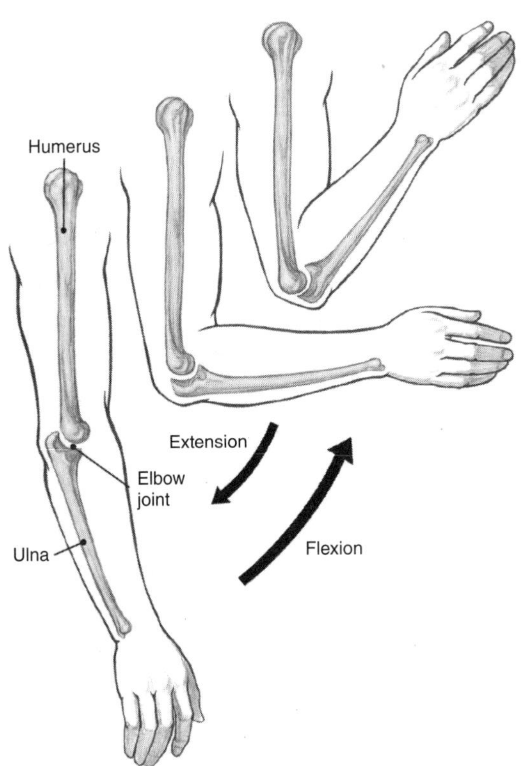

Figure 9.1 The hinge joint at the elbow allows flexion and extension of the forearm.

Reprinted by permission from CLASSIC HUMAN ANATOMY IN MOTION: THE ARTISTS GUIDE TO THE DYNAMICS OF FIGURE DRAWINGS by Valerie L. Winslow, copyright © 2015 by Valerie L. Winslow. Used by permission of Watson-Guptill Publications, in imprint of Random House, a division of Penguin Random House LLC. All rights reserved.

Although stretching is mainly addressed within the joints and tendons, the bones and muscles are also involved throughout the related movement of the specific body part. As we travel through the upper body, it would be beneficial to explore how all components harmonize in order to synchronize each movement successfully.

Understanding that most joints are complex, the neck muscles, called the suboccipital muscles, collectively extend and rotate the head, which is stabilized mainly by the cervical spine. The four joints—*glenohumeral, acromioclavicular, scapulothoracic, and sternoclavicular*—are all connected by their associated ligaments and make up the shoulder. The shoulder muscles are *supraspinatus, infraspinatus, teres minor,* and the *subscapularis,* which is commonly referred to as the rotator cuff. These are the main stabilizers of the shoulder and deltoids, giving the shoulder its rounded shape. The major back muscles are the *trapezius, latissimus dorsi, levator scapulae,* and the *rhomboids,* which are mostly attached to the backbone. Their partnering

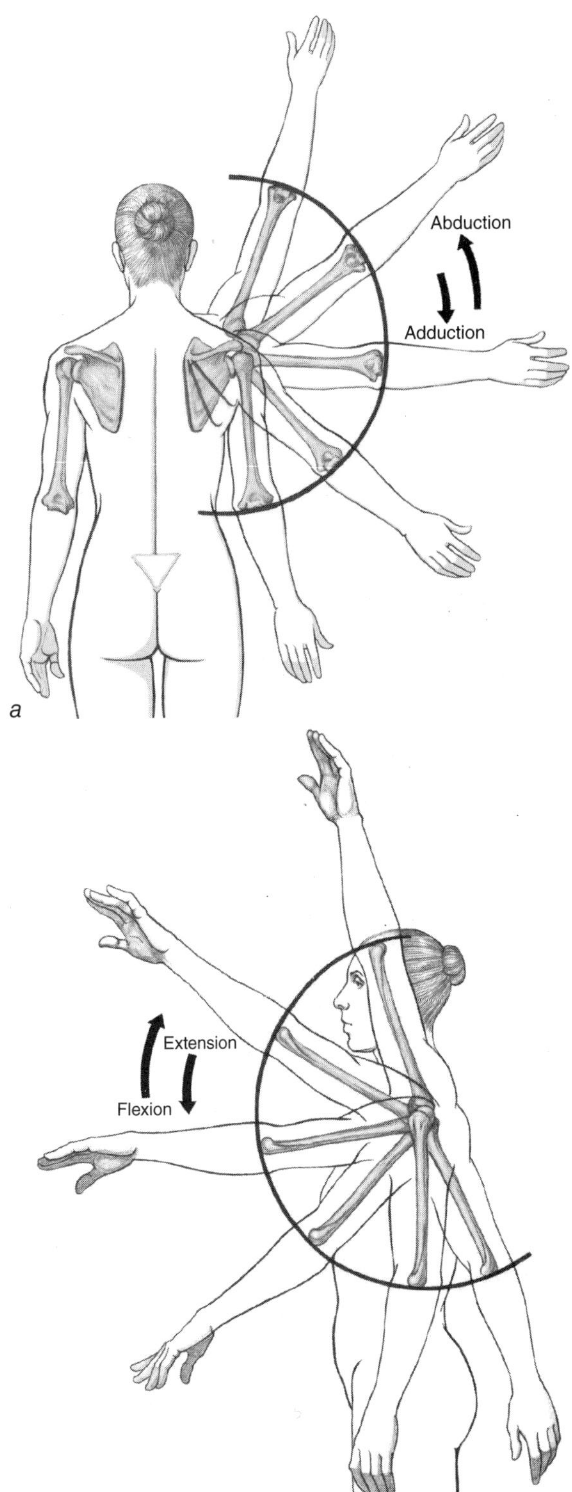

Figure 9.2 The shoulder's ball-and-socket joint allows a large ROM, including abduction and adduction (*a*) and flexion and extension (*b*).

Reprinted by permission from CLASSIC HUMAN ANATOMY IN MOTION: THE ARTISTS GUIDE TO THE DYNAMICS OF FIGURE DRAWINGS by Valerie L. Winslow, copyright © 2015 by Valerie L. Winslow. Used by permission of Watson-Guptill Publications, in imprint of Random House, a division of Penguin Random House LLC. All rights reserved.

chest muscle is made up of the *pectoralis major* and *minor, serratus anterior,* and *subclavius*. These muscles stretch from the *clavicles* (collar bones) to each side of the *sternum* (breastbone). The *humerus, ulna,* and *radius* together form the elbow, and the movement of this hinge joint happens with the help of the major muscles of the *biceps* and *triceps* of the upper arm and the *flexors, extensors, pronators,* and *supinators* of the forearm.

Upper-body stretches are not only an important part of our daily lives and physical activities but also necessary in the majority of sports as well. For example, increasing upper-body flexibility in swimming is integral for increasing speed, by maximizing the pull for each stroke. The same exists for increasing the ROM; the full potential of the joint, in reference to flexion and extension; and power in throwing events, such as javelin, baseball, softball, and football and in gymnastics events, such as swinging on bars and floor exercises. In tennis, a large ROM around the shoulder is a clear advantage because the sport requires movement in many directions (see figure 9.3).

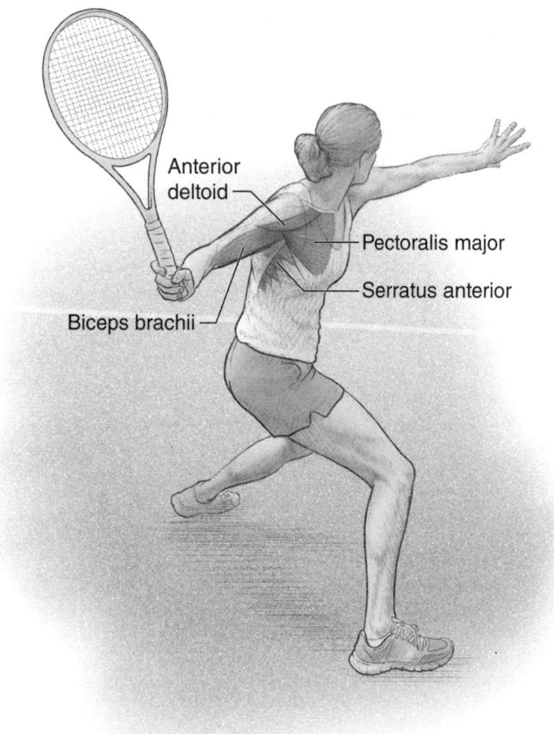

Figure 9.3 Tennis players need a large range of motion in the shoulder to execute different swings, such as the forehand.

This is not about how strong or weak a person is, but rather about a person's ability to move the body freely and painlessly. If we plan to use that muscle, we need to consider all the connecting parts. Therefore, as we engage in an exercise routine of the upper body muscles in this chapter, it is necessary to address those same joint movements through stretching. It is also important to note that, although this chapter focuses on the importance of stretching as an entity in itself, to increase flexibility, many of the exercises described here will also be used as warm-up and cool-down exercises in subsequent chapters.

As the physical education teacher, you can use the exercises in this chapter as part of a warm-up or cool-down, lesson on upper-body stretching, or routine. Each exercise has a description and illustration, with notes about the type of stretch, the body part and muscle groups worked, steps for safely executing the stretch with good form, and accommodations and modifications for those unable to perform the stretch as described. Many stretches are illustrated with video in HK*Propel*. Teach each exercise separately, ensuring that students are performing the stretch correctly, emphasizing the type of stretch (static or dynamic) and the muscle group being engaged. This is extremely important because what students learn during this initial instruction will enable them to use the appropriate stretch for subsequent physical activities, as well as enable them to safely engage in routines and circuits throughout the class. We include guidelines for developing routines for the beginner, intermediate, and advanced levels after the exercises, along with further teaching tips.

As you develop your daily lesson plans, align each lesson with the National Standards and your own state and local standards so that every student taught in your class can participate in the activities. The following sample lesson overview shows the National Standards and Grade-Level Outcomes (GLOs) relevant to this material, lesson objectives, and accommodations and modifications to be kept in mind when teaching a lesson on stretching. All of the exercises in this book are designed to provide accommodations and modifications as needed. This ensures equity, opportunity, and access for all students. Additionally, as you progress through your fitness education course, your students should be able to identify which stretching activities will be required for the daily activity you present.

LESSON OVERVIEW

Upper-Body Stretching Routine

Lesson length: 5 to 20 minutes

Grade level: 9th to 12th

National Standards and GLOs: S1.H3, S2.H2, S3.H9, S3.H11, S4.H5

Grade level: 6th to 8th

National Standards and GLOs: S3.M9, S3.M11, S3.M12, S3.M14, S3.M15, S3.M16, S4.M7, S5.M1

Lesson objectives: By the end of the lesson, students will be able to do the following:

- Perform a warm-up cardiorespiratory activity prior to a stretching routine.
- Perform an upper-body muscle stretching routine, showing proper technique throughout each movement.
- Perform a cool-down including cardiorespiratory activity and hydration.
- Perform a cool-down routine using static stretching showing ROM in muscle-joint areas.

Accommodations and modifications: It is important for all movements and exercises to be modified to meet the individual needs of every student in order for them to engage in full participation. Implementing universal design for learning (UDL) will assist teachers in ensuring that all students can reach their full potential. Follow the general instructional recommendations, as discussed in chapter 3, for all activities.

WARM-UP DYNAMIC AND STATIC STRETCHES FOR THE UPPER BODY

HEAD SIDE-TO-SIDE ROTATION

Dynamic Stretch

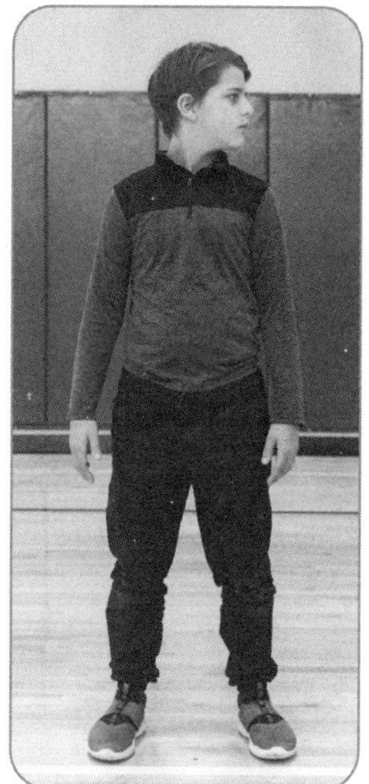

Body part: Neck

Muscle group: Trapezius

1. Stand with back straight, feet hip-width apart, and arms relaxed at sides.
2. Slowly rotate the head to one side.
3. Reverse motion by rotating to opposite direction.
4. Continue movement in both directions 10 to 30 seconds.
5. Stop, relax, and repeat 2 to 3 more times.

Accommodations and modifications: For students unable to perform this movement, while seated, have them slowly rotate their heads from side to side. Tell them they should not tilt their head back. Have students repeat movement for time or repetitions.

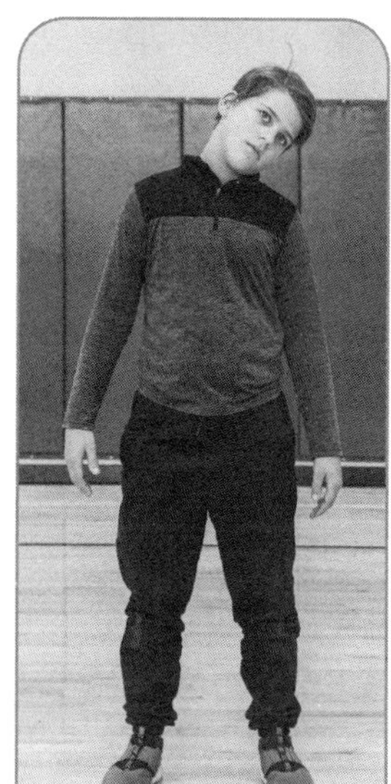

HEAD TILT

Static Stretch

Body part: Neck

Muscle group: Trapezius

1. Stand with back straight, feet hip-width apart, and arms relaxed at sides.
2. Slowly tilt the head toward the shoulder.
3. Hold position for 15 to 30 seconds.
4. Return head back to original position.
5. Slowly tilt the head toward opposite shoulder.
6. Stop, relax, and repeat 2 to 3 more times.

Accommodations and modifications: For students unable to perform this movement, while seated, have them slowly tilt their head toward their shoulders. Tell them they should not tilt their head back. Repeat movement for time and repetitions.

ARM CIRCLES

Dynamic Stretch

Body part: Shoulders

Muscle group: Deltoids

1. Stand with feet shoulder-width apart.
2. Extend arms out to sides and parallel to ground.
3. Slowly perform small circles by rotating at the shoulder.
4. Reverse motion moving in opposite direction.
5. Gradually increase size of circular movement in both directions.
6. Repeat movement 15 to 20 times.

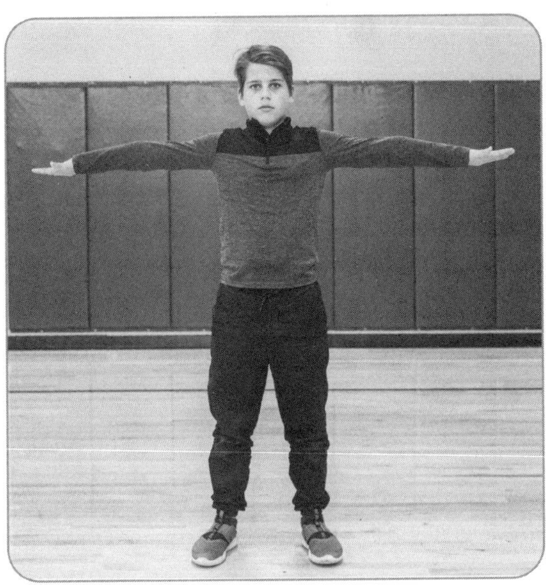

Accommodations and modifications: For students unable to perform this movement, have students maintain small and slow rotating movements. Repeat movement for time and repetitions. This activity can also be performed in a seated position.

SHOULDER ROTATION: GOAL POST

Dynamic Stretch

Body part: Shoulders

Muscle group: Deltoids

1. Stand with back straight and feet hip-width apart.
2. Bring both arms up and flex elbows to 90 degrees.
3. Align shoulders and elbows, palms facing forward.
4. Keeping arm position, rotate at shoulder, one arm downward, while opposite remains stationary.
5. Slowly reverse movement, rotating opposite arm downward, and return opposite arm upward to starting position.
6. Repeat up-and-down movement in a controlled fashion.
7. Continue movement in both directions 10 to 30 seconds.
8. Stop, relax, and repeat 2 to 3 more times.

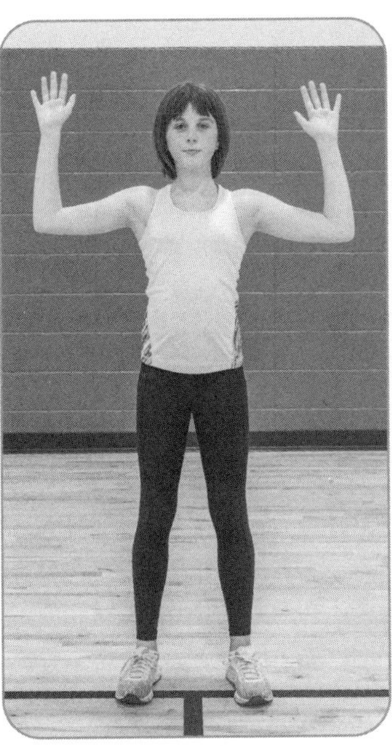

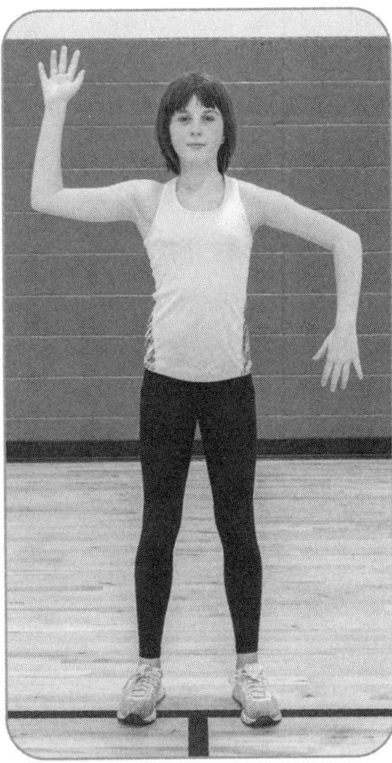

Accommodations and modifications: Students may partner, back-to-back, for more support. For students unable to perform this movement, the exercise can be performed from a seated position. Repeat movement for time and repetitions.

FRONT-CROSS SHOULDER STRETCH

Static Stretch

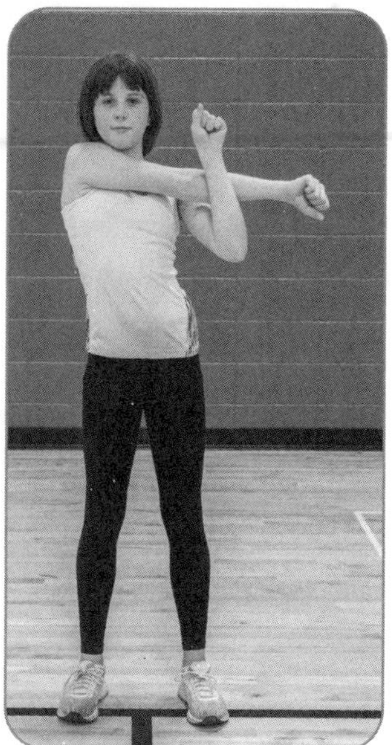

Body part: Shoulders

Muscle group: Deltoids

1. Stand with back straight and feet hip-width apart.
2. Cross one arm in front of chest.
3. Grab elbow with opposite hand, gently pulling elbow toward chest.
4. Hold position for 15 to 30 seconds.
5. Return to original position.
6. Repeat with opposite arm.
7. Stop, relax, and repeat 2 to 3 more times.

Accommodations and modifications: For students unable to perform this movement, this exercise can be performed from a seated position. Repeat movement for time and repetitions.

Progression: To progress this stretch, try the following shoulder extensor and adductor stretch.

PROGRESSION: SHOULDER EXTENSOR AND ADDUCTOR STRETCH

Static Stretch

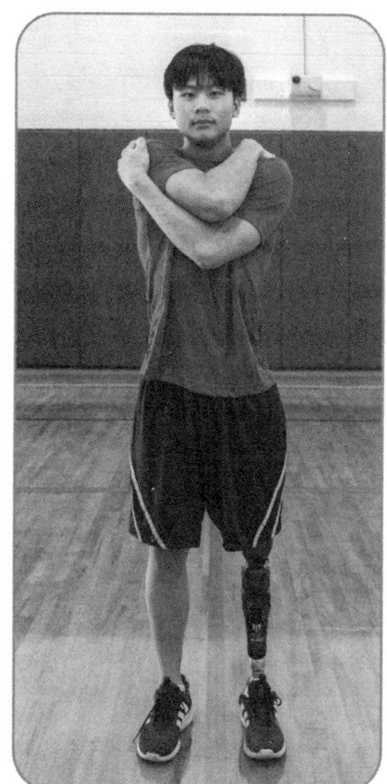

Body part: Upper body

Muscle group: Latissimus dorsi and deltoids

1. Stand with feet shoulder-width apart.
2. Wrap arms around body at shoulder height.
3. Give yourself a hug.
4. Pull shoulders forward in order to place hands behind them.
5. Hold position for 10 to 30 seconds.
6. Stop, relax, and repeat 2 to 3 more times.

SIDE-ARM SWING

Dynamic Stretch

Body part: Chest and shoulders

Muscle group: Pectorals and deltoids

1. Stand with back straight and feet hip-width apart.
2. Extend arms out to sides.
3. While keeping arms straight, swing arms in and out, crossing in front of the chest.
4. Slowly continue movement for 10 to 30 seconds.
5. Stop, relax, and repeat 2 to 3 more times.

Accommodations and modifications: For students unable to perform this movement, this exercise can be performed from a seated position. Repeat movement for time and repetitions.

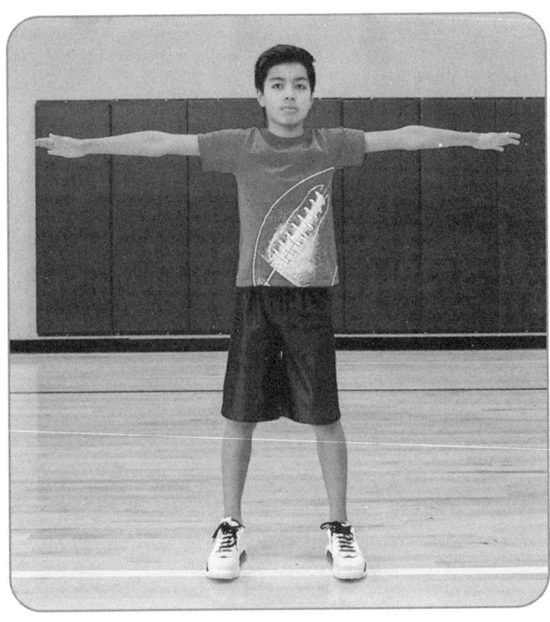
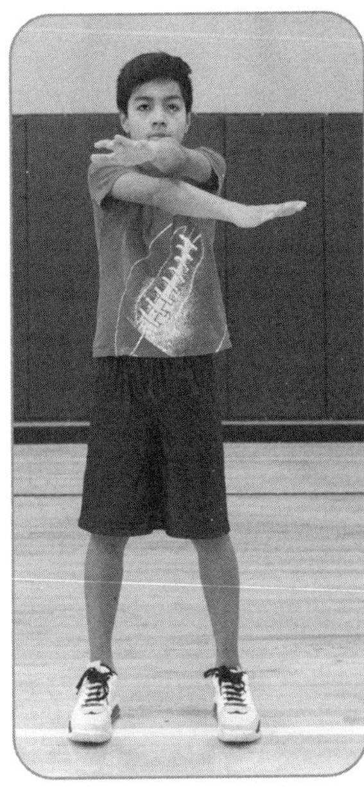

ARM FLEXION AND EXTENSION SWING

Dynamic Stretch

Body part: Chest and shoulders

Muscle group: Pectorals and deltoids

1. Stand with feet shoulder-width apart.
2. Extend arms down to sides.
3. Swing arms forward and back.
4. Begin with small pendulum movements from the shoulder.
5. Gradually increase the range of movement.
6. Repeat the movement 15 to 20 times.

Accommodations and modifications: For students unable to perform this movement, this exercise can be performed from a seated position. Repeat movement for time and repetitions.

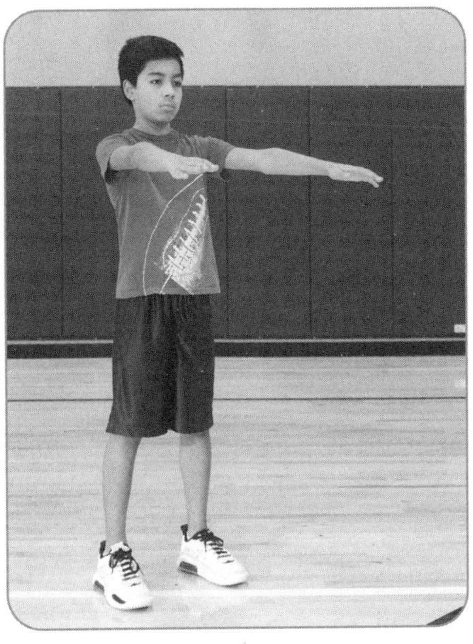
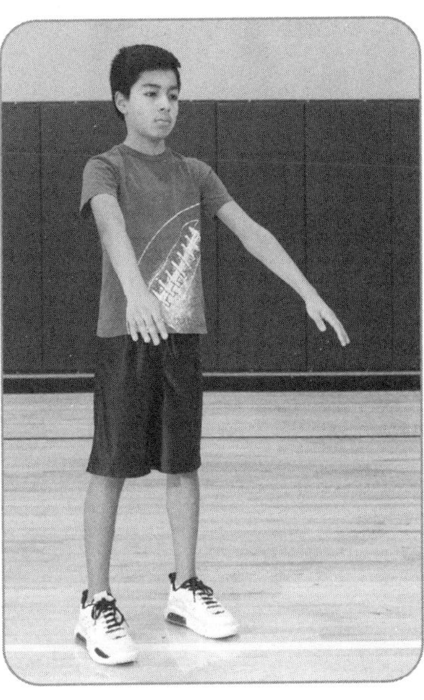

CHEST STRETCH

Static Stretch

Body part: Chest

Muscle group: Pectorals

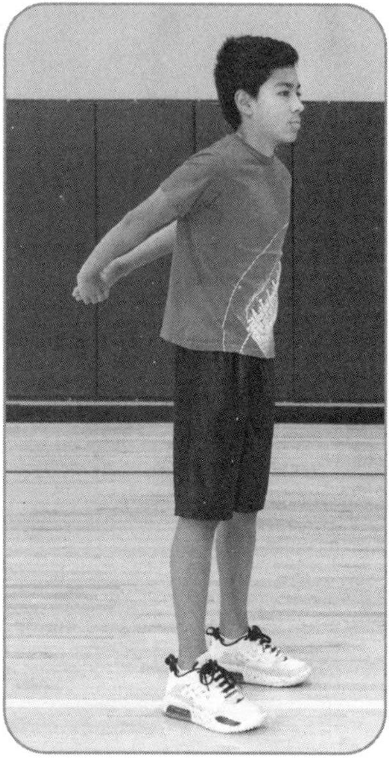

1. Stand with back straight, feet hip-width apart, and arms relaxed at sides.
2. Clasp hands and palms together behind back.
3. Keeping arms straight, slowly raise arms.
4. Keep shoulders back and do not lead forward.
5. Hold position for 15 to 30 seconds.
6. Return to original position.
7. Stop, relax and repeat 2 to 3 more times.

Accommodations and modifications: For students unable to perform this movement, this exercise can be performed from a seated position. The seated model is demonstrating the Chest Expansion stretch.

1. Stretch arms out in front with palms together.
2. Slowly bring straight arms back.
3. Bring back to center position with palms touching.
4. Repeat movement for time and repetitions.

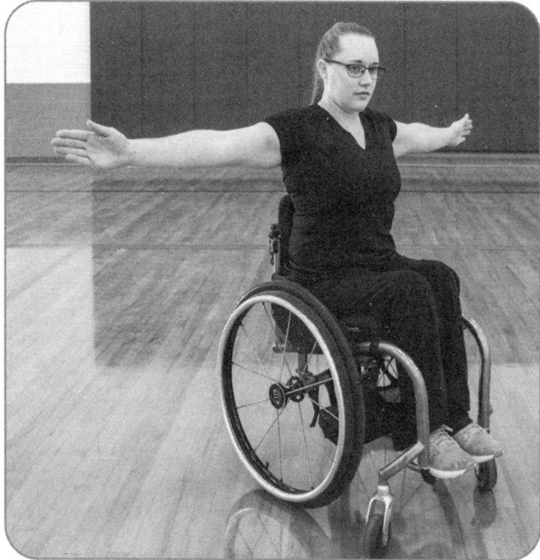

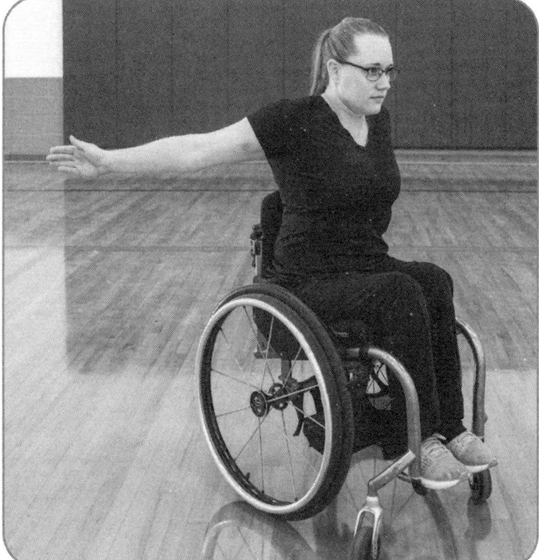

TOE TOUCHES

Dynamic Stretch

Body part: Back

Muscle group: Latissimus dorsi

1. Stand with back straight, feet hip-width apart, and arms relaxed at sides.
2. Slowly bend at waist to touch toes.
3. Keeping knees straight, flex as far as possible, then pause.
4. Slowly stand up tall.

5. Reach up with straight arms over head.
6. Slowly bend back down to touch toes.
7. Continue controlled movement for 10 to 30 seconds.
8. Stop, relax, and repeat 2 to 3 more times.

Accommodations and modifications: For students unable to perform this movement, this exercise can be performed from a seated position (shown). Repeat movement for time and repetitions.

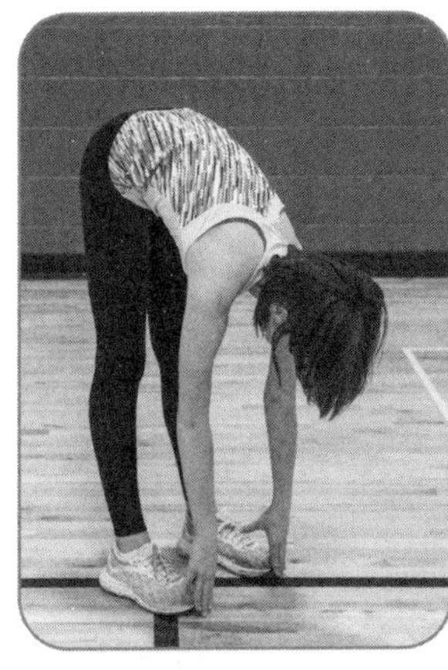

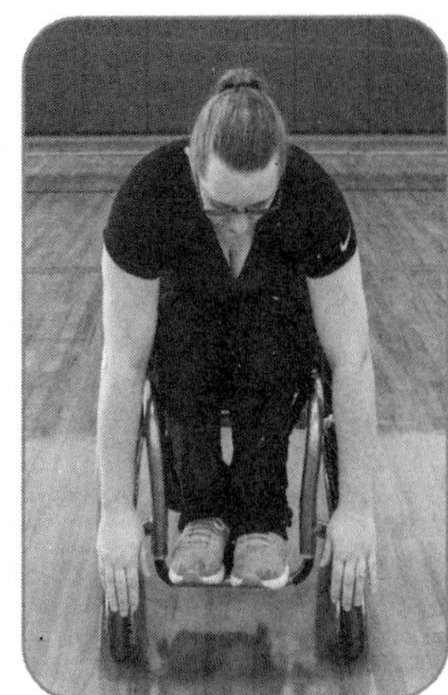

UPPER-BACK STRETCH

Static Stretch

Body part: Back

Muscle group: Latissimus dorsi

1. Stand with back straight and feet hip-width apart.
2. Clasp hands together in front of you.
3. Rotate wrists so the thumbs are pointing down.
4. With arms straight and parallel to ground, roll shoulders and reach forward.
5. Hold position for 15 to 30 seconds.
6. Return to original position.
7. Stop, relax and repeat 2 to 3 more times.

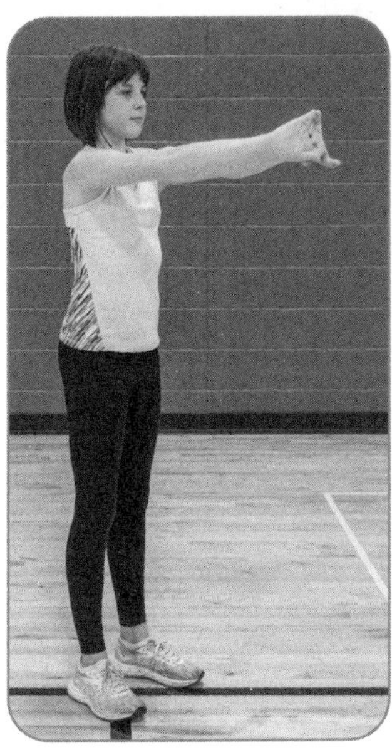

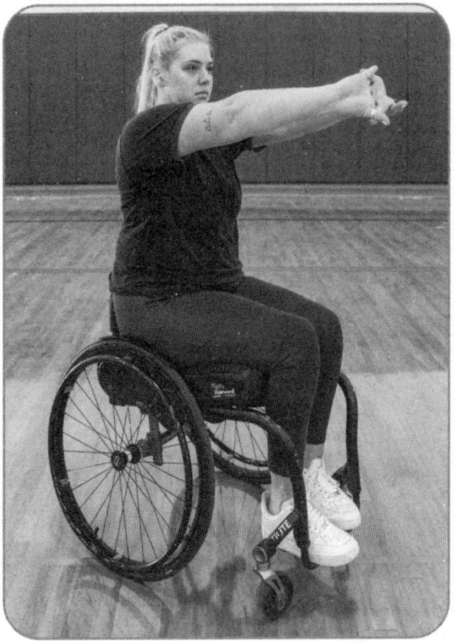

Accommodations and modifications: For students unable to perform this movement, this exercise can be performed from a seated position. Repeat movement for time and repetitions.

SEATED BICEPS STRETCH

Dynamic Stretch

Body part: Arms

Muscle group: Biceps

1. Sit with knees bent, feet hip-width and flat on ground.
2. Place hands on ground behind and fingers facing away from body.
3. Distribute weight evenly between feet, buttocks, and arms.
4. Keeping hands stationary, slide buttocks forward toward feet.
5. Pause and return.
6. Slowly continue movement 10 to 30 seconds.
7. Stop, relax, and repeat 2 to 3 more times.

Accommodations and modifications: For students unable to perform this movement, while seated, have them perform these steps.

1. Straighten arm and place it on the wall at a slightly lower level from shoulder.
2. Turn body away from arm.
3. Hold for 15-30 seconds.
4. Stop, relax, and repeat for time and repetitions.

This stretch helps lengthen the biceps.

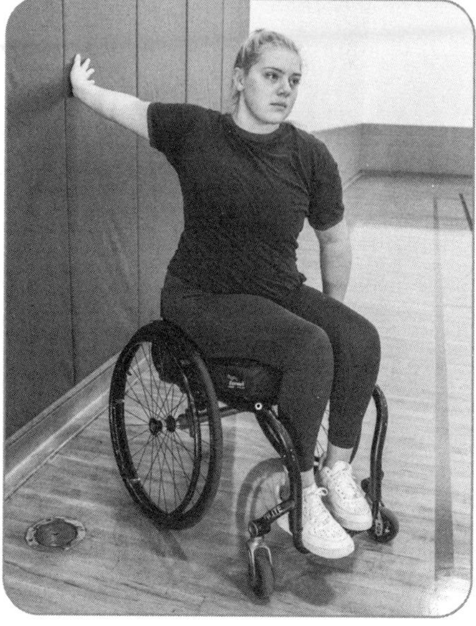

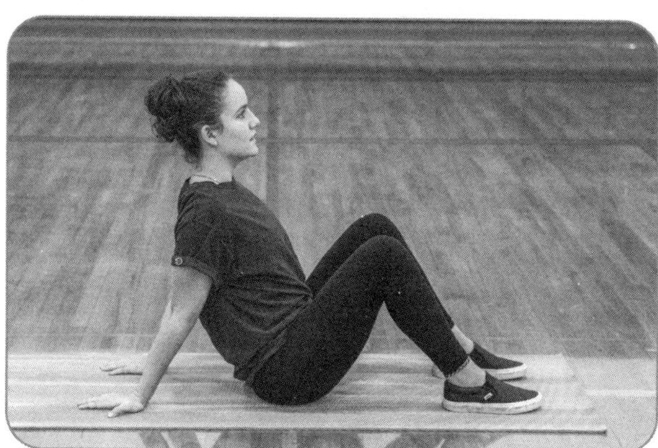

STANDING BICEPS STRETCH

Static Stretch

Body part: Arms

Muscle group: Biceps

1. Stand with back straight and feet hip-width apart.
2. Interlace hands behind at base of spine.
3. Slowly straighten arms and turn palms facedown.
4. Raise arms up until stretch is felt.
5. Hold position for 15 to 30 seconds.
6. Return back to original position.
7. Stop, relax, and repeat 2 to 3 more times.

Accommodations and modifications: This stretch can be performed from a standing or seated position and can use a wall to further stretch your chest, shoulders, and arms. Repeat movement for time and repetitions.

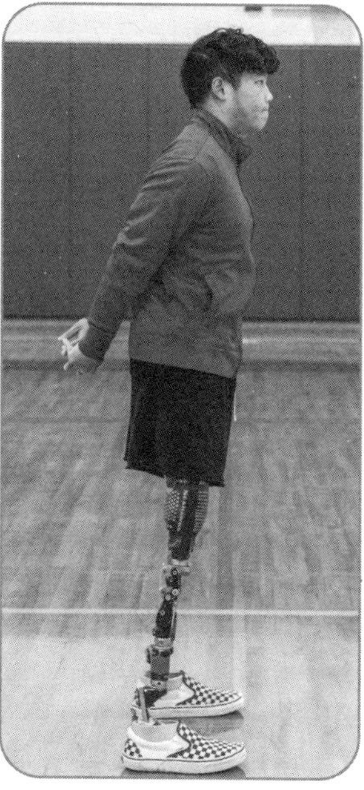

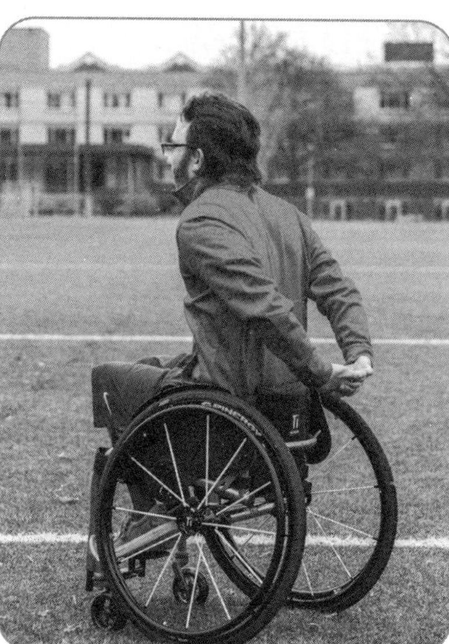

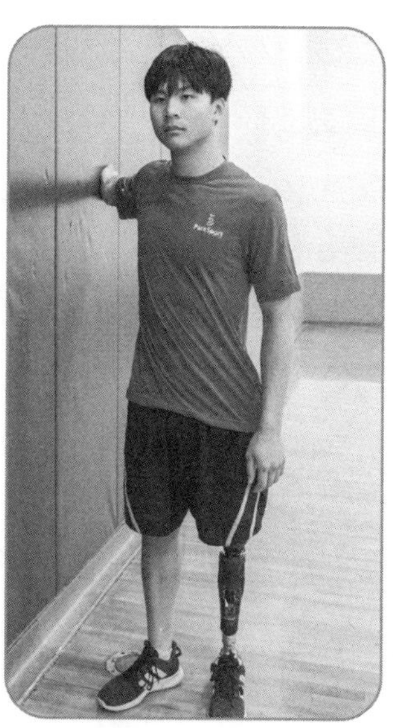

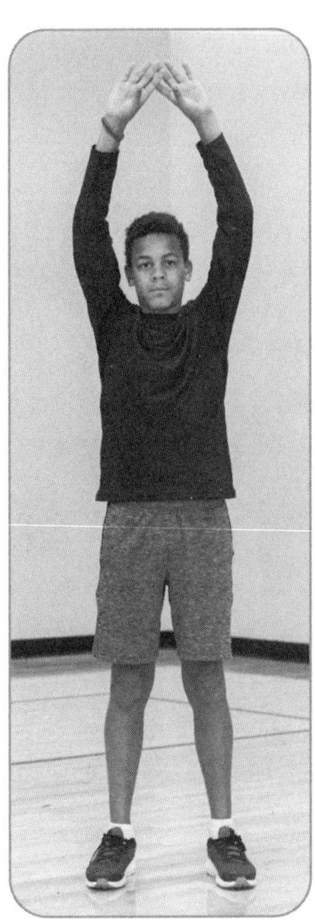

OVERHEAD ARM SWING

Dynamic Stretch

Body part: Arms

Muscle group: Triceps

1. Stand with back straight, feet hip-width apart, and arms relaxed at sides.
2. Slowly raise arms out to side, then overhead.
3. Reverse motion and bring arms back down.
4. At a controlled pace, continue movement for 10 to 30 seconds, mimicking jumping jacks without moving legs.
5. Stop, relax, and repeat 2 to 3 more times.

Accommodations and modifications: For students unable to perform this movement, this exercise can be performed from a seated position. Repeat movement for time and repetitions.

TRICEPS HORIZONTAL STRETCH

Static Stretch

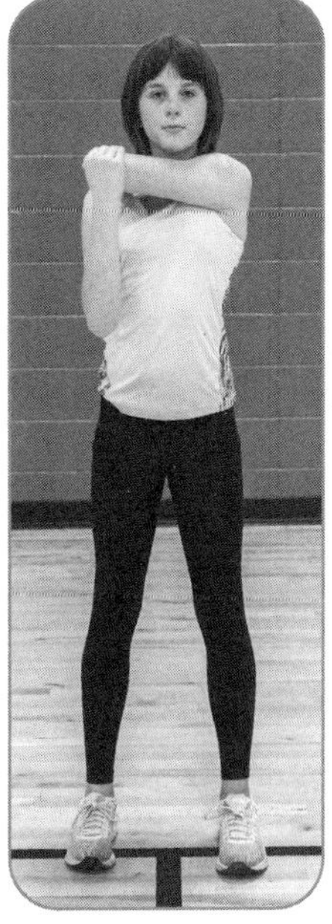

Body part: Arms

Muscle group: Triceps

1. Stand with back straight and feet hip-width apart.
2. Bring one arm across body (chest height).
3. Slightly bend elbow, placing opposite hand below elbow (forearm).
4. Assist by pressing arm into chest.
5. Hold position for 15 to 30 seconds.
6. Return to original position.
7. Repeat with opposite arm.
8. Stop, relax, and repeat 2 to 3 more times.

Accommodations and modifications: For students unable to perform this movement, this exercise can be performed from a seated position. Repeat movement for time and repetitions.

TRICEPS STRETCH

Static Stretch

Body part: Arms

Muscle group: Triceps

1. Stand with feet shoulder-width apart.
2. Raise arm overhead and flex at elbow until hand reaches middle of upper back.

3. Reach over with opposite hand to grasp opposite elbow.
4. Gently pull toward midline of back or until stretch is felt in the triceps.
5. Hold position for 15 to 30 seconds.
6. Stop, relax, and repeat 2 to 3 times on each side.

Accommodations and modifications: For students unable to perform this movement, this exercise can be performed from a seated position. Repeat movement for time and repetitions.

WRIST CIRCLES

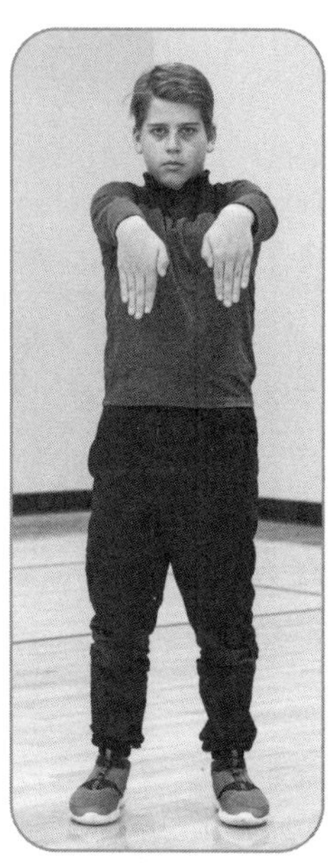

Dynamic Stretch

Body part: Wrists and forearms

Muscle group: Flexors and extensors

1. Stand with back straight and feet hip-width apart.
2. Hold both arms out in front of body at shoulder height with palms facing down (pronated).
3. Rotate wrists clockwise.
4. Reverse motion by rotating counterclockwise.
5. Continue movement in both directions for 10 to 30 seconds.
6. Stop, relax, and repeat 2 to 3 more times.

Accommodations and modifications: For students unable to perform this movement, this exercise can be performed from a seated position. Repeat movement for time and repetitions.

WRIST EXTENSOR STRETCH

Static Stretch

Body part: Forearms

Muscle group: Forearm extensors

1. Stand with feet shoulder-width apart.
2. Extend arms out in front, palms up.
3. Flex one wrist, pointing fingers to the ground.
4. With opposite hand, gently assist the stretching of the wrist farther until a moderate stretch in forearm is felt.
5. Hold position for 15 to 30 seconds time.
6. Stop, relax, and repeat 2 to 3 times on both sides.

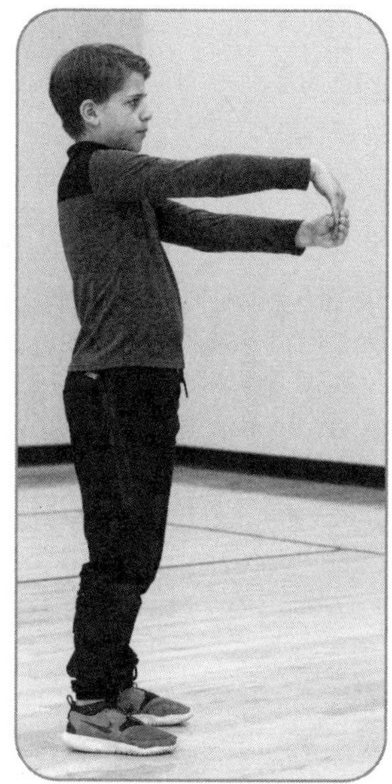

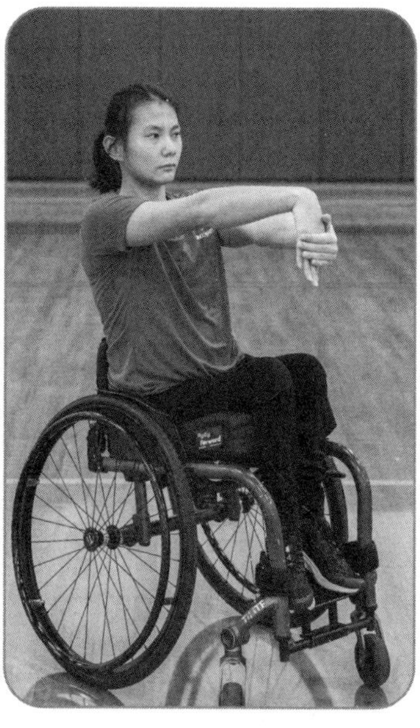

Accommodations and modifications: For students unable to perform this movement, this exercise can be performed from a seated position. Repeat movement for time and repetitions.

FORFARMS STRETCH

Static Stretch

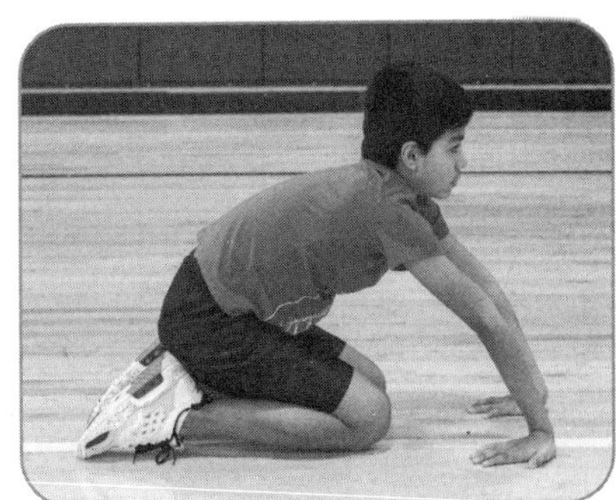

Body part: Wrists and forearms

Muscle group: Flexors and extensors

1. Kneel on ground, legs together, with buttocks resting on heels.
2. Bend torso forward.
3. Place palms on ground with fingers pointed toward knees.
4. Hold position for 15 to 30 seconds.
5. Return to original position.
6. Stop, relax, and repeat 2 to 3 more times.

Accommodations and modifications: For students unable to perform this movement, this exercise can be performed from a seated position. Repeat movement for time and repetitions.

ROUTINES: STRINGING THEM TOGETHER

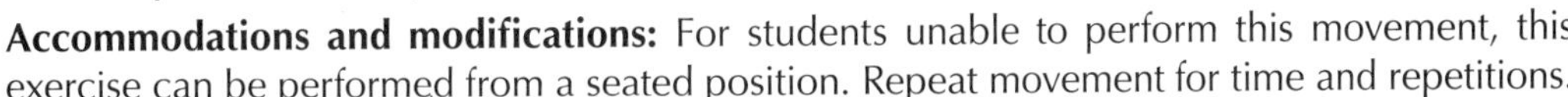

As students become more comfortable with and attuned to their own bodies and how they work, they will be able to adjust to various movements within each stretching routine. This is just the start, so it is important to slowly integrate not only each body part but also each movement that goes along with it. Remind students that everything is a progression, and we do not need to advance any movement before maintaining readiness. With time, both teacher and students will notice and understand the purpose of each stretch.

As we go through the progression routines of beginner, intermediate, and advanced levels, you will notice that they differ in relation to the muscular and endurance routines covered in the following chapters. Always aligning the body parts and joints is key to avoiding discomfort and preventing injury. These movements will improve with practice as your students begin to realize that having better flexibility and mobility will enhance their everyday tasks and performance. Use the following recommendations to get started.

BEGINNER ROUTINE

Introduction

- Review of body parts
- Review of types of joints and muscles and limitations of movements

Warm-up: Brisk walk or slow jog for 5 to 10 minutes

Routine: The beginner's level is to get bodies familiar with the various stretching exercises and techniques. This is where the teacher, possibly with the assistance of a select student, will model the correct positioning and alignment of the body parts and joints, allowing students to replicate the movement.

- Model and practice each specific stretch, making sure that proper form and alignment is being performed.
- Verbalize the body parts, joints, and muscles being stretched.
- Travel through the area, visiting each student and making corrections, if needed.
- Review and perform both dynamic and static stretches of each body part until students feel comfortable doing them.
- Through time and repetitiveness, students will show their level of readiness to proceed to the next level.

Cool-down: Cardiorespiratory activity and hydration

INTERMEDIATE ROUTINE

Introduction

- Review of body parts
- Review of types of joints and limitations of movements

Warm-up: Brisk walk or slow jog for 5 to 10 minutes

Routine: The intermediate level is a bit more intense, and students will be able to execute more of a routine with a limited number of body parts and joints involved. Constant emphasis on the proper alignment of all joints within each stretch is still necessary.

- Choose 2 to 3 body parts to practice a short routine that will allow flowing movements from one stretch to another. Choosing partnering body parts, such as back and chest or biceps and triceps of the arms, will keep students focused on a specific area.
- Practice all dynamic stretches first, followed by static stretches. Be sure that both routines follow the same order of chosen stretches.
- Within this intermediate routine, consistently remind students of the importance of alignment and focus on their own degree of stretch.
- Remember that all students do not have an equal degree of stretching points due to age, gender, joint structure, activity level, muscular frame, or previous experience.

Cool-down: Cardiorespiratory activity and hydration

ADVANCED ROUTINE

Introduction

- Review of body parts
- Review of types of joints and limitations of movements

Warm-up: Brisk walk or slow jog for 5-10 minutes

Routine: This level allows students to engage in various stretches, having the comfort and ability to focus on balance and proper positioning needed for success. Students at this level will be able to perform a routine of stretches from head to toe, placing emphasis on preparing for the following daily activities assigned. Knowing their own limitations and points of discomfort, students will be able to successfully perform the following:

- Complete an entire stretching routine.
- Show knowledge of alignment and joint positioning.
- Execute each stretch freely and painlessly.
- Show improved flexibility.
- Create a personalized stretching routine and be able to lead class.

Cool-down: Cardiorespiratory activity and hydration

Upon completion of each stage, slowly introduce the following advanced techniques or increase the length of time of the hold of the stretch:

- *Passive stretching.* While in a stretch, having a partner or an accessory, such as a towel or resistance band, intensifies the stretch by placing pressure on that body part.
- *Ballistic stretching.* Using momentum or a bouncing movement forces joints beyond their normal ROM.
- *Proprioceptive neuromuscular facilitation (PNF).* This is another partnering technique to improve the elasticity and ROM.

Be aware that although many of these techniques are often performed by fitness specialists, they can be a great way to challenge students to perform research on various modes of stretching while staying within their level of readiness.

TEACHING TIPS

It is a best practice to end the lesson where you began. Why is stretching so important? Always relating what students are doing to their daily lives will, in most cases, answer the question of "why." For example: "What is the first thing we do in the morning? That's right, stretch. We put our arms up, hands over our head; twist our torso; and rotate our neck. Movements like this allow us to stretch the muscles and bring the joints through their full range of motion, preparing them to take on and accomplish the tasks that are planned for the day."

Remind students that proper form and technique are required for stretches to be effective and to avoid injuries, such as excessive strain on the joints and connective tissues. Through the improvement of flexibility, all movements will become less taxing on the body, both physically and mentally, especially as students get older.

Students should further be reminded to

- warm up before stretching,
- not stretch to the point where it is painful,
- avoid overstretching the ligaments and capsules,
- incorporate stretching before and after each exercise session or activity,
- be specific in the stretches they initiate for the activity they are preparing to perform,
- take extra time if needed to perform the stretch,
- breathe evenly while stretching, and
- do not hold breath while stretching.

CONCLUSION

As seen throughout this chapter, a variety of stretching exercises can be incorporated into your daily lesson plans and exercise routines. Though too often overlooked or minimized, stretching is an important tool in enhancing health-related fitness. Incorporating stretching into our daily lives not only will yield immediate benefits but also could provide benefits for later in life since flexibility and mobility can be easily lost over time.

The benefits of stretching are the increase in blood flow to make muscles more flexible, release of stress and tension, easing of muscle stiffness, and enhanced sport performance, to name just a few. Preparing the muscles will better equip students for participation in physical activities, allowing them to move smoothly through full range of motion. This will, in turn, prevent injuries and pain in both the muscles and joints.

Stretching not only is a technique for muscle toning and strengthening but also gives the body the ability to relax and focus, both mentally and physically. Stretching is a form of exercise that improves a person's well-being. Therefore, it is necessary that stretching is included in weekly workouts. As a teacher, it is critically important to motivate your students to see the importance of flexibility through stretching; ensure that they stay on task; and keep them focused through questioning, guidance, and inspiration.

Review Questions

1. Explain the importance of stretching the upper-body muscles in relation to injury prevention.
2. Explain how increasing the range of motion enhances athletic performance.
3. Select one exercise and identify the muscles that are engaged in that exercise.
4. Describe the everyday benefits of increasing your flexibility through stretching.
5. Identify a specific sports activity and explain how stretching your upper-body muscles will affect that sport.

Visit HK*Propel* for additional material related to this chapter.

CHAPTER 10

Core Stretching Exercises

Chapter Objective

After reading this chapter, you will understand the role that proper stretching technique plays on increasing flexibility in the core to increase the range of motion (ROM), which improves performance during activities, increases blood flow to the muscles, reduces the risk of injuries, and assists in the pre- and post exercise cool-down; know how to develop lessons that teach these concepts to secondary school students; be able to effectively demonstrate a series of exercises and exercise routines designed to stretch the core muscles; and employ best teaching practices that enhance student learning.

Key Concepts

- Stretching the muscles of the core is essential to enhanced physical activity performance as well as everyday activities by increasing the range of motion.
- The exercises presented will help you teach students to identify the muscles, tendons, ligaments, and joints involved in stretching exercises to increase flexibility.
- Warm-up and cool-down stretches should be performed prior to and after implementing core exercises.
- Accommodations and modifications are recommended so that all activities can be modified and performed by all students in the class.

INTRODUCTION

The core, or torso, is the conduit between the upper and lower body that is responsible for maintaining the stability and balance, which allows us to stand upright. It also enables us to do the simple tasks such as tying our shoelaces and more complex tasks such as being able to lift heavy objects.

Because the midsection of the body includes several different muscles in the front, back, and sides, as a teacher, you need to be conscious of incorporating a variety of movements in different directions. Therefore, it is important to maintain the flexibility of this area, acknowledging that, although we try to isolate a certain muscle group, there is overall interconnectedness of the muscles and tendons in this region. All too often, we have a tendency to visualize the torso as being sedentary for the most part, but in reality, it is the body's center of power—meaning, it has the responsibility of supporting the spine and pelvis during physical activity while controlling the movements we make with our arms and legs in order to use them to our advantage. Being aware of the core's functions is the first step of ensuring that ample time and effort are provided in delivering evidence-based instruction in taking the necessary steps to take advantage of the benefits of proper stretching protocols. Students should also be taught that the intent of the exercises in this chapter is to build and develop flexibility, which is more extensive and aligned with one of the fitness components as discussed in chapter 2, while stretching would be performed prior to starting any physical activity or athletic competition. Students should be observed during instruction to avoid improper techniques that could lead to detrimental outcomes.

The components of the skeletal system involved within the core are the spine, ribs, and pelvis. These are kept aligned by the core musculature of the trunk, which includes the *transverse abdominis*, a muscle that wraps around from the back of the spine to the front of the waist, *multifidus*, a deep muscle located along the midline of the back of the spine, *internal and external obliques*, a pair of muscles that lie on the lateral sides of the body, *rectus abdominis*, a pair of long muscles that run vertically up the front of the abdomen, and *erector spinae*, a group of muscles that run along the length of the spine on both sides. Anatomically, all reside in the abdomen and lower back of the torso (see figure 10.1).

Now that we understand what is really behind the muscles that comprise the core, let's go deeper to learn the benefits of them all working together. Stretching your abdominal muscles is an important factor for overall performance and better health. Along with preparation for a successful workout, increasing the range of motion in both the abdominal and lower-back area will decrease risk of lower-back pain, increase flexibility, improve posture, and boost recovery, so that you are able to successfully continue with your workout. The core is also critical in sports performance. For example, all movements in dance are generated by the torso, which serves as the foundation (figure 10.2).

As we begin to provide appropriate exercises involved in the stretching of the core muscles, it is important to also review with your students the principle of specificity, as well as the definitions of a *static stretch, dynamic stretch, proprioceptive neuromuscular facilitation* (PNF), and *ballistic stretch* as discussed in chapter 9. Although each type of stretch serves a specific purpose, according to the ACSM (2017, p. 156),

> dynamic stretching should be performed prior to the workout, as these activities encourage large movements that raise the heart rate and increase blood flow to the muscles, tendons, and ligaments . . . and reduce injury while preparing the body for the upcoming workout.

Conversely, static stretches should be performed post exercise. Students should continuously be reminded that, when beginning a stretching routine, it is important to listen to their body and be cautious not to overstretch the ligaments and capsules that surround the joints, as this could cause damage to tissues. Stretching should be performed with slow, continuous, and controlled movements.

It is also important to note that although this chapter focuses on the importance of stretching as an entity in itself, many of the exercises described here will also be used as warm-up and cool-down exercises in subsequent chapters.

As the physical education teacher, you can use the exercises in this chapter as part of a warm-up or cool-down, lesson on core stretching exercises, or routine. Each exercise has a description and illustration, with notes about the type of stretch, the body part and muscle groups worked, steps for safely executing the stretch with good form, and accommodations and modifications for those unable to perform the stretch as described. Many stretches are illustrated with video in HK*Propel*. Teach each exercise separately, ensuring that students are

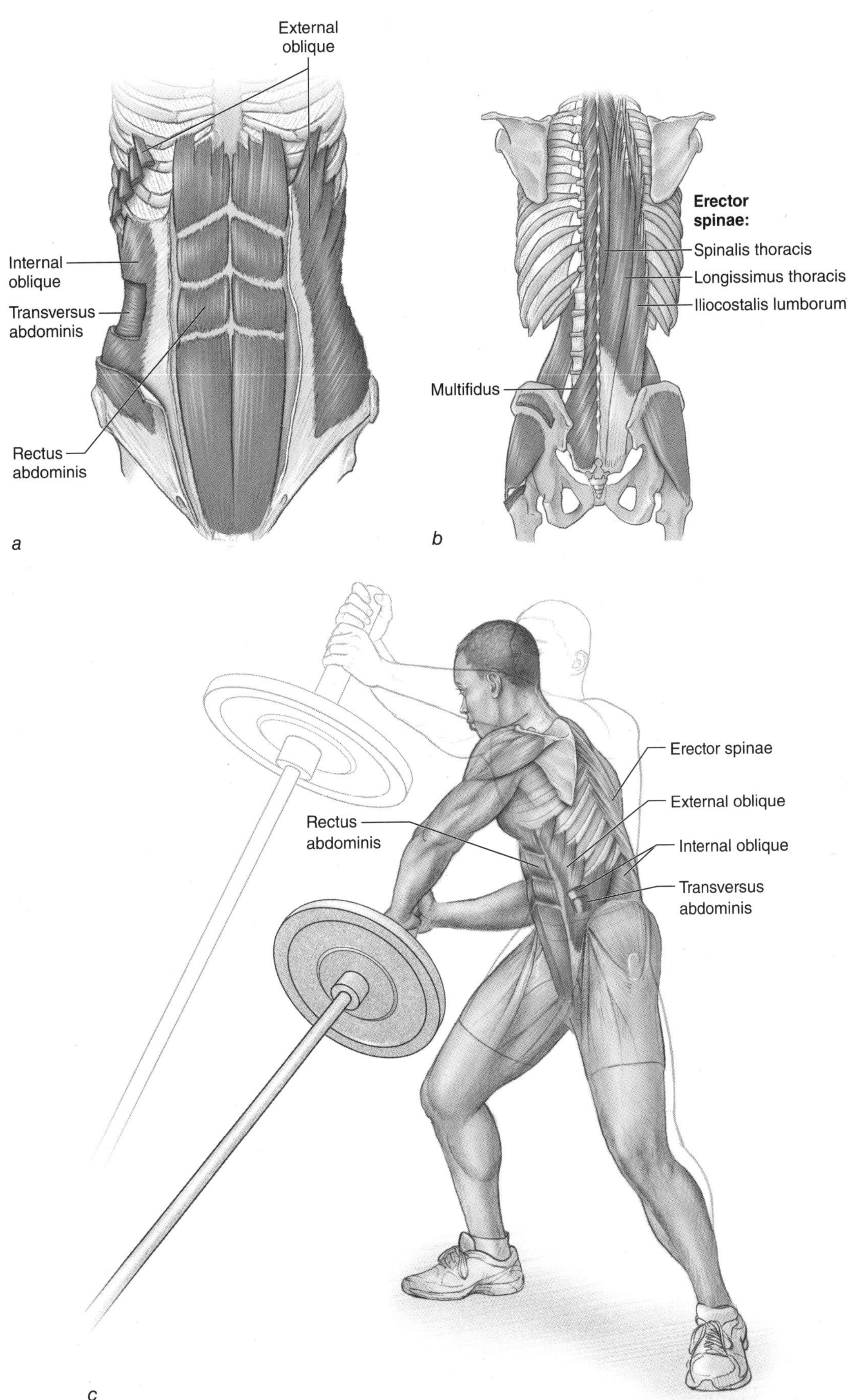

Figure 10.1 Anterior (*a*), posterior (*b*), and lateral (*c*) view of the core muscles.

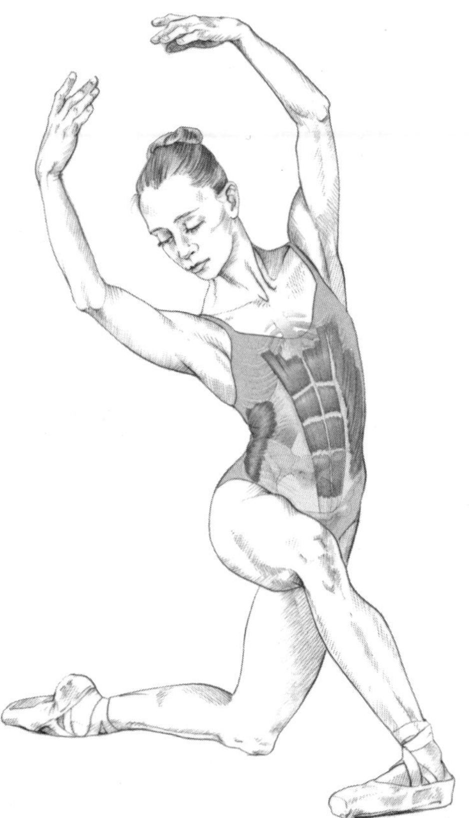

Figure 10.2 Dancers, like all athletes, need strong core muscles to perform at their best.

performing the stretch correctly, emphasizing the type of stretch (static or dynamic) and the muscle group being engaged. This is extremely important because what students learn during this initial instruction will enable them to use the appropriate stretch for subsequent physical activities, as well as enable them to safely engage in routines and circuits throughout the class. We include guidelines for developing routines for the beginner, intermediate, and advanced levels after the exercises, along with further teaching tips.

As you develop your daily lesson plans, align each lesson with the National Standards and your own state and local standards so that every student taught in your class can participate in the activities. The following sample lesson overview shows the National Standards and Grade-Level Outcomes (GLOs) relevant to this material, lesson objectives, and accommodations and modifications to be kept in mind when teaching a lesson on core stretching exercises. All of the exercises in this book are designed to provide accommodations and modifications as needed. This ensures equity, opportunity, and access for all students. Additionally, as you progress through your fitness education course, your students should be able to identify which stretching activities will be required for the daily activity you present.

LESSON OVERVIEW

Core Stretching Routine

Lesson length: 5 to 20 minutes

Grade level: 9th to 12th

National Standards and GLOs: S1.H3, S2.H2, S3.H9, S3.H11, S4.H5

Grade level: 6th to 8th

National Standards and GLOs: S3.M9, S3.M11, S3.M12, S3.M14, S3.M15, S3.M16, S4.M7, S5.M1

Lesson objectives: By the end of the lesson, the students will be able to do the following:

- Perform a warm-up cardiorespiratory activity prior to your stretching routine.
- Perform core muscles stretching routine, showing proper technique throughout each movement.
- Perform a cool-down including cardiorespiratory activity and hydration.
- Perform a cool-down routine using static stretching showing ROM in muscle-joint areas.

Accommodations and modifications: It is important for all movements and exercises to be modified to meet the individual needs of every student in order for them to engage in full participation. Implementing universal design for learning (UDL) will assist teachers in ensuring that all students can reach their full potential. Follow the general instructional recommendations, as discussed in chapter 3, for all activities.

WARM-UP DYNAMIC AND STATIC STRETCHES FOR THE CORE

TRUNK LATERAL FLEXION

Dynamic Stretch

Body part: Trunk

Muscle group: Abdominals and obliques

1. Stand upright with feet shoulder-width apart, arms relaxed at sides.
2. Bend laterally side to side with each arm sliding down each thigh toward the knee.
3. Alternate between right and left sides.
4. Continue movement in both directions 10 to 30 seconds, or
5. Repeat the movement from right to left 10 to 20 times.

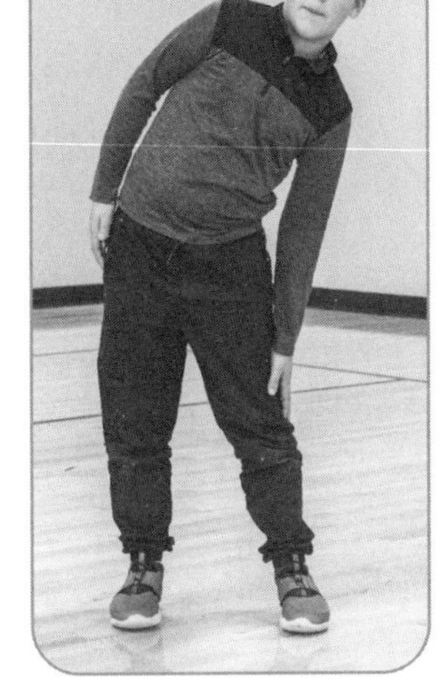

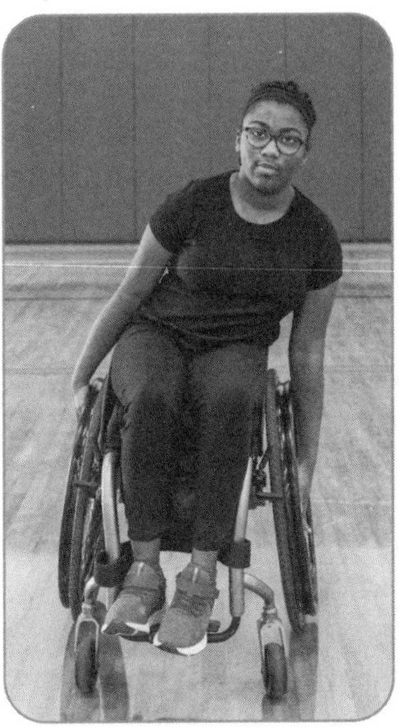

Accommodations and modifications: For students unable to perform this movement, encourage them to slowly bend laterally as far as they are able to. Adjust time and repetitions for movement as needed. This activity can be performed while seated, slowly moving arms down the sides of the chair.

Progression: To progress the exercise, use the standing oblique stretch.

PROGRESSION: OBLIQUE STRETCH

1. Stand upright with feet shoulder-width apart.
2. Raise one arm up over the head while leaning to the opposite side.
3. Bend laterally side to side with the opposite arm sliding down the thigh toward the knee.
4. Alternate between right and left sides.
5. Repeat the movement from right to left 10 to 20 times.

Accommodations and modifications: This activity can be performed while seated (shown).

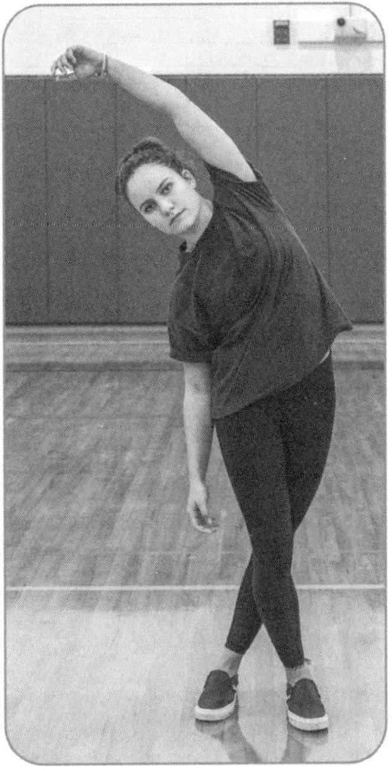

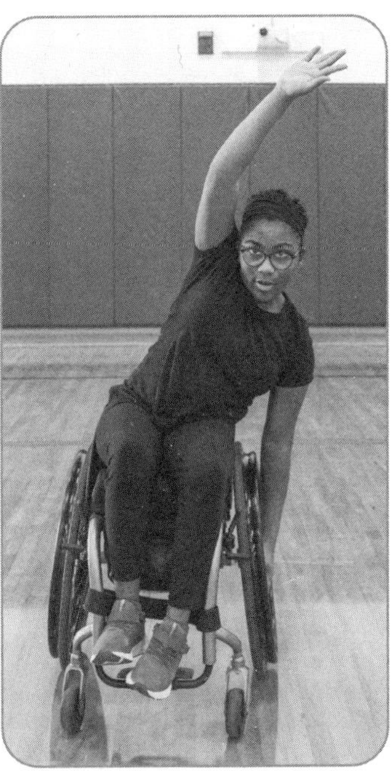

FORWARD BEND STRETCH

Static Stretch

Body part: Lower back

Muscle group: Erector spinae

1. Stand upright with feet together.
2. Bend knees slightly and bend or flex at hips, lowering torso downward.
3. Keeping the head in neutral position, loosely hang arms down over the head, toward the ground.
4. Gently straighten legs without hyperextending.
5. Maintain a straight back by rolling shoulders back.
6. Hold position for 15 to 30 seconds.
7. Slowly reverse movement and return to original position.
8. Stop, relax, and repeat 2 to 3 more times.

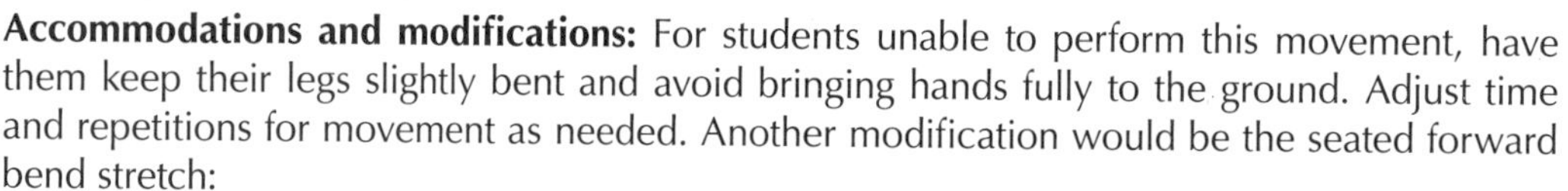

Accommodations and modifications: For students unable to perform this movement, have them keep their legs slightly bent and avoid bringing hands fully to the ground. Adjust time and repetitions for movement as needed. Another modification would be the seated forward bend stretch:

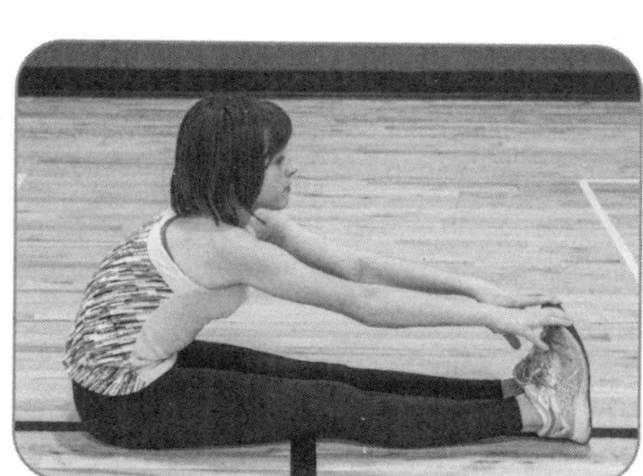

1. Sit on the ground with feet together.
2. Bend knees slightly and bend or flex at hips.
3. Keeping the head in a neutral position, with arms straight, reach toward feet.
4. Gently straighten legs without hyperextending.
5. Maintain a straight back by rolling shoulders back.
6. Hold position for 15 to 30 seconds.
7. Slowly reverse movement and return to original position.
8. Stop, relax, and repeat 2 to 3 more times.

TRUNK ROTATOR

Dynamic Stretch

Body part: Core

Muscle group: Abdominals and obliques

1. Stand upright with feet shoulder-width apart.
2. Bend elbows and place hands close to chest.
3. Rotate torso toward each side, right and left.
4. Keep trunk upright and turn head to each side, following the movement from right to left.
5. Continue movement in both directions 10 to 30 seconds, or
6. Repeat the movement from right to left 10 to 20 times

Accommodations and modifications: For students unable to perform this movement, encourage students to rotate as far as they can. Adjust time or repetitions for movement as needed. This exercise can also be performed seated.

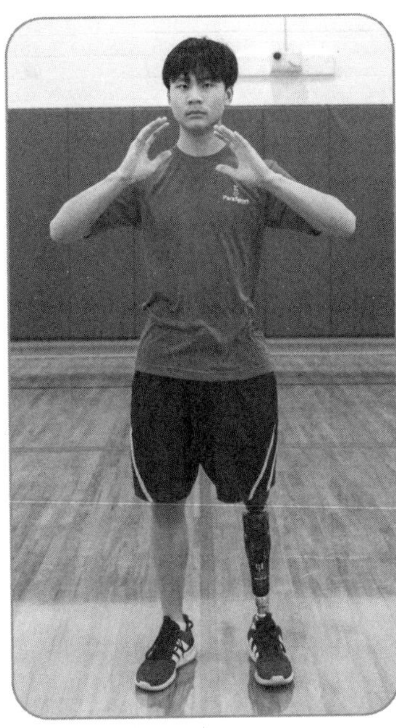

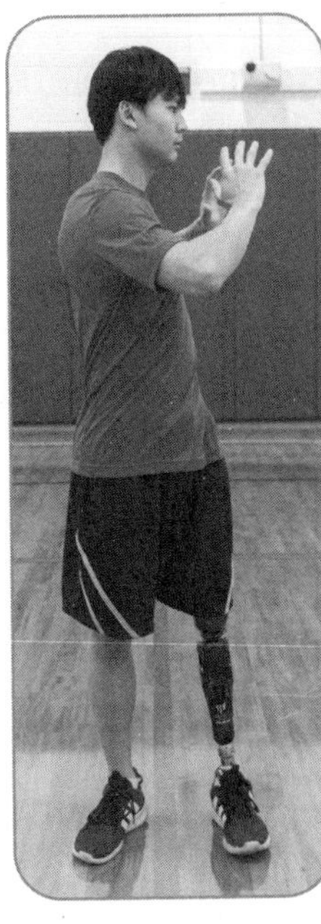

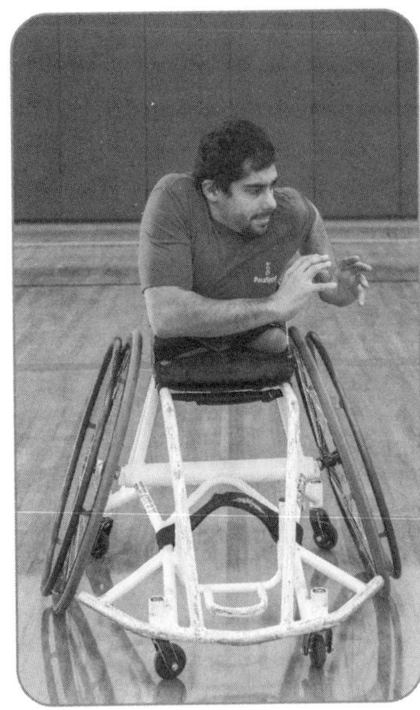

SEATED SPINAL TWIST

Static Stretch

Body part: Lower back

Muscle group: Erector spinae, gluteals, and obliques

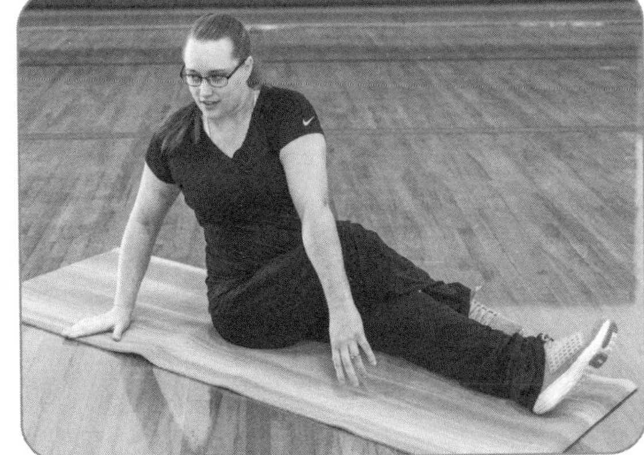

1. Sit on floor, legs crossed with right leg on top.
2. With right leg crossing over the left leg, place right foot on the ground against the outside of the left knee.
3. Gently twist shoulders toward the right, pushing against right leg, using left elbow against the right knee for leverage.
4. Twist as far as comfortable and hold position for 10 to 30 seconds.
5. Repeat on other side.
6. Repeat on both sides 3 to 4 times.

Accommodations and modifications: For students unable to perform this movement, encourage them to rotate as far as they are able to. Adjust time and repetitions for movement as needed.

KNEE DROP

Dynamic Stretch

Body part: Core

Muscle group: Obliques

1. Lie on back, with knees bent at 90 degrees, hips and knees aligned, and arms straight and out to the sides.
2. Slowly rotate torso to one side, lowering the knees down to the ground.

3. Pause, keeping shoulders in contact with the ground.
4. Slowly, reverse motion by rotating to the opposite direction.
5. Pause, keeping shoulders in contact with the ground.
6. Continue movement in both directions for 10 to 30 seconds.
7. Stop, relax, and repeat 2 to 3 more times.

Accommodations and modifications: For students unable to perform this movement, encourage them to rotate as far as they are able to, for some may not be able to reach the ground at first. Adjust time and repetitions for movement as needed.

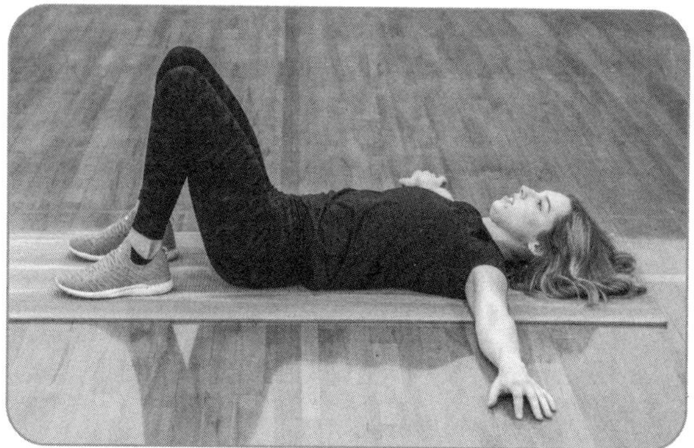

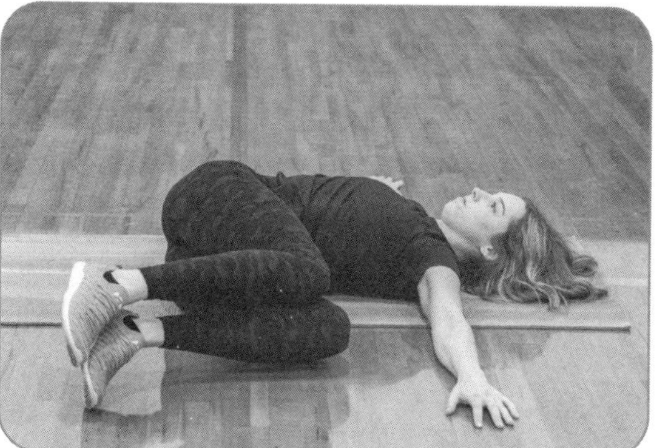

DOWNWARD DOG STRETCH

Static Stretch

Body part: Core

Muscle group: Rectus abdominis and erector spinae

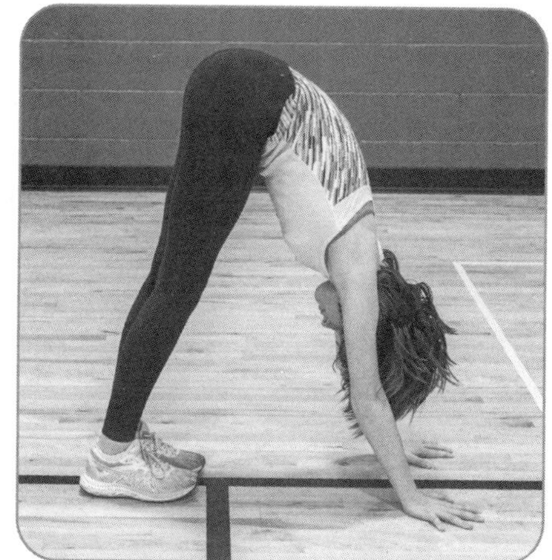

1. Begin in a straight-arm plank position.
2. Position hands slightly in front of shoulders and knees on ground.
3. Align shoulders, elbows, wrists, hips, and knees, with toes tucked.
4. Slowly press back on the ground with hands to lift body, lifting glutes upward, and straighten knees, forming a V shape.
5. Hold position for 15 to 30 seconds.
6. Return to the original position.
7. Relax and repeat 2 to 3 more times.

Accommodations and modifications: For students unable to perform this movement, instruct them to focus on the order of progression of the motions, leaving the straightening as a last priority. Adjust time and repetitions for movement as needed.

SPINE TWIST

Dynamic Stretch

Body part: Core

Muscle group: Abdominals

1. Lie on the ground with legs straight and hips, knees, and ankles aligned.
2. Hold arms straight and out to the sides.

3. Slowly rotate torso to one side.
4. Guide a knee to the floor and gently place the same foot on the opposite straight knee.
5. Pause, keeping shoulders in contact with the ground.
6. Slowly reverse motion by rotating to opposite direction.
7. Pause, keeping shoulders in contact with the ground.
8. Continue movement in both directions for 10 to 30 seconds.
9. Stop, relax, and repeat 2 to 3 more times.

Accommodations and modifications: For students unable to perform this movement, encourage them to make individual adjustments as needed. Adjust time and repetitions for movement as needed. This exercise can be performed in the seated position (shown).

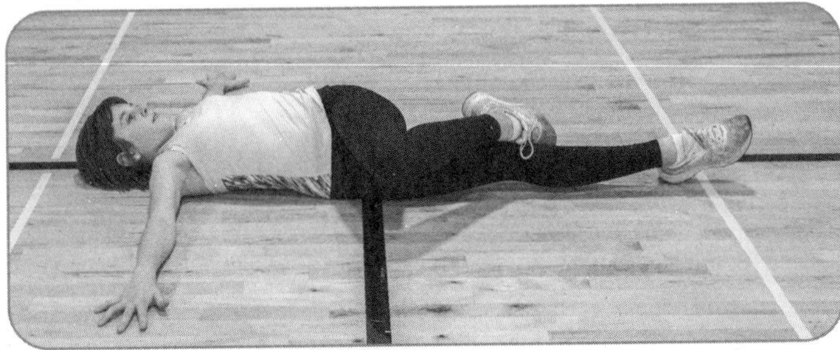

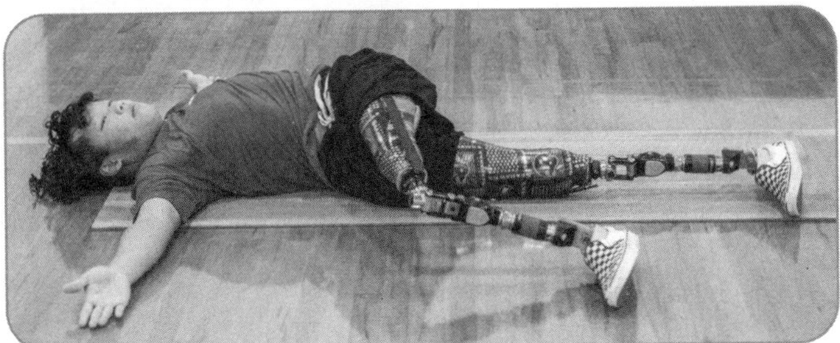

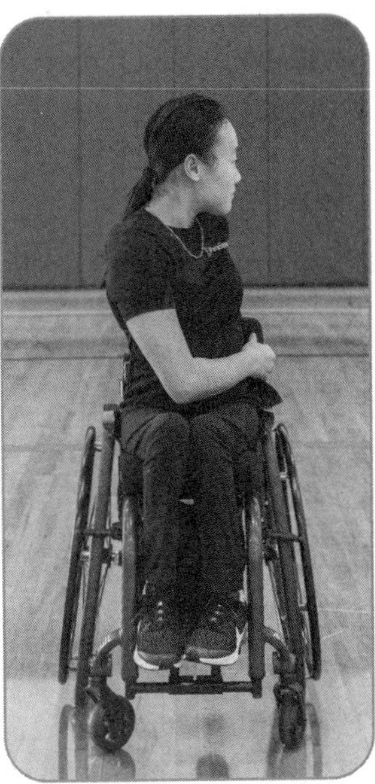

SEATED SIDE-STRADDLE STRETCH

Static Stretch

Body part: Core

Muscle group: Obliques and erector spinae

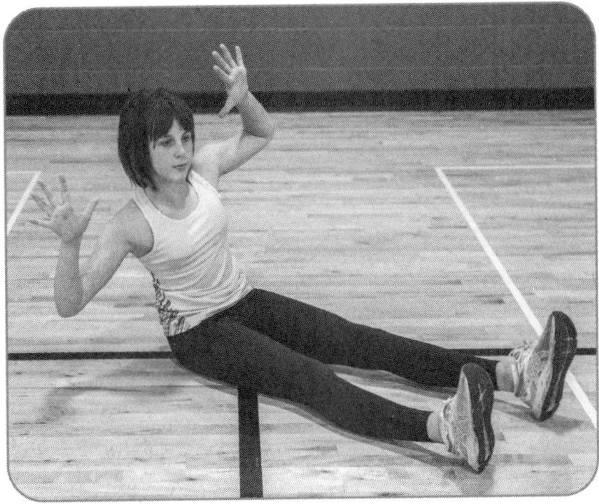

1. Sit upright on the ground with legs apart in a V-shape position.
2. Raise arms, bending elbows, with fingers pointed up.
3. Slowly bend to one side, bringing elbow toward the ground.
4. Do not bend forward or rotate trunk.
5. Hold position for 15 to 30 seconds.
6. Return to original position.
7. Slowly repeat on the opposite side.
8. Relax and repeat 2 to 3 more times on each side.

Accommodations and modifications: For students unable to perform this movement, they may need to slightly bend their knee while reaching their elbow to ground. Adjust time and repetitions for movement as needed.

CAT–COW STRETCH

Dynamic Stretch

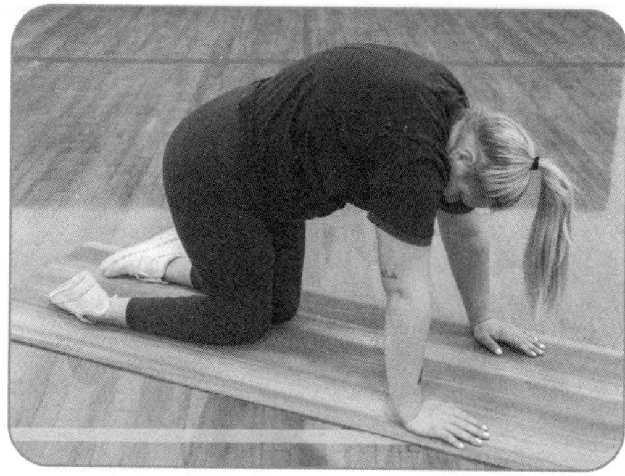

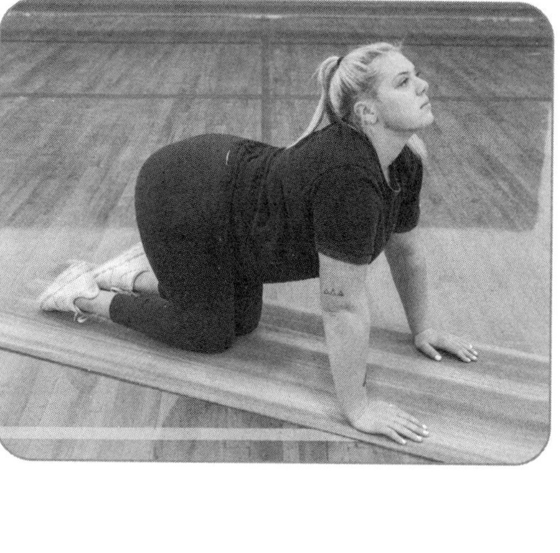

Body part: Core

Muscle group: Abdominals and erector spinae

1. Place hands and knees on the ground.
2. Align shoulders, elbows, wrists, hips, and knees, with toes tucked.
3. Slowly tuck head downward while arching back.
4. Pause.
5. Reverse motion while extending neck upward.
6. Drop belly downward toward the ground.
7. Pause.
8. Continue movement in both directions for 10 to 30 seconds.
9. Stop, relax, and repeat 2 to 3 more times.

Accommodations and modifications: For students unable to perform this movement, break down the progression of the movement. Adjust time and repetitions for movement as needed. The cat pose can be executed in the seated position by doing the following (KD Smart Chair, 2019):

1. Place hands on thighs or grip a chair.
2. Round upper body forward on exhale.
3. Arch the spine like a cat and drop chin toward chest.
4. Hold position for a few deep breaths, then release.

The cow pose can be executed in the seated position (shown) by doing the following (KD Smart Chair, 2019):

1. Hold the chair or place hands on thighs.
2. Slowly lift head toward the ceiling on inhale, then exhale through the front of chest, carefully arching the back.
3. Continue breathing while holding the pose for a few deep breaths.

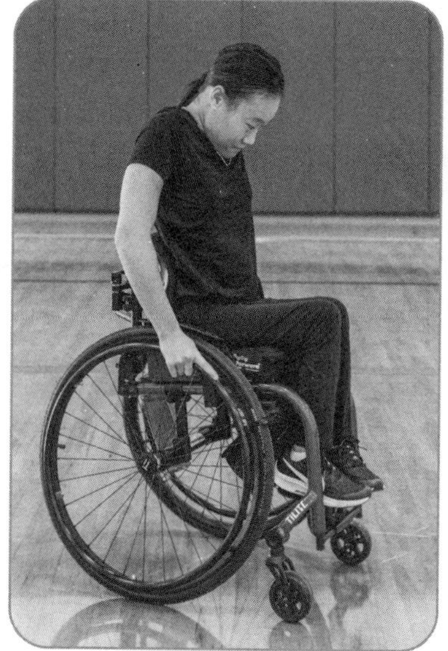

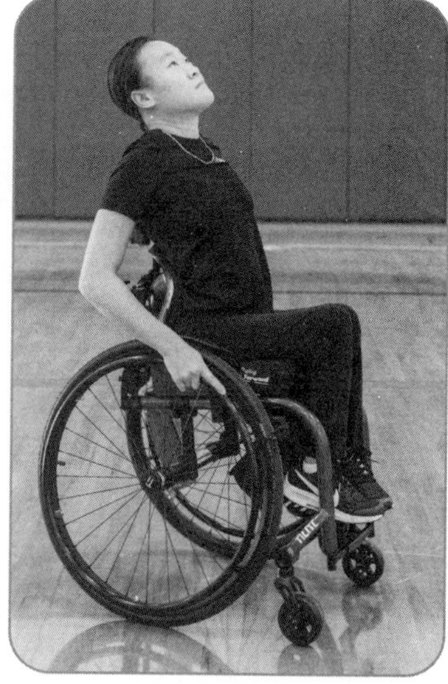

ABDOMINAL STRETCH

Static Stretch

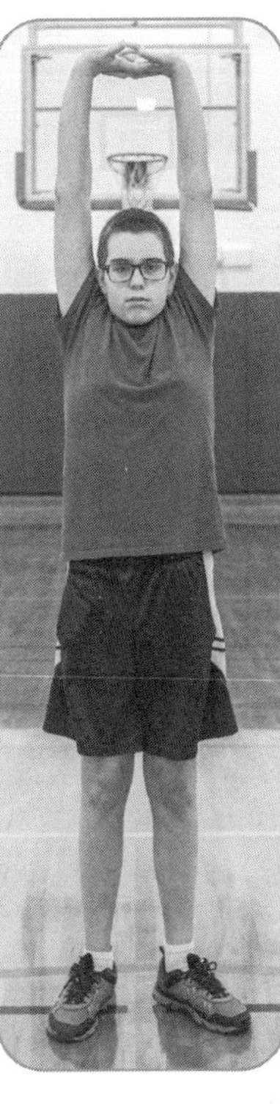

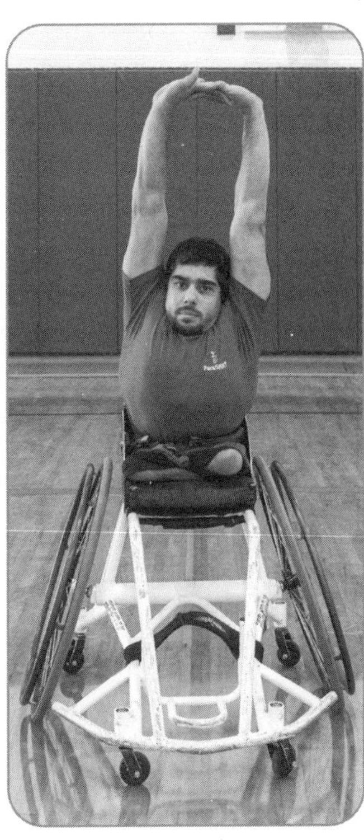

Body part: Core

Muscle group: Rectus abdominis, pectoralis major, erector spinae

1. Standing up straight with feet hip-width apart, reach arms straight above the head.
2. Slowly lean back and arch spine.
3. Hold position for 15 to 30 seconds.
4. Return to original position.
5. Stop, relax, and repeat 2 to 3 more times.

Accommodations and modifications: For students unable to perform this movement, have them slowly perform the stretch from a seated position on the ground or in a chair (shown), as balance may be a factor for some. Tell students to avoid tilting their head back and have them repeat the movement for time and repetitions.

WINDMILLS

Dynamic Stretch

Body part: Core

Muscle group: Abdominals, obliques, erector spinae

1. Stand upright with feet slightly wider than shoulder-width apart.
2. Raise arms straight out to either side.
3. Keep arms in this position while reaching down with one arm toward the opposite toe.
4. Rise back up to starting position.
5. Continue movement for other side.
6. Repeat movement from right to left 10 to 20 times.

Accommodations and modifications: For students unable to perform this movement, have them remain seated on the ground with legs straight and in a V-shape position. Have students follow the same sequence slowly, for balance may be a factor for some. Repeat the movement for time and repetitions.

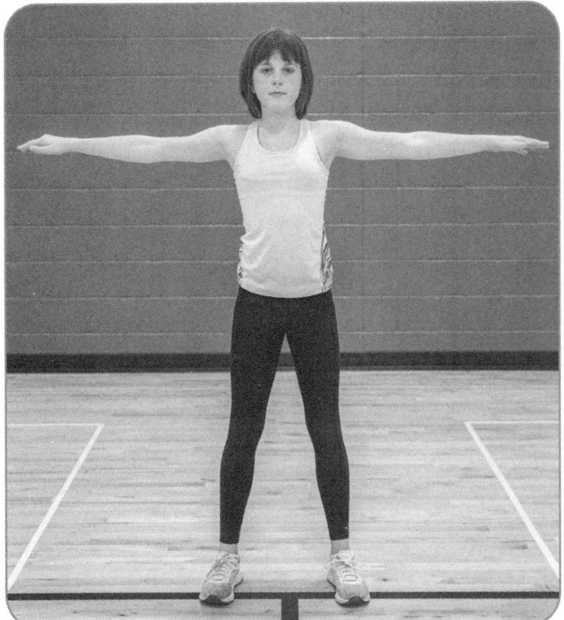

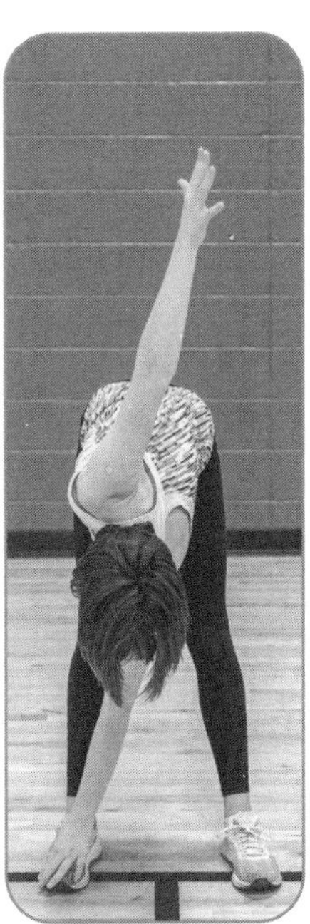

DOUBLE KNEES-TO-CHEST STRETCH

Static Stretch

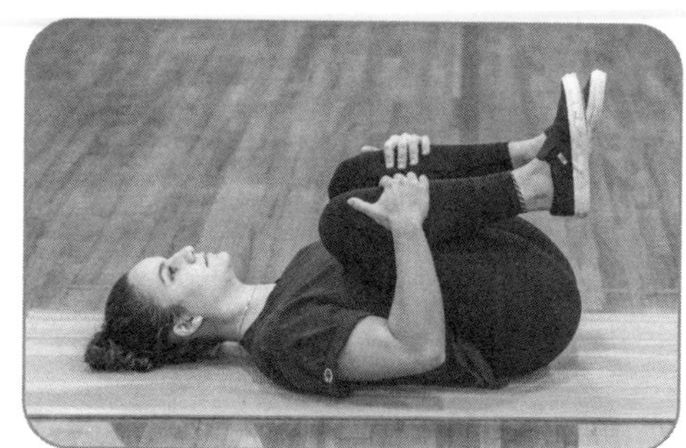

Body part: Core

Muscle group: Lower latissimus dorsi and erector spinae

1. Start by lying face up, legs straight, and both heels on the floor.
2. Bring both knees to chest.
3. Place hands below the knee area on top of the shin.
4. Hold position for 15 to 20 seconds.
5. Repeat position on the opposite side.
6. Stop, relax, and repeat 2 to 3 more times.

Accommodations and modifications: For students unable to perform this movement, have the students remain seated on the ground or in a chair with legs straight and in a V-shape position. Have students follow the same sequence slowly, as balance may be a factor for some. Repeat movement for time/repetitions.

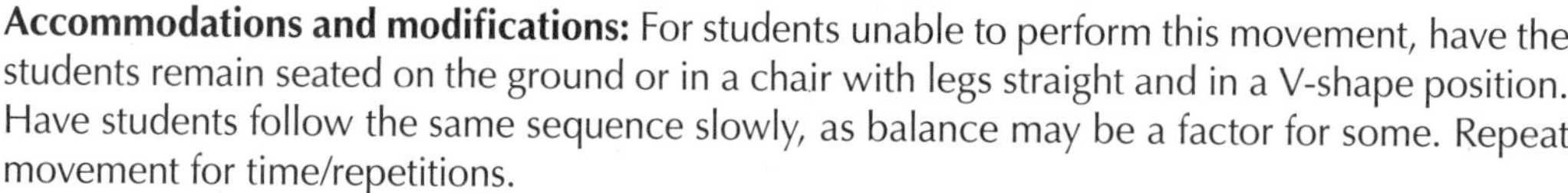

SINGLE KNEE-TO-CHEST STRETCH

Static Stretch

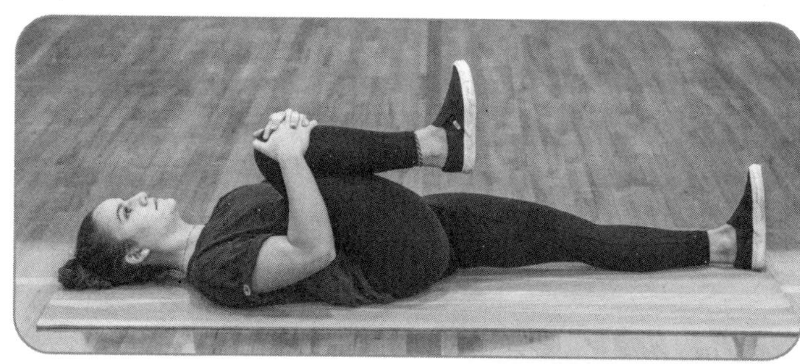

Body part: Core

Muscle group: Lower latissimus dorsi and erector spinae

1. Start by lying face up, legs straight, and both heels on the floor.
2. Bring one knee to chest, keeping the opposite leg in the original position.
3. Place hands below the knee area on top of the shin.
4. Slowly bring knee toward chest and hold for time.
5. Return to starting position and slowly do the same with opposite leg.
6. Hold position for 15 to 30 seconds.
7. Repeat position on the opposite side.
8. Relax and repeat 2 to 3 more times.

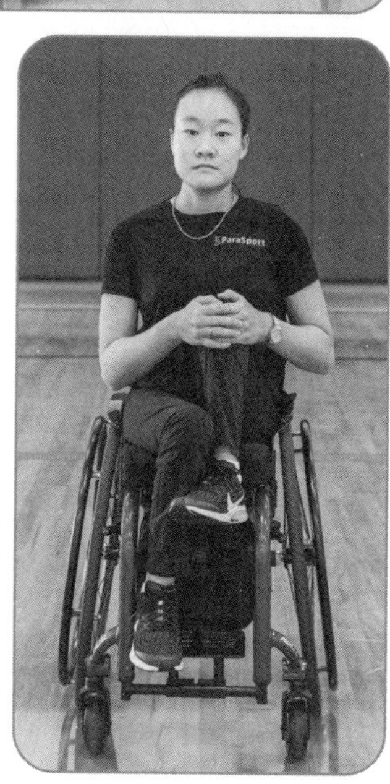

Accommodations and modifications: Single knee-to-chest stretches can be performed from the seated position (shown). This movement can also be performed as a seated crunch while in a chair:

1. Sit with the spine straight while crossing arms across chest.
2. Pull belly button in to engage core muscles.
3. Press lower back against the wheelchair.
4. Twist to the right.

5. Straighten the spine and come back to the starting position.
6. Twist to the left.
7. Straighten the spine and come back to the starting position.
8. Repeat on both sides 3 to 4 times.

PELVIC TILT

Dynamic Stretch

Body part: Core

Muscle group: Abdominals and erector spinae

1. Lie on back, with knees bent, feet flat on ground, and hands relaxed behind head.
2. Contract abdominal muscles and flatten back against ground.
3. Tighten glutes and slightly raise pelvis off ground toward the ceiling.
4. Hold position for 15 to 30 seconds.
5. Repeat movement 3 to 5 times.
6. Stop, relax, and repeat 2 to 3 more times.

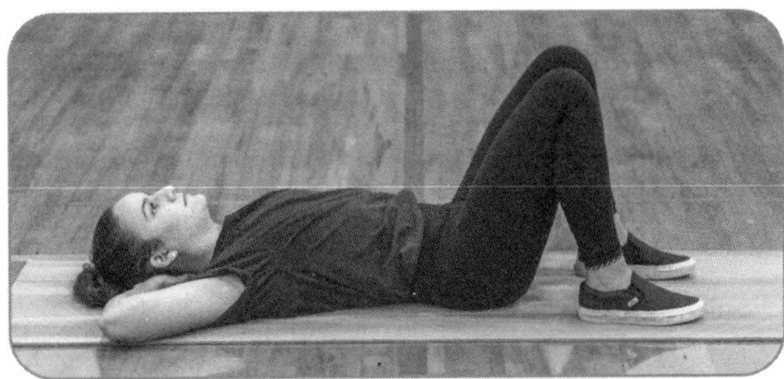

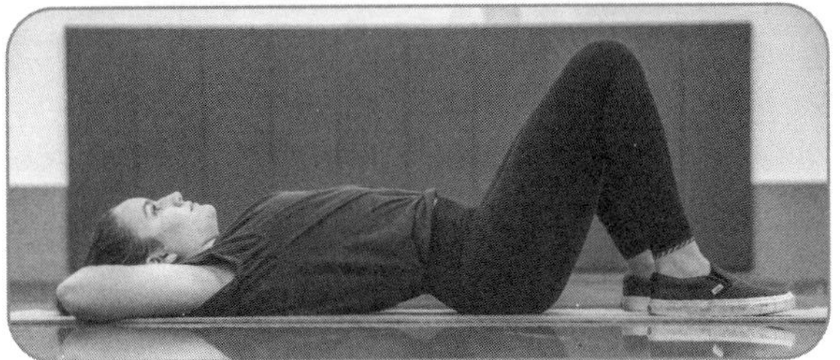

Accommodations and modifications: For students unable to perform this movement, have them focus on contracting the muscles of the gluteals and abdominals prior to the movement. Adjust time and repetitions for movement as needed.

COBRA STRETCH

Static Stretch

Body part: Trunk and hips

Muscle group: Rectus abdominis and obliques

1. Start by lying face down on the floor.
2. Keeping hips flat on the ground and using both arms, push upper body upward.
3. Hold position for 10 to 30 seconds, then return to starting position.
4. Stop, relax, and repeat 3 to 4 times.

Accommodations and modifications: For students unable to perform this movement, have them focus solely on increasing range of motion and the progression of the stretch and monitoring the alignment of each joint. Adjust time and repetitions for movement as needed. For modification of this movement, decreasing the range of motion may be more comfortable at first. For other progressions and modifications, incorporate the following movements.

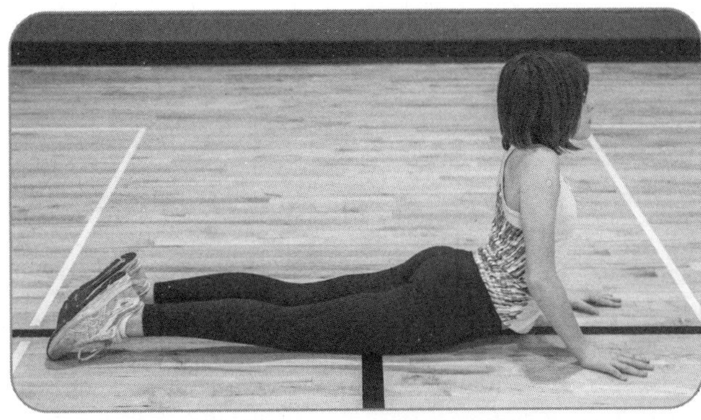

SPHINX STRETCH

Static Stretch

Body part: Core

Muscle group: Abdominals and erector spinae

1. Lie on stomach with forearms on the ground and elbows and shoulders aligned.
2. Extend hands in the front with palms facing down (pronated).
3. Keep legs straight, feet slightly apart, and toes pointing away from body.
4. Gently lift head and chest while pressing pelvis into the ground.
5. Keeping forearms on the ground, look straight ahead.
6. Hold position for 15 to 30 seconds.
7. Return to original position.
8. Stop, relax, and repeat 2 to 3 more times.

Accommodations and modifications: For students unable to perform this movement, have them focus on the progression of the stretch, monitoring the alignment of each joint. Adjust time and repetitions for movement as needed.

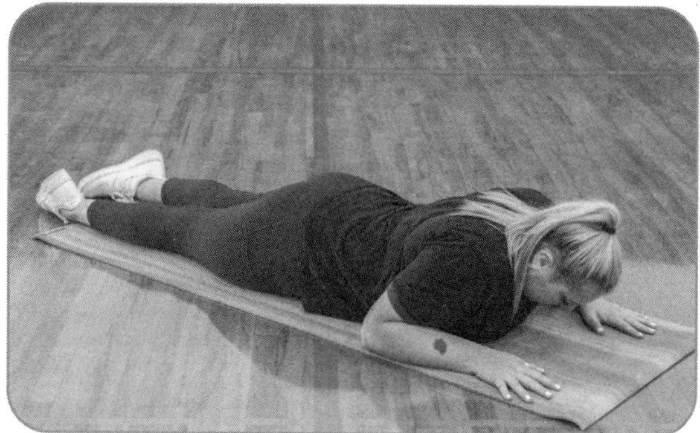

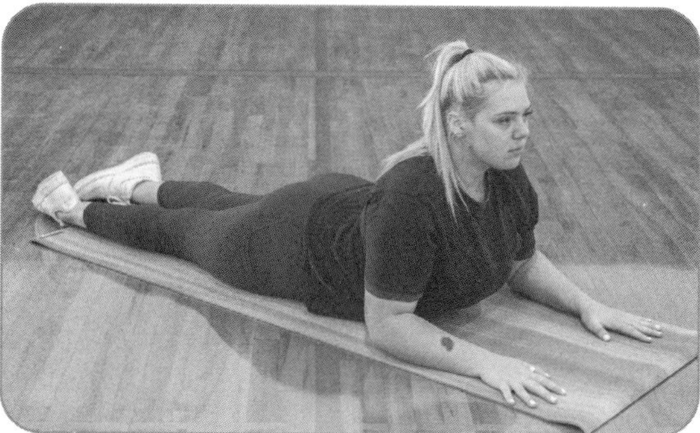

CHILD'S POSE

Static Stretch

Body part: Trunk and hips

Muscle group: Abdominals and erector spinae

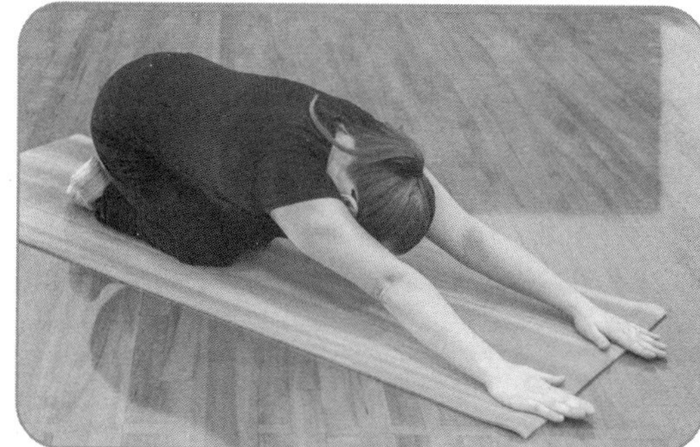

1. Place hands and knees on the ground.
2. Keep knees and hips aligned and top of feet on the ground.
3. Push gluteal back as torso will come to rest on thighs.
4. Keep arms straight in front, over the head with palms pronated.
5. Hold position for 10 to 30 seconds, then return to starting position.
6. Repeat 3 to 4 times.

Accommodations and modifications: The child's pose can be performed from the seated position. Sitting comfortably in a chair, students should lean forward, stretching their arms out in front of them with their head facing down. This should be a relaxing stretch.

Progression: To progress the exercise, use the threading-the-needle stretch.

PROGRESSION: THREADING-THE-NEEDLE STRETCH

Static Stretch

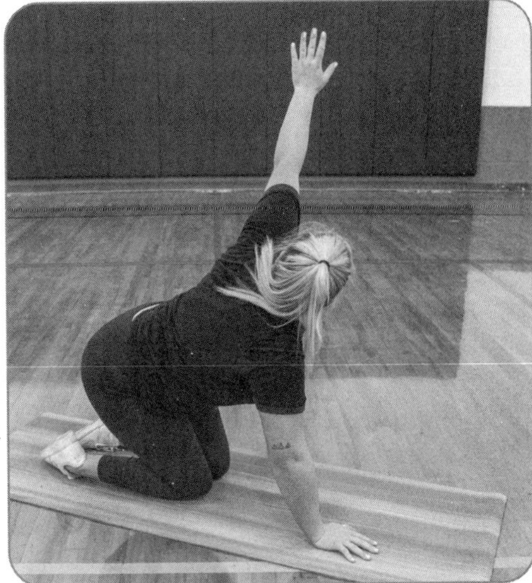

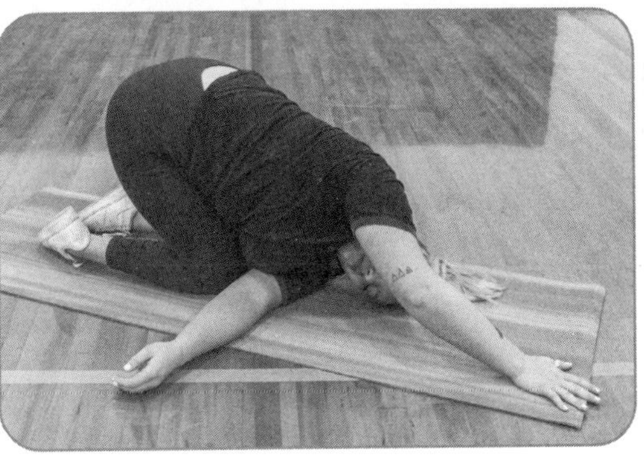

Body part: Trunk and hips

Muscle group: Abdominals and erector spinae

1. Place hands and knees on the ground.
2. Align shoulders, elbows, wrists, hips, and knees, with feet extended and toes pointed to the rear, away from body.
3. Raise and extend one arm upward.
4. Turn head in the same direction with eyes focused upward.
5. Slowly lower arm down across chest under the opposite armpit.
6. Keeping both knees and arm on the ground for support, continue sliding arm under the body, allowing the shoulder to rest on the ground.
7. Follow the arm and hand movement with head and eyes, lying with head on the ground.
8. Extend opposite arm over head with hand and fingertips touching the ground.
9. Hold position for 15 to 20 seconds.
10. Return to original position.
11. Repeat movement on the opposite side.
12. Alternating between right and left sides.
13. Repeat 2 to 3 more times.

Accommodations and modifications: For students unable to perform this movement, have them focus on the progression of the stretch, monitoring the alignment of each joint. Adjust time and repetitions for movement as needed.

ROUTINES: STRINGING THEM TOGETHER

The focus of developing routines is to provide for an emphasis on student progression, not perfection, since perfecting the stretch should be part of the instructional program. Although form, alignment, and consistency are important, it will take practice and time before students feel a comfortable level of accomplishment. It is not just about doing the stretches; it's more about the proper performance of each stretch. *Quality* versus *quantity* is the major consideration in this activity, and *quality* needs to prevail.

- Model and practice each specific stretch, making sure that proper form and alignment is being performed.
- Verbalize the body parts, joints, and muscles being stretched.
- Travel through the area, visiting each student and making corrections, if needed.
- Review and perform both dynamic and static stretches of each body part until students feel comfortable doing them.
- Through time and repetitiveness, students will show their level of readiness to proceed to the next level.

BEGINNER ROUTINE

Introduction

- Review of body parts
- Review of types of joints and muscles and limitations of movements

Warm-up: Brisk walk or slow jog for 5 to 10 minutes

Routine: The beginner's level is to get bodies familiar with the various stretching exercises and techniques. This is where the teacher, possibly with the assistance of a select student, will model the correct positioning and alignment of the body parts and joints, allowing students to replicate the movement.

Cool-down: Cardiorespiratory activity and hydration

INTERMEDIATE ROUTINE

Introduction

- Review of body parts
- Review of types of joints and limitations of movements

Warm-up: Brisk walk or slow jog for 5 to 10 minutes

Routine: The intermediate level is a bit more intense, and students will be able to execute more of a routine with a limited number of body parts and joints involved. Constant emphasis on the proper alignment of all joints within each stretch is still necessary.

- Choose 2 to 3 body parts to practice a short routine that will allow flowing movements from one stretch to another. Choosing partnering body parts, such as back and chest or biceps and triceps of the arms, will keep students focused on a specific area.
- Practice all dynamic stretches first, followed by static stretches. Be sure that both routines follow the same order of chosen stretches.
- Within this intermediate routine, consistently remind students of the importance of alignment and focus on their own degree of stretch.
- Remember that all students do not have an equal degree of stretching points due to age, gender, joint structure, activity level, muscular frame, or previous experience.

Cool-down: Cardiorespiratory activity and hydration

ADVANCED ROUTINE

Introduction

- Review of body parts
- Review of types of joints and limitations of movements

Warm-up: Brisk walk or slow jog for 5-10 minutes

Routine: This level allows students to engage in various stretches, having the comfort and ability to focus on balance and proper positioning needed for success. Students at this level will be able to perform a routine of stretches from head to toe, placing emphasis on preparing for the following daily activities assigned. Knowing their own limitations and points of discomfort, students will be able to successfully perform the following:

- Complete an entire stretching routine.
- Show knowledge of alignment and joint positioning.
- Execute each stretch freely and painlessly.
- Show improved flexibility.
- Create a personalized stretching routine and be able to lead class.

Cool-down: Cardiorespiratory activity and hydration

Upon completion of each stage, slowly introduce the following advanced techniques or increase the length of time of the hold of the stretch:

- *Passive stretching.* While in a stretch, having a partner or an accessory, such as a towel or resistance band, intensifies the stretch by placing pressure on that body part.
- *Ballistic stretching.* Using momentum or a bouncing movement forces joints beyond their normal ROM.
- *Proprioceptive neuromuscular facilitation (PNF).* This is another partnering technique to improve the elasticity and ROM.

Be aware that although many of these techniques are often performed by fitness specialists, they can be a great way to challenge students to perform research on various modes of stretching while staying within their level of readiness.

TEACHING TIPS

Does having a six-pack dictate good health? Not in this case. Remember, many factors, such as genetics, diet, and body fat percentage that may be low enough to reveal these muscles, come into play when it comes to our physique. While working toward improving all aspects of fitness, we cannot ignore genetic constructs such as our age, gender, and joint structure. However, we can work on the things we do have control over—our activity level, muscle mass, and flexibility.

Assisting students in gaining a knowledge and understanding of their own bodies is a key element in making individual changes. Students should be taught that comparing their body to others is not going to lead to success, and, in return, it will probably only lead to frustration and an end result of quitting. Students should be empowered to understand that reaching their full potential can only be achieved within themselves and with their willingness to work toward a specific goal, always aiming higher once that goal is attained. This is all possible if some key concepts are followed. Remind students of the following:

- Go at your own pace—this is not a race to the finish line. The importance of avoiding quick motions is essential to keep from straining involved muscles.
- Stretch as far as you can and do not be afraid to decrease the range of motion if you feel discomfort..
- Lastly, inhale and exhale through every movement in a controlled tempo. Never hold your breath while stretching or exercising.

Frequency and patience, as in every task, are two components in the recipe for success. The more practice and tolerance that is given to each stretching movement, the greater the probability is of leading to a better performance overall.

CONCLUSION

With the core muscles representing another major muscle group, to both enhance performance and prevent injuries, it is crucial to stretch these muscles on a regular basis, especially before or after specific physical activity or sport experiences. Having a thorough understanding of the anatomical makeup of the core, as well as an understanding of the benefits of stretching the core muscles, will provide the students the knowledge and skills necessary to maintain a healthier lifestyle.

Being cognizant of the role that the support and stability of the trunk plays in order to accomplish our daily routines is also magnified throughout many athletic activities. As an example, in the case of runners, having a strong core will result in better posture and mechanical efficiency, thus resulting in a faster speed. Possessing a flexible and strong torso will give runners the ability to move all of their limbs smoothly throughout each stride. Golfers, tennis players, and surfers also rely on core strength and stability; therefore, enhancing flexibility and maximizing the range of motion within the core region is most favorable.

Although stretching is often overlooked and may not be the most exciting part of a workout, it is an important element of every fitness routine. Including stretching into the schedule will help improve flexibility, reduce back pain, and help make workouts more efficient and safe. Optimal mobility will also relieve muscle stress and tension, allowing us to move freely throughout the day. Stretching is not difficult to perform; it just takes time.

Review Questions

1. Explain the importance of stretching the core muscles in balance and stability.
2. Identify the benefits of an increased range of motion.
3. Select one exercise and identify the muscles that are engaged in that exercise.
4. Describe the difference between a dynamic stretch and a static stretch.
5. Identify a specific sports activity and explain how increasing the flexibility of your core muscles will impact that sport.

Visit HK*Propel* for additional material related to this chapter.

CHAPTER 11

Lower-Body Stretching Exercises

Chapter Objective

After reading this chapter, you will understand how proper stretching technique enhances flexibility and improves range of motion (ROM) in the lower body. Better ROM can improve performance during activities, increase blood flow to the muscles, reduce the risk of injuries, and assist in the cool-down after exercise. You will also know how to develop lessons that teach these concepts to secondary school students; be able to effectively demonstrate a series of exercises and exercise routines designed to stretch the upper-body muscles, tendons, ligaments, and joints; and employ best teaching practices that enhance student learning.

Key Concepts

- Stretching the lower-body muscles is essential to enhanced physical activity performance as well as everyday activities for increasing the range of motion.
- The exercises presented will help you teach students to identify the muscles, tendons, ligaments, and joints involved in stretching exercises that increase flexibility.
- Warm-up and cool-down stretches should be performed before and after lower-body exercises.
- Accommodations and modifications are recommended so that all activities can be modified and performed by all students in the class.

INTRODUCTION

Stretching is an important part of any workout, and flexibility is one of the health-related components of fitness. Improved flexibility enables the body to move effectively and painlessly through full range of motion. This flexibility is particularly important for the lower body simply because it carries the majority of the body's weight and maintains balance and stability while participating in a variety of physical activities. Therefore, to avoid the possible risks of joint pain, strains, and muscle damage, it's important to understand how daily stretches will enhance a healthy workout routine.

As we enter the last third of the body's stretching routine, having started with the upper body and moving through the core to the lower body, the teacher must maintain the knowledge and continuously share the concepts from those prior chapters. The movements of these joints will include flexion, extension, abduction, adduction, and rotation. All of these body parts and joints are surrounded by large, strong muscles of the *quadriceps, hamstrings,* and *gluteals,* along with the smaller muscles of the lower leg, the *gastrocnemius* and *soleus,* all of which play a major role in performing daily activities.

When teaching students stretching activities in reference to the lower body, they should comprehend that reference is made to the hips, thighs, lower legs, and feet. The range of motion of each body part will depend on the degree of freedom of movement within the specific joint. The ball-and-socket joint of the hip allows flexion, extension, abduction, adduction, and rotation of the thigh. The hinge joint of the knee allows flexion and extension of the lower leg. And finally, the ellipsoidal joint of the ankle allows dorsiflexion, plantarflexion, inversion, eversion, and medial and lateral rotation of the foot. Figure 11.1 illustrates how the bones move during various movements of lower-body joints. As stated in the previous chapters, each specific joint type has its limitations of movement; therefore, the need to prepare each muscle-tendon is crucial to prevent discomfort.

As we move through the lower body and examine the functional anatomy, it is noteworthy to observe how efficiently the joints and muscles work together: from the hips to the knees, then down to the ankles and feet. Starting with the hip, a ball-and-socket joint formed by the connection of two bones—the *pelvic acetabulum* and the head of the *femur,* the longest bone in the body—this strong, weight-bearing joint is joined by the *iliofemoral, pubofemoral,* and *ischiofemoral ligaments*. The main muscle of hip flexion, in fact, the only muscle that attaches the upper and lower body is the *psoas major.*

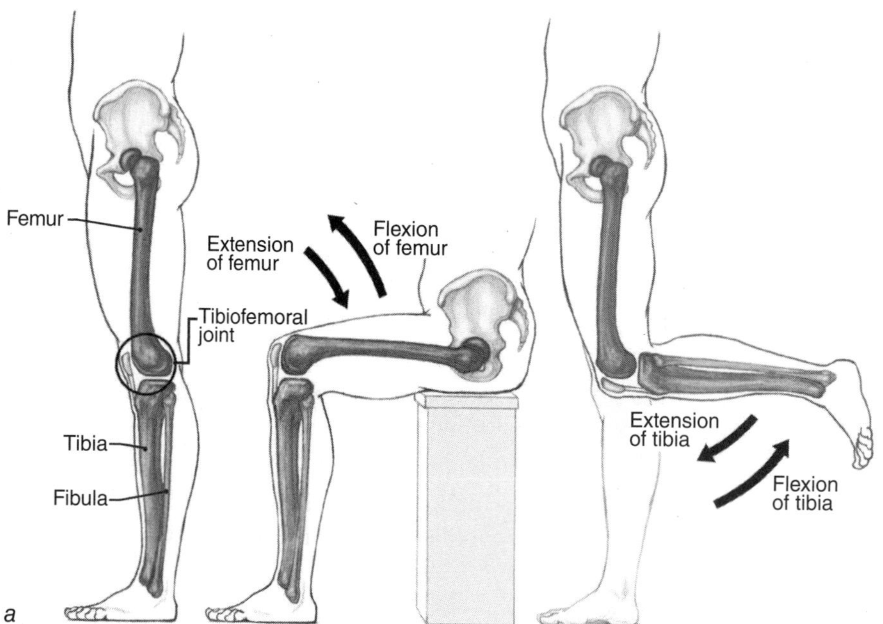

Figure 11.1 Movement of the bones during flexion and extension of the knee and hip (*a* and *b*), during adduction and abduction of the hip (*c*), and during plantarflexion and dorsiflexion of the ankle (*d*).

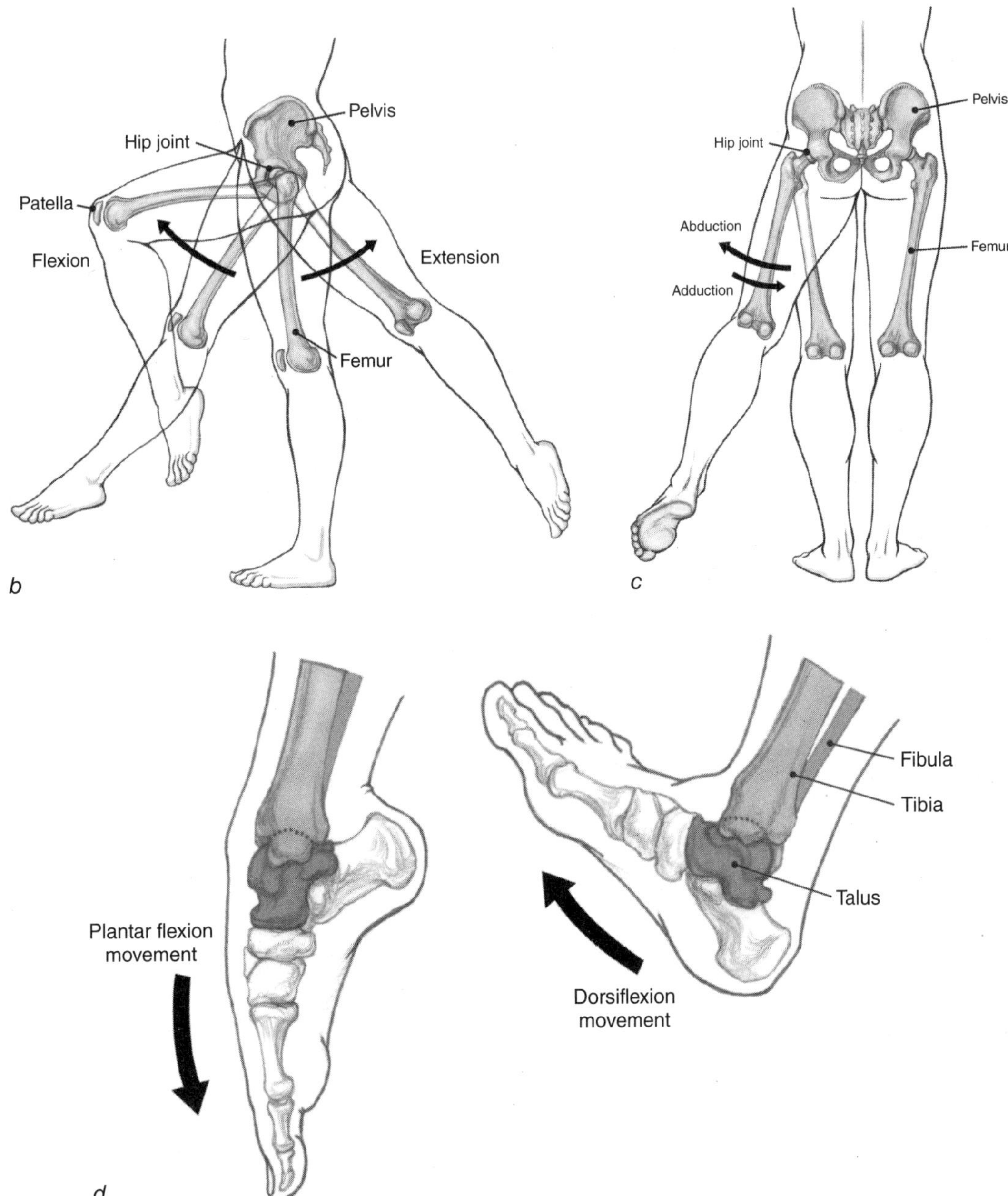

Figure 11.1 *(continued)*

Working along with other major muscles of the hip are the largest muscles in the body, the *gluteal muscles,* which comprise the *gluteus maximus, gluteus medius,* and *gluteus minimus.*

Next, we consider the thigh muscles, which are engaged in the movement of the hip as well as the knee. The quadriceps comprises a group of four muscles, the *rectus femoris, vastus lateralis, vastus medialis,* and *vastus intermedius.* Moving downward is the connection to the knee joint, the union of the *femur, tibia, fibula,* and the *patella,* the kneecap. This hinge joint allows for flexion and extension through the connection of the *patellar ligament, collateral ligaments,* and *cruciate ligaments.* The two *menisci,* the cartilages, complete the complexity of the knee joint. Although not a ligament, they play a crucial role as a shock absorber within the joint, a cushion between the femur and tibia. The knee is a very vulnerable joint and common to injuries.

Whether an athlete, or an active or inactive person, the most common injuries that may be unavoidable, if not careful, are the *collateral ligament injury,* caused by damage to the ligaments on each side of the knee; *anterior cruciate ligament*

(ACL) injury, caused by hyperextension of the knee; *bursitis*, inflammation of the bursae, caused by kneeling on hard surfaces; or *patella tendonitis*, "jumper's knee," caused by inflammation of the tendon connecting the kneecap (patella) and the shin bone (tibia), due to stress, tight leg muscles, running, or jumping.

Last, but not least, is the ankle joint, which is formed by the *tibia*, the shinbone; *fibula*, the lateral bone of the leg; *talus*, the ankle bone; *calcaneus*, the heel bone; and the *tarsal bones* of the foot. The *gastrocnemius muscle* and *soleus muscle* of the calves mainly accommodate the movements of the foot. As a hinge joint, the main movements of the ankle are *plantar flexion*, bending the ankle, pointing toes away from the body, and *dorsiflexion*, bending the ankle, pointing toes toward the shin. The *subtalar joint* allows for *inversion*, turning the foot inward, and *eversion*, turning the foot outward.

As many of us have experienced the common ankle *sprain*, a stretch or tear of a ligament, damage from eversion and inversion sprains occurs in two sets of ligaments: the *medial* or *deltoid ligaments*, and the *lateral ligaments*, the *anterior talofibular*, *posterior talofibular*, and *calcaneofibular*. The stability of the *subtalar joint* of the ankle is dependent on the *posterior talocalcaneal*, *medial talocalcaneal*, and *lateral talocalcaneal ligaments*. Although sprains can occur in various parts of the body, the most common site of sprains is in the ankle, by simply causing the joint to move out of its normal range of motion. Since many sports, such as basketball, soccer, and tennis, involve speed; sudden changes of direction; and powerful, explosive movements, maintaining flexibility and strength in the lower body is crucial to injury prevention. For example, soccer players are prone to groin strains, which can occur while blocking or defending a pass or shot, while taking a very hard shot, or during a rapid reactive change of direction (see figure 11.2). Therefore, it is necessary to implement fitness plans into a well-rounded fitness education program that incorporate strength and flexibility to avoid such injuries.

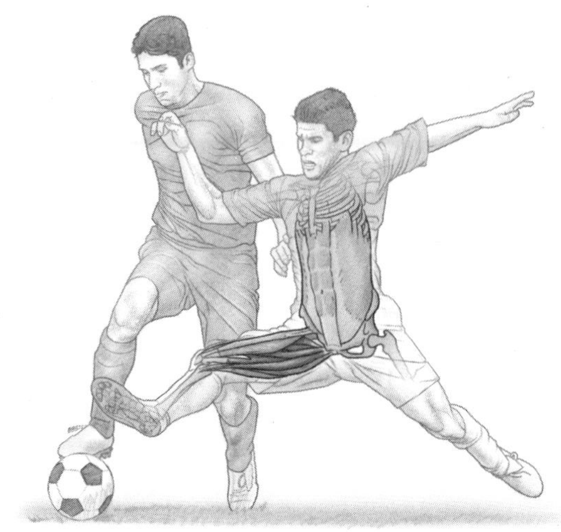

Figure 11.2 Soccer players can protect themselves against groin strains and other lower-body injuries by increasing ROM in the lower-body joints.

As briefly stated, several of the largest and most powerful muscles in the body are housed in the lower body. Almost every move we make, from getting out of bed, sitting in a chair, climbing stairs, or going for a walk, is the responsibility of all these bones, muscles, and joints combined. Acknowledging the undertaking that the lower extremities endure, it is the obligation of each person to maintain the mobility and flexibility of this area. It is also important to note that, although this chapter focuses on the importance of stretching as an entity in itself, many of the exercises described here will also be used as warm-up and cool-down exercises in subsequent chapters.

As the physical education teacher, you can use the exercises in this chapter as part of a warm-up or cool-down, lesson on lower-body stretching exercises, or routine. Each exercise has a description and illustration, with notes about the type of stretch, the body part and muscle groups worked, steps for safely executing the stretch with good form, and accommodations and modifications for those unable to perform the stretch as described. Many stretches are illustrated with video in HK*Propel*. Teach each exercise separately, ensuring that students are performing the stretch correctly, emphasizing the type of stretch (static or dynamic) and the muscle group being engaged. This is extremely important because what students learn during this initial instruction will enable them to use the appropriate stretch for subsequent physical activities, as well as enable them to safely engage in routines and circuits throughout the class. We include guidelines for developing routines for the beginner, intermediate, and advanced levels after the exercises, along with further teaching tips.

As you develop your daily lesson plans, align each lesson with the National Standards and your own state and local standards so that every student taught in your class can participate in the activities. The following sample lesson overview shows the National Standards and Grade-Level Outcomes (GLOs) relevant to this material, lesson objectives, and accommodations and modifications to be kept in mind when teaching a lesson on lower-body stretching exercises. All of the exercises in this book are designed to provide accommodations and modifications as needed. This ensures equity, opportunity, and access for all students. Additionally, as you progress through your fitness education course, your students should be able to identify which stretching activities will be required for the daily activity you present.

LESSON OVERVIEW

Lower-Body Stretching Routine

Lesson length: 5 to 20 minutes

Grade level: 9th to 12th

National Standards and GLOs: S1.H3, S2.H2, S3.H9, S3.H11, S4.H5

Grade level: 6th to 8th

National Standards and GLOs: S3.M9, S3.M11, S3.M12, S3.M14, S3.M15, S3.M16, S4.M7, S5.M1

Lesson objectives: By the end of the lesson, students will be able to do the following:

- Perform a warm-up cardiorespiratory activity prior to your stretching routine.
- Perform lower-body muscle stretching routine, showing proper technique throughout each movement.
- Perform a cool-down including cardiorespiratory activity and hydration.
- Perform a cool-down routine using static stretching showing ROM in muscle-joint areas.

Accommodations and modifications: It is important for all movements and exercises to be modified to meet the individual needs of every student in order for them to engage in full participation. Implementing universal design for learning (UDL) will assist teachers in ensuring that all students can reach their full potential. Follow the general instructional recommendations, as discussed in chapter 3, for all activities.

WARM-UP DYNAMIC AND STATIC STRETCHES FOR THE LOWER BODY

LEG SWINGS

Dynamic Stretch

Body part: Hips

Muscle group: Hip flexors

1. Stand upright on one foot with hands on hips or arms out to sides for balance.
2. Gently swing opposite leg forward and backward.
3. Alternate between right and left sides.
4. Continue movement in both directions 10 to 30 seconds, or
5. Repeat the movement with each leg 10 to 20 times.
6. Stop, relax, and repeat 2 to 3 more times.

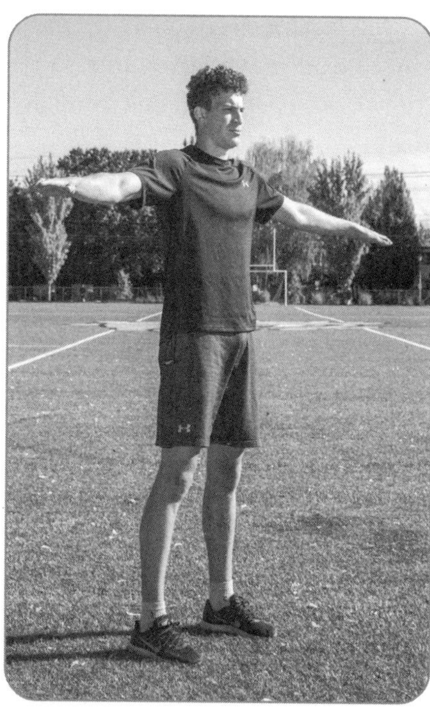

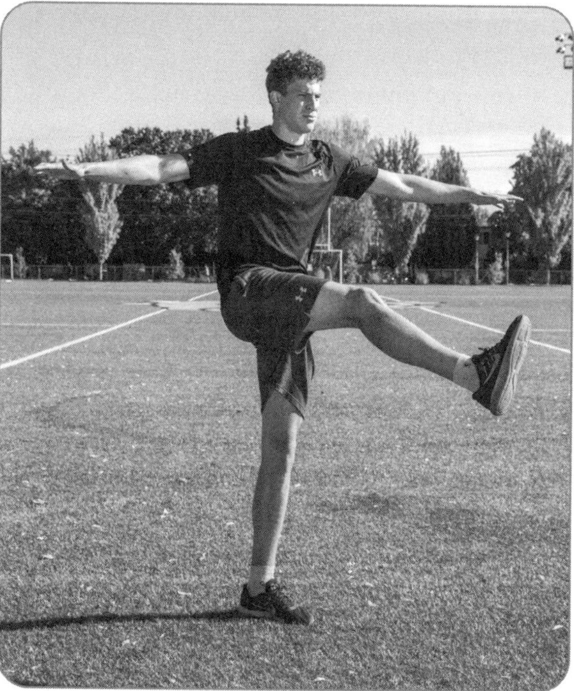

Accommodations and modifications: For students unable to perform this movement, have them begin with small pendulum swings and gradually increase when comfortable. Repeat movement for time or repetitions. For students with balance problems, have them put the opposite arm on a wall as they swing the opposite leg.

STANDING QUADRICEPS STRETCH

Static Stretch

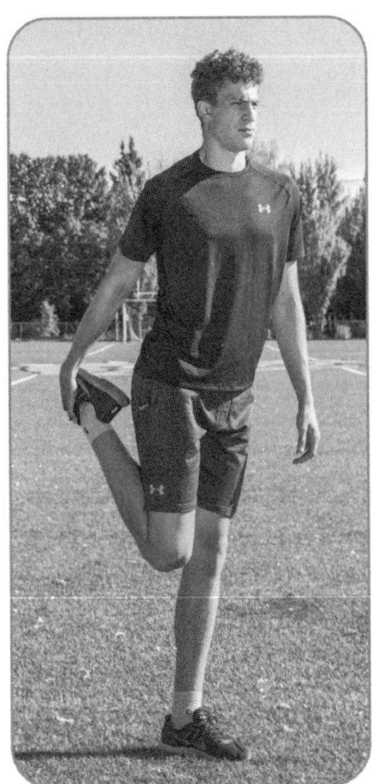

Body part: Lower body

Muscle group: Quadriceps, adductors, gluteals

1. Standing upright with feet shoulder-width apart and feet pointed forward, bend one knee and use same hand to grasp foot toward buttocks.
2. Keep knees together.
3. Maintain upright position with shoulders back, eyes forward.
4. Hold position for 10 to 30 seconds.
5. Return to starting position.
6. Repeat with opposite leg.
7. Stop, relax, and repeat 2 to 3 more times.

Accommodations and modifications: For students unable to perform this movement, have them hold onto a stationary object (chair, wall, bleachers) with opposite hand to maintain balance. Stretch may also be performed while lying on one side on the ground.

ABDUCTION AND ADDUCTION LEG SWINGS

Dynamic Stretch

Body part: Hips

Muscle group: Hip flexors

1. Stand upright on one foot, with hands on hips or arms out to sides for balance.
2. Gently swing one leg side to side in front of body, alternating between right and left sides.
3. Repeat the movement with each leg 10 to 20 times.
4. Stop, relax, and repeat 2 to 3 more times.

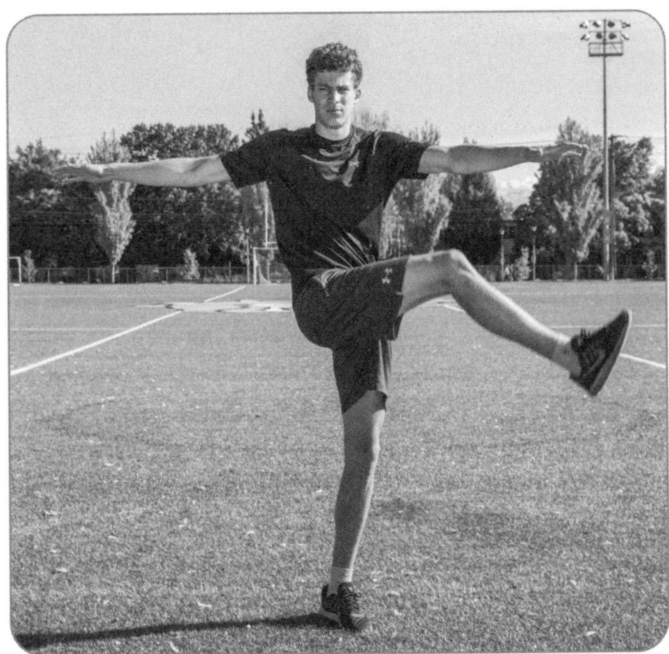

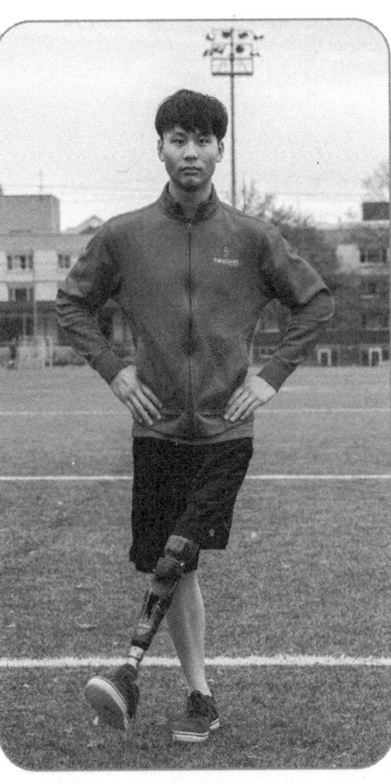

Accommodations and modifications: For students unable to perform this movement, have them begin with small pendulum swings and gradually increase when comfortable. Students could also hold onto a stationary object (chair, wall, bleachers) with opposite hand to maintain balance. Repeat movement for time/repetitions.

STANDING IT-BAND STRETCH

Static Stretch

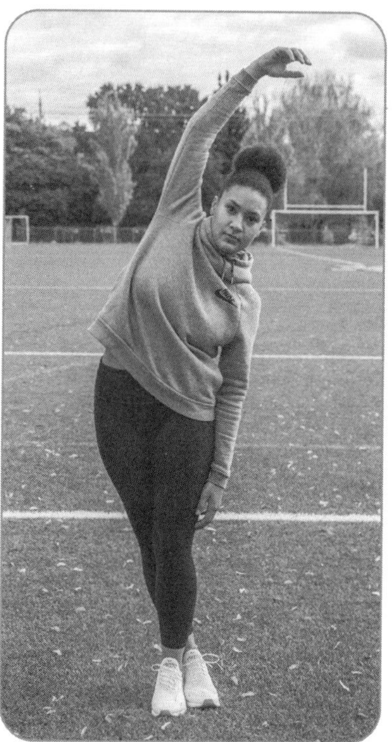

Body part: Hips and knees

Muscle group: Iliotibial band

1. Standing upright with one leg crossed behind the opposite leg, lean to one side until stretch is felt.
2. Raise arm that is on the same side of the crossed leg over the head and reach to opposite side.
3. Hold position for 10 to 30 seconds.
4. Return to starting position.
5. Repeat with opposite leg.
6. Stop, relax, and repeat 2 to 3 more times.

Accommodations and modifications: For students unable to perform this movement, have them minimize the degree of the stretch and avoid twisting at the hip.

HIGH KICKS

Dynamic Stretch

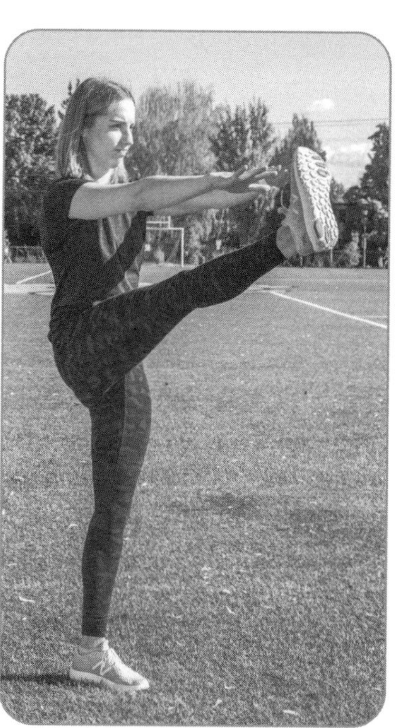

Body part: Thighs

Muscle group: Hamstrings

1. Stand upright on one foot.
2. Extend one arm up in front of body, parallel to the ground.
3. Kick leg up to palm of hand of extended arm.
4. Alternate leg kicks and extended arm.
5. Keep trunk upright and opposite foot stationary on the ground.
6. Repeat the movement from right to left 10 to 20 times.
7. Stop, relax, and repeat 2 to 3 more times.

Accommodations and modifications: For students unable to perform this movement, have them kick as high as they feel comfortable. Have students hold onto a stationary object (chair, wall, bleachers) with their opposite hand to maintain balance.

CROSSOVER HAMSTRING STRETCH

Static Stretch

Body part: Thighs

Muscle group: Hamstrings and gluteals

1. Standing upright with one leg crossed over the other, bend forward at the hips (hip flexion).
2. Attempt to touch the ground with hands, keeping back knee straight.
3. Place hands on knees.
4. Hold position for time.
5. Return to starting position.
6. Repeat with opposite leg.
7. Stop, relax, and repeat 2 to 3 more times.

Accommodations and modifications: For students unable to perform this movement, have them refrain from touching ground or straightening the back leg. This stretch may be performed while sitting on the ground or in a chair, with legs extended outward in front of their body.

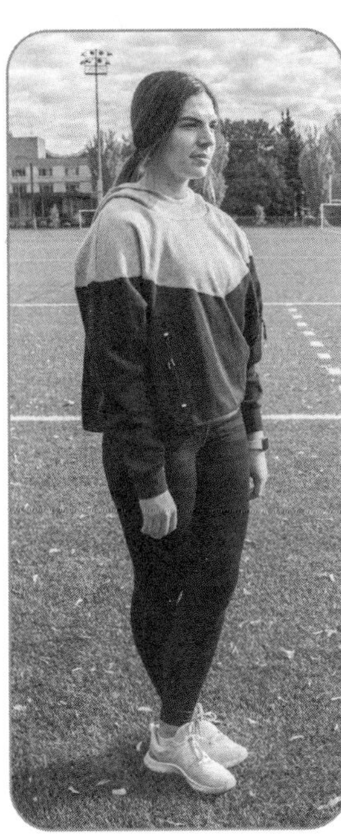

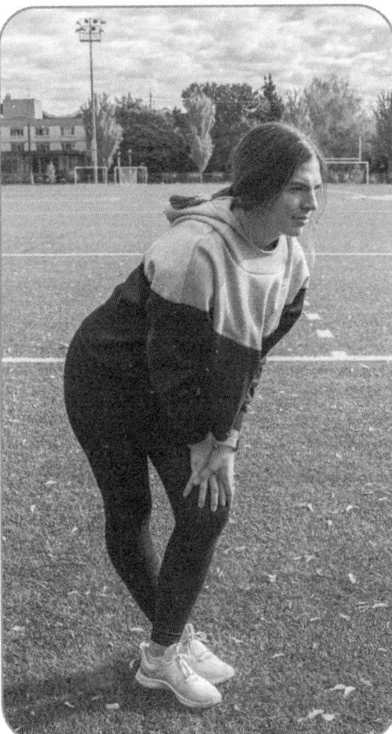

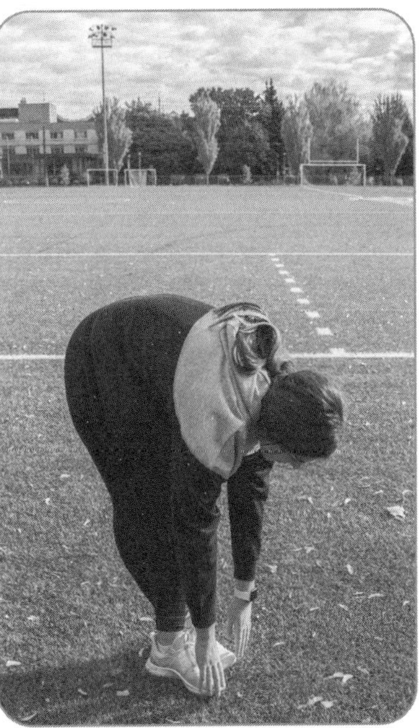

BENT-KNEE SIDE-LUNGE STRETCH

Dynamic Stretch

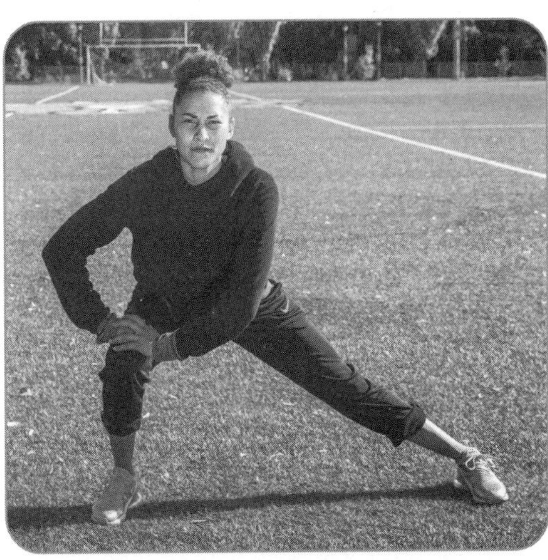

Body part: Thighs

Muscle group: Quadriceps, hamstrings, adductors

1. Stand upright with feet slightly wider than shoulder-width apart.
2. While bending at one knee in a squat position, extend opposite leg straight out to the side.
3. Place both hands on the top of the thigh of the bent knee.
4. Hold position for 10 to 30 seconds.
5. Raise back up to starting position.

6. Repeat the movement slowly, alternating from right to left 10 to 20 times.
7. Stop, relax, and repeat 2 to 3 more times.

Accommodations and modifications: For students unable to perform this movement, have them try going one quarter of the way down, and shortening the stride, while maintaining balance during the stretch. Students can also modify the exercise by placing their hands on the ground for balance until they feel comfortable placing their hands on their thighs.

SUMO SQUAT STRETCH

Static Stretch

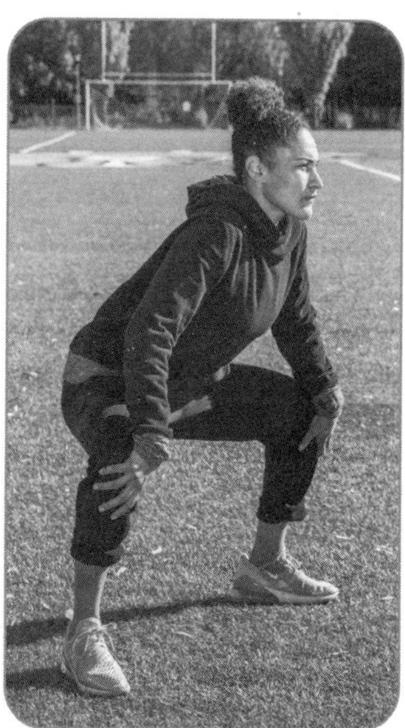

Body part: Lower body

Muscle group: Quadriceps, adductors, gluteals

1. Stand upright with feet more than shoulder-width apart and feet pointed outward.
2. While keeping trunk straight, lower torso until thighs are horizontal to the ground.
3. Place one hand on each knee.
4. Hold position for 10 to 30 seconds.
5. Return to starting position.
6. Stop, relax, and repeat 2 to 3 more times.

Accommodations and modifications: For students unable to perform this movement, have them hold onto a stationary object (chair, wall, bleachers) with their opposite hand to maintain balance.

INTERNAL AND EXTERNAL HIP-ROTATOR STRETCHES

Dynamic Stretch

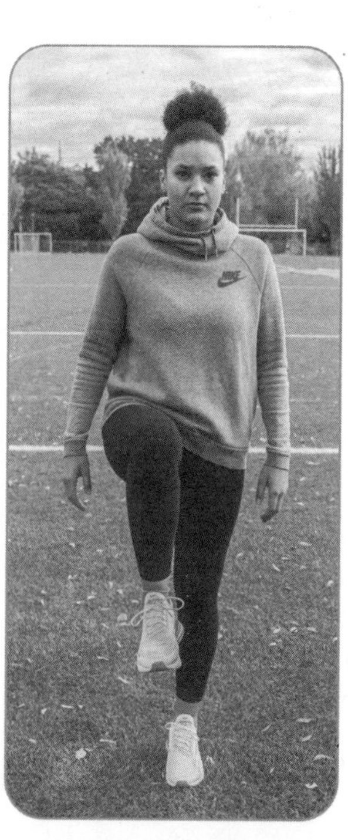

Body part: Hips and thighs

Muscle group: Gluteals and hip rotators

1. Stand upright on one leg with knee straight.
2. Flex at opposite hip, bringing bent knee in line with the same hip.
3. Swing and rotate (bent leg) at hip in a circular motion.
4. Rotate circular movements in both directions.
5. Repeat the movement slowly, 10 to 20 times.
6. Keep trunk upright; circular motion takes place at hip joint.
7. Repeat stretch with opposite leg.
8. Stop, relax, and repeat 2 to 3 more times.

Accommodations and modifications: For students unable to perform this movement, have them hold onto a stationary object (chair, wall, bleachers) with their opposite hand to maintain balance.

HIP ROTATOR AND EXTENSOR STRETCH

Static Stretch

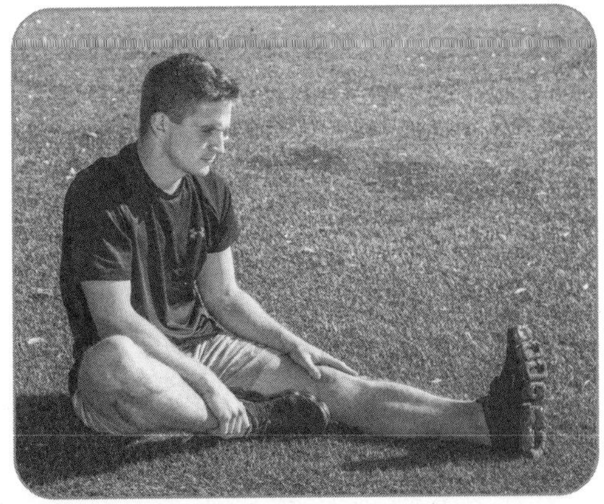

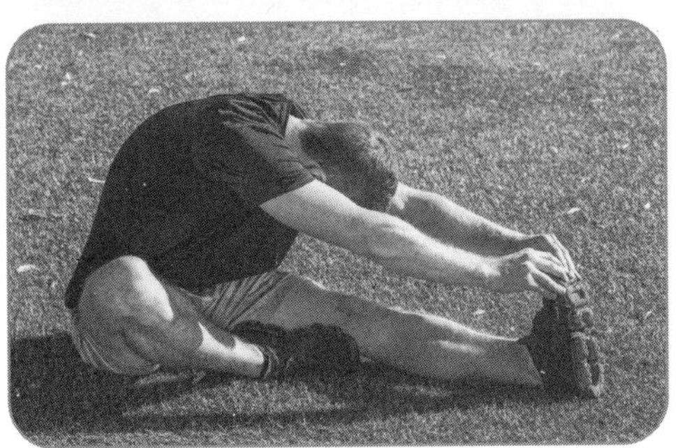

Body part: Lower body

Muscle group: Gluteals, quadriceps, gastrocnemius

1. Sit with one leg extended straight out in front.
2. Bend opposite leg, placing the bottom of the foot against the inner thigh of the straight leg.
3. Reach up with both arms, bend over toward the foot of the straight leg.
4. Reach as far as comfortable and hold position for 10 to 30 seconds.
5. Return to starting position.
6. Repeat on other side.
7. While holding position, dorsiflex foot (pull toes toward knee) to engage a stretch in the gastrocnemius muscle (calf).
8. Stop, relax, and repeat 2 to 3 more times.

Accommodations and modifications: For students unable to perform this movement, have them slightly bend their extended leg until they feel comfortable to straighten it.

KNEELING-KNEE HIP-THRUST STRETCH

Dynamic Stretch

Body part: Hips and thighs

Muscle group: Quadriceps

1. Kneel on both knees on the ground, keeping toes tucked, upper body in upright position, and shoulders back.
2. Slowly drop buttocks down toward calves and pop back up.
3. Return to upright position and push hips forward.
4. Continue a controlled rocking motion.
5. Repeat the movement slowly.
6. Stop, relax, and repeat 2 to 3 more times.

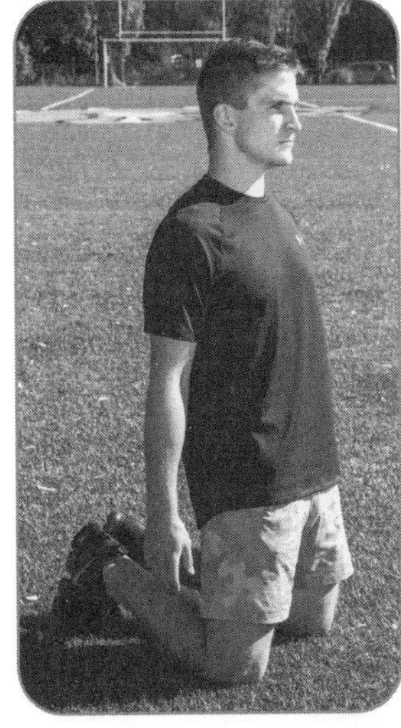

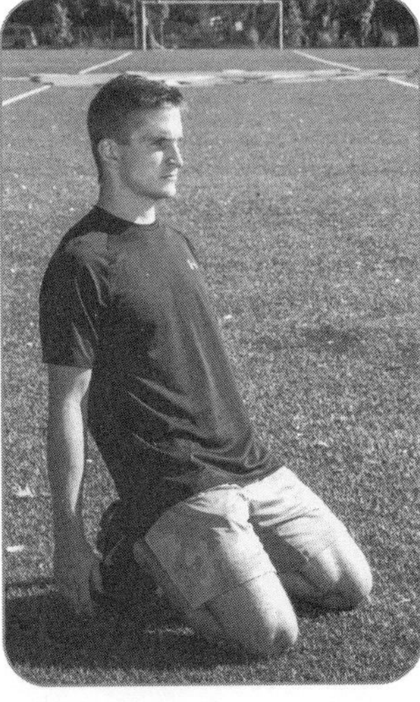

Accommodations and modifications: For students unable to perform this movement, have them eliminate the full rocking motion, buttocks to calves, and direct them to remain in an upright position while pushing hips forward.

LUNGING PSOAS STRETCH

Static Stretch

Body part: Thighs

Muscle group: Quadriceps and psoas major

1. Kneel on one knee on the ground.
2. Place opposite foot flat in front of body (bent knee at 90-degree angle).
3. Place both hands on bent knee for balance.
4. Maintain upper body in an upright position (straightening back leg).
5. Slowly move hips forward toward bent leg to push knee over ankle into dorsiflexion.
6. Reach as far as comfortable and hold position for 10 to 30 seconds.
7. Return to starting position.
8. Repeat on opposite side.
9. Stop, relax, and repeat 2 to 3 more times.

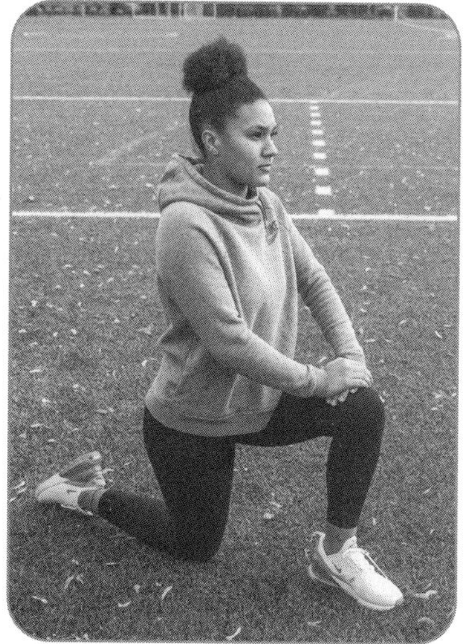

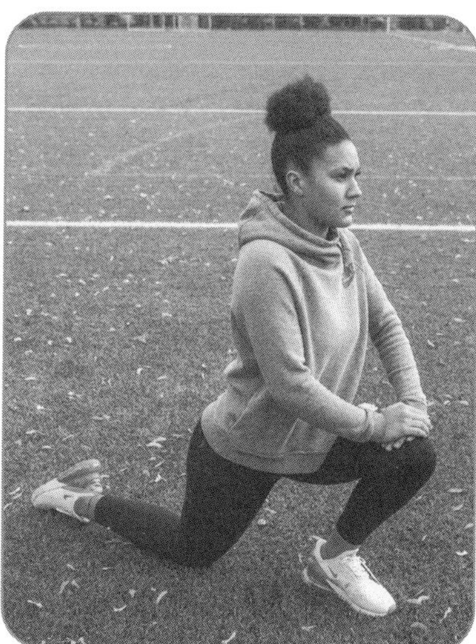

Accommodations and modifications: For students unable to perform this movement, have them minimize the degree of the stretch until comfortable. Direct students to remain in an upright position while moving their hips forward.

ANKLE CIRCLE STRETCH

Dynamic Stretch

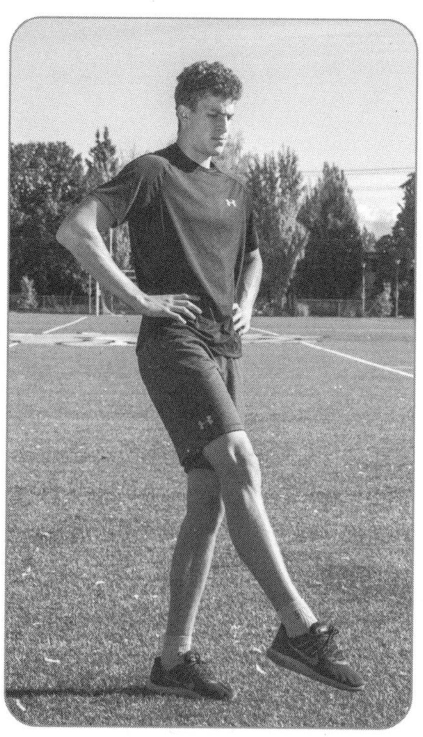

Body part: Lower Leg

Muscle group: Quadriceps, calves (gastrocnemius), tibialis anterior

1. Slowly begin rotating ankle in a circular motion.
2. Circle to each direction and then reverse movement.
3. Repeat the movement slowly, alternating from right to left 10 to 20 times.
4. Stop, relax, and repeat 2 to 3 more times.

Accommodations and modifications: For students unable to perform this movement, have them perform the movement on the ground or in a chair.

STANDING TOE EXTENSOR STRETCH

Static Stretch

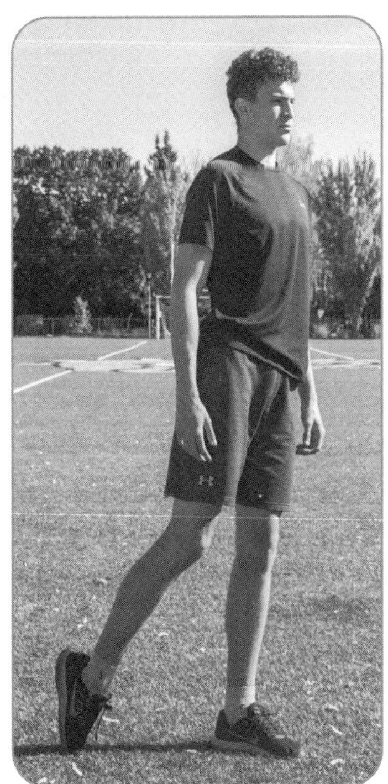

Body part: Lower legs

Muscle group: Tibialis anterior

1. Stand upright with feet shoulder-width apart.
2. Point one foot backward (plantar flexion) away from the body.
3. While the top of the foot is touching the ground, gently lean body weight onto that foot, feeling pressure.
4. Hold stretched position for 10 to 30 seconds.
5. Maintain upper body in an upright position.
6. Return to starting position.
7. Repeat on opposite side.
8. Stop, relax, and repeat 2 to 3 more times.

Accommodations and modifications: For students unable to perform this movement, have them perform the movement on the ground or in a chair. Placing the top side of their foot on towel or soft ground may be more comfortable.

HIP ADDUCTOR STRETCH

Static Stretch

Body part: Lower body

Muscle group: Adductors and gluteals

1. Sit on the floor with knees bent, bringing the bottoms of both feet together.
2. Slide the heels of both feet in toward the body.
3. While grasping both feet, position each elbow outward and touching each leg below the knees.
4. Flex and bend at hips, leaning toward feet.
5. Gently press the thighs down with elbows.
6. Stop, relax, and repeat 2 to 3 more times.
7. Do not bounce (ballistic).

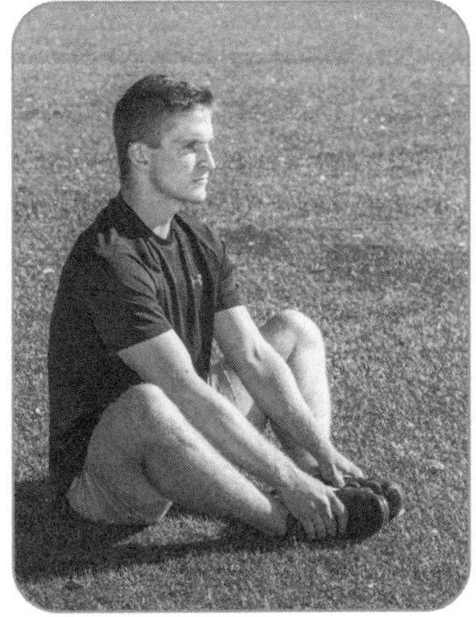

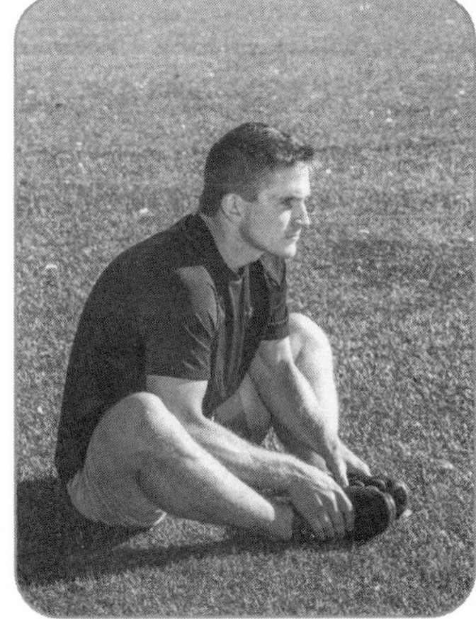

Accommodations and modifications: For students unable to perform this movement, have them refrain from bringing the heels of their feet so close toward their body until they are comfortable.

SEATED KNEE FLEXOR STRETCH

Static Stretch

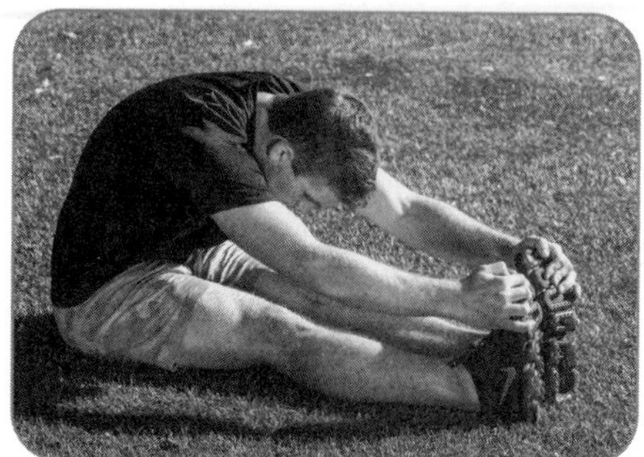

Body part: Lower body

Muscle group: Gluteals, hamstrings, gastrocnemius

1. While seated, extend both legs, bringing feet together.
2. Place hands on each side of thighs.
3. While keeping legs straight, slowly bend at the waist, lowering the head toward legs.
4. At the same time, slide hands toward feet and hold for 10 to 30 seconds.
5. Return to starting position and repeat 3 to 4 times.
6. While holding position, dorsiflex foot (pull toes toward knee) to engage a stretch in the gastrocnemius muscle (calf).
7. Relax and repeat 2 to 3 more times.

Accommodations and modifications: For students unable to perform this movement, have them refrain from dorsiflexing their foot, relieving the stretch in their calf.

ROUTINES: STRINGING THEM TOGETHER

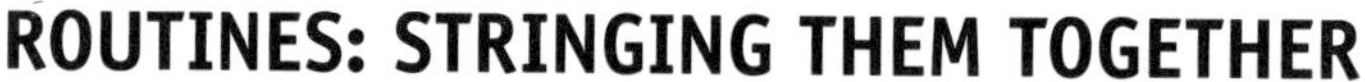

As we go through the routines of beginner, intermediate, and advanced levels, you will notice that they differ in relation to the muscular and endurance routines covered in the following chapters. Always aligning the body parts and joints is key to avoiding discomfort and preventing injury. These movements will improve with practice as your students will begin to realize that having better flexibility and mobility will enhance their everyday tasks and performance. Use the following recommendations to get started.

BEGINNER ROUTINE

Introduction

- Review of body parts
- Review of types of joints and limitations of movements

Warm-up: Brisk walk or slow jog for 5 to 10 minutes

Routine: The beginner's level is to get bodies familiar with the various stretching exercises and techniques. This is where the teacher, possibly with the assistance of a select student, will model the correct positioning and alignment of the body parts and joints, allowing students to replicate the movement.

- Model and practice each specific stretch making sure that proper form and alignment is being performed.
- Verbalize the body parts, joints, and muscles being stretched.
- Travel through the area, visiting each student and making corrections, if needed.
- Review and perform both dynamic and static stretches of each body part until students feel comfortable doing them.
- Through time and repetitiveness, students will show their level of readiness to proceed to the next level.

Cool-down: Cardiorespiratory activity and hydration

INTERMEDIATE ROUTINE

Introduction

- Review of body parts
- Review of types of joints and limitations of movements

Warm-up: Brisk walk or slow jog for 5 to 10 minutes

Routine: The intermediate level is a bit more intense, and students will be able to execute more of a routine with a limited number of body parts and joints involved. Constant emphasis on the proper alignment of all joints within each stretch is still necessary.

- Choose 2 to 3 body parts to practice a short routine that will allow flowing movements from one stretch to another. Choosing partnering body parts, such as back and chest or biceps and triceps of the arms, will keep students focused on a specific area.
- Practice a dynamic stretch first, followed by a static stretch. Be sure that both stretches are given the same intensity.
- Within this intermediate routine, consistently remind students of the importance of alignment and focus on their own degree of stretch.
- Remember that all students do not have an equal degree of stretching points due to age, gender, joint structure, activity level, muscular frame, or previous experience.

Cool-down: Cardiorespiratory activity and hydration

ADVANCED ROUTINE

Introduction

- Review of body parts
- Review of types of joints and limitations of movements

Warm-up: Brisk walk or slow jog for 5-10 minutes

Routine: This level allows students to engage in various stretches, having the comfort and ability to focus on balance and proper positioning needed for success. Students at this level will be able to perform a routine of stretches of the lower body, placing emphasis on preparing for the following daily activities assigned. Knowing their own limitations and points of discomfort, students will be able to be successfully perform the following:

- Complete an entire stretching routine.
- Show knowledge of alignment and joint positioning.
- Execute each stretch freely and painlessly.
- Show improved flexibility.
- Create a personalized stretching routine and be able to lead class.

Cool-down: Cardiorespiratory activity and hydration

Upon completion of each stage, slowly introduce the following advanced techniques or increase the length of time of the hold of the stretch:

- *Passive stretching.* While in a stretch, having a partner or an accessory, such as a towel or resistance band, intensifies the stretch by placing pressure on that body part.
- *Ballistic stretching.* Using momentum or a bouncing movement forces joints beyond their normal ROM.
- *Proprioceptive neuromuscular facilitation (PNF).* This is another partnering technique to improve the elasticity and ROM.

Be aware that although many of these techniques are often performed by fitness specialists, they can be a great way to challenge students to perform research on various modes of stretching while staying within their level of readiness.

TEACHING TIPS

As teachers, we may be in pursuit of excellence, but, at the same time, have the ability to adapt to different scenarios, understanding individual differences in students. From the environment in which we teach and the inclement weather we may endure, to the level of readiness of the students within our classrooms, guiding students to their fullest potential in the safest way possible is a commitment of physical education teachers that is everlasting.

As we come to the end of the stretching sequence, it is the job of the teacher to review, recall, and remind students of the benefits of stretching the lower body and how essential it is when preparing for or recovering from an activity. Stretching is a part of the equation of a well-rounded fitness program. Therefore, no matter what type of stretching the students execute, the benefits are monumental. Whether is it *static stretching,* the act of holding a stretch for a period of time; d*ynamic stretching,* a stretch that uses sport-specific movements; *ballistic stretching,* a stretch that involves bouncing movements rather than the holding of the stretch; or *proprioceptive neuromuscular facilitation (PNF) stretching,* a technique that stretches a contracted muscle through the joint's range of motion, everyone needs to be involved in a regular stretching routine in order to be effective in the other health-related components as well.

Let's not forget to practice what we preach. Knowing the benefits, both mentally and physically, of stretching regularly will help you, the teacher, and help you to be a positive role model for the students. Sharing your experience and movements with the class will allow students to feel more comfortable, knowing and seeing that you are not asking them to do anything that you will not do yourself, but also acknowledging your state of fitness and ability as well.

As flexibility brings positive benefits to our muscles and joints, it may also bring soreness to our bodies. Upon the onset of students' complaints of aches and pains, quickly turn that negative into a positive, explaining that it is only a temporary side effect, as long as students start at the point of where they are and not move too fast through the progressions. Through exercise or movement, the muscle fibers begin to break down and then begin to repair themselves. This is good news! It is a sign that the muscles are getting stronger and will be better prepared for the next workout routine. Recommend that the best care for muscles soreness is a gentle massage and the application of ice.

CONCLUSION

Remember that exercise recovery, *anything that repairs the damage or impact to the body,* is another important part of the workout by bringing the body back to where it was before, through stretching. Athletes stretch before an athletic performance to prepare the muscles and stretch afterward for the prevention of injury. Student and professional athletes understand that flexibility is specific to the type of movement needed for their sports. The key here is to have the correct stretching routine for a particular sport or activity. This will allow athletes to perform to their fullest potential with the least amount of strain. For example, cyclists may require less hip flexibility than hurdlers, and swimmers need more shoulder flexibility than runners do.

Overall, flexibility and stretching go hand in hand, whether you consider yourself an athletic person or moderately active person. In reality, every active person is at risk of injury, but having the knowledge to prevent that risk is essential. Being aware that most common injuries treated are found to be in the hip, knee, ankle, or foot, taking the preventative track would be nothing less than proactive. Stretching not only feels good but is also a way of deliberately increasing the range of motion of the joint, allowing us to move freely and painlessly throughout the day.

Review Questions

1. Explain the importance of stretching the lower-body muscles in terms of flexion and extension of the ankle joint.
2. Identify the role that stretching the ligaments and tendons plays in injury prevention.
3. Select one exercise and identify the muscles that are engaged in that exercise and what their roles are.
4. Describe the types of joints associated with the lower body and the movements associated with those joints.
5. Identify a specific sports activity and explain how increasing the flexibility of your lower body will impact that sport.

Visit HK*Propel* for additional material related to this chapter.

CHAPTER 12

Upper-Body Muscular Strength and Endurance Exercises

Chapter Objective

After reading this chapter, you will understand the role that the upper-body muscles play in the development of muscular strength and endurance for good posture, bone strength, force production, reduction in the risk of injuries, body balance, and stability when combined with the core and lower body; know how to develop lessons that teach these concepts to secondary school students; be able to effectively demonstrate a series of exercises and exercise routines designed to strengthen the upper-body muscles; and employ best teaching practices that enhance student learning.

Key Concepts

- The strength of the upper-body muscles is essential to enhanced physical activity performance as well as everyday activities.
- The exercises presented will help you teach students to identify the muscles involved, understand the specificity principle, learn tips for executing the exercise, and gain the ability to strengthen their upper-body muscles.
- Warm-up and cool-down activities should be performed before and after upper-body strengthening exercises.
- Accommodations and modifications are recommended so that all activities can be modified and performed by all students in the class.

INTRODUCTION

When you ask any child or adult to show how strong they are, they will immediately raise their arms and flex at their elbows to display their biceps. Although magnified at times, this display of muscular strength is just a small means of epitomizing the perception of the importance of building strength and endurance in the upper body, just as it is when middle school or high school students stand in front of a mirror flexing their muscles as a sign of strength and power.

Every inch of our bodies plays a part in the overall movement of the next, for we function as a well-synchronized beings. As we start at the top, the upper body, and move down to the core and lower body, as the teacher, you will enable your students to learn and experience how each and every muscle group, as well as individual muscles, are important. From the smallest to the largest, the weakest to the strongest, every muscle is like a building block that needs to be properly developed in order to maintain our bodies' daily routines.

Many movements of the upper body are simple ones that may be taken for granted, such as reaching, pulling, pushing, and lifting. Raising a hand in class or casting a fishing pole are movements of the upper body that people have been doing for decades. As we explore the following chapters, acquiring strength in the abdominals, core muscles, and legs are important for overall fitness. Through the implementation of specific exercises and workout routines in this chapter, you will see that most of the workouts require the use of the shoulders, chest, back, and arms. Therefore, the upper body completes this fitness equation; a strong upper body not only prevents slouching but also decreases the risk of shoulder, elbow, and wrist injuries. Developing the muscles of the upper body and implementing proper mechanics can prevent common injuries, such as rotator cuff tear, tennis elbow, or carpal tunnel syndrome.

The primary muscles of the upper body are the *deltoids,* which are located in the shoulders and comprise a group of three muscles, the *anterior, lateral,* and *posterior deltoids* (see figure 12.1*a*); the *pectoralis major and minor,* which are located in the chest (figure 12.1*b*); the *trapezius,* the upper-back muscle, the *latissimus dorsi,* the largest upper-body back muscle (figure 12.1*c*); the *biceps,* which is located in the front (anterior) of the upper arms; and the *triceps,* which is located in the back (posterior) of the upper arms (figure 12.1*d-e*).

Although developing strength and endurance in the upper body is critically important to perform everyday physical activities, it is especially important for reaching optimal performance in a variety

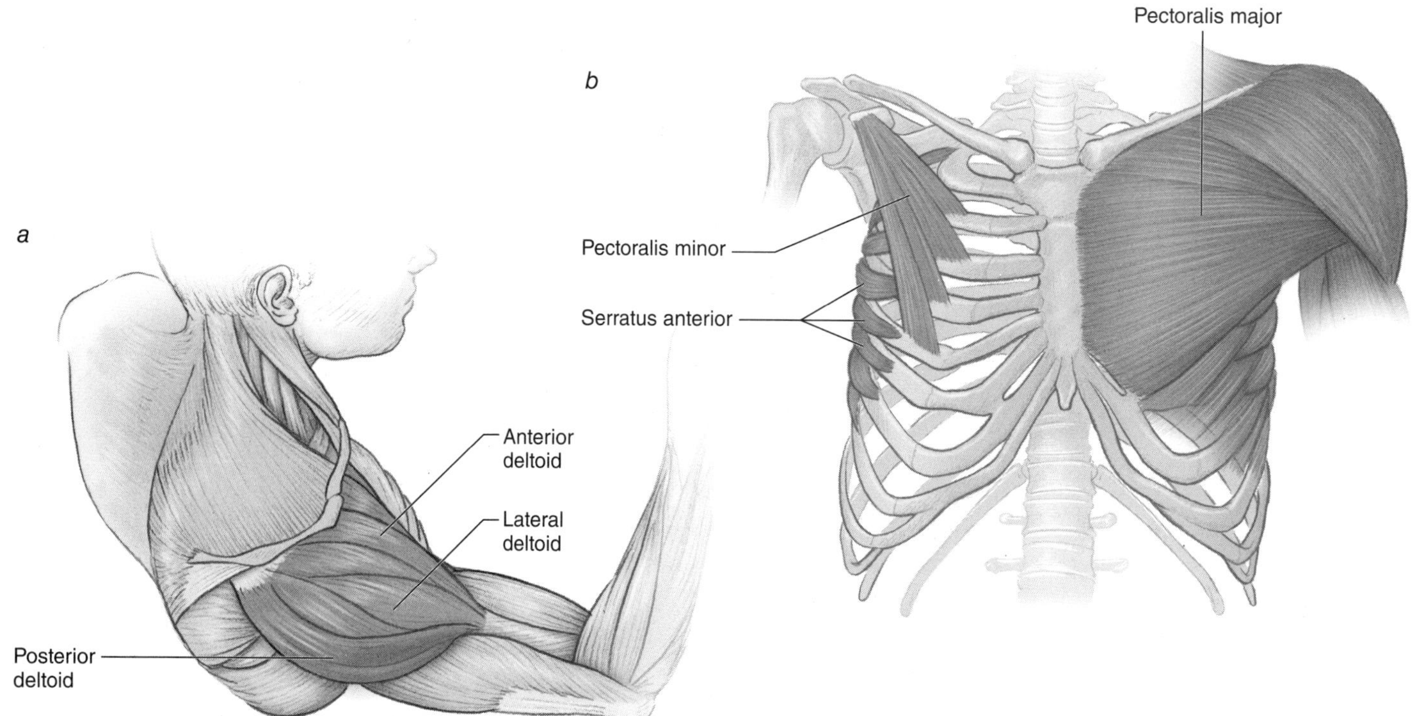

Figure 12.1 The muscles of the upper body include the deltoids (*a*), pectoralis major and minor (*b*), trapezius and latissimus dorsi (*c*), and the biceps (*d*) and triceps (*e*).

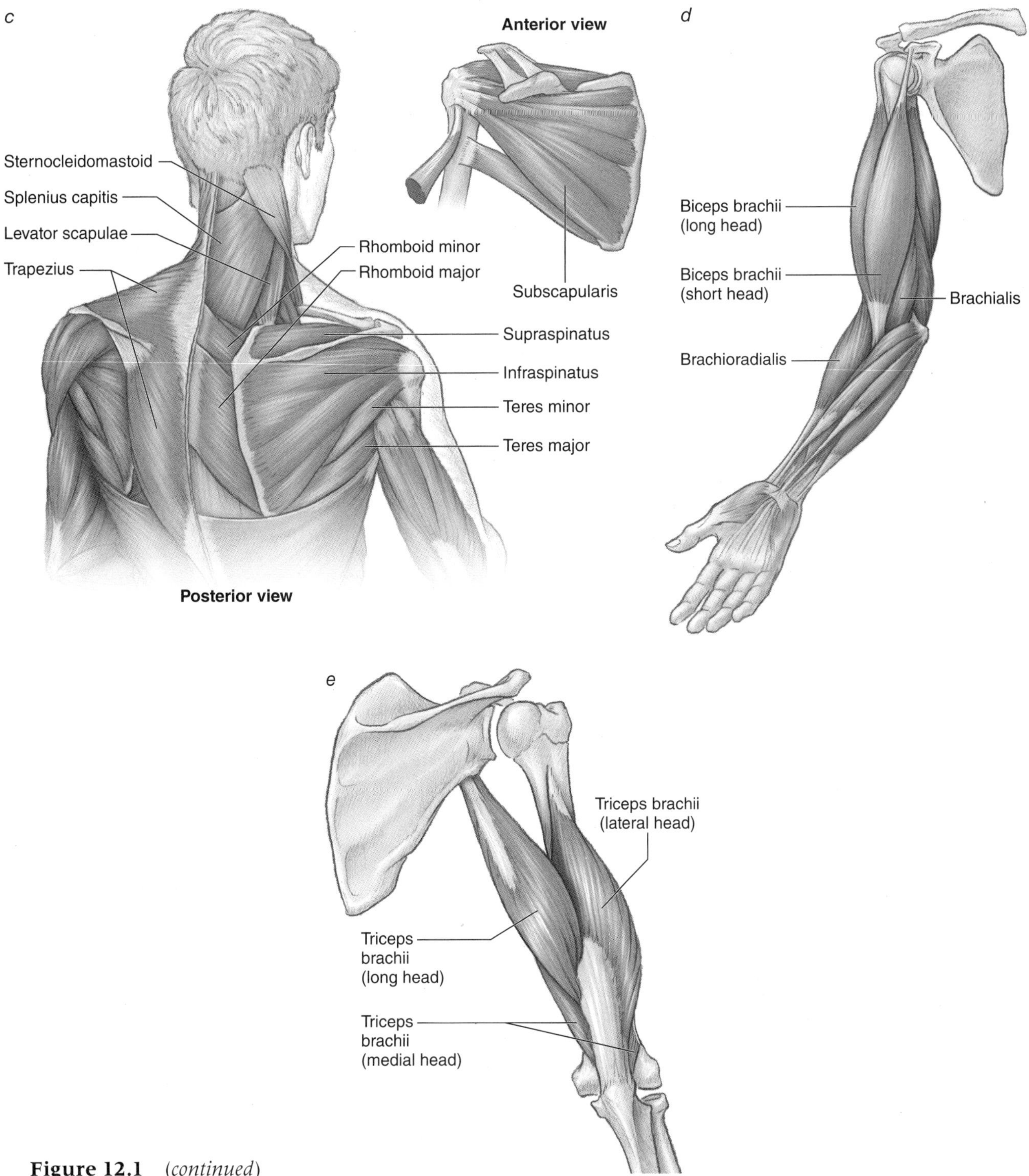

Figure 12.1 *(continued)*

of sports as well, especially when performing repetitive movements for longer periods of time. For example, baseball and softball players need to develop upper-body strength for throwing and batting; swimming strokes, such as the freestyle, butterfly, backstroke, and breaststroke are fueled by strong muscle development and integral to speed in competitions (see figure 12.2); and gymnasts in particular depend on the development of a strong upper body for most events, including the rings, high bar, floor exercise, and vaulting to name a few. Recreational sports such as rowing, kayaking, and canoeing further require the development of upper-body strength and endurance, enabling participants to enjoy such activities without experiencing premature fatigue or injury.

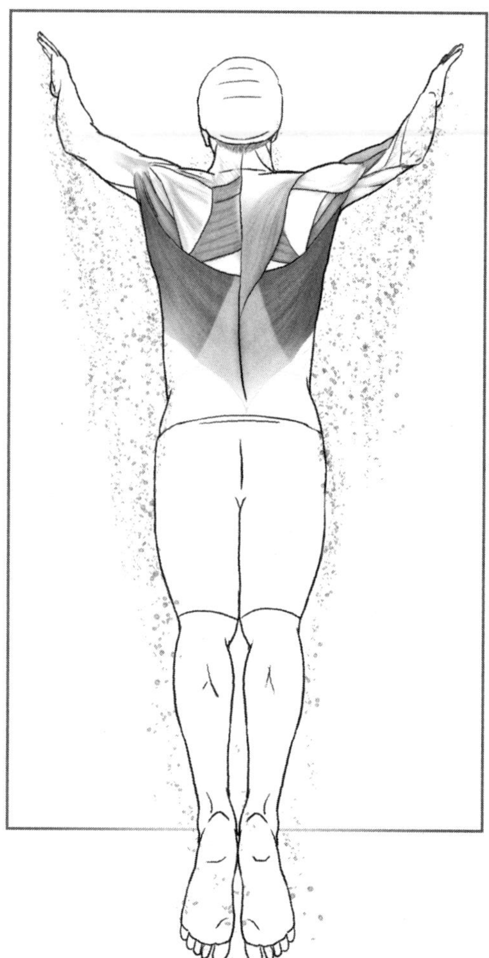

Figure 12.2 The arms are extremely important in swimming because they are the link between the primary force-generating muscles of the upper extremity, the latissimus dorsi and pectoralis major, and the hands and forearms, which are the anchor points that propel the swimmer through the water.

It is important to take into account that large and small muscles comprise the upper body. However, more importantly, the smaller muscles are needed when working the larger muscle group. Therefore, be mindful when developing routines to ensure that the larger muscles are addressed prior to smaller muscles in order to have an effective workout.

As the physical education teacher, you can use the exercises in this chapter as part of a warm-up or cool-down, lesson on upper-body muscular strength and endurance exercises, or routine. Each exercise has a description and illustration, with notes about the type of stretch, the body part and muscle groups worked, steps for safely executing the stretch with good form, and accommodations and modifications for those unable to perform the stretch as described. Many stretches are illustrated with video in HK*Propel*. Teach each exercise separately, ensuring that students are performing the stretch correctly, emphasizing the type of stretch (static or dynamic) and the muscle group being engaged. This is extremely important because what students learn during this initial instruction will enable them to use the appropriate stretch for subsequent physical activities, as well as enable them to safely engage in routines and circuits throughout the class. We include guidelines for developing routines for the beginner, intermediate, and advanced levels after the exercises, along with further teaching tips.

As you develop your daily lesson plans, align each lesson with the National Standards and your own state and local standards so that every student taught in your class can participate in the activities. The following sample lesson overview shows the National Standards and Grade-Level Outcomes (GLOs) relevant to this material, lesson objectives, and accommodations and modifications to be kept in mind when teaching a lesson on upper-body muscular strength and endurance exercises. All of the exercises in this book are designed to provide accommodations and modifications as needed. This ensures equity, opportunity, and access for all students. Additionally, as you progress through your fitness education course, your students should be able to identify which stretching activities will be required for the daily activity you present.

LESSON OVERVIEW

Upper-Body Muscular Strength and Endurance Routine

Lesson length: 15 to 30 minutes

Grade level: 9th to 12th

National Standards and GLOs: S1.H3, S2.H2, S3.H7, S3.H9, S3.H12, S4.H5

Grade level: 6th to 8th

National Standards and GLOs: S3.M6, S3.M7, S3.M8, S3.M10, S3.M11, S3.M12, S3.M14, S3.M16, S4.M7, S5.M1

Lesson objectives: By the end of the lesson, students will be able to do the following:

- Perform a warm-up routine using dynamic stretching showing ROM in preparation for activity.
- Perform upper-body muscle strength and endurance routine, showing proper technique throughout each movement.
- Perform a cool-down including cardiorespiratory activity and hydration.
- Perform a cool-down routine using static stretching showing ROM in muscle-joint areas.

Accommodations and modifications: It is important for all movements and exercises to be modified to meet the individual needs of every student in order for them to engage in full participation. Implementing universal design for learning (UDL) will assist teachers in ensuring that all students can reach their full potential. Follow the general instructional recommendations, as discussed in chapter 3, for all activities.

WARM-UP DYNAMIC STRETCHES

For students in wheelchairs, these warm-up exercises can be performed from the seated position. Ensure that the wheels are in the locked position before starting any activity and that there is appropriate space provided for assistive mobility.

ARM CIRCLES

Dynamic Stretch

Body part: Shoulders

Muscle group: Deltoids

1. Stand with feet shoulder-width apart.
2. Extend arms out to sides and parallel to the ground.
3. Slowly perform small circles by rotating at the shoulder.
4. Reverse motion, moving in the opposite direction.
5. Gradually increase size of circular movement in both directions.
6. Repeat the movement 15 to 20 times.

Accommodations and modifications: For students unable to perform this movement, have students maintain small and slow rotating movements. Repeat movement for time and repetitions. This activity can also be performed in a seated position.

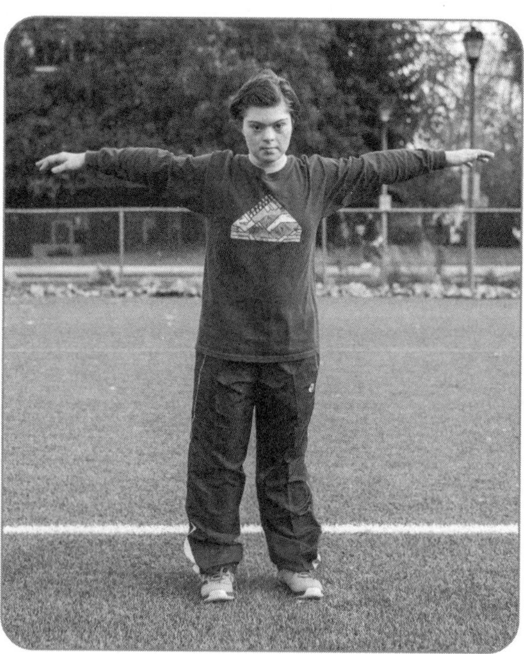

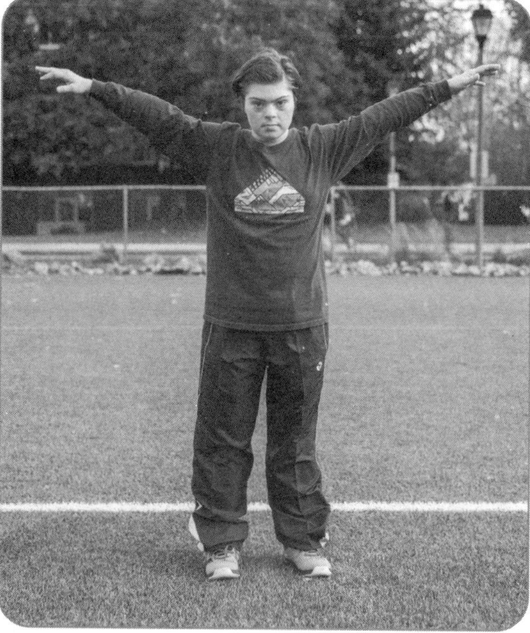

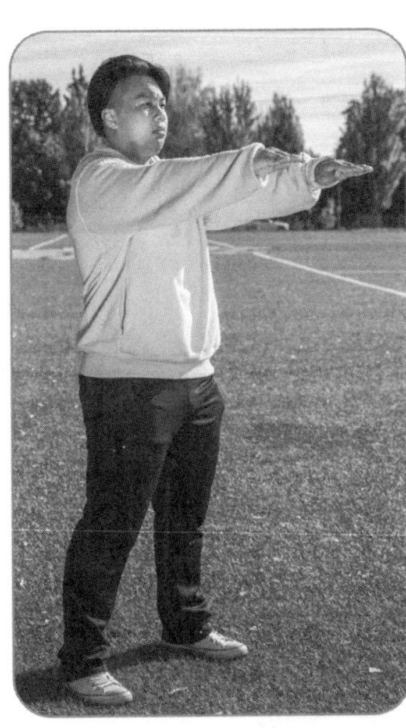

ARM FLEXION AND EXTENSION SWINGS

Dynamic Stretch

Body part: Shoulders

Muscle group: Deltoids

1. Stand with feet shoulder-width apart.
2. Extend arms down to sides.
3. Swing arms forward and back.
4. Begin with small pendulum movements from the shoulder.
5. Gradually increase the range of movement.
6. Repeat the movement 15 to 20 times.

Accommodations and modifications: For students unable to perform this movement, this exercise can be performed from a seated position. Repeat movement for time and repetitions.

ARM ADDUCTION AND ABDUCTION SWINGS

Dynamic Stretch

Body part: Shoulders

Muscle group: Deltoids

1. Stand with feet shoulder-width apart.
2. Extend arms out to sides, parallel to the ground.
3. Swing arms toward the midline of the body until arms cross over each other.
4. Return to original position.
5. Slowly continue lateral movement.
6. Repeat the movement 15 to 20 times.

Accommodations and modifications: For students unable to perform this movement, this exercise can be performed from a seated position. Repeat movement for time and repetitions.

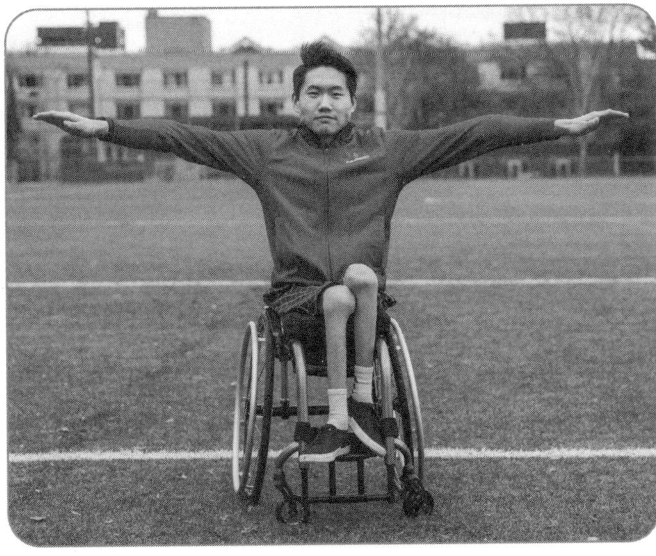

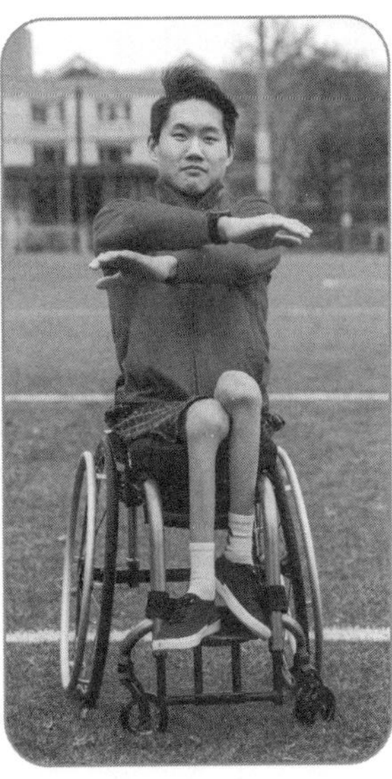

UPPER-BODY MUSCULAR STRENGTH AND ENDURANCE EXERCISES

Students will perform each exercise for 30 to 60 seconds per exercise with equal rest time between each exercise, or the traditional exercise consisting of 10 to 15 repetitions per exercise with ample time between exercises. For progression, students should increase the number of repetitions as their fitness level improves.

Y SUPERMAN

Body part: Back

Muscle group: Latissimus dorsi, trapezius, rhomboid

1. Lie prone (facedown) with legs straight.
2. Keep ankles flexed with toes touching the ground.
3. Hold head and neck in neutral position, with arms straight out in front to form a Y shape.
4. Point thumbs up toward the sky.
5. Squeeze shoulder blades together.
6. Raise arms and chest off the ground slightly above the head.
7. Hold at top of movement briefly.
8. Slowly lower to the ground and repeat.
9. Continue movement for time or repetitions.
10. Increase time and repetitions as fitness level improves.

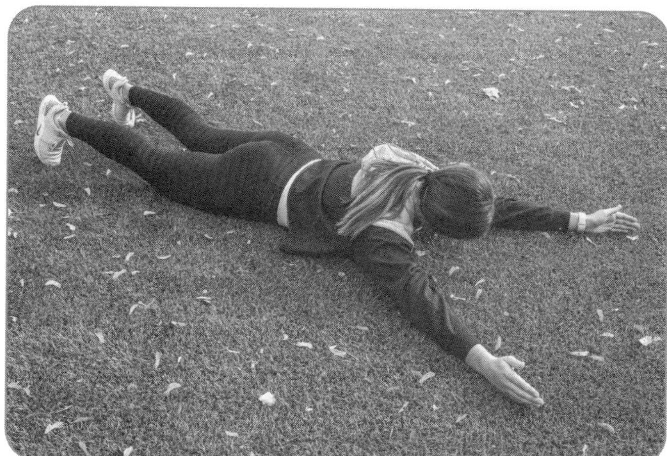

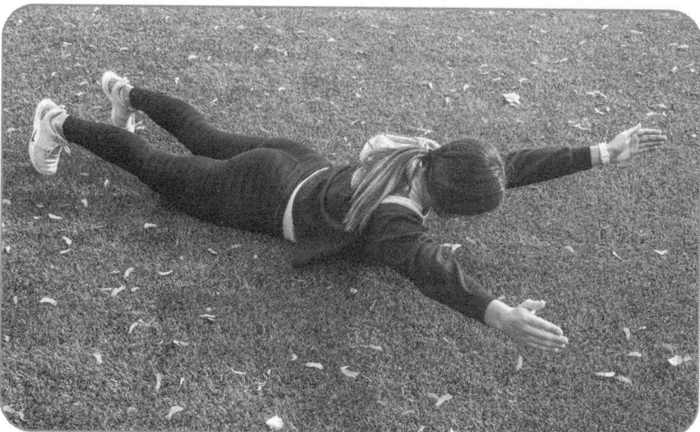

Accommodations and modifications: For students unable to perform this movement, have them remain on ground without lifting their chest and only lifting their arms. Repeat movement for time or repetitions.

W SUPERMAN

Body part: Back

Muscle group: Latissimus dorsi, trapezius, rhomboid

1. Lie prone (facedown) with legs straight.
2. Keep ankles flexed and toes touching the ground.
3. Hold head and neck in neutral position.
4. Bend (flex) arms at elbows, slightly below the shoulders, with palms facing toward head to form a W shape.
5. Point thumbs up toward the sky.
6. Squeeze shoulder blades together.

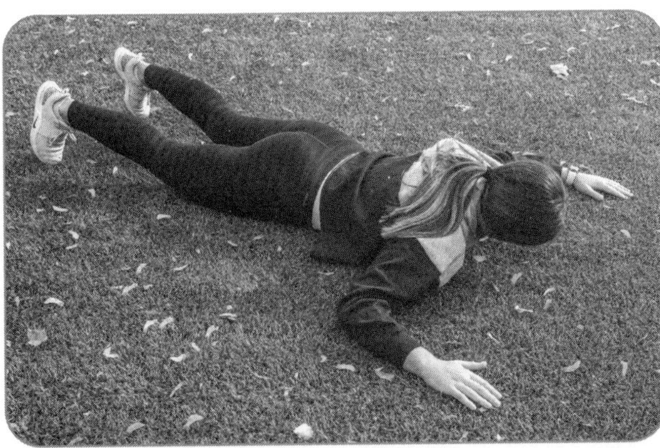

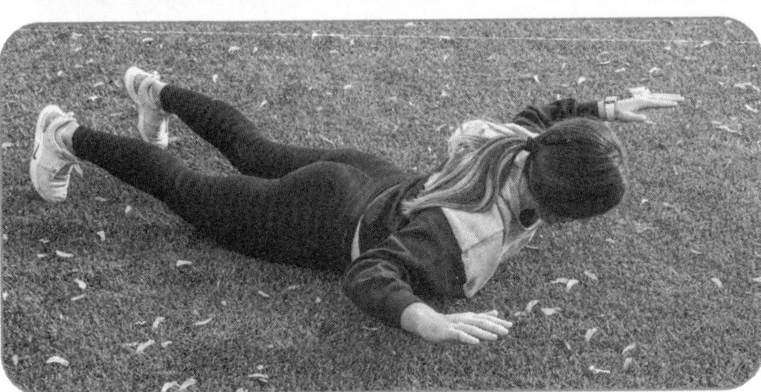

7. Raise arms and chest off the ground.
8. Squeeze at the upper body muscles while lifting to maintain shape.
9. Hold at top of movement briefly.
10. Slowly lower to the ground and repeat.
11. Continue movement for time or repetitions.
12. Increase time and repetitions as fitness level improves.

Accommodations and modifications: For students unable to perform this movement, have them remain on ground without lifting their chest and only lifting their arms. Repeat movement for time or repetitions.

Progression: To progress the exercise, try the Y–W pull-up superman.

PROGRESSION: Y–W PULL-UP SUPERMAN

For students able to master the Y and W superman movements, progress the move by introducing the Y–W circuit, a combination of both the Y and W movements. At the peak of the raise of the chest and arms, students will hold the Y position, pause, and move arms into the W position, mimicking a pull-up motion. Slowly continue pull-up movement for time or repetitions.

T SUPERMAN

Body part: Back

Muscle group: Latissimus dorsi, trapezius, rhomboid

1. Lie prone (facedown) with legs straight.
2. Keep ankles flexed and toes touching the ground.
3. Hold head and neck in neutral position.
4. Extend arms out to the sides and aligned with shoulders.
5. Keep palms on the ground and aligned with head to form a T shape.
6. Squeeze shoulder blades together.
7. Raise arms and chest off the ground.
8. Squeeze at the upper body muscles while lifting to maintain shape.
9. Hold at top of movement briefly.
10. Slowly lower to the ground and repeat.
11. Continue movement for time or repetitions.
12. Increase time and repetitions as fitness level improves.

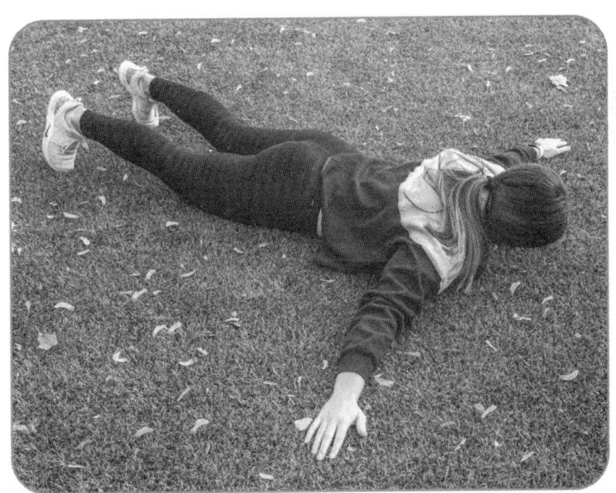

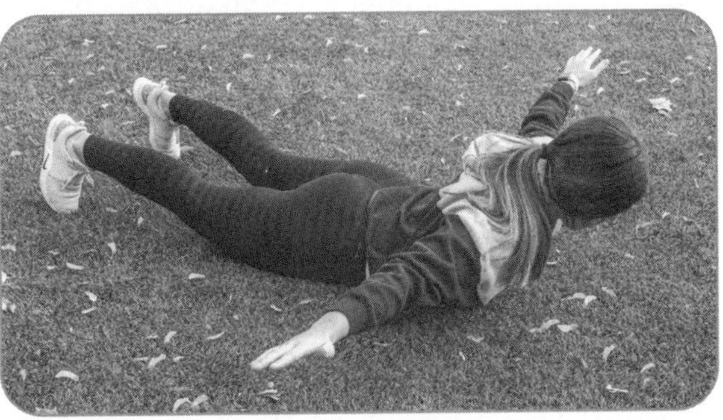

Accommodations and modifications: For students unable to perform this movement, have them remain on ground without lifting the chest and only lifting the arms. Repeat movement for time or repetitions.

Progression: To progress the exercise, try the Y–W–T superman.

PROGRESSION: Y–W–T SUPERMAN

For students able to master the T superman, progress the move by introducing the Y–W–T circuit, a combination of all three Y–W–T movements. At the peak of the raise of the chest and arms, students will hold the Y position, pause, move arms into the W position, pause, and finally, move arms into the T position. Slowly continue circuit movement for time or repetitions.

ISOMETRIC PRESS

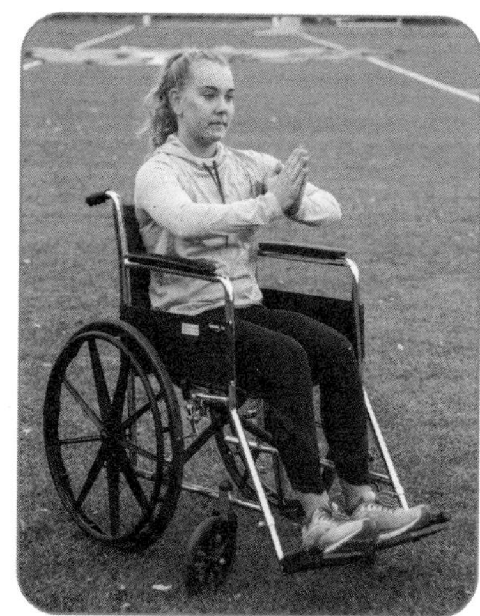

Body part: Chest

Muscle group: Pectoralis (major and minor)

1. Stand with feet hip-width apart.
2. Extend arms in front of body with slight flexion in elbows.
3. Press hands forcefully together.
4. Hold contraction for time and repeat.
5. Continue movement for time or repetitions.
6. Increase time and repetitions as fitness level improves.

Accommodations and modifications: For students unable to perform this movement, have them increase flexion at the elbows, allowing hands to be closer to their chest. This exercise can be done in the seated position as well. Repeat movement for time or repetitions.

PUSH-UP

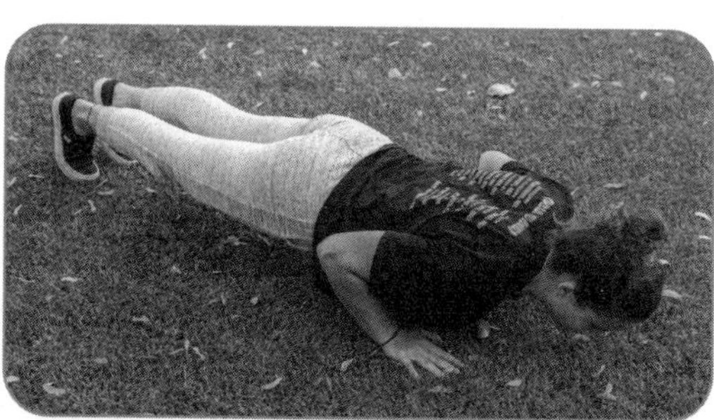

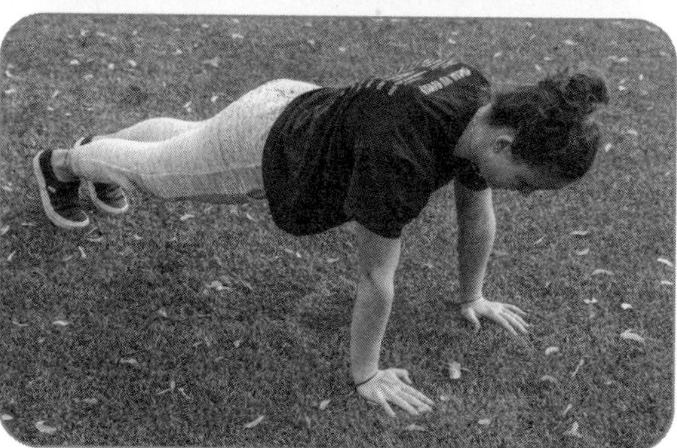

Body part: Chest

Muscle group: Pectoralis (major and minor)

1. Lie prone on the ground with hands slightly wider than shoulder width.
2. Keep legs straight and feet close together.
3. Raise chest, legs, and thighs simultaneously off the ground, raising body into a high plank position.
4. Lower body to return to starting position.
5. Raise total body quickly again.
6. Repeat up-and-down movement.
7. Continue movement for time or repetitions.
8. Increase time and repetitions as fitness level improves.

Accommodations and modifications: For students unable to perform this movement, have them place bent knees on the ground to perform movement. Repeat movement for time or repetitions.

Progression: To progress the exercise, try the wide push-ups or diamond push-ups.

PROGRESSION: WIDE PUSH-UPS OR DIAMOND PUSH-UPS

For students able to master the push-up, increase the difficulty by having them progress the move by introducing the wide push-up or the diamond push-up. Each of these movements changes the base from wide to narrow, challenging the different areas of the chest. Keeping correct form, slowly continue movement for time or repetitions.

SWIMMER'S ARM JACKS

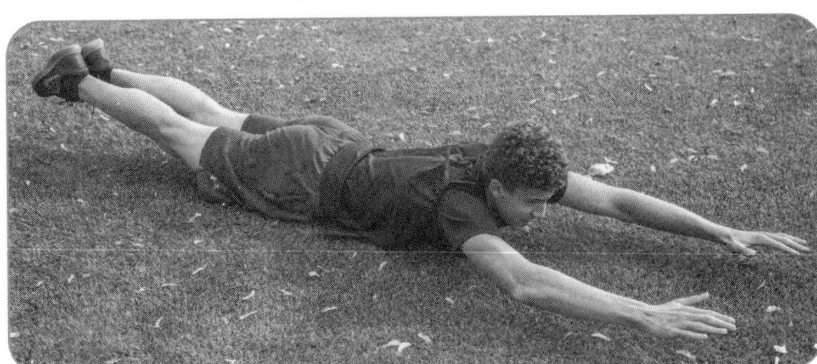

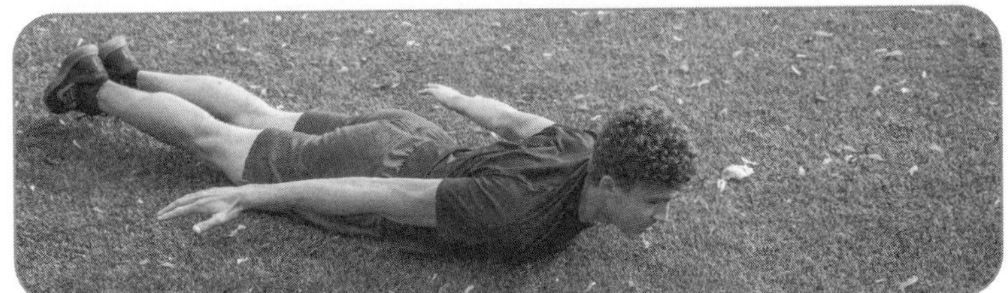

Body part: Shoulders

Muscle group: Deltoids (anterior, medial, posterior)

1. Lie prone on the ground with arms stretched forward in front of the body, palms down, and knees slightly bent and hip-width apart.
2. Raise chest, legs, and thighs simultaneously off the ground.
3. Keeping arms straight and off the ground, bring down to sides.
4. Reverse movement to return to starting position.
5. Hold position for time.
6. Increase time and repetitions as fitness level improves.

Accommodations and modifications: For students unable to perform this movement, have them keep their lower extremities on the ground while performing the arm movements. Repeat movement for time or repetitions.

SHOULDER TAP

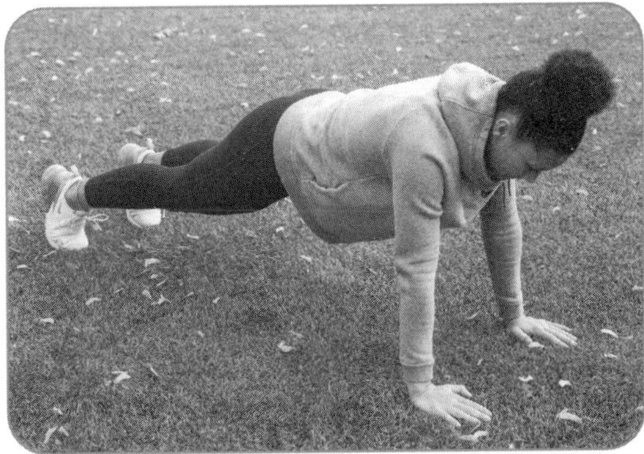

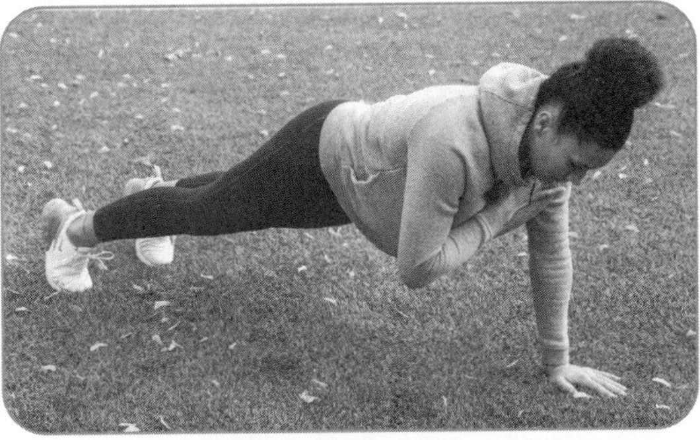

Body part: Shoulders

Muscle group: Deltoids (anterior, medial, posterior)

1. Start in a high plank position, prone to the ground.
2. Hold head and neck in neutral position.
3. Keep shoulders, elbows, and wrists aligned and feet wider than shoulder width.
4. Keep hips square to the ground.
5. Tap one hand to opposite shoulder and return to the ground.
6. Tap other shoulder with opposite hand.
7. Slowly repeat, alternating shoulder taps.
8. Continue movement for time or repetitions.
9. Increase time and repetitions as fitness level improves.

Accommodations and modifications: For students unable to perform this movement, have them bend knees to the ground to use as a support for balance. This exercise can also be performed from a seated position. Repeat movement for time or repetitions.

ALTERNATE PLANK PUSH-UPS

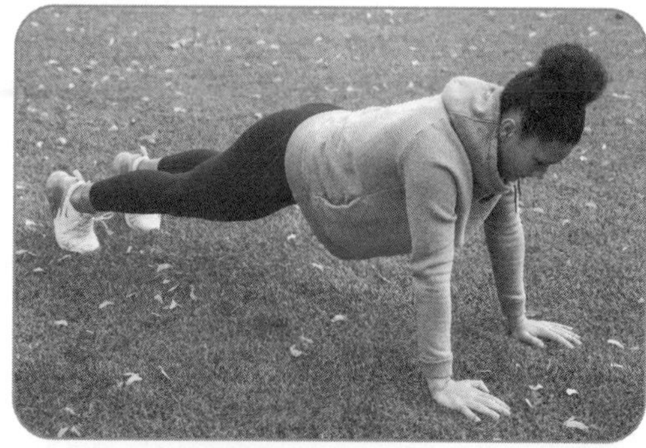

Body part: Arms

Muscle group: Biceps (biceps brachii, brachialis)

1. Start in a high plank position with legs straight and feet close together.
2. Slowly lower one arm until forearm and elbow are resting on the ground.
3. Gently lean on that forearm to bring opposite arm down to rest on the ground the same way.
4. Raise body into a high plank position using one arm at a time.
5. Repeat up-and-down movement.
6. Continue movement for time or repetitions.
7. Increase time and repetitions as fitness level improves.

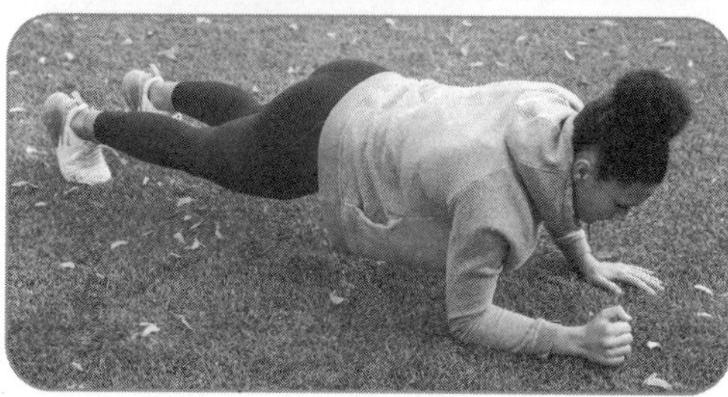

Accommodations and modifications: For students unable to perform this movement, have them bend knees to the ground to use as a support for balance. Repeat movement for time or repetitions.

Progression: To progress the exercise, try the plank push-up.

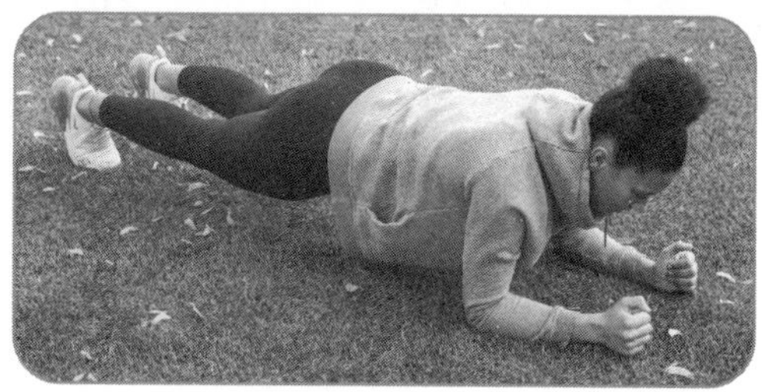

PROGRESSION: PLANK PUSH-UPS

For students able to master the alternate plank push-up, progress the move by introducing the plank push-ups. This movement changes the lowering and rising of the body from alternating the arm movements to the ground to using both arms simultaneously. Keep correct form and slowly continue movement for time or repetitions.

CHATURANGA

Body part: Arms

Muscle group: Biceps (biceps brachii, brachialis), triceps, latissimus dorsi, rhomboids

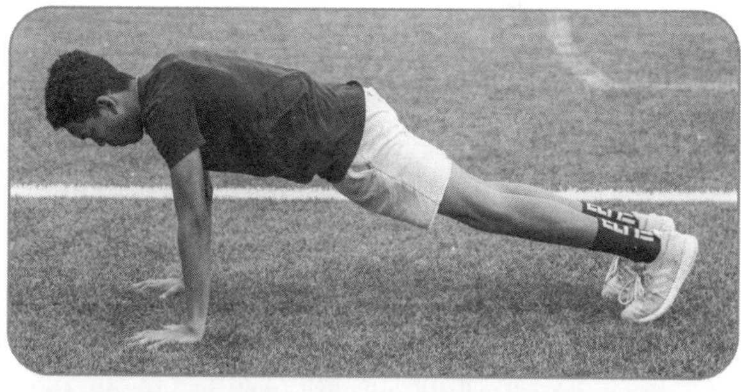

1. Start in a high plank position with legs straight and feet close together.
2. Lower body until elbows are even with sides, keeping chest, shoulders, and elbows aligned.
3. Do not allow body to touch the ground.
4. Push body up to high plank position.
5. Repeat controlled movement.
6. Continue movement for time or repetitions.
7. Increase time and repetitions as fitness level improves.

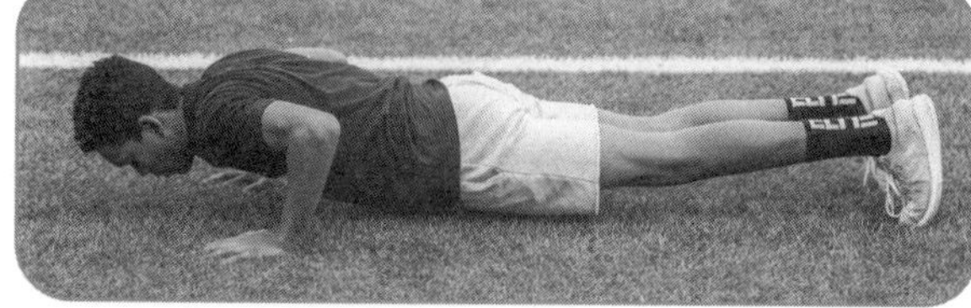

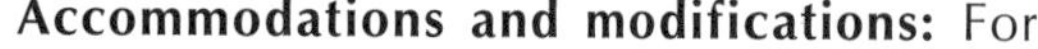

Accommodations and modifications: For students unable to perform this movement, have them bend knees to the ground to use as a support for balance. Repeat movement for time or repetitions.

TRICEPS DIP

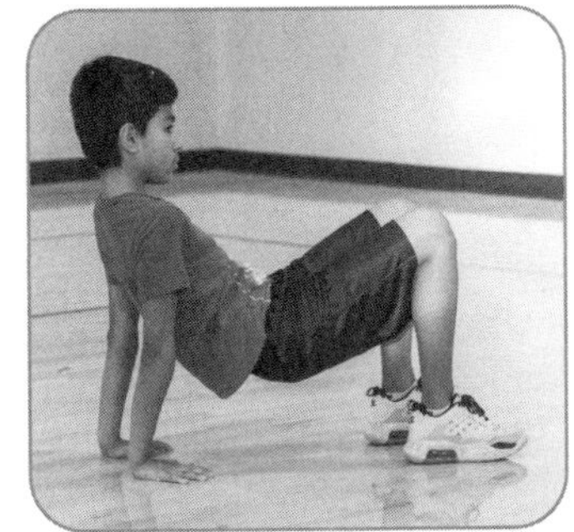
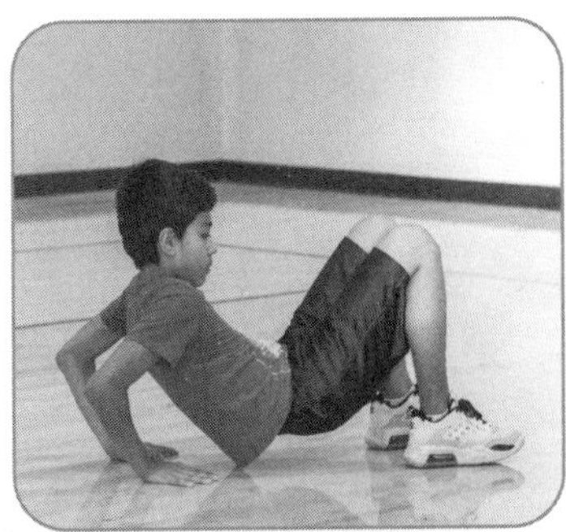

Body part: Arms

Muscle group: Triceps

1. In a seated position on the ground, position hands under and aligned with shoulders, flat on ground and fingers pointing toward buttocks.
2. Stretch legs out in front of body with feet placed hip-width apart and flat on ground.
3. Straighten arms, lifting upper body and buttocks off the ground.
4. Pause.
5. Bend arms at elbows and lower upper body and buttocks toward the ground.
6. Slowly press off with hands to raise upper body and buttocks to starting position, in a 1-2 second count.
7. Repeat to slowly lower body in a 3-4 second count to the ground.
8. Pause and repeat.
9. Continue movement for a time or repetitions.
10. Increase time and repetitions as fitness level improves.

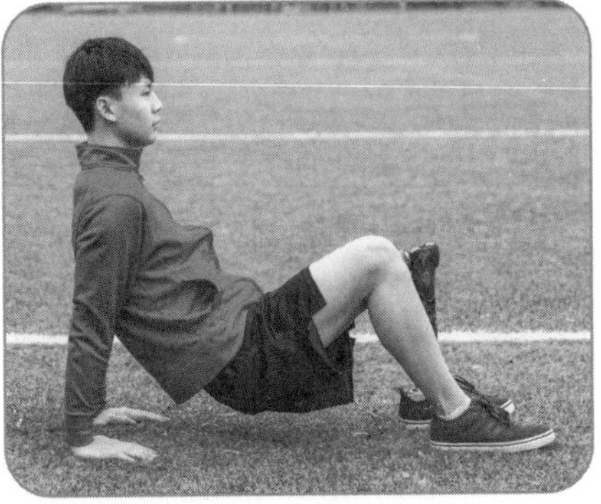

Accommodations and modifications: For students unable to perform this movement, have them keep buttocks on the ground to use as a support for balance. They can perform the same triceps dip movement by lifting and lowering the upper body. Repeat movement for time or repetitions.

Progression: To progress the exercise, try the advanced triceps dip.

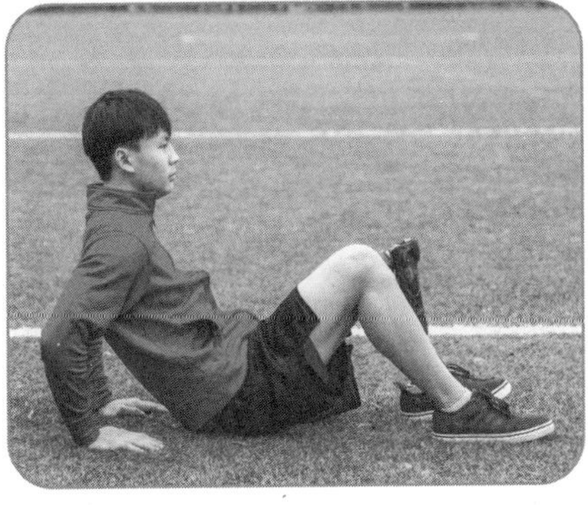

PROGRESSION: ADVANCED TRICEPS DIP

For students able to master this movement, progress the move by introducing one of the following options:

- Option 1: Keep only one foot stationary on the ground while the other is extended and straight, or:
- Option 2: Perform movement on a secured bench:
    1. Place hands on a bench rather than the floor.
    2. While keeping back close to bench, lower the upper body toward the floor until elbow is flexed to approximately 90 degrees.
    3. Pause.
    4. Slowly press off the bench with hands and push back up to starting position.

One foot may also be lifted off the ground when performing this movement to further challenge students. Be sure they maintain correct form and slowly continue movement for time or repetitions.

REVERSE PUSH-UP

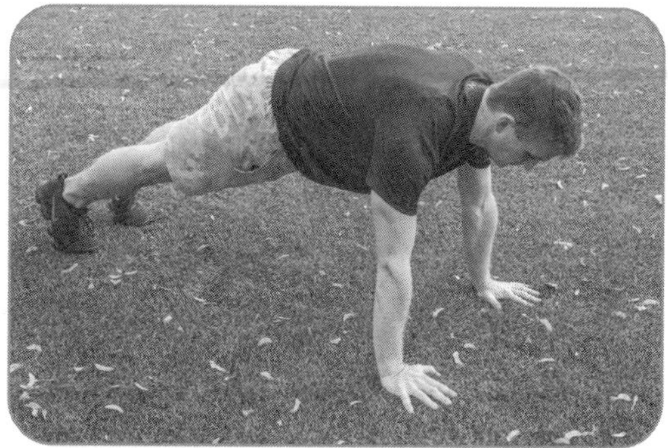

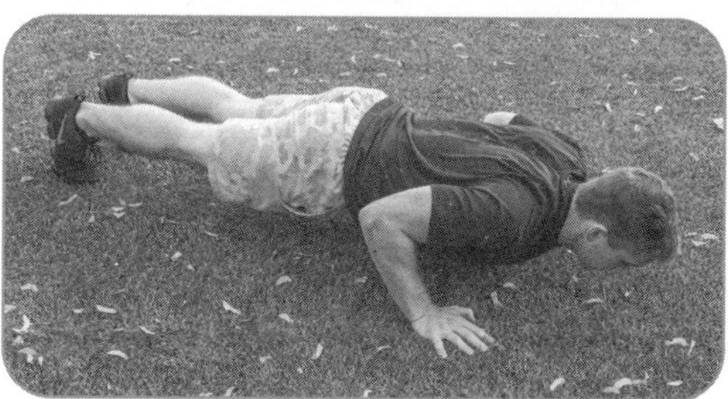

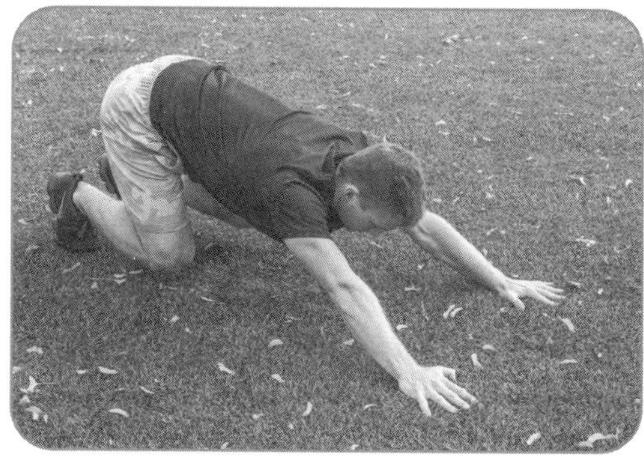

Body part: Arms

Muscle group: Triceps

1. Start in a high plank position, prone to the ground with hands aligned with shoulders.
2. Keep legs straight and feet close together.
3. Keeping body straight, bend elbows to lower body until chest is slightly above the ground.
4. Simultaneously, bend knees and push buttocks toward ankles and slightly up in the air.
5. Continue movement until knees are at a 90-degree angle and remain off the ground.
6. Pause.
7. Reverse movement by sliding body forward and up to the original high plank position.
8. Pause and repeat.
9. Continue movement for time or repetitions.
10. Increase time and repetitions as fitness level improves.

Accommodations and modifications: For students having difficulty, start slowly with one full rep prior to continuing. Have students bend their knees to the ground to use as support for balance. Perform the same reverse movement and repeat movement for time or repetitions. Be sure each movement is executed correctly.

PROGRESSION: ADVANCED REVERSE PUSH-UP

For students able to master this movement, progress by repeating each movement in a more rapid pace, gradually increasing to 8 to 12 repetitions per set.

COOL-DOWN STATIC STRETCHES

SHOULDER EXTENSOR AND ADDUCTOR STRETCH

Static Stretch

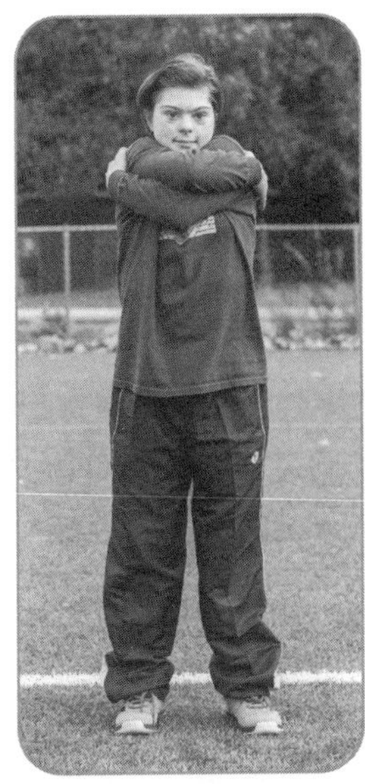

Body part: Upper body

Muscle group: Latissimus dorsi and deltoids

1. Stand with feet shoulder-width apart.
2. Wrap arms around body at shoulder height.
3. Give yourself a *hug.*
4. Pull shoulders forward in order to place hands behind them.
5. Hold position for 10 to 30 seconds.
6. Relax and repeat as needed.

TRICEPS STRETCH

Static Stretch

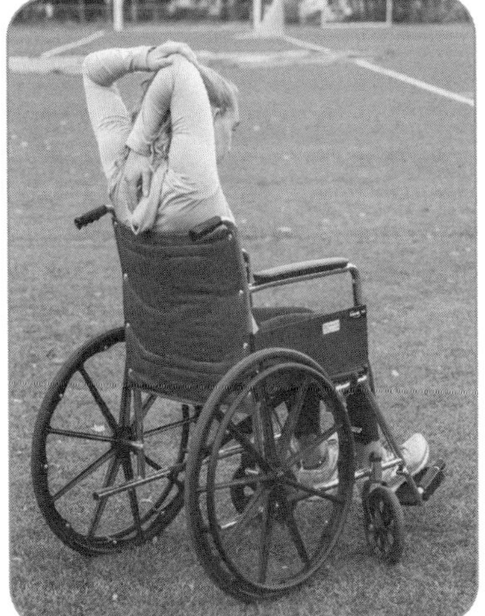

Body part: Upper body

Muscle group: Triceps

1. Stand with feet shoulder-width apart.
2. Raise arm over head and flex at elbow until hand reaches middle of upper back.
3. Reach over with opposite hand to grasp opposite elbow.
4. Gently pull toward midline of back or until stretch is felt in the triceps.
5. Hold position for 10 to 30 seconds.
6. Relax and repeat on opposite side.

WRIST EXTENSOR STRETCH

Static Stretch

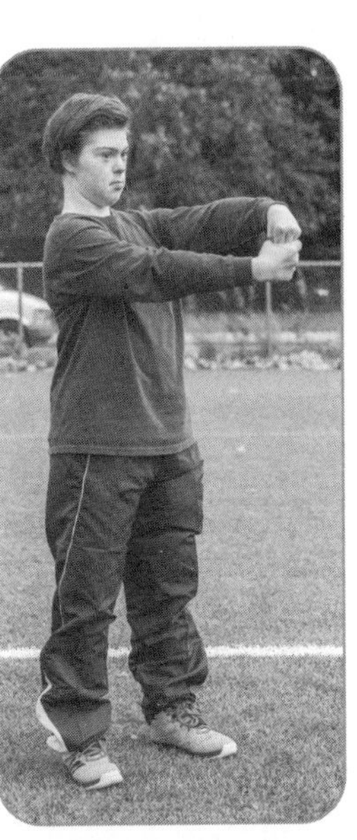

Body part: Forearm

Muscle group: Forearm extensors

1. Stand with feet shoulder-width apart.
2. Extend arms out in front of body with palms up.
3. Flex one wrist, pointing fingers to the ground.
4. With opposite hand, gently assist with stretching the wrist farther, feeling a moderate stretch in forearm.
5. Hold position for 10 to 30 seconds.
6. Relax and repeat on opposite side.

ROUTINES: STRINGING THEM TOGETHER

After evaluating the variety of fitness levels within each class, teachers will then need to make a decision as to how they will proceed with the upper-body lesson regarding progression and routines. Keeping routines short and simple will promote form, focus, and concentration throughout the exercises. The following sample routines will assist you in getting your classes progressing through the process of building upper-body strength and endurance.

- Model and practice each specific exercise, making sure that proper form and alignment is being performed.
- Verbalize the body parts, joints, and muscles being strengthened and stretched.
- Travel through the area, visiting each student and making corrections, if needed.
- Review and perform both dynamic and static stretches and muscular strength and endurance exercises of each body part until students feel comfortable doing them.
- Through time and repetitiveness, students will show their level of readiness to proceed to the next level.

Cool-down: Cardiorespiratory activity, stretching, and hydration.

BEGINNER ROUTINE

Introduction

- Review of body parts
- Review of muscle groups

Warm-up: Dynamic stretches

Routine: These particular exercises keep the body in the same position. The movements are primarily in the shoulders and arms, which allows students to focus on each movement and gives the teacher an aerial view for corrections. Keep the duration of movement short or repetitions minimal.

- Y superman: Observe and correct
- W superman: Observe and correct
- T superman: Observe and correct
- Cool-down: Static stretches
- Closure

INTERMEDIATE ROUTINE

Introduction

- Review of body parts
- Review of muscle groups

Warm-up: Dynamic stretches (increase time)

Routine: These specific exercises will introduce different muscles groups of the upper body. Each exercise will give students the experience of the contract and movement of each body part. While enhancing their strength, students will also need to focus on their form and balance throughout.

- Isometric presses: Observe and correct
- Push-ups: Observe and correct
- Alternate plank push-ups: Observe and correct
- Shoulder taps: Observe and correct

ADVANCED ROUTINE

Introduction

- Review of body parts
- Review of muscle groups

Warm-up: Dynamic stretches (increase time)

Routine: This grouping of exercises will challenge students with a variety of muscles as well as provide the experience working them out in a non-traditional way. During these exercises, proper form of movements is not only crucial but also difficult to accomplish. Therefore, be sure to slowly introduce the movements, keeping repetitions to a minimum.

- Wide push-ups: Observe and correct
- Diamond push-ups: Observe and correct
- Plank push-ups: Observe and correct
- Eccentric dips: Observe and correct
- Reverse push-ups: Observe and correct
- Cool-down: Static stretches
- Closure

Upon completion of each stage, slowly introduce an additional exercise following a progression or increase the number of repetitions. Keep in mind that various types of workouts can also be incorporated, such as HIIT, as explained in chapter 2 or Tabata and a stacker, as explained in chapter 15. Such exercises will challenge students, staying within their level of readiness and also gradually increasing their fitness levels.

TEACHING TIPS

As both the teacher and students begin to embark into the muscular strength and endurance exercises, it is imperative that students strive to discipline themselves throughout this journey while the teacher focuses on preparation in providing quality instruction.

As the journey begins, be prepared to interact, engage, motivate, and relate to each student's experiences. Not everyone will react nor benefit at the same pace. In many cases, this will be very foreign for them. Therefore, a slow and steady start will be the best path to take. Soon after, students will begin to feel safe, see a change in their bodies, and feel more comfortable to engage in advanced movements throughout the course.

As previously mentioned, the upper body comprises both large and small muscle groups, and both are equally important. For muscles to become stronger, they need to be engaged in movements that will demand more force from them. We rely on our bodies to use force daily, for example, carrying our book bags, walking up the stairs, dancing, or playing a sport. After each activity, our bodies will be tired and our muscles will feel fatigued. Therefore, they need to rest or recover. The teacher needs to take this into consideration when planning any routine. Keep in mind that each and every muscle cannot be heavily engaged each and every day. Each muscle needs to go through a recovery period, a time for muscles to strengthen and reconstruct. This window may differ depending on age and fitness level. Allowing 24 to 48 hours of rest time to repair and rebuild is a good rule to follow. This means that a body part or muscle group should never be specifically worked out two days in a row.

In addition, the overall healthy habits of adequate sleep, hydration, and nutrition all play an important part in maintaining a safe and healthy lifestyle. Therefore, the challenge of developing the muscular system will take time, patience, and consistency. As the teacher, being that positive role model is invaluable. Cheering students through that next plank push-up or shoulder tap will give them the motivation, confidence, and trust that you believe they can do it. Remind your students that their future self will thank them for what they are doing now.

As a teacher, be prepared for each lesson and choose routines carefully. Progression is key. Being able to guide students through this journey successfully will dictate their future growth in your class. Choose which way you will point your compass each day as you carefully monitor progress!

CONCLUSION

As we complete the first part of the muscular strength and endurance journey, take advantage of reviewing the concepts and terms. Monitoring the routines and making adjustments or corrections along the way will dictate the future chapters. The upper body is just the beginning, so how you reflect and review, watch and listen, and react and discipline will carry over when the core and lower body are addressed.

The feeling of students' soreness or inabilities cannot be ignored. The decision to make modifications, accommodations, and progressions needs to be immediate to avoid students feeling awkward, embarrassed, or, more importantly, injured. Understanding that every child does not develop at the same pace, you, as the teacher, may feel overwhelmed at first, so be prepared to show empathy and understanding as this is a new experience for all involved.

Repeat, review, and *reflect* are words to remember throughout the chapter. As steps are taken to advance to the next movement, the teacher must constantly repeat instructions and commands while students are performing the exercise, review what students did, and reflect on how the students felt and why the activities were important. Asking students the relevance of the exercise in everyday life may spark a reaction to work harder because they can see relevance and make real-life connections. The use of terms and vocabulary is important, as well. This will allow students to not only perform the task but also be able to share the exercise with peers and family members while making connections to other subjects, such as science.

As we begin to navigate through these next chapters of muscular strength and endurance, you may need to review and revamp lesson plans based on your students' levels. Don't stress! Re-evaluating each day must become a common practice with all lesson planning. Whether a beginning or veteran teacher, your student body is forever changing and therefore, you will, too. Do not be afraid to try new things as you begin to expand the opportunities in your curriculum and classes because, at times, expanding our own mindset means stepping outside of our own comfort zone as well. Remember, it is all about raising the fitness levels of your students!

Review Questions

1. Explain the importance of developing upper-body muscles in relation to injury prevention.
2. Identify the muscle groups that comprise the upper-body muscles.
3. Select one exercise and identify the muscles that are engaged in that exercise.
4. Describe the negative impact of weak upper-body muscles.
5. Identify a specific sports activity and explain how strengthening your upper-body muscles will impact that sport.

Visit HK*Propel* for additional material related to this chapter.

CHAPTER 13

Core Muscular Strength and Endurance Exercises

Chapter Objective

After reading this chapter, you will understand the role that core muscles play in the development of muscular strength and endurance, know how to develop lessons that teach these concepts to secondary school students, be able to effectively demonstrate a series of exercises and exercise routines designed to strengthen the core muscles, and employ best teaching practices that enhance student learning.

Key Concepts

- The strength of the core muscles is essential to enhanced physical activity performance as well as everyday activities.
- The exercises presented will help you teach students to identify the muscles involved, understand the specificity principle, learn tips for executing the exercise, and gain the ability to strengthen their core muscles.
- Warm-up and cool-down activities should be performed before and after core-strengthening exercises.
- Accommodations and modifications are recommended so that all activities can be adjusted and performed by all students in the class.

INTRODUCTION

The ability to bend, reach, twist, and lift are all essential daily movements that involve the core muscle group. Therefore, the strength and endurance of the core muscles improve balance and physical stamina, helping make daily physical activities easier and seem effortless. The core muscles initiate everyday activities, such as sitting up in bed in the morning, bending over to tie your shoes, reaching up to grab a book off the top shelf, lifting a child, and swinging a golf club. Strong core muscles also help improve performance in athletic competitions, recreational activities, and physically demanding jobs after high school graduation. In addition, strong core muscles lessen the chance of lower back pain, poor posture, and other related injuries.

Along with the importance of strength, endurance, and flexibility, the total body cannot properly function or move without core stability and structural balance, with the goal being to keep the center of gravity over the base of support while performing the exercise (McGill & Montel, 2017), as well as impacting your posture (Corbin & LeMasurier, 2014). Essentially, all movements are executed from the core, the body's center of gravity. With so many abdominal exercises to be found, where do we begin and which are the best? Remember, in support of the individuality principle (SHAPE America, 2020), exercises that meet the goals, interests, and fitness levels of students are the best!

Students and the general public alike frequently refer to the core muscles as the six-pack, chiseled abs, washboard abs, or those unwanted love handles. Many envy and strive for the "perfect" abs, but it is difficult to achieve. Although they may look great, core muscles are not for appearances only. These muscles have an important function and are much needed for fitness workouts, sports, and activities in our everyday lives. Understanding each muscle and its function will assist you in creating a proper and effective training program that will meet individual goals. The type of exercise employed to provide the greatest impact on the core muscles will determine the physiological outcome expected, also known as the specificity principle (McGill & Montel, 2017).

Identifying the actual core area may be a bit confusing, and many professional opinions may vary. Keeping it simple is best. Imagine the area on which a corset would cover your body: the area approximately located from the rib cage to the top of the hips, including the lower back (see figure 13.1). The major muscles involved are the *rectus abdominis*, a pair of long muscles that run vertically up the front of the abdomen. The *external* and *internal obliques* are a pair of muscles that lie on the lateral sides of the body. *Transverse abdominis* is a muscle that wraps around from the back of the spine to the front of the waist. *Multifidus* is a deep muscle located along the midline of the back of the spine. The *erector spinae* is a group of muscles that run along the length of the spine on both

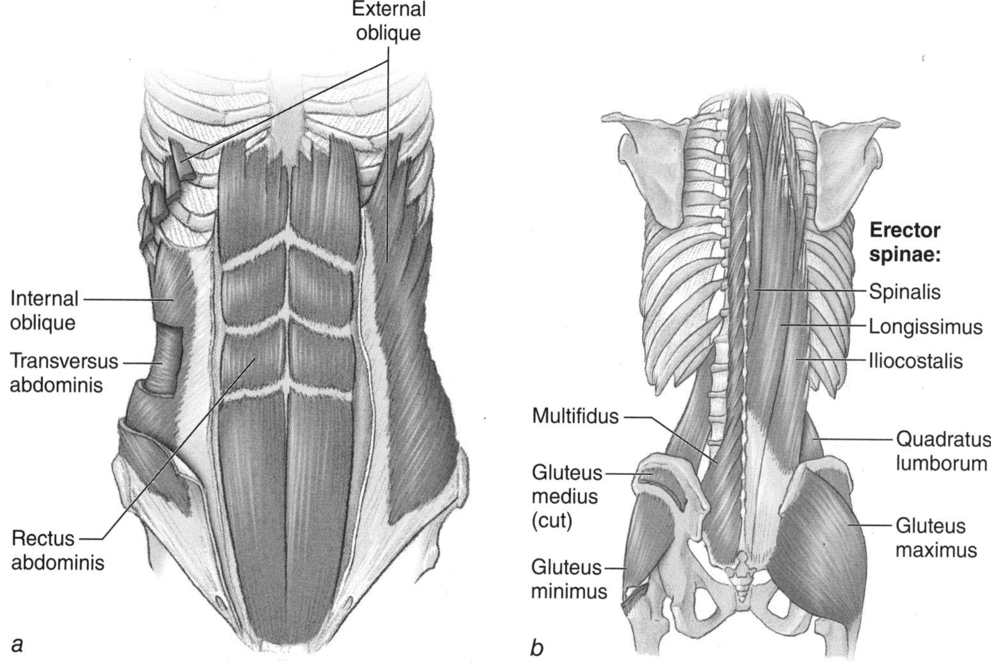

Figure 13.1 Anterior (*a*) and posterior (*b*) view of the muscles of the core.

sides and form a cylinder around the trunk of the body, protecting and supporting the spinal column and allowing the torso the ability to safely move through flexion, extension, and rotation.

With the understanding of the benefits of the core area and the primary muscle group involved, it is time to set goals and take action. Understanding how the fitness education course is aligned with the National Physical Education Standards, coupled with the Grade-Level Outcomes for K-12 Physical Education (SHAPE America, 2014) will further assist you to develop and deliver a course that comprises sound curricular content, teaching concepts and skills, and appropriate alignments that successfully meets the intended outcomes of the class. Having knowledge of the specific criteria, goals can then be set and a fitness improvement plan can then be created. Additionally, at the middle and high school levels, focus should also be on the health-related fitness assessments required of your county or state. Knowledge of the specific assessment, an understanding of the correct technique, and the ability to execute the exercise correctly are key to success.

After identifying those specific strength and endurance exercises of the core, choose other abdominal exercises within a workout plan that will complement and trigger those same muscles. Remember that all classes are very diverse, and you may find some exercises seem to be easier or more difficult than others simply because of your students' current levels of fitness. Be sure to choose a workout that can easily accommodate everyone, can be modified for students with physical disabilities to ensure an inclusive environment, and is challenging but not an impossible task. Therefore, implementing such exercises in a circuit routine that are efficient, effective, and modifiable will maximize the workout time allotted within minimum classroom time.

Proper form is the main key to success when performing these exercises. Although each movement is small and simple, it requires a great deal of muscle control and execution. However, if proper form is compromised, it may negate the benefits and increase the chance of injury. Attention to proper form also helps with performance in sport, especially highly skilled sports such as golf. Strong back muscles are needed to maintain a precise, straight spinal posture during the backswing (see figure 13.2). Without this strength, the upper back and shoulders round forward, making it nearly impossible to return the club face square for impact on the ball.

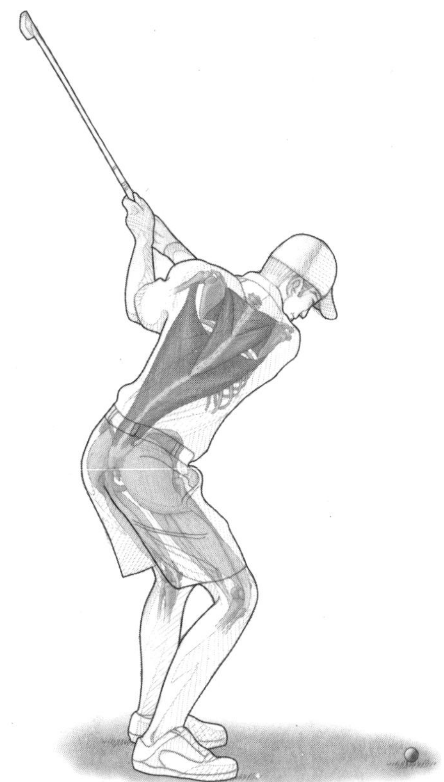

Figure 13.2 A strong core is critical to a successful backswing.

As the physical education teacher, you can use the exercises in this chapter as part of a warm-up or cool-down, lesson on core muscular strength and endurance exercises, or routine. Each exercise has a description and illustration, with notes about the type of stretch, the body part and muscle groups worked, steps for safely executing the stretch with good form, and accommodations and modifications for those unable to perform the stretch as described. Many stretches are illustrated with video in HK*Propel*. Teach each exercise separately, ensuring that students are performing the stretch correctly, emphasizing the type of stretch (static or dynamic) and the muscle group being engaged. This is extremely important because what students learn during this initial instruction will enable them to use the appropriate stretch for subsequent physical activities, as well as enable them to safely engage in routines and circuits throughout the class. We include guidelines for developing routines for the beginner, intermediate, and advanced levels after the exercises, along with further teaching tips.

As you develop your daily lesson plans, align each lesson with the National Standards and your own state and local standards so that every student taught in your class can participate in the activities. The following sample lesson overview shows National Standards and Grade-Level Outcomes (GLOs) relevant to this material, lesson objectives, and accommodations and modifications to be kept in mind when teaching a lesson on core muscular strength and endurance exercises. All of the exercises in this book are designed to provide accommodations and modifications as needed. This ensures equity, opportunity, and access for all students. Additionally, as you progress through your fitness education course, your students should be able to identify which stretching activities will be required for the daily activity you present.

LESSON OVERVIEW

Core Muscular Strength and Endurance Exercises

Lesson length: 15 to 30 minutes

Grade level: 9th to 12th

National Standards and GLOs: S1.H3, S2.H2, S3.H7, S3.H9, S3.H12, S4.H5

Grade level: 6th to 8th

National Standards and GLOs: S3.M6, S3.M7, S3.M8, S3.M10, S3.M11, S3.M12, S3.M14, S3.M16, S4.M7, S5.M1

Lesson objectives: By the end of the lesson, students will be able to do the following:

- Perform a warm-up routine using dynamic stretching that shows ROM in preparation for activity.
- Perform an abdominal muscle strength and endurance routine, showing proper technique throughout each movement.
- Perform a cool-down including cardiorespiratory activity and hydration.
- Perform a cool-down routine using static stretching that shows ROM in muscle-joint areas.

Accommodations and modifications: It is important for all movements and exercises to be modified to meet the individual needs of every student in order for them to engage in full participation. Implementing universal design for learning (UDL) will assist teachers in ensuring that all students can reach their full potential. Follow the general instructional recommendations, as discussed in chapter 3, for all activities.

WARM-UP DYNAMIC STRETCHES

TRUNK LATERAL FLEXION

Dynamic Stretch

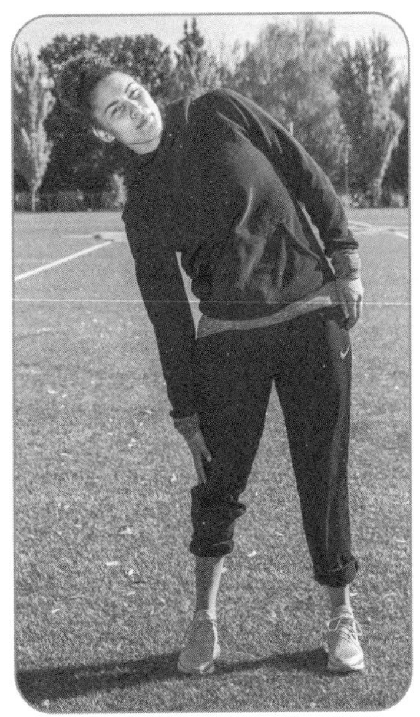

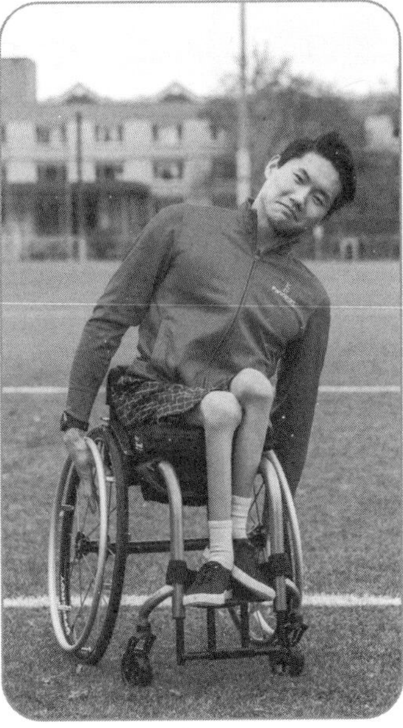

Body part: Trunk

Muscle group: Abdominals and obliques

1. Stand upright with feet shoulder-width apart and arms hanging down by sides.
2. Bend laterally side to side with each arm sliding down each thigh toward knee.
3. Alternate between right and left sides.
4. Repeat the movement from right to left 10 to 20 times.

Accommodations and modifications: Encourage students who are unable to perform this movement to slowly bend laterally as far as they can. Adjust time and repetitions for movement as needed. This activity can be performed from a seated position, with students slowly moving their arms down the sides of a chair.

TRUNK ROTATOR

Dynamic Stretch

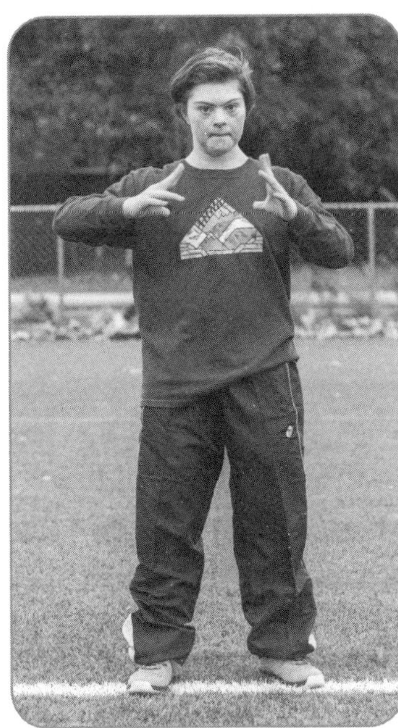

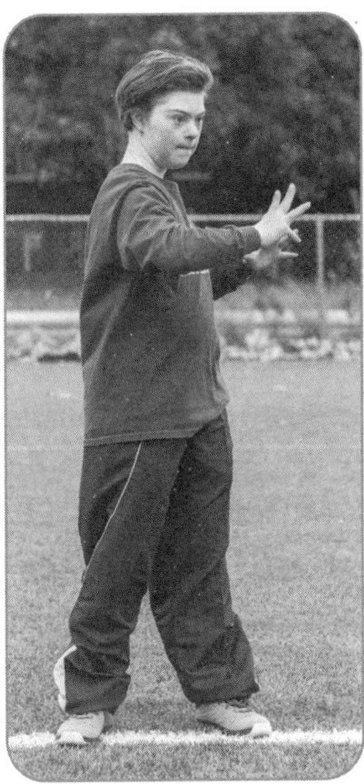

Body part: Trunk

Muscle group: Abdominals and obliques

1. Stand upright with feet shoulder-width apart.
2. Bend elbows and place hands close to chest.
3. Rotate torso toward each side, right and left.
4. Keep trunk upright and turn head to each side, following the movement from right to left.
5. Repeat the movement from right to left 10 to 20 times.

Accommodations and modifications: Encourage students who are unable to perform this movement to rotate as far as they can. Adjust time and repetitions for movement as needed. An additional modification may be performed from the seated position.

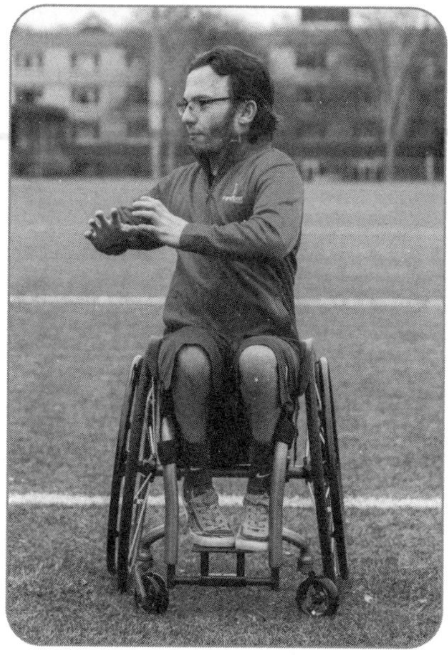

WINDMILLS

Dynamic Stretch

Body part: Trunk

Muscle group: Abdominals, obliques, erector spinae

1. Stand upright with feet slightly wider than shoulder-width apart.
2. Raise arms straight out to either side.
3. Keep arms in this position while reaching down with one arm toward opposite toe.
4. Raise back up to starting position.
5. Continue movement to other side.
6. Repeat the movement from right to left 10 to 20 times.

Accommodations and modifications: For students unable to perform this movement, have the students remain seated on ground or in a chair with legs straight and in a V-shape position. Have students follow the same sequence slowly, as balance may be a factor for some. Repeat movement for time and repetitions.

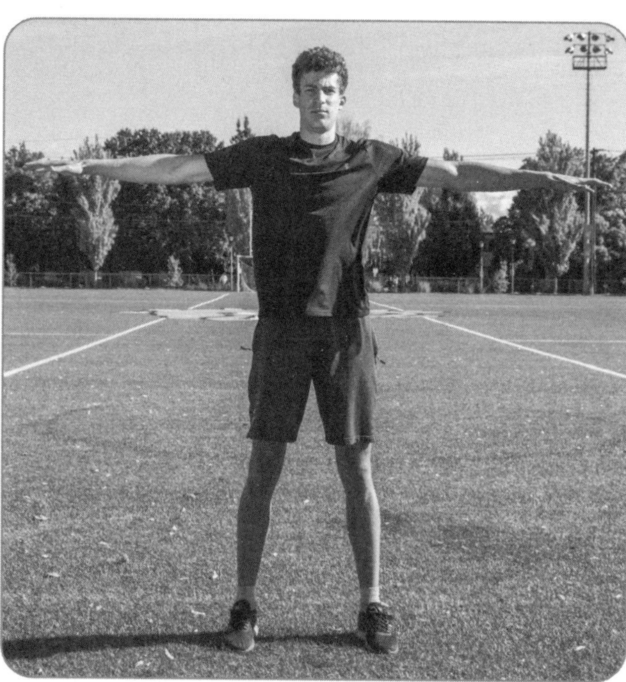

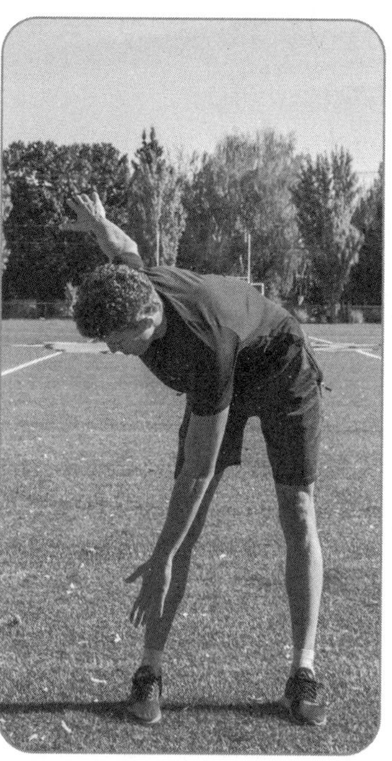

CORE MUSCULAR STRENGTH AND ENDURANCE EXERCISES

Students will perform exercises consisting of 30 to 60 seconds per exercise with equal rest time between each exercise or the traditional routine consisting of 10 to 20 repetitions per exercise with ample time between exercises, increasing the number of repetitions as their fitness level improves.

CRUNCHES

Body part: Trunk

Muscle group: Abdominals and obliques (rectus abdominis, external and internal obliques)

1. Lie supine (face up) with knees bent, feet flat on ground, and hands behind ears.
2. Hold head and neck in neutral position with eyes to the sky.
3. Flex spine to 30 degrees flexion.
4. Hold at top of movement briefly.
5. Slowly lower the trunk and repeat.
6. Continue movement for time, 30 to 60 seconds, or repetitions, 10 to 20.
7. Increase time or repetitions as fitness level improves.

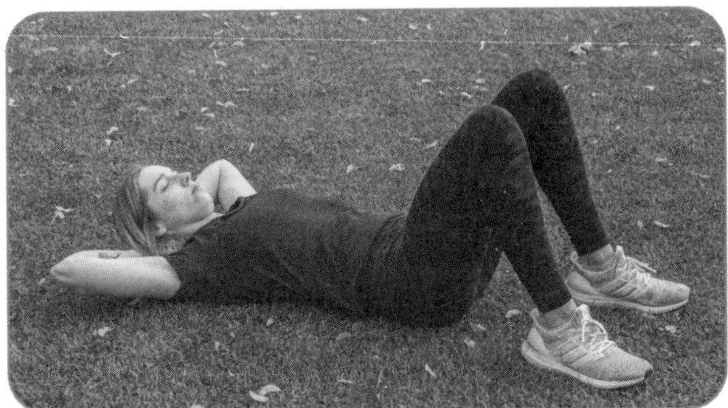

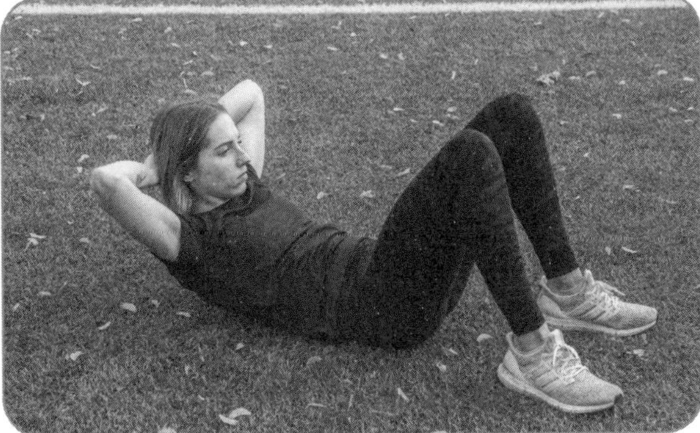

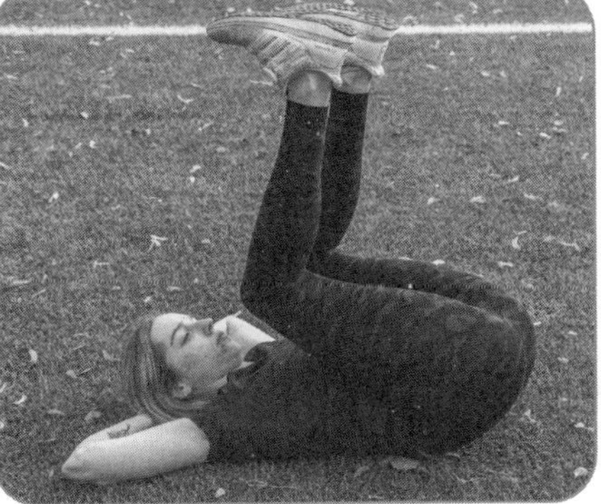

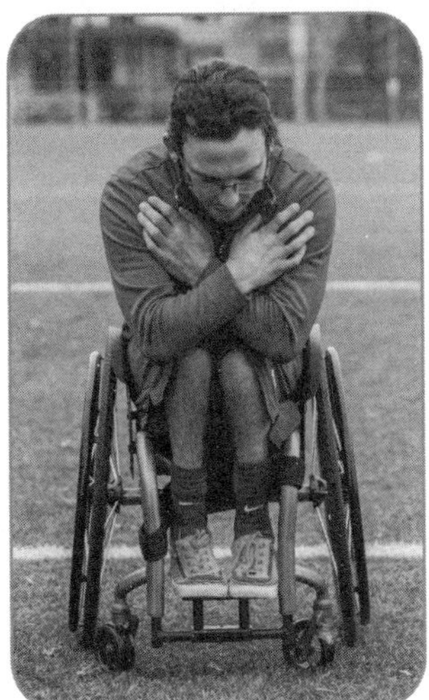

Accommodations and modifications: For students unable to perform this movement, have them do the opposite movement, the reverse crunch, by pulling their knees into their chest while keeping their upper body flat in the original supine position. Repeat movement for time or repetitions. This movement can also be performed as a seated crunch (shown) while in a chair.

1. Sit with spine straight and cross arms over chest.
2. Pull belly button in to engage core muscles.
3. Press lower back against chair.
4. Curl shoulders, head, and chest toward thighs.
5. Straighten spine and come back to a starting position.

BICYCLE CRUNCHES

Body part: Trunk

Muscle group: Abdominals and obliques (rectus femoris and abdominis, external and internal obliques)

1. Lie supine (face up) with hips flexed at 90 degrees and hands at ears.
2. Flex and rotate upper body by raising the upper body and twisting while flexing opposite hip until elbow and opposite knee meet.
3. Reverse movements and twist to opposite side as if riding a bicycle.
4. Continue movement for time and increase as fitness level improves.

Accommodations and modifications: Some students may find it difficult to balance. Allow them to perform the movement unilaterally while keeping the opposite heel of their foot on the ground.

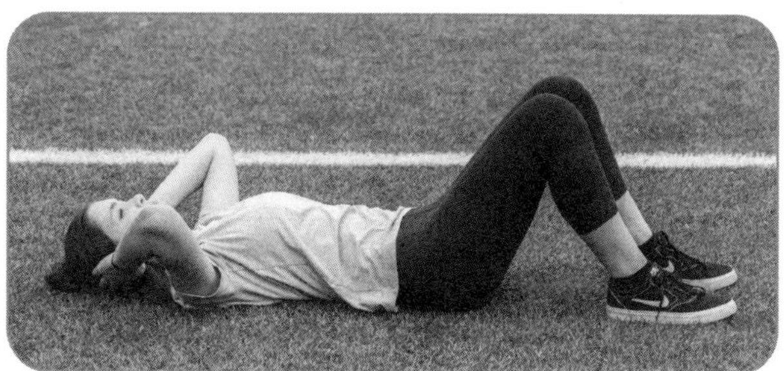

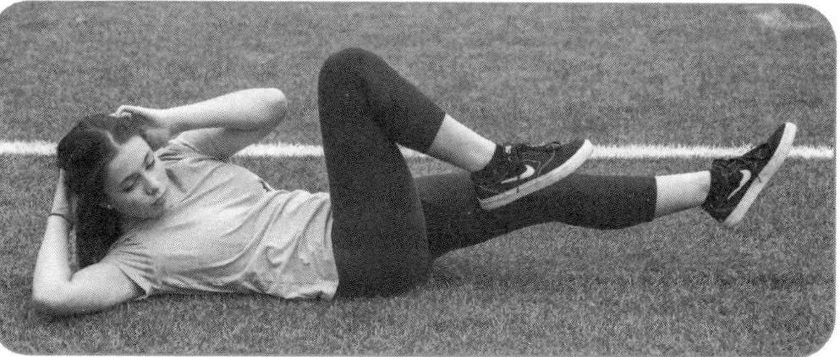

DOUBLE STRAIGHT-LEG RAISES

Body part: Trunk

Muscle group: Abdominals and obliques (rectus femoris and abdominis)

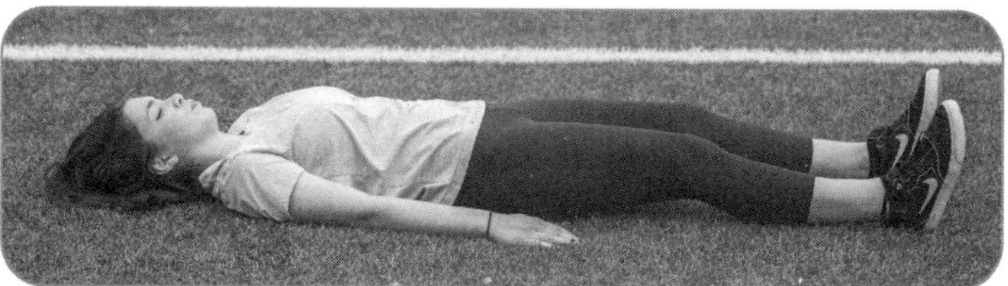

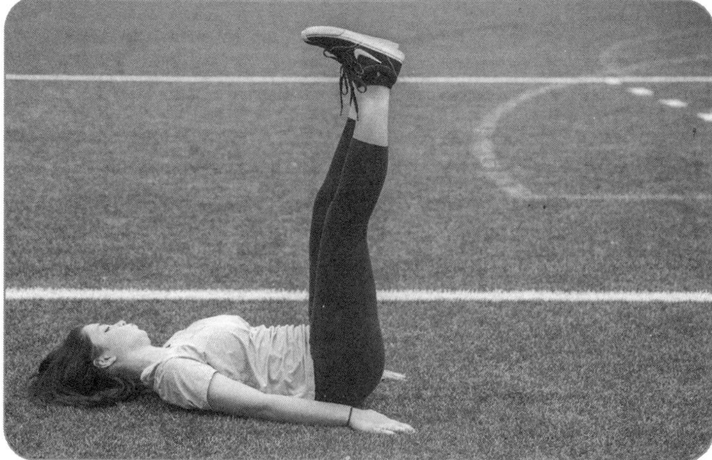

1. Lie supine with palms down, legs straight, feet together, and neck in neutral position.
2. Raise both legs, placing hips in a flexed position, then slowly lower legs to hip extension.
3. Perform movement slowly and under control.
4. Continue movement for time and increase as fitness level improves.

Accommodations and modifications: Due to the slight curvature of the lower back when lying in this position, students may experience some discomfort. If so, adjust their straight legs to bent while they continue flexing at the hips and lifting their thighs toward their chest.

ALTERNATE STRAIGHT-LEG RAISES

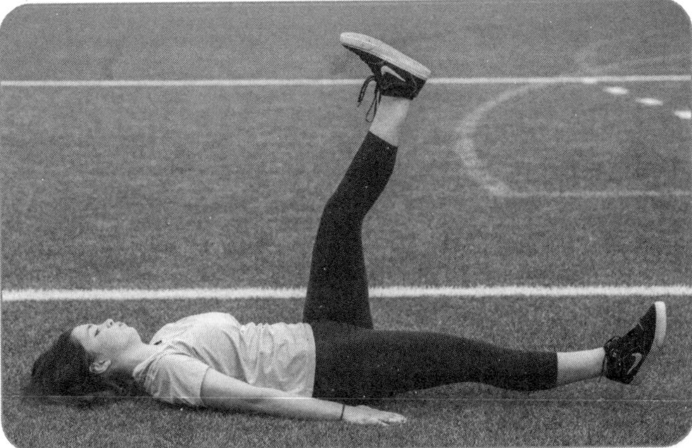

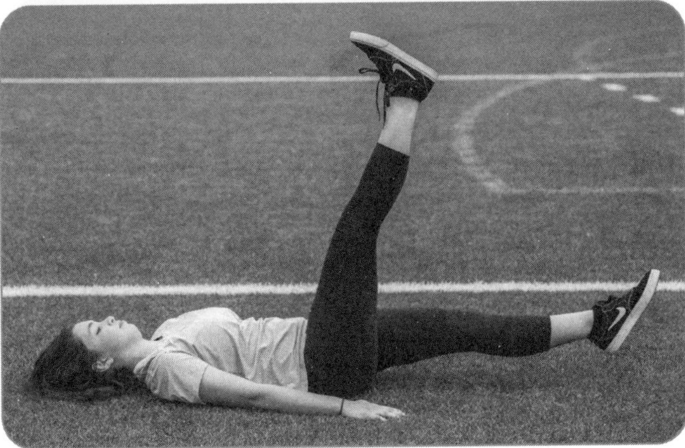

Body part: Trunk

Muscle group: Abdominals and obliques (rectus femoris and abdominis)

1. Lie supine with palms down, legs straight, feet together, and neck in neutral position.
2. Raise both legs, placing hips in a flexed position and slowly lower one leg to hip extension.
3. Focus on keeping other leg straight and hip in original flexed position.
4. Alternate each leg, performing movement slowly and under control.
5. Continue movement for time and increase as fitness level improves.

Accommodations and modifications: Follow the same modifications as the double straight-leg raise, having students bend at the knees and flex at the hips, lifting each thigh to their chest alternately.

HEEL TAPS

Body part: Trunk

Muscle group: Abdominals and obliques (rectus abdominis, external and internal obliques)

1. Lie on back with knees bent and arms next to side.
2. Raise shoulders slightly off ground.
3. Reach right hand to tap right heel, then repeat on left side.
4. Keep core tight throughout movement.
5. Continue movement for time and increase as fitness level improves.

Accommodations and modifications: If students are unable to reach heels, allow them to comfortably bend their knees at a tighter angle and attempt to reach as far as they can.

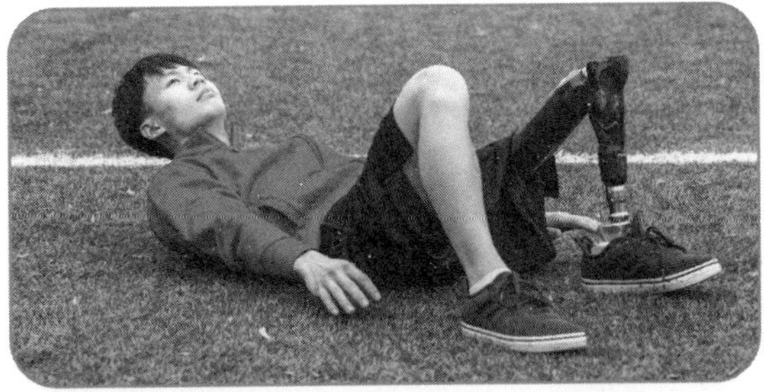

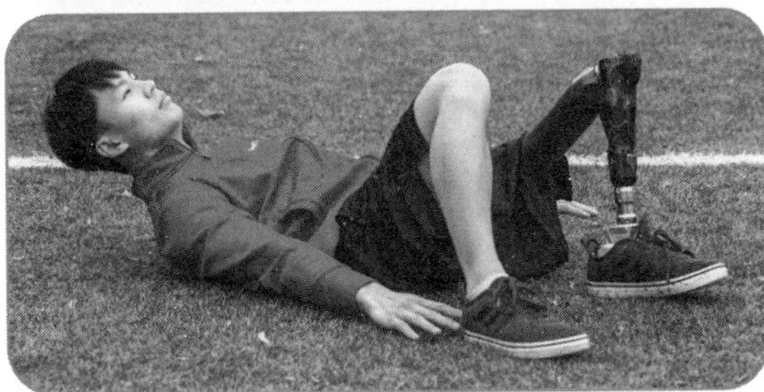

LOW PLANK

Body part: Trunk

Muscle group: Abdominals and obliques (rectus abdominis, external and internal obliques)

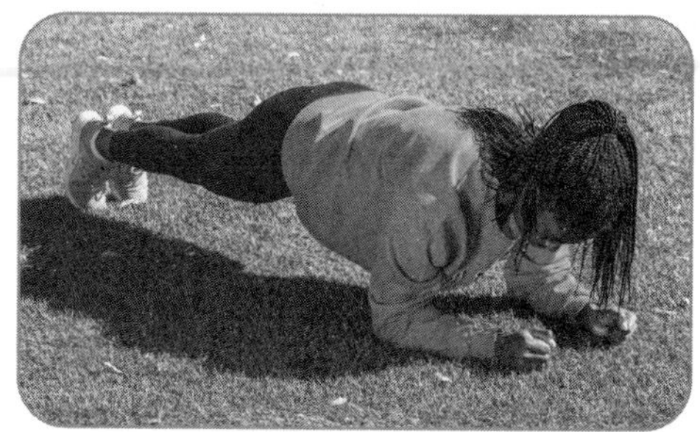

1. Support the body in a prone (facedown) position with only the toes and forearms touching the ground.
2. With the elbows directly beneath the shoulders and hands flat on the ground, keep the body in a straight line while looking down at the ground.
3. Hold position through the contraction of the abdominals, quadriceps, and gluteal muscles.
4. Hold position for time and increase as fitness level increases.

Accommodations and modifications: You may need to incorporate high plank, where straight, not bent, arms support the body. Be sure that the wrists, elbows, and shoulders are aligned. As always, adapt to students' needs and modify the movement to their comfort level.

SIDE PLANK

Body part: Trunk

Muscle group: Abdominals and obliques (gluteals, rectus abdominis, external and internal obliques)

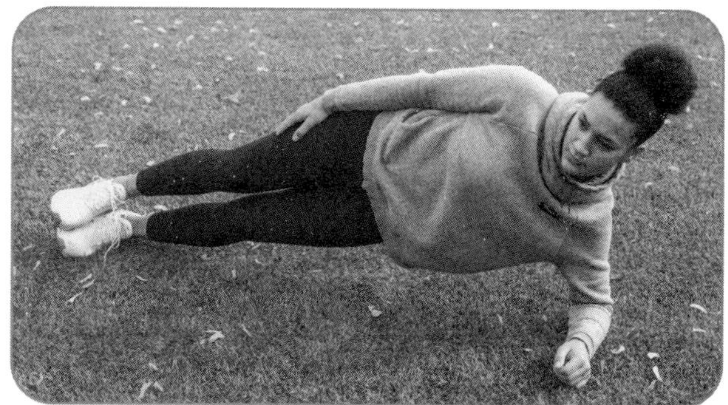

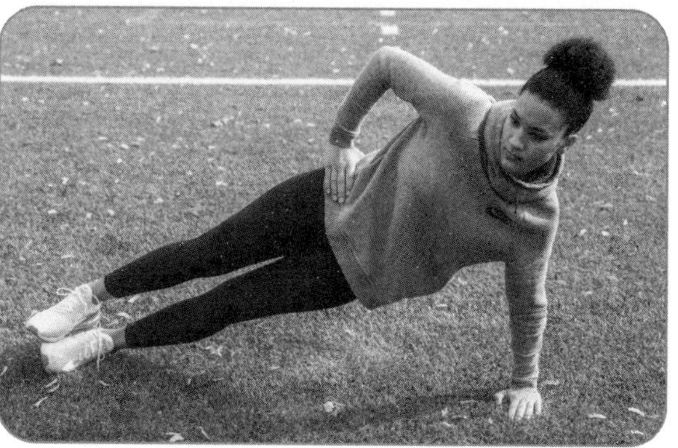

1. Form a side bridge by supporting body in a side-lying position with one foot and forearm touching the ground.
2. Stack the feet, keeping legs straight, and place hand of the free arm on hip.
3. Keep body in a straight line from head to foot with forearm of the lower arm pointed forward.
4. Keep elbow under shoulder and squeeze glutes.
5. Hold position for 30 seconds and increase as fitness level improves.

Accommodations and modifications: You may need to incorporate high plank, where straight, not bent, arms support the body. Be sure that the wrists, elbows, and shoulders are aligned. As always, adapt to students' needs and modify the movement to their comfort level.

MOUNTAIN CLIMBERS

Body part: Trunk

Muscle group: Abdominals and obliques (rectus abdominis, external and internal obliques)

1. Start in a high plank position (arms straight and body in a straight line from head to ankles).
2. While holding that high plank position, bring right knee to chest.
3. Quickly switch knee positions by bringing left knee to chest while pushing right leg back.
4. Continue movement for time and increase as fitness level improves.

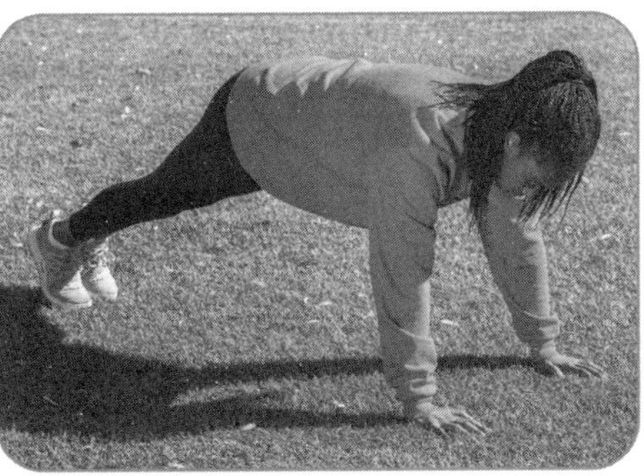
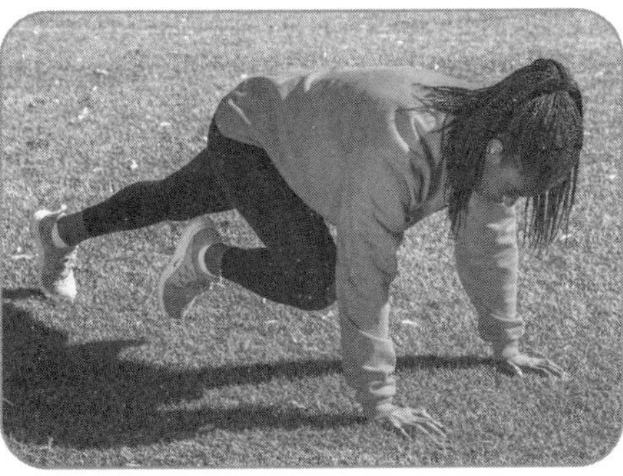
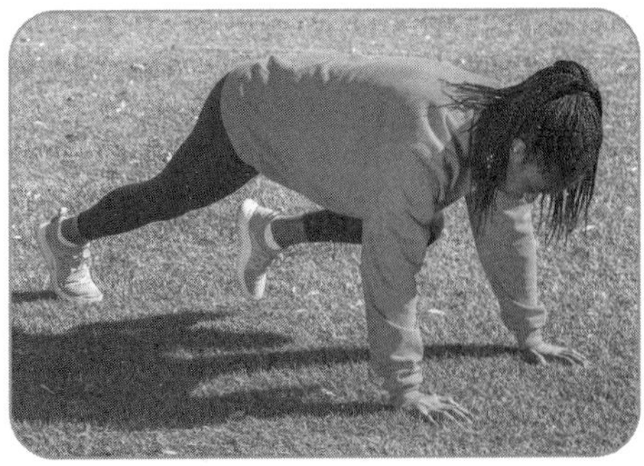

Accommodations and modifications: Again, students may feel uncomfortable switching knees due to instability or lack of balance. Have them perform the movement unilaterally, on one side, while keeping one foot on the ground. Continue movement for time and then change to the opposite side.

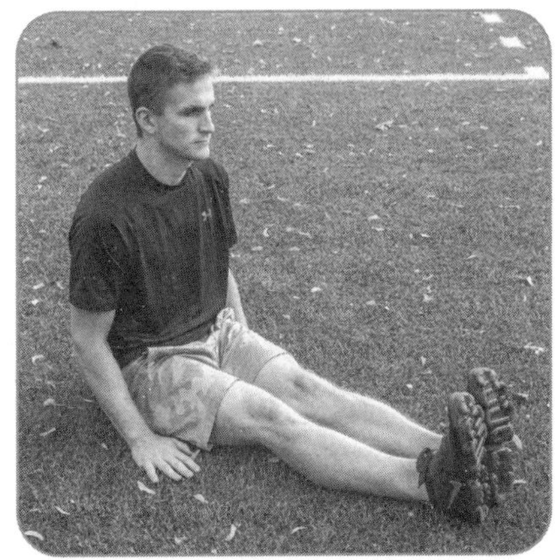

V-SITS

Body part: Trunk

Muscle group: Abdominals and obliques (rectus and transverse abdominis, external and internal obliques)

1. Begin in a seated position with hands and feet on the floor.
2. Contract core and straighten knees while lifting legs up to a 45-degree angle with torso.
3. Keep arms straight, reaching forward and up toward shins.
4. Hold position for 5 to 10 seconds.
5. Return to starting position and repeat.

Accommodations and modifications: Due to balance, the modification for this movement is to keep both hands on the ground while straightening legs and hold. This will give students more support.

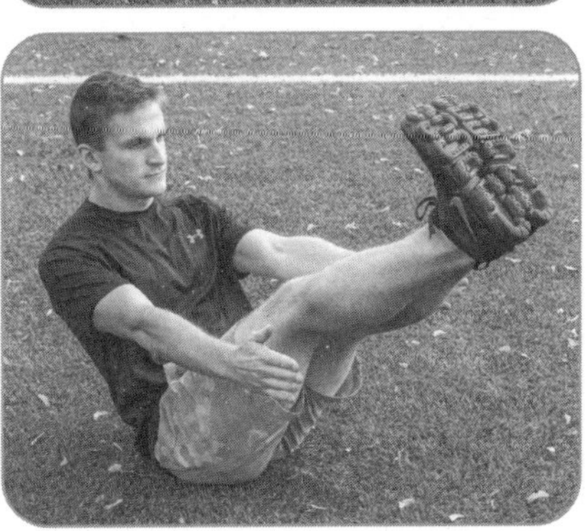

BRIDGES

Body part: Trunk

Muscle group: Abdominals and obliques (rectus abdominis, external and internal obliques, erector spinae)

1. Lie on back (supine position), keeping knees bent and feet flat on the floor.
2. Raise hips off the floor, aligning hips with knees and shoulders.
3. Hold for 10 to 30 seconds.
4. Return to starting position and repeat.

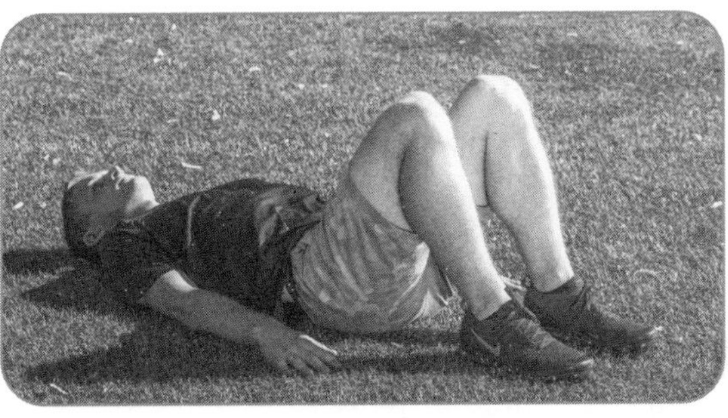
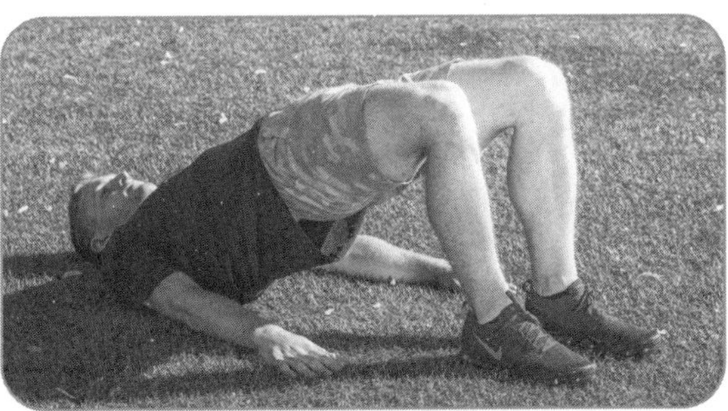

Accommodations and modifications: As students gain more stability in their lumbar region, advance the movement by having them do single-leg bridges (shown), raising their hips off the floor, using one leg while the other leg is straight.

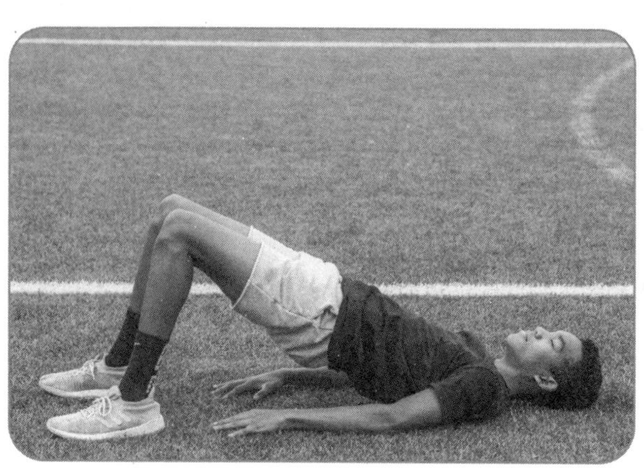

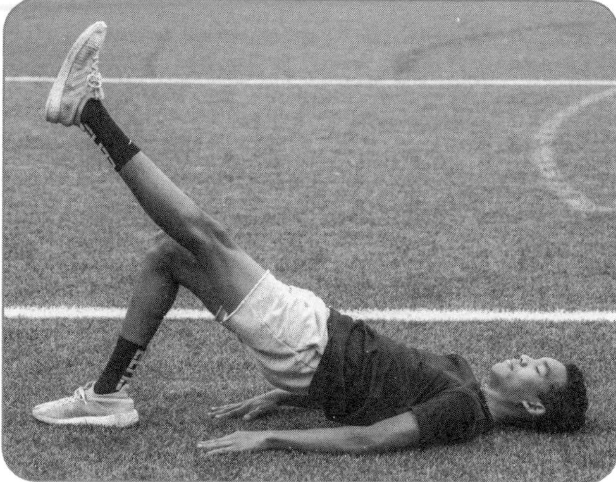

SPIDERMAN CRUNCHES

Body part: Trunk

Muscle group: Abdominals and obliques (rectus abdominis, external and internal obliques, erector spinae)

1. Begin in high plank position.
2. Pull knee toward the outside of elbow, then push knee back to return to plank position.
3. Keep inner thigh parallel to the ground throughout movement.
4. Alternate knees from right to left.
5. Continue movement for time and increase as fitness level improves.

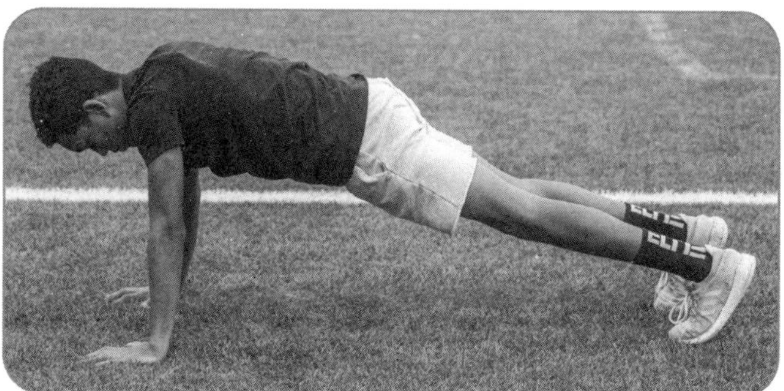

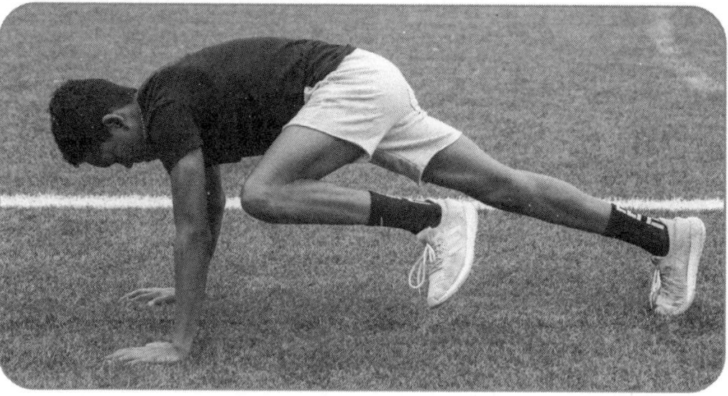

Accommodations and modifications: Again, students may feel uncomfortable switching knee due to instability or lack of balance. Have them perform the movement unilaterally, on one side, while keeping one foot on the ground. Continue movement for time and then change to the opposite side.

SUPERMAN

Body part: Trunk

Muscle group: Abdominals and obliques (erector spinae, rectus abdominis, gluteals)

1. Lie prone on the ground with arms stretched forward in front of body, palms down, and knees slightly bent and shoulder-width apart.
2. Raise torso, legs, and thighs simultaneously off the ground, hyperextending at the hips while squeezing gluteal muscles and contracting the abdominals.
3. Hold position for time and increase as fitness level improves.

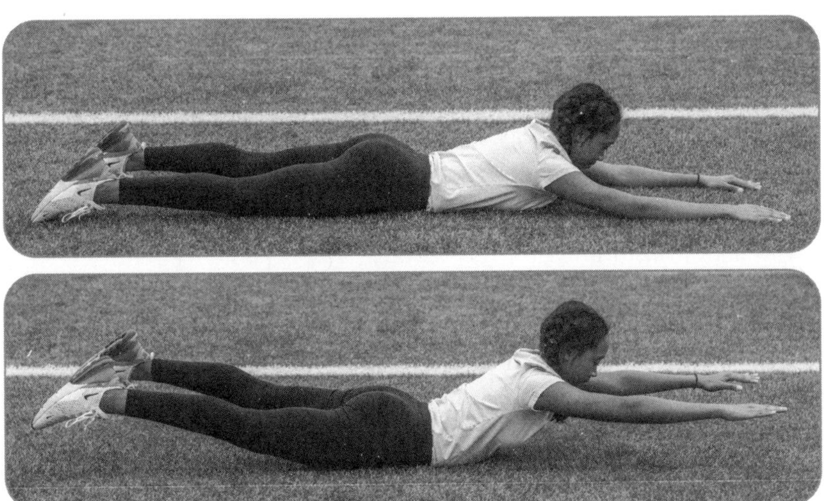

Accommodations and modifications: Some students may not have both the control and stability of their lumbar region early in the year. To modify the movement, have them lift only the upper body, chest, shoulders and arms, leaving the lower body, legs, thighs, and feet on the ground.

BIRD DOGS

Body part: Trunk

Muscle group: Abdominals and obliques (rectus abdominis, external and internal obliques, erector spinae)

1. Begin on all fours (hands aligned below shoulders and knees aligned below hips).
2. Lift and straighten right leg back to hip level.
3. Lift and extend left arm simultaneously up and forward to shoulder level.
4. Hold for 5 to 10 seconds.
5. Return to starting position and repeat with opposite limbs.

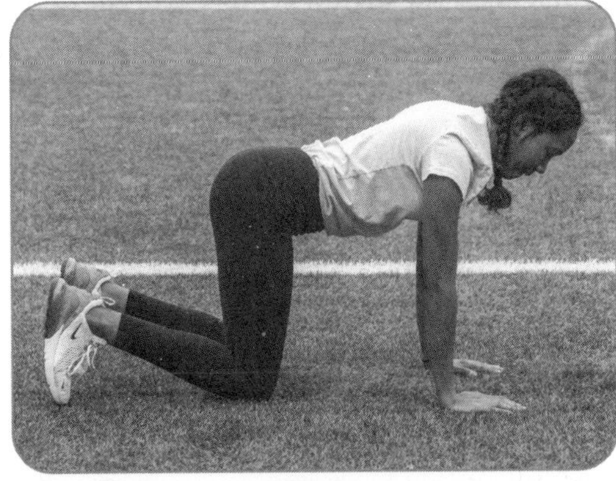

Accommodations and modifications: Having both the control and stability of their lumbar region is challenging for some students. To modify this movement, have them lift only one limb off the ground at a time, which will still allow them to work on their balance and confidence while strengthening their lumbar region.

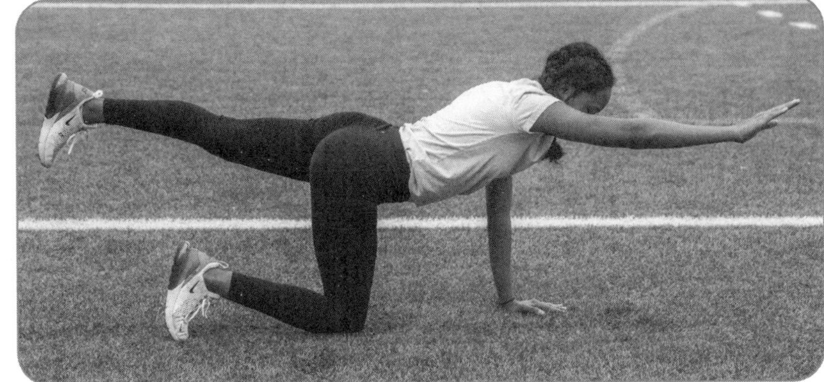

COOL-DOWN STATIC STRETCHES

Students with disabilities should engage in all cool-down activities as well. The spinal twist can be performed from the seated position.

1. Sit with spine straight and cross arms over chest.
2. Pull belly button in to engage core muscles.
3. Press lower back against the wheelchair.
4. Twist to the right.
5. Straighten spine and come back to starting position.
6. Twist to the left.
7. Straighten spine and come back to starting position.
8. Repeat on both sides 3 to 4 times.

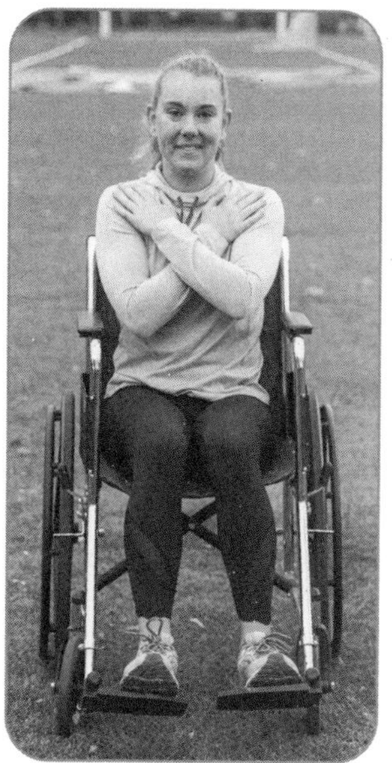

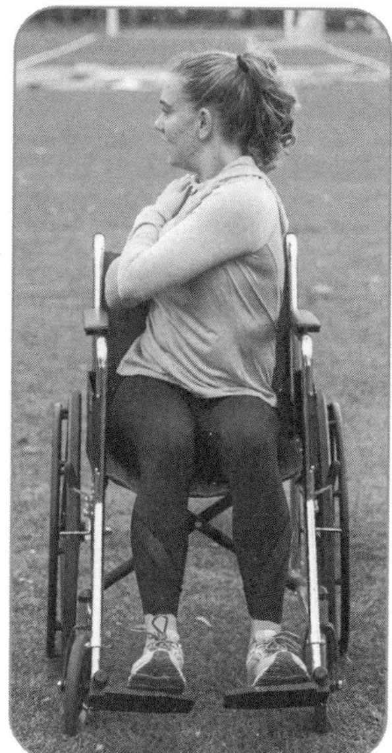

COBRA STRETCH

Static Stretch

Body part: Trunk and hips

Muscle group: Rectus abdominis and obliques

1. Start by lying face down on the floor.
2. Keeping hips flat on the ground, use both arms to push upper body upward.
3. Hold position for time, then return to starting position.
4. Repeat 3 to 4 times.

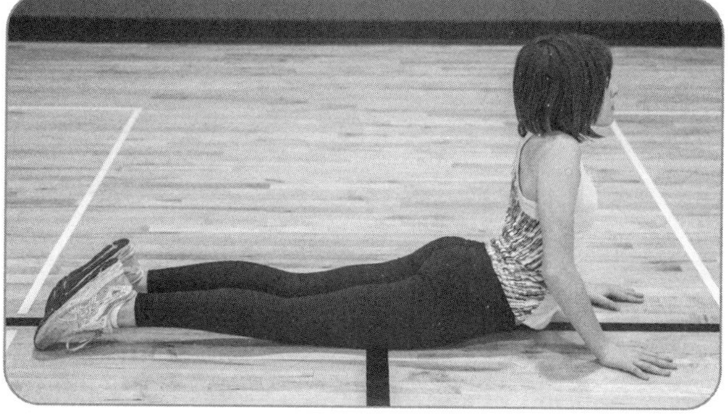

CHILD'S POSE

Static Stretch

Body part: Trunk and hips

Muscle group: Abdominals and erector spinae

1. Place hands and knees on the ground.
2. Keep knees and hips aligned and top of feet on the ground.
3. Push gluteal back as torso will come to rest on thighs.
4. Keep arms straight in front, over the head with palms pronated.

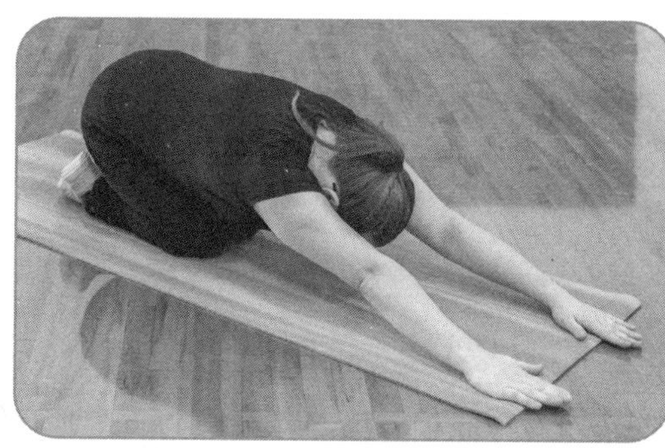

5. Hold position for 10 to 30 seconds, then return to starting position.
6. Repeat 3 to 4 times.

SEATED SPINAL TWIST

Static Stretch

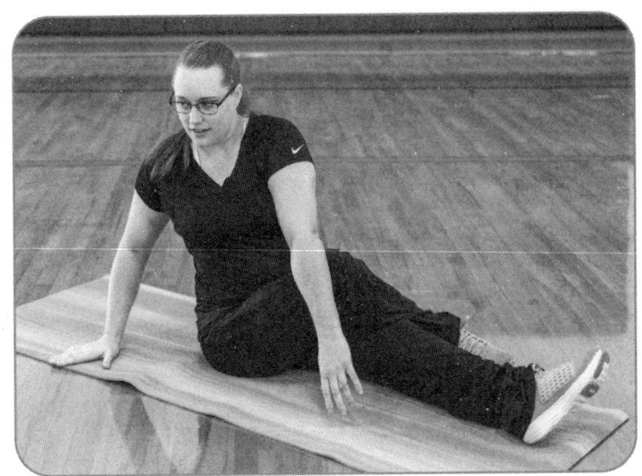

Body part: Lower back

Muscle group: Erector spinae, gluteals, obliques

1. Sit cross-legged on floor with right leg on top.
2. Keeping right leg crossed over left leg, place right foot on the ground against the outside of the left knee.
3. Gently twist shoulders toward the right, pushing against the right leg, using the left elbow against the right knee for leverage.
4. Twist as far as comfortable and hold for time.
5. Repeat on other side.
6. Repeat on both sides 3 to 4 times.

SINGLE KNEE-TO-CHEST STRETCH

Static Stretch

Body part: Trunk

Muscle group: Lower latissimus dorsi and erector spinae

1. Start by lying face up with legs straight and both heels on the floor This stretch may also be done from a seated position (shown).
2. Bring one knee to chest, keeping opposite leg in original position.
3. Place hands below the knee area on top of the shin.
4. Bring knee slowly toward chest and hold for 10 to 30 seconds.
5. Return to starting position and slowly do the same with opposite leg.
6. Repeat 3 to 4 times.

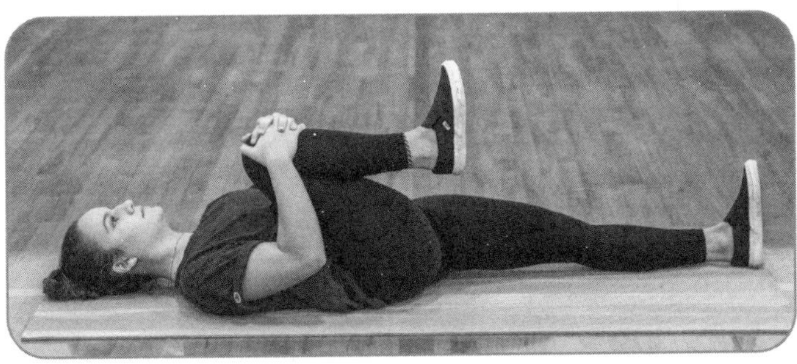

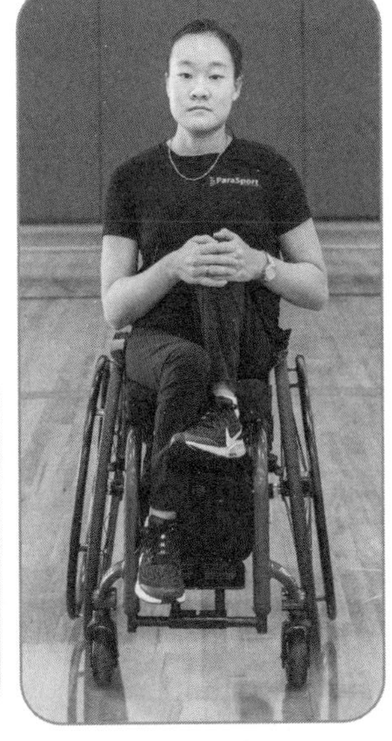

ROUTINES: STRINGING THEM TOGETHER

As your class progresses through the semester, greater strength and endurance outcomes will be achieved by further implementing a progressively challenging exercise program through appropriate routines. For beginners, it's best to meet them where they are to ensure students stay motivated as they begin to gain strength and endurance. As students progress through the class, you should guide them through more progressively difficult exercises by either increasing the repetitions or time engaged in an exercise or increasing the difficulty level of the routine. Use the following recommendations to get started.

- Model and practice each specific exercise, making sure that proper form and alignment are being performed.
- Verbalize the body parts, joints, and muscles being strengthened and stretched.
- Travel through the area, visiting each student and making corrections, if needed.
- Review and perform both dynamic and static stretches and muscular strength and endurance exercises of each body part until students feel comfortable doing them.
- Through time and repetition, students will show their level of readiness to proceed to the next level.

Cool-down: Cardiorespiratory activity, stretching, and hydration.

BEGINNER ROUTINE

Introduction

- Review of body parts
- Review of muscle groups

Warm-up: Dynamic stretches

Routine: At this stage, full-body movement is limited, allowing students to focus on each exercise. Keep the duration of movement short or repetitions minimal.

- Double straight-leg raise: Observe and correct
- Alternate straight-leg raise: Observe and correct
- Heel tap: Observe and correct
- Cool-down: Static stretches
- Closure

INTERMEDIATE ROUTINE

Introduction

- Review of body parts
- Review of muscle groups

Warm-up: Dynamic stretches (increase time)

Routine: Although students maintain the prone position while engaging in these exercises, they will need to focus not only on form but also proper movement of other body parts while keeping in the plank position.

- Low plank: Observe and correct
- Side plank: Observe and correct
- Mountain climbers: Observe and correct
- Spiderman crunches: Observe and correct
- Superman: Observe and correct
- Bird dogs: Observe and correct
- Cool-down: Static stretches
- Closure

ADVANCED ROUTINE

Introduction

- Review of body parts
- Review of muscle groups

Warm-up: Dynamic stretches (increase time)

Routine: This grouping of exercises are all in the supine position but will challenge students with the importance of keeping proper form and maintaining the ability to balance and stabilize their trunk. During these exercises, proper form of movements is not only crucial but also difficult to accomplish. Therefore, be sure to slowly introduce the movements, keeping repetitions to a minimum.

- Crunches: Observe and correct
- Bicycle crunches: Observe and correct
- V-sits: Observe and correct
- Bridges: Observe and correct
- Cool-down: Static stretches
- Closure

Upon completion of each stage, slowly introduce an additional exercise following a progression or increase the number of repetitions. Keep in mind that various types of workouts can also be incorporated, such as HIIT, as explained in chapter 2 or Tabata or a stacker, as explained in chapter 15. Such exercises will challenge students, staying within their level of readiness and also gradually increasing their fitness levels.

TEACHING TIPS

After receiving instruction in understanding the roles of the core, body parts, muscle groups, and exercises and their implementation, it is essential that student are successful in learning the fitness concepts. Whether the teaching environment is traditional, set up as a five-day instructional format, or is an alternative block schedule plan, it is necessary that all aspects of the core exercises are performed properly. Therefore, it is imperative that you become proficient when teaching them. Due to the nature and vulnerability of the trunk region, the prevention of unforeseen injuries needs to be addressed. When introducing each movement, be sure to emphasize what makes strengthening this area important, how it relates to everyday life, and what future implications it has for leading to a healthy lifestyle.

When introducing a core movement, each movement must be correctly introduced, properly modeled, and fully experienced. The gradual release educational approach of "I do it, we do it, you do it" is a great teaching method to implement. As the teacher, and due to the variety of levels of readiness, introducing a core movement may prove very challenging. Therefore, repetition and the ability to make corrections on an individual basis are important. Remember that form and technique are key, so students need to be slowly engaged into a routine. Based on their present fitness levels, be conscious of choosing movements that will easily flow from one movement to the next. Simplicity is what will keep students engaged and successful.

After close evaluation of students' capabilities, carefully choose a couple of core exercises that students can easily perform, utilizing minimal moving parts. For example, starting with double straight-leg raises and moving into alternate straight-leg raises will allow students to focus on the movement of one body part, the legs, executed from one position, lying on back, supinated. You will then be able to circulate through the class, observing the correct arm placements and providing continuous feedback of keeping the head and neck in a neutral position. As students go through the movements, you will also be able to visualize the proper ROM of the hips during flexion throughout the lowering and raising of the legs. As students perfect each exercise, continue to introduce another.

Keep in mind that the core muscle group is complex, and contraction of the abdominal region is difficult. Therefore, following some best teaching practices of simplicity, repetition, technique, flow, creativity, and engagement is key to success. Be patient, and soon students will be able to perform a full routine with proper execution and results.

CONCLUSION

Throughout this chapter, we emphasized the importance of developing core muscles to enhance athletic performance, physical activity performance, and activities involving everyday movements. As we introduced the essential core muscles integral to postural stability and balance, along with the age- and ability-appropriate exercises to strengthen these muscles, it should be noted that all of these exercises were performed without any weights or external equipment. If additional funds become available, items such as stability balls, resistance bands, and TRX bands can be included in the class activities without needing, or having access to, the school's weight room.

Upon completion of each core routine, it is always a best instructional practice to review the lesson taught from beginning to end, the information covered, and body parts and muscles involved. Emphasize that there is a possibility of soreness throughout the next couple of days, especially in the areas of the abdominals, lower back, and lateral sides of the trunk. Reassure students that this is a normal side effect from exercising any muscle, especially in the beginning stages of exercising. Recommend stretching and massaging those muscles as needed.

Be conscious that not all students enroll in a fitness education course for the same reasons, train with the same levels of intensity, or are at the same starting points. Whether physical, emotional, or psychological, make individual modifications and accommodations as soon as you see it necessary or when students feel that it is necessary. Any slight change in the movement will make students more comfortable and lead them toward success without feeling different from their classmates.

For extended learning opportunities, always attempt to guide your students to use concepts and principles outside the classroom. Reflect upon the relevance of the lesson and why this specific workout is important not just for today but also for the long-term. Review with students and probe for questions and answers through proper questioning techniques, both formal and informal. For example, "How would the core- and back-strengthening exercises assist you or your parents in everyday life?" It is important for students to understand the concepts and the importance of the workout instead of simply just going through the motions of the workout.

As teachers, we must have a continuous growth mindset and evaluate ourselves along with our students! We do that through the success and observation of students with the underlying belief that, through their efforts and hard work, they will reach higher levels of achievement. Throughout any lesson, the teacher should focus on whether or not they met their objectives, as well as the goals and challenges of students. Be mindful when planning a routine, making sure that the movements flow easily for students to transition from one to the next. If movements lack easy transitions, students may become frustrated or quickly fatigued and quit. In addition, engaging students in creating a routine or inviting them to implement some of their favorite movements will allow them to feel more comfortable and confident to try new movements and take part more consistently throughout the year.

Review Questions

1. Explain the importance of core muscles in balance and stability.
2. Identify the muscle groups that comprise the core muscles.
3. Select one exercise and identify the muscles that are engaged in that exercise.
4. Describe the negative impact of weak core muscles.
5. Identify a specific sports activity and explain how strengthening your core muscles will impact that sport.

Visit HK*Propel* for additional material related to this chapter.

CHAPTER 14

Lower-Body Muscular Strength and Endurance Exercises

Chapter Objective

After reading this chapter, you will understand the role that the muscles in the lower body play in the development of muscular strength and endurance for stabilization, agility, and power; know how to develop lessons that teach these concepts to secondary school students; be able to effectively demonstrate a series of exercises and exercise routines designed to strengthen the lower-body muscles; and employ best teaching practices that enhance student learning.

Key Concepts

- The strength of the lower-body muscles is essential to enhanced physical activity performance as well as everyday activities.
- The exercises presented will help you teach students to identify the muscles involved, understand the specificity principle, learn tips for executing the exercise, and gain the ability to strengthen their lower-body muscles.
- Warm-up and cool-down activities should be performed before and after lower-body strengthening exercises.
- Accommodations and modifications are recommended so that all activities can be modified and performed by all students in the class.

INTRODUCTION

Building strength and endurance in our lower body is essential for functional movements such as balance, agility, and overall stabilization of the body. Since our lower body comprises the largest muscle groups in the body, developing strong lower-body musculature provides for our base of support and gives us the ability to stand, walk, run, jump, and dance. Additionally, since the muscles of the lower body are essential for locomotor movements, they further serve to maintain healthy bones and joints, thus leading to the prevention of injury. Incorporating resistance training using basic body-weight techniques as part of a well-rounded fitness education program will contribute to the development of muscular strength and endurance of youth and adolescents (Lloyd et al., 2014).

The muscles of the lower body (see figure 14.1) comprise the anterior and posterior muscles; the largest muscle, *gluteus maximus*; the longest muscle, the *sartorius*; and one of the most powerful muscles, the *soleus*. The primary muscles in this simple locomotive movement are the *quadriceps*, located in the front (anterior) of the thighs, made up of a group of four separate muscles, the *rectus femoris*, *vastus lateralis*, *vastus intermedius*, and *vastus medialis*. The *hamstrings*, located in the back (posterior) of the thighs, are made up of a group of muscles, the *biceps femoris*, the *semitendinosus*, and the *semimembranosus*. It is important to note that, since there are four muscles in the quadriceps and three muscles in the hamstrings, in order to avoid an imbalance in strength, each muscle group must be addressed when developing a fitness routine. The largest muscle group of the *gluteals* comprises a group of three muscles that make up the buttocks, the *gluteus maximus*, *gluteus medius*, and the *gluteus minimus*. Finally, the *gastrocnemius*, the calf muscle, located in the back (posterior) of the lower legs, is primarily responsible for movements involving walking, running, sprinting, skipping, jumping, hopping, and sliding. The sartorius muscle, a hip and knee flexor, is also engaged to assist with these movements. As previously stated, the sartorius is the longest muscle in the human body, helping us to flex and adduct and rotate the hip. The sartorius works in tandem with the soleus muscle, allowing us to push off the ground when we walk.

These movements are incorporated not only in our daily lives and physical activities but also in the majority of sports. Although the legs are utilized in most athletic activities, it is the synchronization and strength of multi-muscular movements that are important. For example, sprinting and jumping are two base components in performing the long jump. Being able to gain the speed of running and the power and force (National Strength and Conditioning Association, 2015) to jump in order to propel the body is necessary in this particular competition. Volleyball is another example of a sport where lower-body strength, endurance, and power are needed to jump, spike, and block balls through quick and explosive movements. In soccer, players with a strong lower body are at an advantage during tackling and other player-to-player challenges (see figure 14.2).

Although several muscles comprise the lower body, enabling concise and gross movements, one of the beneficial functions tasked to these muscles groups is the prevention of injuries. As the body goes through numerous movements of flexion, extension, adduction, and abduction, to name a few, the area of vulnerability is the *joint*, the union of two or more bones. Specifically, the hip, the knee, and the ankle are the most commonly injured joints throughout our daily lives. Therefore, the knowledge of what each muscle does and how it does it plays an important role in planning exercise routines. It must be taken into consideration that the simplest adjustment in the foot placement changes the angle of that specific muscle, which, in turn, could be the difference of building the strength of that body part or injuring it at the same time. With that in mind, beginning with the easier movements of the larger muscles will protect the vulnerability of the involved joint.

As the physical education teacher, you can use the exercises in this chapter as part of a warm-up or cool-down, lesson on lower-body muscular strength and endurance exercises, or routine. Each exercise has a description and illustration, with notes about the type of stretch, the body part and muscle groups worked, steps for safely executing the stretch with good form, and accommodations and modifications for those unable to perform the stretch as described. Many stretches are illustrated with video in HK*Propel*. Teach each exercise separately, ensuring that students are performing the stretch correctly, emphasizing the type of stretch (static or dynamic) and the muscle group being engaged. This is extremely important because what students learn during this initial instruction will enable them to use the appropriate stretch for subsequent physical activities, as well as enable them to safely engage in routines and circuits throughout the class. We include guidelines for developing routines for the beginner, intermediate, and advanced levels after the exercises, along with further teaching tips.

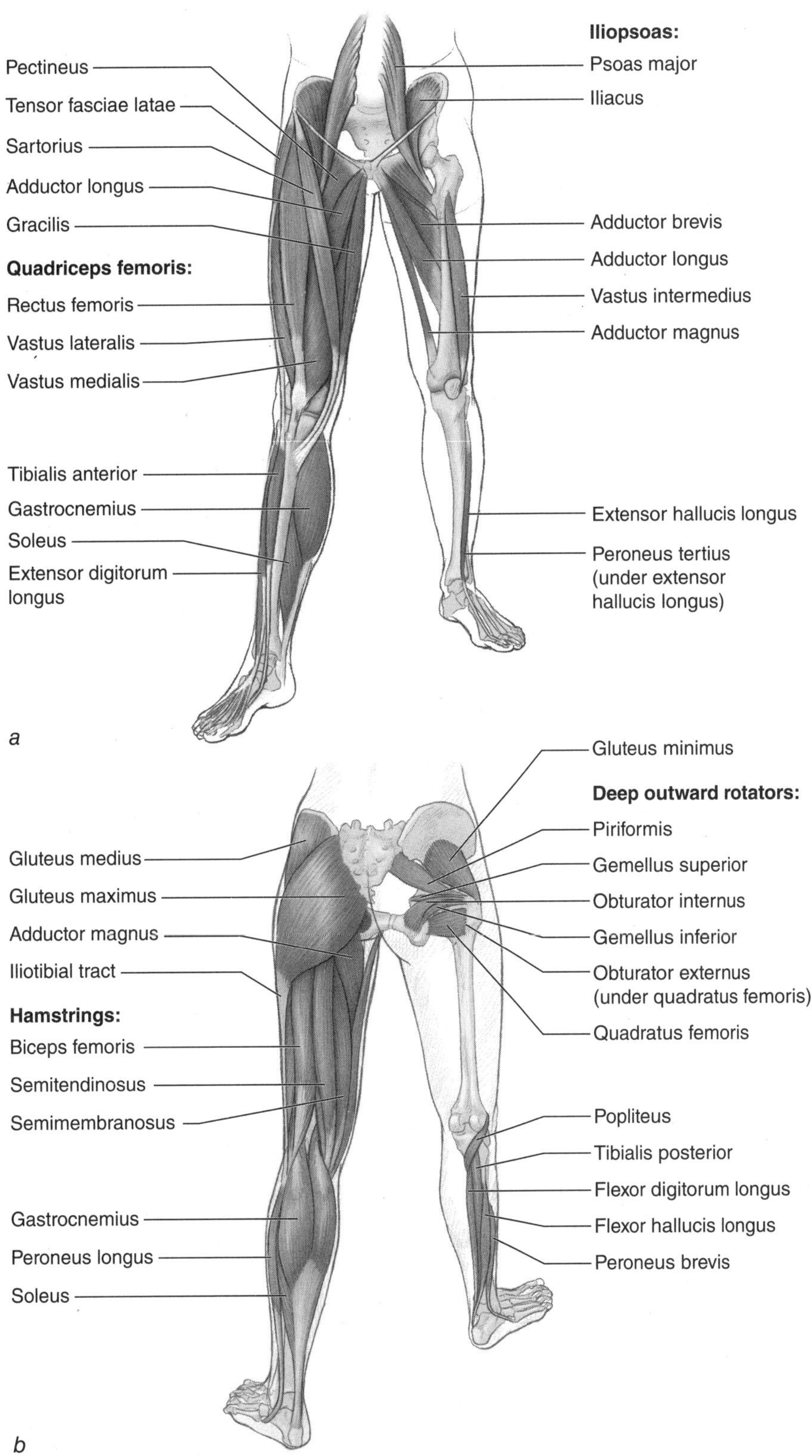

Figure 14.1 Anterior (*a*) and posterior (*b*) views of the lower-body muscles.

As you develop your daily lesson plans, align each lesson with the national standards and your own state and local standards so that every student taught in your class can participate in the activities. The following sample lesson overview shows National Standards and Grade-Level Outcomes (GLOs) relevant to this material, lesson objectives, and accommodations and modifications to be kept

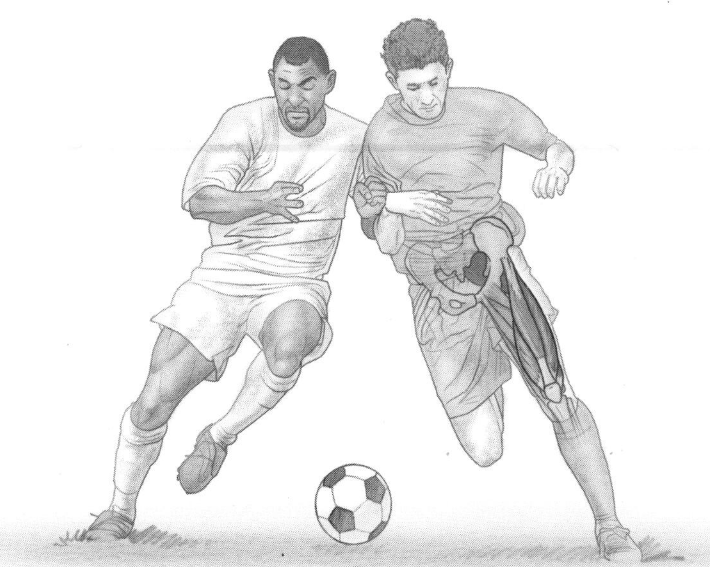

Figure 14.2 Increasing strength in the lower body will enhance performance in soccer, as well as many other sports.

in mind when teaching a lesson on lower-body muscular strength and endurance exercises. All of the exercises in this book are designed to provide accommodations and modifications as needed. This ensures equity, opportunity, and access for all students. Additionally, as you progress through your fitness education course, your students should be able to identify which stretching activities will be required for the daily activity you present.

LESSON OVERVIEW

Lower-Body Muscular Strength and Endurance Exercises

Lesson length: 15 to 30 minutes

Grade level: 9th to 12th

National Standards and GLOs: S1.H3, S2.H2, S3.H7, S3.H9, S3.H12, S4.H5

Grade level: 6th to 8th

National Standards and GLOs: S3.M6, S3.M7, S3.M8, S3.M10, S3.M11, S3.M12, S3.M14, S3.M16, S4.M7, S5.M1

Lesson objectives: By the end of the lesson, students will be able to do the following:

- Perform a warm-up routine using dynamic stretching that shows ROM in preparation for activity.
- Perform a lower-body muscle strength and endurance routine, showing proper technique throughout each movement.
- Perform a cool-down including cardiorespiratory activity and hydration.
- Perform a cool-down routine using static stretching that shows ROM in muscle-joint areas.

Accommodations and modifications: It is important for all movements and exercises to be modified to meet the individual needs of every student in order for them to engage in full participation. Implementing universal design for learning (UDL) will assist teachers in ensuring that all students can reach their full potential. Follow the general instructional recommendations, as discussed in chapter 3, for all activities.

WARM-UP DYNAMIC STRETCHES

LEG SWINGS

Dynamic Stretch

Body part: Hips

Muscle group: Hip flexors

1. Stand upright on one foot with hands on hips or arms out to sides for balance.
2. Gently swing opposite leg forward and backward.
3. Alternate between right and left sides.
4. Continue movement in both directions 10 to 30 seconds, or repeat the movement with each leg 10 to 20 times.
5. Stop, relax, and repeat 2 to 3 more times.

Accommodations and modifications: For students unable to perform this movement, have them begin with small pendulum swings and gradually increase when comfortable. Repeat movement for time or repetitions. For students with balance problems, have them put the opposite arm on a wall as they swing the opposite leg.

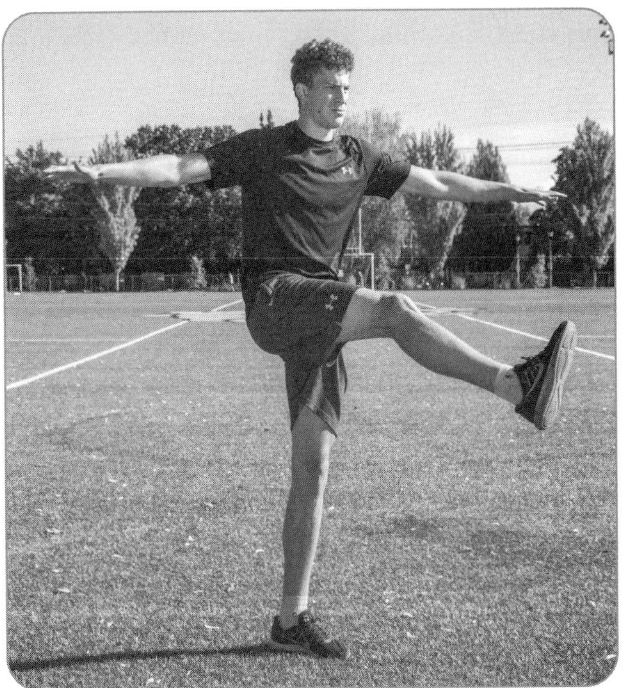

HIGH KICKS

Dynamic Stretch

Body part: Thighs

Muscle group: Hamstrings

1. Stand upright on one foot.
2. Extend one arm up in front of body, parallel to ground.
3. Kick leg up to palm of hand of extended arm.
4. Alternate leg kick and extended arm.
5. Keep trunk upright and opposite foot stationary on ground.
6. Repeat the movement from right to left 10 to 20 times.
7. Stop, relax, and repeat 2 to 3 more times.

Accommodations and modifications: For students unable to perform this movement, have them kick as high as they feel comfortable. Have students hold onto a stationary object (chair, wall, bleachers) with their opposite hand to maintain balance.

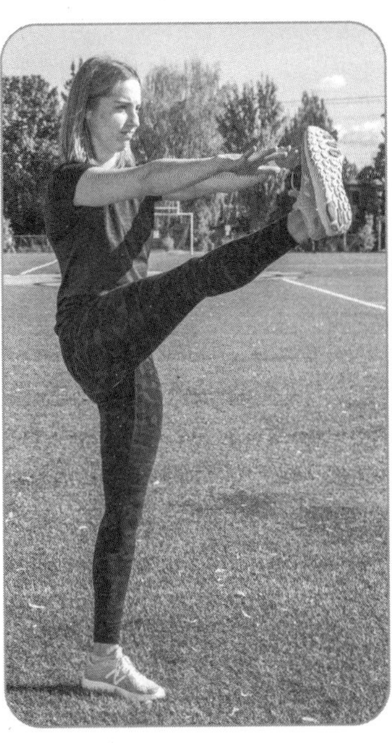

BENT-KNEE SIDE-LUNGE STRETCH

Dynamic Stretch

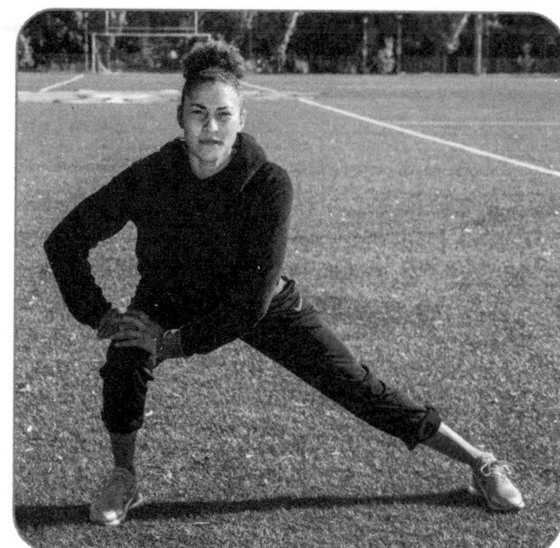

Body part: Thighs

Muscle group: Quadriceps, hamstrings, adductors

1. Stand upright with feet slightly wider than shoulder-width apart.
2. While bending at one knee in a squat position, extend opposite leg straight out to the side.
3. Place both hands on the top of the thigh of the bent knee.
4. Hold position for 10 to 30 seconds.
5. Raise back up to starting position.
6. Repeat the movement slowly, alternating from right to left 10 to 20 times.

Accommodations and modifications: For students unable to perform this movement, have them hold onto a stationary object (chair, wall, bleachers) with their opposite hand to maintain balance.

LOWER-BODY MUSCULAR STRENGTH AND ENDURANCE EXERCISES

Students will perform a routine consisting of 30 to 60 seconds per exercise with equal rest time between each exercise or the traditional routine consisting of 10 to 15 repetitions per exercise with ample time between exercises, increasing the number of repetitions as their fitness level improves.

SQUATS

Body part: Lower body

Muscle group: Quadriceps (rectus femoris; vastus lateralis, medialis, and intermedius)

1. Stand upright with feet shoulder-width apart and toes pointed forward.
2. Squat down slowly until thighs are parallel to ground.
3. Keep knees aligned with the ankles.
4. While keeping trunk in an upright position, extend arms in front for balance.
5. Hold for 10 to 30 seconds and then return to starting position.
6. Continue movement for time or repetitions.
7. Increase time or repetitions as fitness level improves.

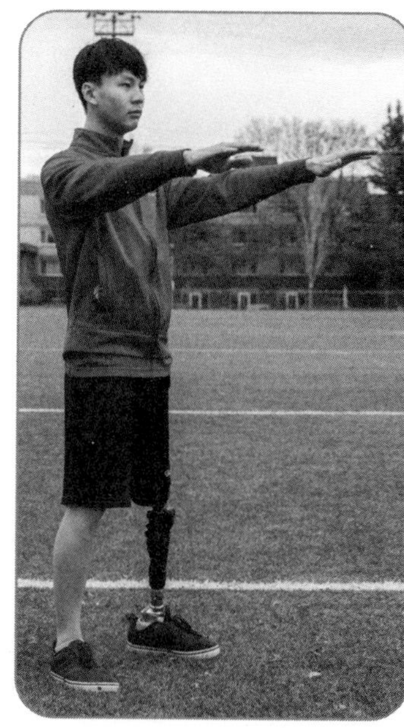

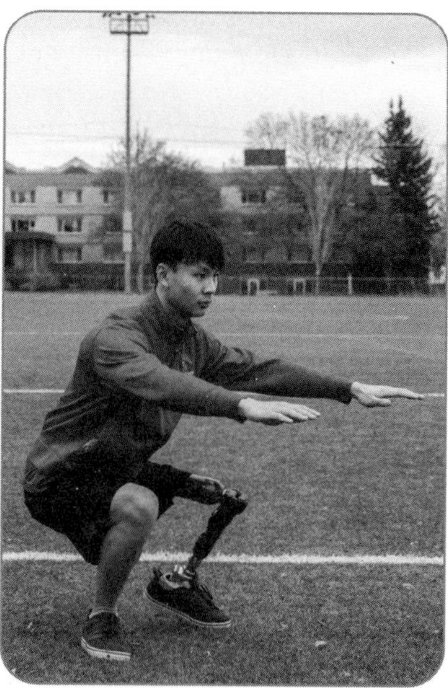

Accommodations and modifications: It may be difficult for some students to maintain the correct form throughout this movement, such as keeping the torso erect, heels in contact with the ground, and knees aligned with the ankles and not the toes. If so, allow students to partner, face to face, grasping hands and squatting together. This will give them the ability to lean slightly back on their heels safely.

JUMP SQUATS

Body part: Lower body

Muscle group: Quadriceps (rectus femoris; vastus lateralis, medialis, and intermedius)

1. Stand upright with feet shoulder-width apart and toes pointed forward or slightly outward.
2. Squat down slowly until thighs are parallel to ground.
3. Keep knees aligned with ankles.
4. While keeping trunk in an upright position, extend arms in front for balance.
5. Hold for 2 to 3 seconds.
6. Return to starting position through a jumping movement, using both legs and arms to explode upward.
7. Continue movement for time or repetitions.
8. Increase time or repetitions as fitness level improves.

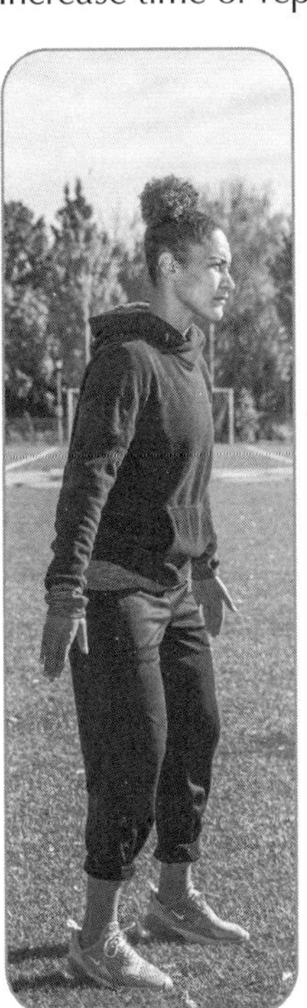
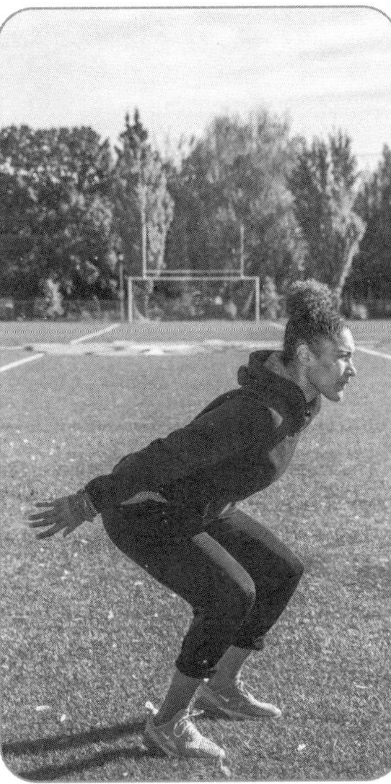
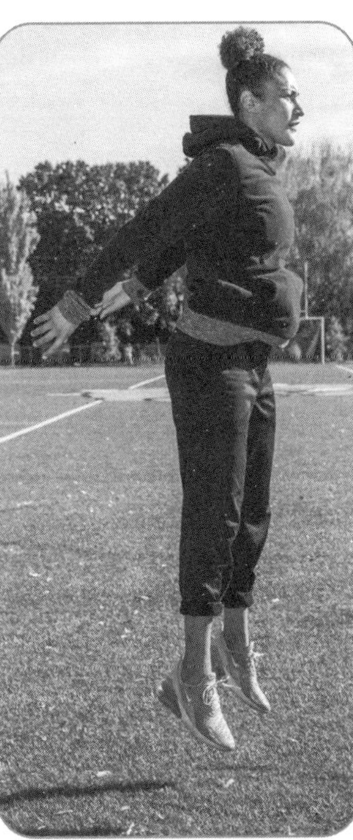

Accommodations and modifications: For students who are unable to perform this movement, follow the accommodations for squats and decrease the height of the jump so that their knees can better absorb the landing and to meet the ability of students.

SUMO SQUATS

Body part: Lower body

Muscle group: Quadriceps (rectus femoris; vastus lateralis, medialis, and intermedius)

1. Stand upright with feet slightly wider than hip-width apart and feet pointed outward.
2. Squat down slowly until thighs are parallel to ground.

3. Keep knees aligned with ankles.
4. While keeping trunk in an upright position, extend arms in front for balance.
5. Hold for 2 to 3 seconds and then return to starting position.
6. Continue movement for time or repetitions.
7. Increase time or repetitions as fitness level improves.

Accommodations and modifications: For students who are unable to perform this movement, follow the accommodations of squats and modify by minimizing the outward angle of the feet or have students go only as low as they can without pain or losing balance.

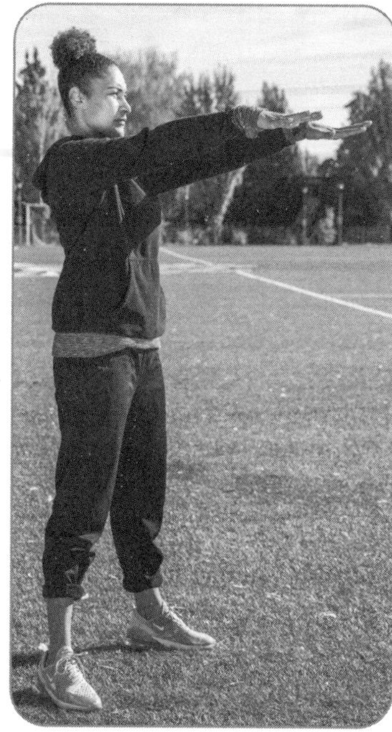

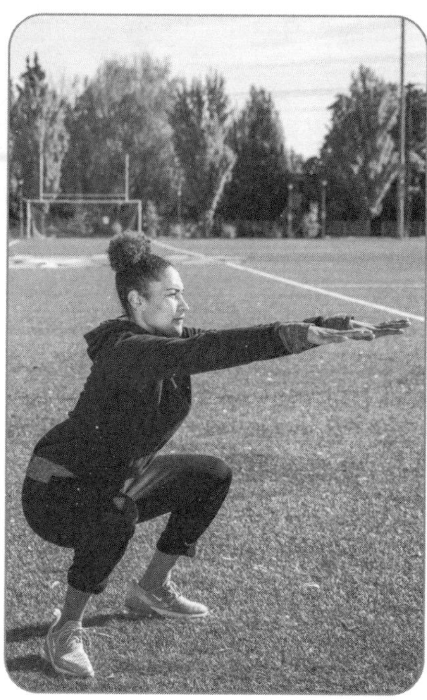

SPLIT SQUATS

Body part: Lower body

Muscle group: Quadriceps and gluteals (rectus femoris; vastus lateralis, medialis, and intermedius; gluteus maximus)

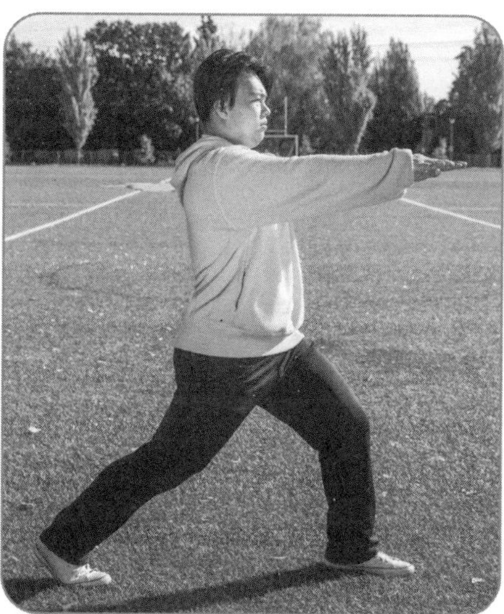

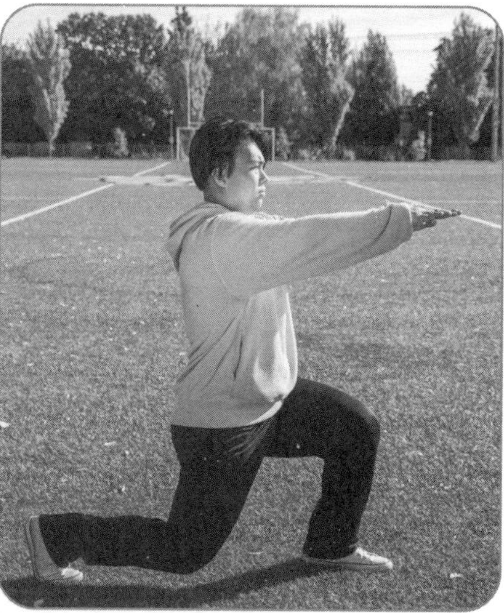

1. Stand upright in a split-stance with one foot forward and opposite back, maintaining shoulder-width apart distance.
2. Point feet forward.
3. Squat down slowly until back bent knee is about 1 to 2 inches (3 to 5 cm) away from the ground.
4. Keep front knee aligned with the ankle.
5. While keeping trunk in an upright position, extend arms in front for balance.
6. Hold for 2 to 3 seconds and then return to starting position.
7. Continue movement for time or repetitions.
8. Increase time or repetitions as fitness level improves.

Accommodations and modifications: For students who are unable to perform this movement, decrease the angle of the squat, without requiring the back knee to touch the ground. Adequate flexion of the hips and balance are necessary for this movement.

CURTSY SQUATS

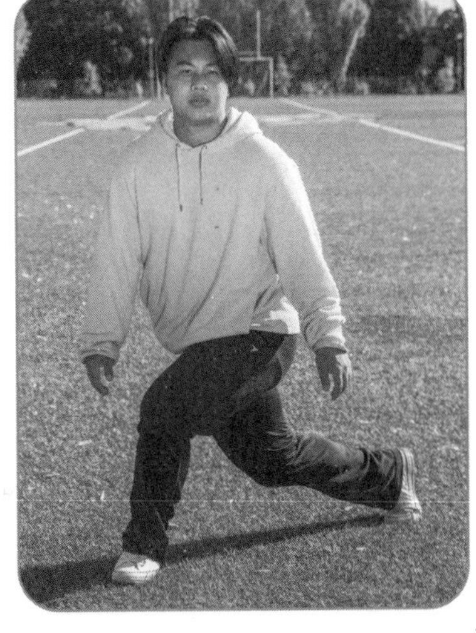

Body part: Lower body

Muscle group: Quadriceps and gluteals (rectus femoris; vastus lateralis, medialis, and intermedius; gluteus maximus)

1. Stand upright with feet shoulder-with apart.
2. Step one leg behind and across the opposite thigh.
3. Bend both knees, as if curtsying.
4. Keep front knee aligned with ankle.
5. Lower the trunk slowly, bending at both knees.
6. Return to standing position and repeat on same side or opposite side.
7. Continue movement for time or repetitions.
8. Increase time and repetitions as fitness level improves.

Accommodations and modifications: For students who are unable to perform this movement, decrease the angle of the squat, without requiring the back knee to touch the ground. Adequate flexion of the hips and balance are necessary for this movement.

Progression: To progress the exercise, try the Bulgarian splits squat.

PROGRESSION: BULGARIAN SPLIT SQUATS

For students who are able to master the curtsy squat, progress the move by introducing the Bulgarian splits squat. The major difference is that the rear foot is elevated, through the use of a bleacher, crate, or box. Adjustment increases the difficulty of the split squat because it challenges students' balance and places more of a weight load on their front leg.

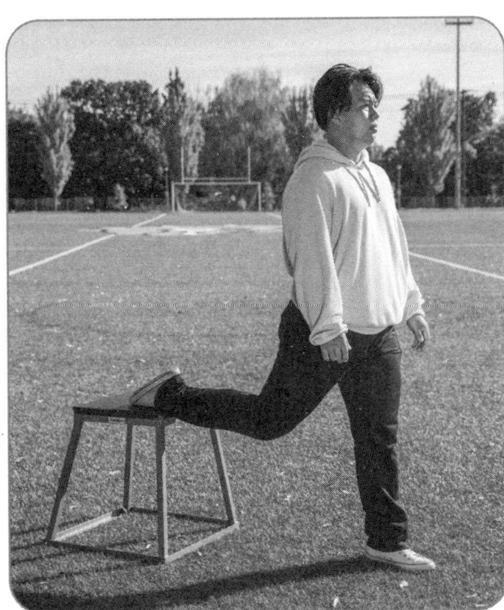

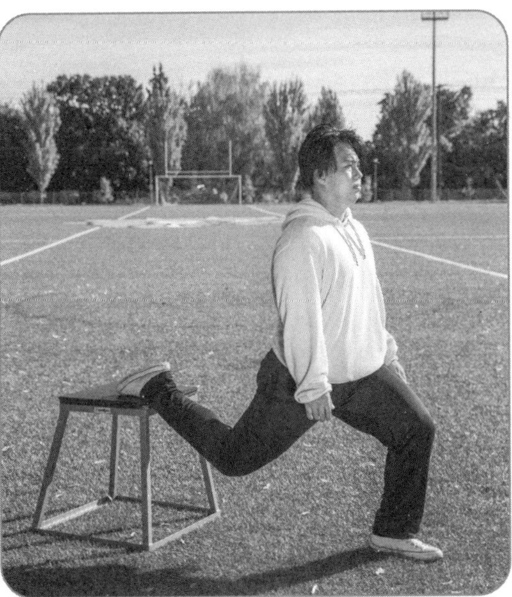

SKI JUMPS

Body part: Lower body

Muscle group: Gluteals, quadriceps, hamstrings (rectus and biceps femoris; vastus lateralis, medialis, and intermedius)

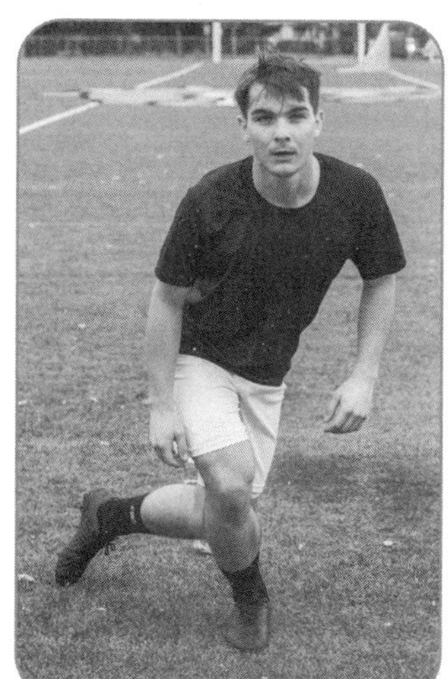

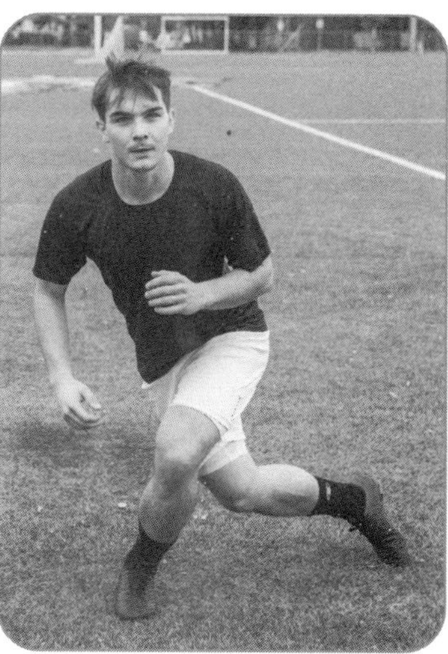

1. Stand upright with feet hip-width apart and toes pointed forward.
2. Slightly bend at knees and lower buttocks.
3. Take an explosion jump to one side, toward front and angled, as if skiing.
4. Land on one foot, lowering the body into a single-leg squat.
5. Take an explosion jump to the other side in the same manner.
6. Repeat movement, alternating sides.
7. Continue movement for time or repetitions
8. Increase time and repetitions as fitness level improves.

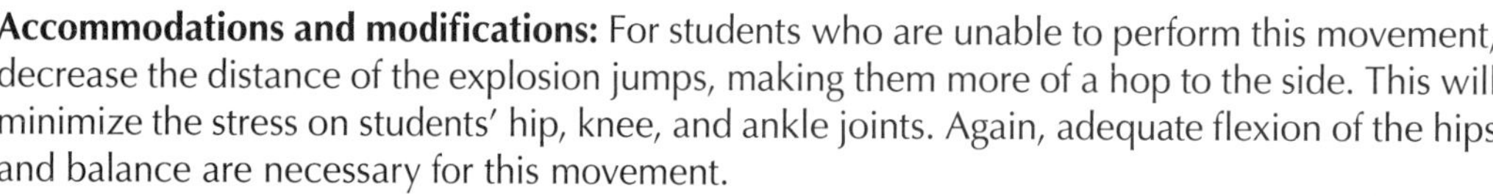

Accommodations and modifications: For students who are unable to perform this movement, decrease the distance of the explosion jumps, making them more of a hop to the side. This will minimize the stress on students' hip, knee, and ankle joints. Again, adequate flexion of the hips and balance are necessary for this movement.

LUNGES

Body part: Lower body

Muscle group: Quadriceps and gluteals (rectus femoris; vastus lateralis, medialis, and intermedius; gluteus maximus)

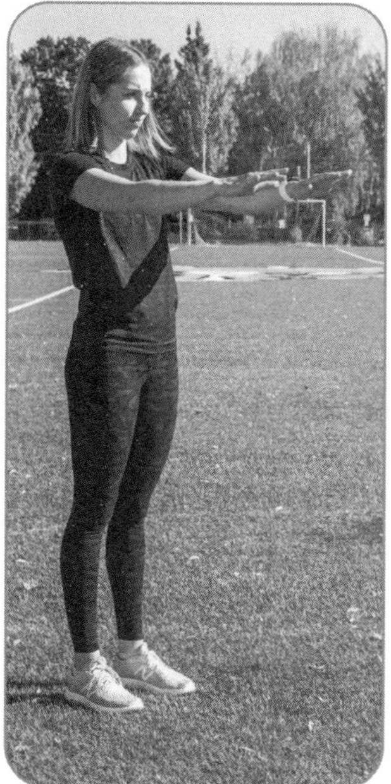

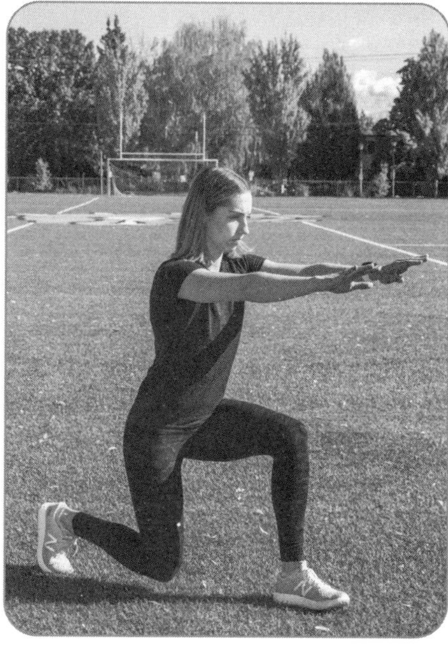

1. Stand upright with feet shoulder width apart and toes pointed forward.
2. Take a step forward with one foot to engage into a split-stance squat.
3. Squat down slowly until back bent knee is about 1 to 2 inches (3 to 5 cm) away from the ground.
4. Keep front knee aligned with ankle.
5. While keeping trunk in an upright position, extend arms in front for balance.
6. Return to starting position by pushing off the heel of the front foot.
7. Repeat with the same foot.
8. Continue movement for time or repetitions.

9. Increase time and repetitions as fitness level improves.

Accommodations and modifications: For students who are unable to perform this movement, shorten the stride length or decrease the depth of the lunge itself.

Progression: To progress the exercise, try the walking lunge.

PROGRESSION: WALKING LUNGES

For students who are able to master the lunge, progress the move by introducing the walking lunge. This movement allows students to transport from one point to another while performing the same exercise. This is a great exercise to implement within a circuit setting, when students need to move from station to station. It is still important to keep correct form and slowly continue movement for time or repetitions

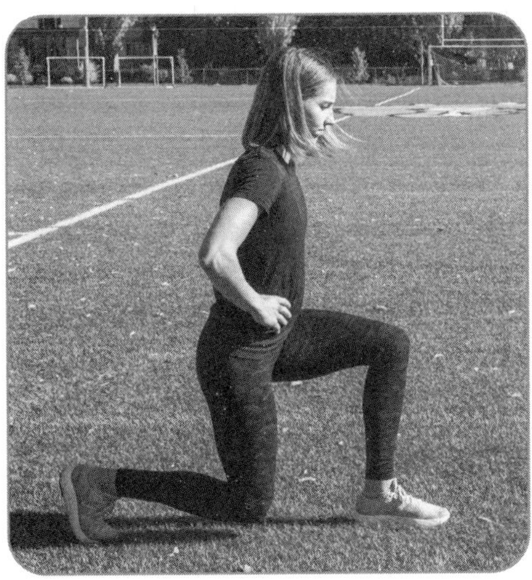

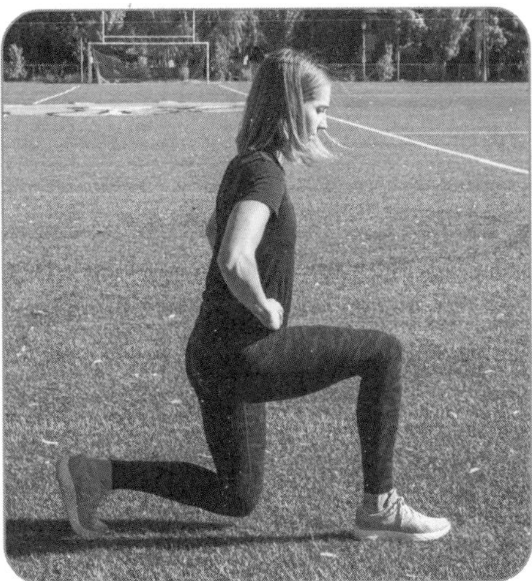

REVERSE LUNGES

Body part: Lower body

Muscle group: Quadriceps, gluteals, hamstrings (rectus femoris; vastus lateralis, medialis, and intermedius; gluteus maximus)

1. Stand upright with feet shoulder-width apart and toes pointed forward.
2. Take a step backward with one foot to engage into a split-stance squat.
3. Squat down slowly until back bent knee is about 1 to 2 inches (3 to 5 cm) away from the ground.
4. Keep front knee aligned with the ankle.
5. While keeping trunk in an upright position, extend arms in front for balance.
6. Return to starting position by pushing off the heel of the front foot.

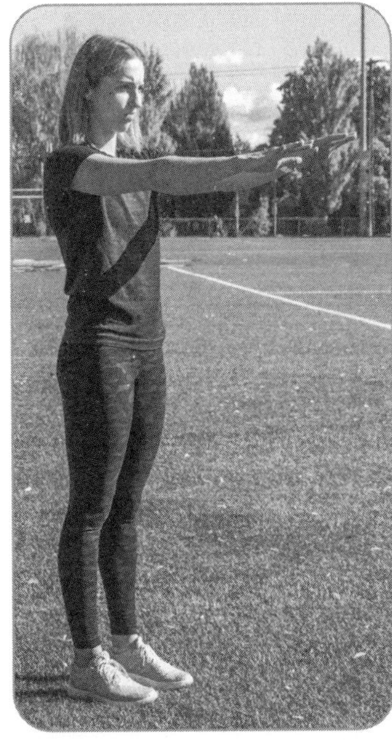

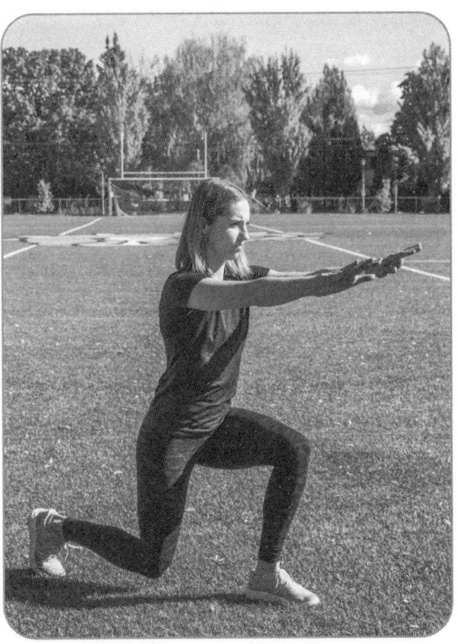

7. Repeat with the same foot or alternating opposite feet.
8. Continue movement for time or repetitions.
9. Increase time and repetitions as fitness level improves.

Accommodations and modifications: For students who are unable to perform this movement, shorten the stride length or decrease the depth of the lunge itself.

Progression: To progress the exercise, try the pulsing lunge.

PROGRESSION: PULSING LUNGES

For students who are able to master the reverse lunge, progress the move by introducing the pulsing lunge. This movement involves lowering and raising the body repetitively while staying in a lunge position, one side at a time. Keep correct form and slowly continue movement for time or repetitions. Repeat movement on opposite side.

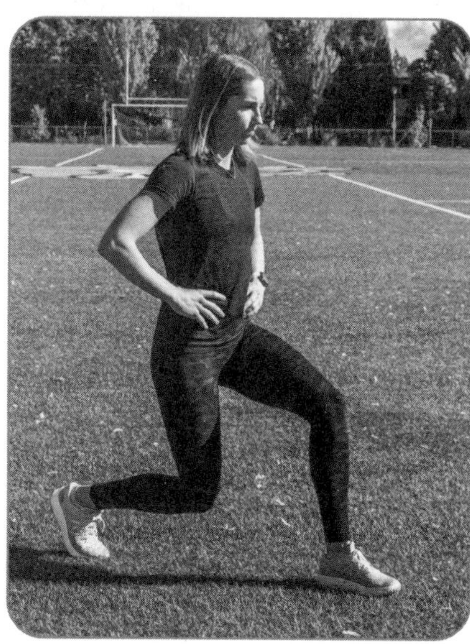

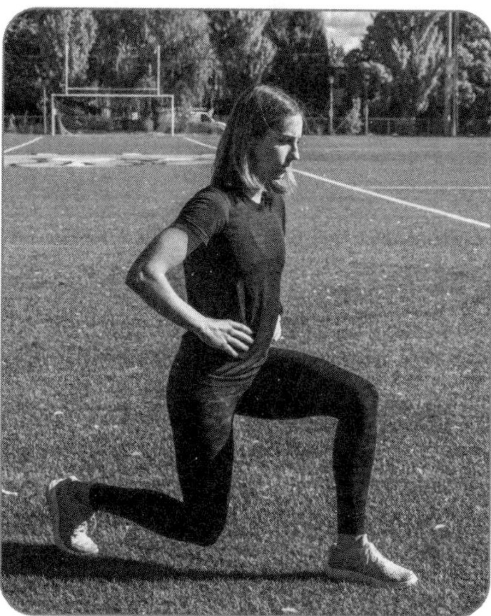

ALTERNATE LUNGES

Body part: Lower body

Muscle group: Quadriceps, gluteals, hamstrings (rectus and biceps femoris; vastus lateralis, medialis, and intermedius; gluteus maximus)

1. Stand upright with feet shoulder-width apart and toes pointed forward.
2. Take a step forward with one foot to engage into a split-stance squat.
3. Squat down slowly until back bent knee is about 1 to 2 inches (3 to 5 cm) away from the ground.
4. Keep front knee aligned with ankle.
5. While keeping trunk in an upright position, extend arms in front for balance.
6. Return to starting position by pushing off the heel of the front foot.
7. Repeat with opposite foot.
8. Continue alternating movements for time or repetitions.
9. Increase time and repetitions as fitness level improves.

Accommodations and modifications: For students who are unable to perform this movement, shorten the stride length or decrease the depth of the lunge itself. To increase the challenge, students can perform jumping lunges by jumping off the ground and landing on the opposite foot that they jumped from.

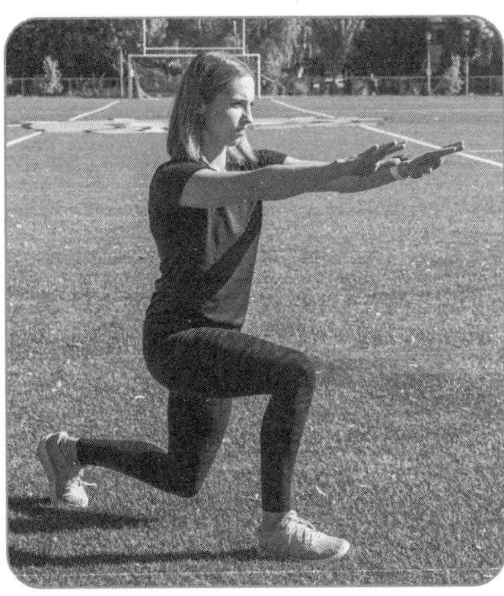
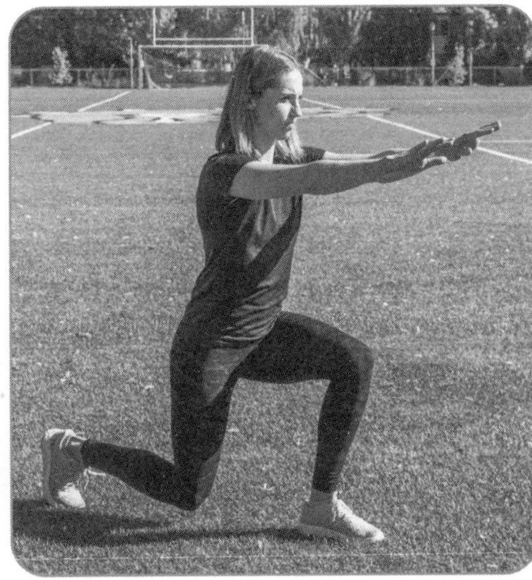

KICKSTAND DEADLIFTS

Body part: Lower body

Muscle group: Hamstrings and gluteals (biceps femoris, semitendinosus, semimembranosus, gluteus maximus)

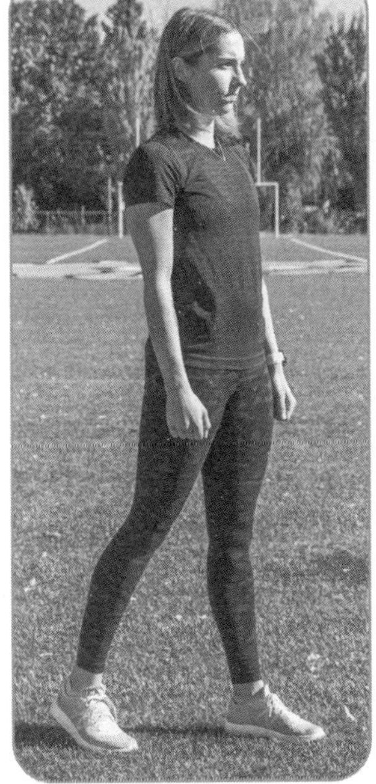
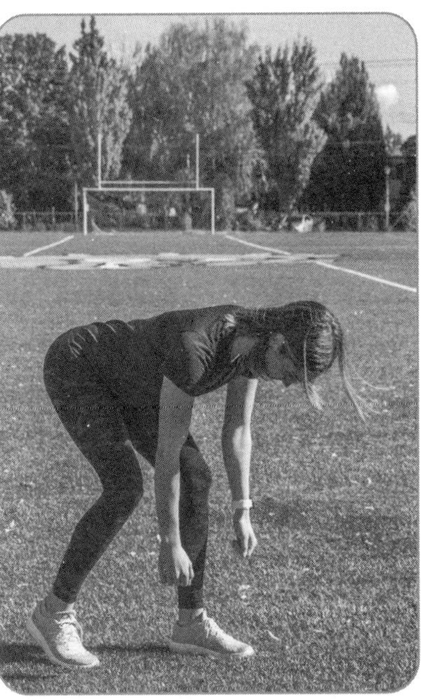

1. Stand upright with feet shoulder-width apart and toes pointed forward.
2. Take one step forward to engage into a split-stance squat while back foot is flexed and ball of foot is placed on the ground and knee is slightly bent.
3. Flex at the hips and slowly lower upper body forward until torso is parallel to the ground.
4. Return to starting position.
5. Repeat with same split-stance for time or repetitions.
6. Repeat movement on opposite side for time or repetitions.
7. Increase time and repetitions as fitness level improves.

Accommodations and modifications: For students who are unable to perform this movement, allow their front knee to flex and decrease the angle of the torso.

SINGLE-LEG DEADLIFTS

Body part: Lower body

Muscle group: Hamstrings, gluteals, erector spinae (biceps femoris, semitendinosus, semimembranosus)

1. Stand upright with feet shoulder-with apart and arms at sides.
2. While shifting weight onto one leg, slowly flex at hips to lower the torso forward, parallel to the ground.
3. Simultaneously swing opposite leg backward until the quadriceps are parallel to the ground.

4. Keep head, neck, spine, and raised leg aligned.
5. Hold at top of movement briefly.
6. Lower leg and raise torso slowly.
7. Repeat movement on same leg for time or repetitions.
8. Repeat movement on opposite leg.
9. Continue movements for time or repetitions.
10. Increase time and repetitions as fitness level improves.

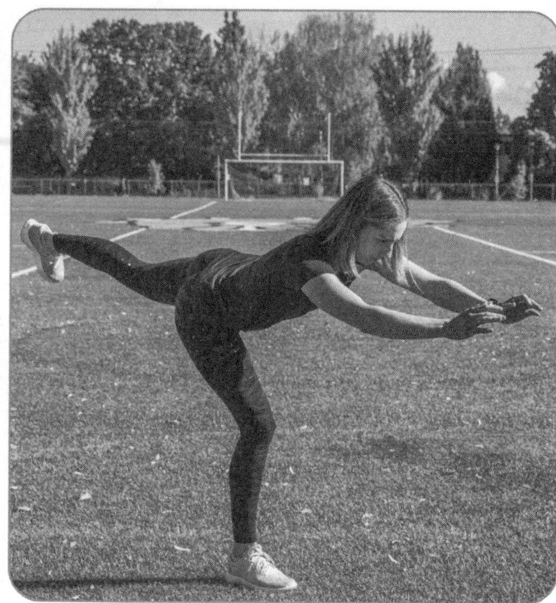

Accommodations and modifications: For students who are unable to perform this movement, increase the flex and decrease the angle of the torso.

HAMSTRING WALKOUT

Body part: Lower body

Muscle group: Hamstrings, gluteals, hip flexors (biceps femoris, semitendinosus, semimembranosus, gluteus maximus)

1. Lie on back (supine position) with knees bent and feet flat on the floor.
2. Keep arms straight and relaxed on sides of body.
3. Raise hips off the floor, aligning with knees and shoulders in a "glute bridge" position.
4. Begin to take small steps, on heels, until legs are in full extension.
5. Hold position for 2 to 3 seconds
6. Take small steps back on heels, returning to the "glute bridge" position.
7. Repeat movement for time or repetitions.
8. Increase time and repetitions as fitness level improves.

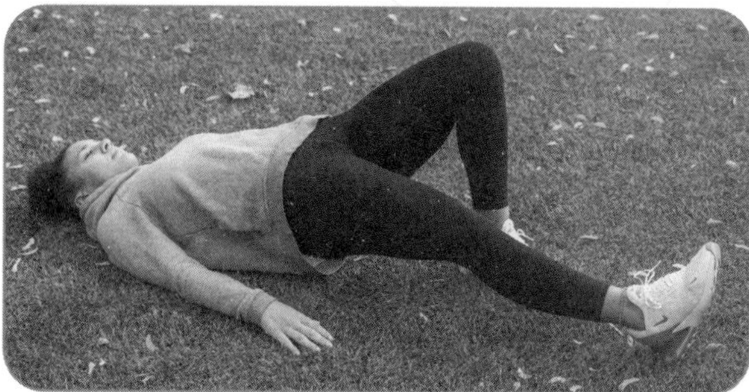

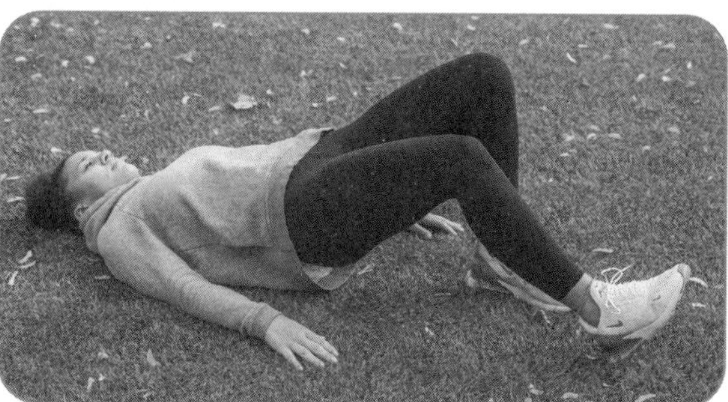

Accommodations and modifications: For students who are unable to perform this movement, break down the exercise into two phases: (1) Have students take small, flat-footed steps and refrain from maintaining the glute bridge position until the gluteals touch ground, and (2) regroup into glute bridge position and continue to take small steps back to starting position.

DONKEY KICKS

Body part: Lower body

Muscle group: Hamstrings, gluteals, hip flexors (biceps femoris, semitendinosus, semimembranosus, gluteus maximus)

1. Begin on all fours (hands aligned below shoulders and knees aligned below hips).
2. Keeping knee bent and same foot flexed, lift knee to hip level.
3. Hold for 2 to 3 seconds.
4. Return to starting position and repeat.
5. Repeat movement on opposite side for time or repetitions.
6. Increase time and repetitions as fitness level improves.

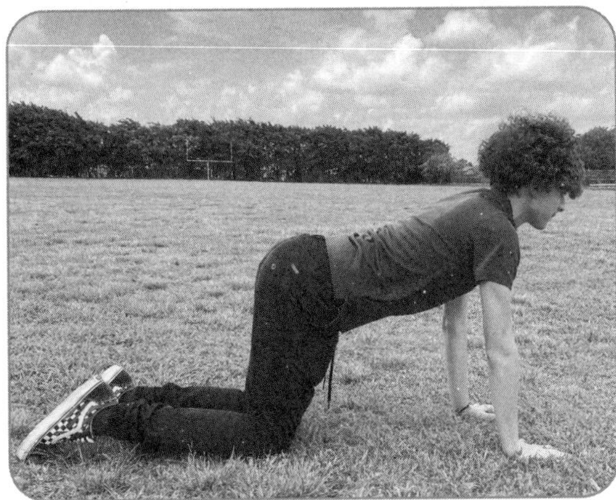

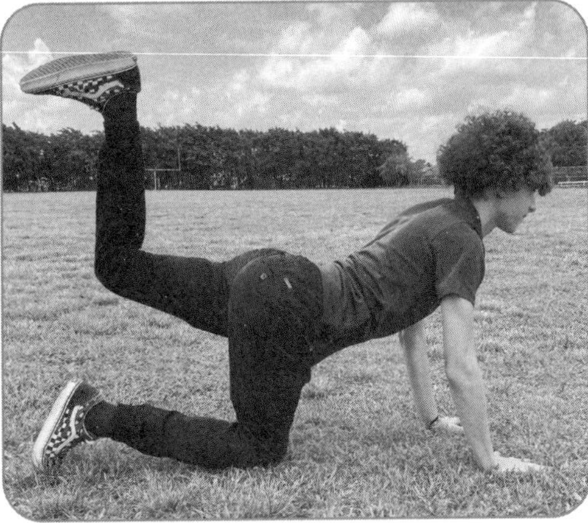

Accommodations and modifications: For students who are unable to perform this exercise, decrease the angle of the lift of the knee or keep the leg extended instead of bent.

Progression: To progress the exercise, try double leg donkey kicks.

CALF RAISES

Body part: Lower body

Muscle group: Calf (gastrocnemius, soleus)

1. Stand upright with feet hip-width apart and toes pointed forward.
2. Push up through the balls of feet.
3. Hold at top of movement briefly.
4. Lower body to return to starting position.
5. Repeat and continue movement for time or repetitions.
6. Increase time and repetitions as fitness level improves.

Accommodations and modifications: For students who are unable to perform this movement, allow students to partner, face to face, grasping hands and performing the movement together. This will provide them with the ability to keep their balance and feel safe.

Progression: To progress the exercise, try the bent-knee calf raise.

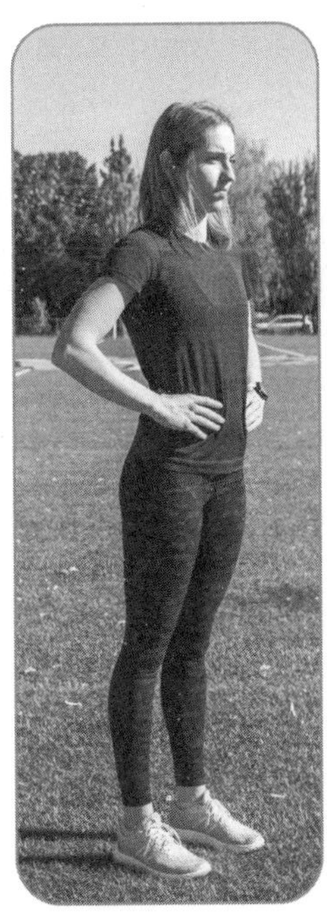

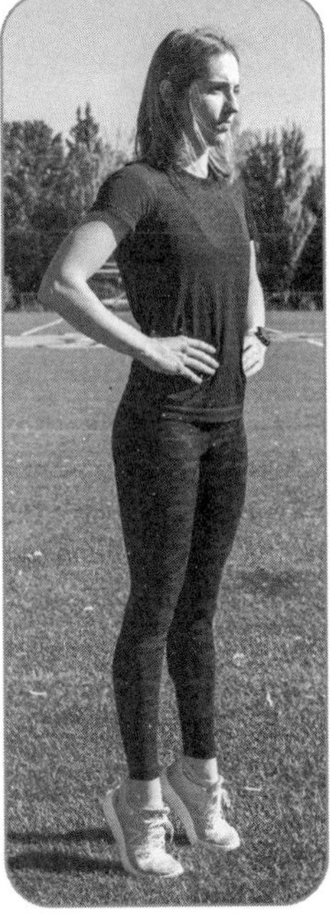

PROGRESSION: BENT-KNEE CALF RAISES

For students who are able to master the calf raise, progress the move by introducing the bent-knee calf raise. Slightly bending or flexing the knees will target the soleus muscle more. Again, balance may be an issue, so it is important to keep correct form and slowly continue movement for time or repetitions.

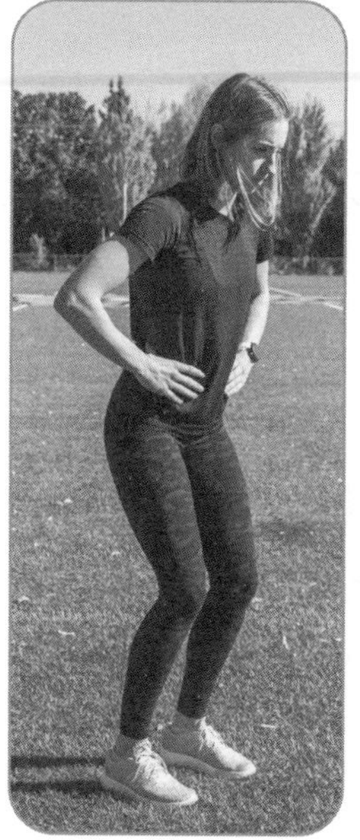

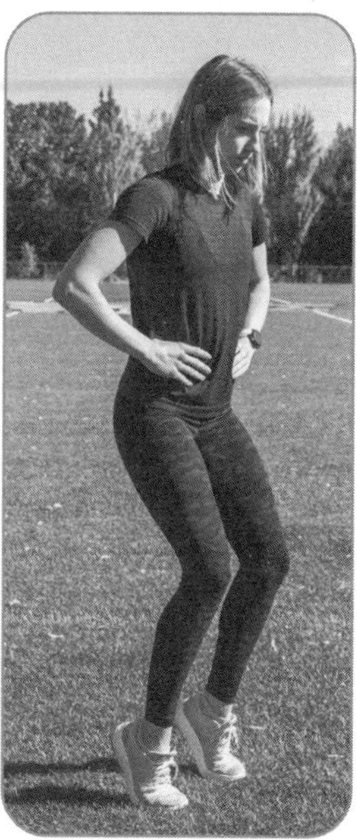

SINGLE-LEG CALF RAISES

Body part: Lower body

Muscle group: Calves (gastrocnemius, soleus)

1. Stand upright with feet hip-width apart and toes pointed forward.
2. Slightly raise one foot off the ground, placing all body weight on opposite leg.
3. Push up through the ball of the foot.
4. Hold at top of movement briefly.
5. Lower body to return to starting position.
6. Repeat movement on opposite leg for time or repetitions.
7. Increase time and repetitions as fitness level improves.

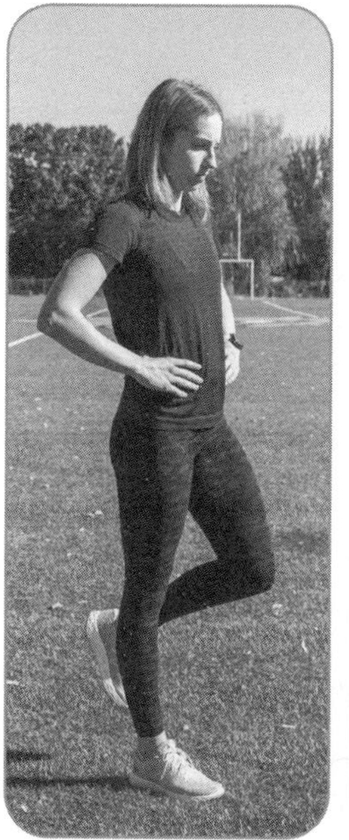

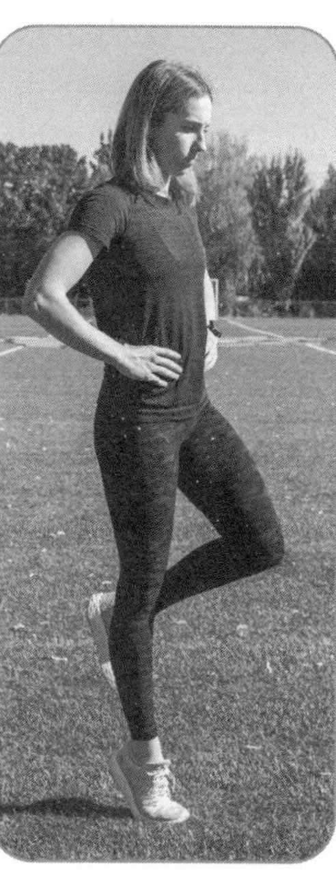

Accommodations and modifications: For students who are unable to perform this movement, allow students to partner, face to face, grasping hands and performing the movement together. This will provide them with the ability to keep their balance and feel safe.

COOL-DOWN STATIC STRETCHES

SUMO SQUAT STRETCH

Static Stretch

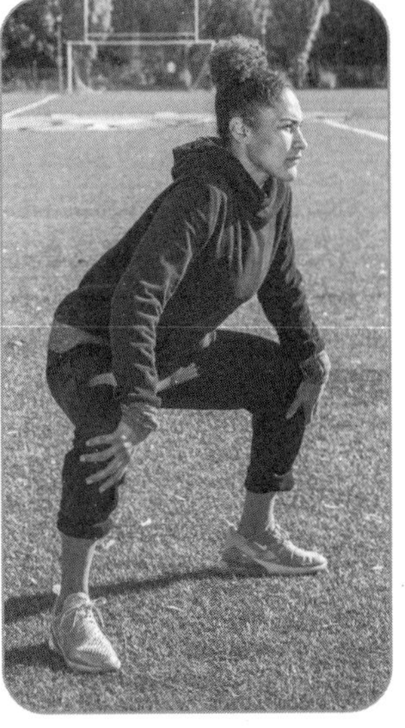

Body part: Lower body

Muscle group: Quadriceps, adductors, gluteals

1. Stand upright with feet more than shoulder-width apart and feet pointed outward.
2. While keeping trunk straight, lower torso until thighs are horizontal to the ground.
3. Place hands on knees.
4. Hold position for time.
5. Return to starting position.
6. Repeat 3 to 4 times.

HIP ROTATOR AND EXTENSOR STRETCH

Static Stretch

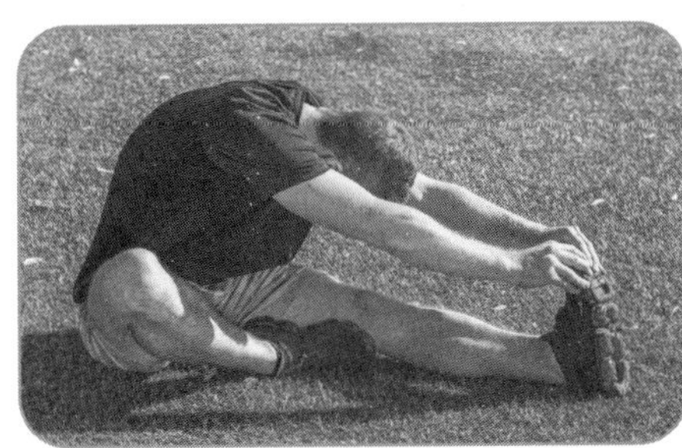

Body part: Lower body

Muscle group: Gluteals, quadriceps, gastrocnemius

1. Sit with one leg extended straight out in front.
2. Bend opposite leg, placing the bottom of foot against inner thigh of the straight leg.
3. Reach up with both arms and bend over toward foot of the straight leg.
4. Reach as far as comfortable and hold position for time.
5. Return to starting position.
6. Repeat on other side.
7. While holding position, dorsiflex foot (pull toes toward knee) to engage a stretch in the gastrocnemius muscle (calf).

HIP ADDUCTOR STRETCH

Static Stretch

Body part: Lower body

Muscle group: Adductors and gluteals

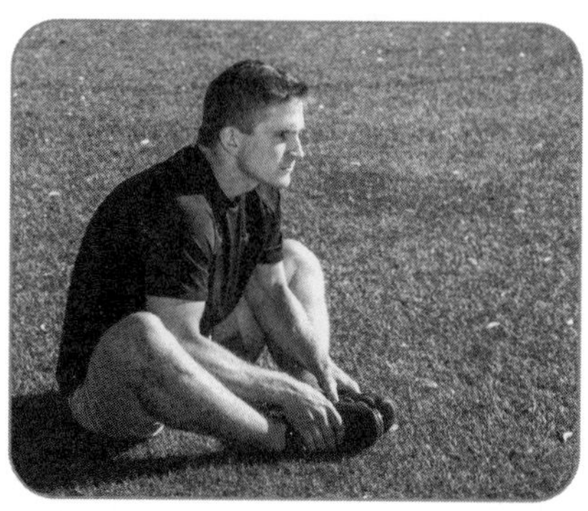

1. Sit on floor with knees bent, bringing the bottoms of both feet together.
2. Slide heels of both feet in toward body.
3. While grasping both feet, position each elbow outward, touching each leg below the knees.
4. Flex and bend at hips while leaning toward feet.
5. Gently press thighs down with elbows.
6. Hold for time and repeat 3 to 4 times.
7. Do not bounce (ballistic).

SEATED KNEE FLEXOR STRETCH

Static Stretch

Body part: Lower body

Muscle group: Gluteals, hamstrings, gastrocnemius

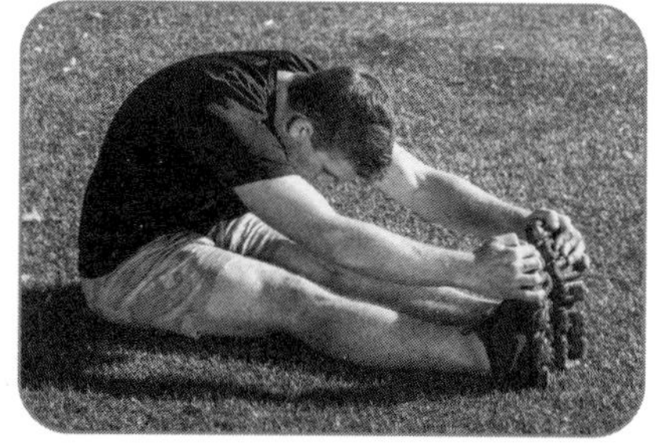

1. While seated, extend both legs, bringing feet together, and place hands on each side of thighs.
2. While keeping legs straight, slowly bend at the waist, lowering head toward legs.
3. At the same time, slide hands toward feet and hold for time.
4. Return to starting position and repeat 3 to 4 times.
5. While holding position, dorsiflex foot (pull toes toward knee) to engage a stretch in the gastrocnemius muscle (calf).

ROUTINES: STRINGING THEM TOGETHER

Upon completion of the lower-body exercises, students have now had some knowledge and practice of each body part and the major muscles taught. With the knowledge that individual students will be at different levels of readiness within the same class, introduce each task in its simplest form as you progress through the beginner, intermediate, and advanced routines. Continuously remind students to maintain structure, proper positioning, alignment, and discipline throughout every lesson. Use the following recommendations to get started.

- Model and practice each specific exercise, making sure that proper form and alignment is being performed.
- Verbalize the body parts, joints, and muscles being strengthened and stretched.
- Travel through the area, visiting each student and making corrections, if needed.
- Review and perform both dynamic and static stretches and muscular strength and endurance exercises of each body part until students feel comfortable doing them.
- Through time and repetitiveness, students will show their level of readiness to proceed to the next level.

Cool-down: Cardiorespiratory activity, stretching, and hydration.

BEGINNER ROUTINE

Introduction

- Review of body parts
- Review of muscle groups

Warm-up: Dynamic stretches

Routine: At this stage, full-body movement is limited, allowing students to focus on each exercise. Keep the duration of movement short or repetitions minimal.

- Squat: Observe and correct
- Jump squat: Observe and correct
- Calf raise: Observe and correct
- Cool-down: Static stretches
- Closure

INTERMEDIATE ROUTINE

Introduction

- Review of body parts
- Review of muscle groups

Warm-up: Dynamic stretches (increase time)

Routine: Students will be engaged in squats that incorporate the repositioning of the feet, while still needing to maintain form and balance.

- Split squat: Observe and correct
- Sumo squat: Observe and correct
- Curtsy squat: Observe and correct
- Lunge: Observe and correct
- Cool-down: Static stretches
- Closure

ADVANCED ROUTINE

Introduction

- Review of body parts
- Review of muscle groups

Warm-up: Dynamic stretches (increase time)

Routine: This grouping of exercises engages students to a level of being able to maintain multiple movements, balance, and proper positioning.

- Kickstand deadlift: Observe and correct
- Single-leg deadlift: Observe and correct
- Alternate lunge and reverse lunge: Observe and correct
- Ski Jump: Observe and correct
- Donkey kick: Observe and correct
- Cool-down: Static stretches
- Closure

Upon completion of each stage, slowly introduce an additional exercise following a progression or increase the number of repetitions. Keep in mind that various types of workouts can also be incorporated, such as HIIT, as explained in chapter 2 or Tabata or a stacker, as explained in chapter 15. Such exercises will challenge students, staying within their level of readiness and also gradually increasing their fitness levels.

TEACHING TIPS

The lower body is often taken for granted; many students assume that because we use these muscle groups every day through simple locomotor activities such as walking, running, jumping, and other basic motor movements, we do not need to work them out as much as the upper body or core. Although this is true to some degree, anatomically, developing strength and endurance in the lower body cannot be ignored. For postural balance and overall strength and endurance, the development of the anterior and posterior muscles groups of the lower body must be developed. When teachers assign their students to run laps for warm-up activities, they are in essence also providing a lower-body workout, which is a simple way for students to comprehend how all of the muscles need to work together to meet the demands of each task. Experiencing less fatigue and faster times will also illustrate to students the importance of developing the muscles of the lower body. The exercises selected do not have to be complicated, so be sure to keep them simple and to the point.

As mentioned throughout this chapter and book, introducing the anatomical properties of the body to students, while addressing the muscles of the lower body, will further enhance students' cognitive understanding of how the body works and how specific exercises will contribute to the quality of everyday activities along with advanced athletic performance. Teachers should continue to emphasize the reasons why the strengthening of the lower body is important and how it relates to lives on a daily basis. Throughout this lesson, it is imperative that each muscle is broken down. For example, the thigh is not just a body part; it is made up of the quadriceps, which comprise four muscles, and the hamstrings, which are made of three muscles. Although it may sound complicated to students at first, it is up to teachers to simplify, practice, and repeat these terms throughout the routines.

Sharing knowledge of the function of the lower body will keep students actively engaged as they perform movements. Remind students that strengthening the muscles in the lower body will bring stability to joints—the hips, knees, and ankles—which may trigger thoughts of a previous injury experience. Therefore, the importance of developing all the individual muscles in the lower body may prevent a common injury, such as meniscus tear in the knee or a sprained ankle.

As always, teachers need to be mindful of the fitness levels of individual students and slowly introduce one movement at a time. Although the movements of the lower body seem simple, be sure to pay close attention to proper form and range of motion throughout each exercise. The incorrect positioning of the feet or misalignment of the knees with the ankles during a squat could cause injury or knee pain. This will discourage students from wanting to revisit the lesson.

Teachers should always begin with the basic exercise and progressively advance to more difficult variations of the exercise when students are ready. Conversely, if students have difficulty performing the exercise, then teachers should allow for accommodations or modifications to ensure that all students have a successful experience while achieving the objectives of the lesson. Teachers should also be cognizant of the size of the class, the class format, and the comfort levels of individual students performing the activity, as discussed in chapter 4.

CONCLUSION

As in every chapter, it is important to review, discuss, and share what was taught, what was experienced, and how the movements will carry over into our daily lives. Remember, although our lower bodies are used as a transportation tool, the breakdown of the muscles worked throughout the routines may lead to soreness within the first few days of implementing the workouts. To keep students motivated, and avoid discouragement, assure them that this is normal and to review the stretches that took place in the lesson. Recommend that additional stretching helps to both prevent and alleviate initial soreness.

Always review and reflect after each lesson. Now that we have come to the last chapter of the strength and endurance unit, continue to make the connections with prior chapters so that students can further understand that the body works in synchronization as well as in isolation with select muscle groups. Probe for prior knowledge and discuss how everything is relevant to what they learned each day. The body is an incredible machine and the more we know about it, the better we can take care of it. Guiding students to utilize concepts and principles outside the classroom will give them the confidence to do it on their own and share it with others, making fitness a lifelong habit.

Although accommodations, modifications, and progressions were addressed in each of these chapters, the accomplishments of every student should be celebrated. As seen thus far, physical readiness varies within the classroom. Whether it is due to age, gender, or lack of confidence or experience, it is the responsibility of teachers to make all students feel good about themselves and successful. This is why the evaluation of each lesson of each class is a major component. Teachers may find that it is not possible to input the exact same routine for each and every class. It is important to individualize the lesson, possibly spending more time on specific areas of the body until students are able to advance to the next level. Implementing a culture of discipline, observation, and correction is imperative and needs to be a constant throughout the course and school year. The quicker the adjustments are made, the sooner students will feel successful. Many times, it ends up being about those little feats that the whole class is cheering about and seeing that particular students are smiling. As teachers, it's seeing the light going on in students acknowledging their own accomplishments toward meeting their individual goals that reminds us that is why we do what we do!

Review Questions

1. Explain the importance of the lower-body muscles in balance and stability.
2. Identify the muscle groups that comprise the quadriceps muscles.
3. Select one exercise and identify the muscles that are engaged in that exercise.
4. Describe the negative impact of weak lower-body muscles.
5. Identify a specific sports activity and explain how strengthening your lower-body muscles will impact that sport.

Visit HK*Propel* for additional material related to this chapter.

CHAPTER 15

Implementing the Fitness Education Program

Chapter Objective

After reading this chapter, you will understand how to incorporate the fitness activities learned in previous chapters into a fitness education program during individual class sessions, identify the different types of fitness-training programs, design age- and developmentally appropriate circuits and routines for student participation, and employ best teaching practices that enhance student learning and comprehension.

Key Concepts

- Implementing a variety of fitness programs and opportunities will expand the fitness education program and keep students motivated.
- Activities selected for routines and circuits should be a part of the individual exercises taught to students in advance.
- Student exercise plans should be individualized and logs should be kept for students to monitor their progress.
- Appropriate warm-up and cool-down activities should be performed before and after exercises.
- Accommodations and modifications should be implemented following previous exercise recommendations when administering fitness routines and circuits.

INTRODUCTION

Regardless of whether you are implementing a fitness education course at the beginning of the school year or during the second semester, it's important for the physical education teacher to think about how to develop the course curriculum, entailing both fitness concepts and activities. It should be designed to be innovative, and motivating, and engaging for students to take responsibility for their own fitness levels while embracing positive fitness habits for lifelong health, fitness, and wellness. Having a solid plan in place to meet students where they are after a sluggish summer of sedentary behavior with limited activity, engaging students with limited fitness knowledge, or empowering the student-athlete to reach higher levels of performance are challenges physical education teachers face when developing a comprehensive fitness education program. Engaging students with something new and innovative, yet challenging, is the first priority.

During your first interaction with students in your new class, your goal is to determine what is making them tick, how they are learning, and what they are learning when it comes to health and fitness. Therefore, setting up a teaching and learning environment in which students will perceive their physical education class to be physically, socially, and emotionally fun and positive takes precedence. In other words, first impressions are crucial.

At this point, it is time to combine concepts and activities from all of the previous chapters, from understanding what a comprehensive fitness education program is and how to incorporate the health- and skill-related fitness components and concepts into it to incorporating ways to assist students in understanding the relationship between good nutritional habits to general health and sports performance. Take what you have learned and implement it into a unit of lessons that students will relate to, feel comfortable with, gain mental and physical results from, and be motivated by while participating in your class. Therefore, first and foremost, preparing students for each class will be beneficial for both the student and the teacher.

In preparation of each day, week, month, or semester, there needs to be an exercise fitness plan that includes the health-related components and training principles. Think of it as preparing students for a total fitness workout. Through daily routines, their bodies will be tested as to how well they are able to perform the fitness components as a whole. These will be applied through stretching (flexibility); fitness circuits and routines (muscular strength and endurance); and jogging, sprinting, or walking (cardiorespiratory endurance).

In a typical class environment, all classes will go through the daily managerial procedures of students lining up, taking roll, entering the locker room to change clothes, and then reconvening back to their teacher. This is where the fun begins. Following the format covered in the previous chapters regarding warm-up, activity, and cool-down, the educational concepts of fitness must be embedded into every lesson. Reviewing and repeating prior material of the principles of specificity, individuality, overload, progression, variation, and regularity is necessary so that students understand and grasp why such workouts are being implemented. How the physical education teacher implements the course will be contingent on a variety of issues to consider, such as the number of days per week the class meets, class size, the level of readiness of individual students and the class as a whole, and the individuality of goals to be met. For example, if the class meets three times per week, then incorporating the FITT principle allows the teacher to incorporate a workout that targets different body parts each day, thereby covering the total body. Whereas, if a particular class only meets one or two days that week, then a total-body workout may be more suitable.

Let's revisit that first day of class. In many cases, students have led a sedentary lifestyle involving little or no physical activity. Therefore, the challenge at the beginning of any semester is to enhance students' physical well-being as well as mental and emotional mindset. If the class is offered at the beginning of the school year, then it may take a bit of reprogramming students to shift them away from sitting around all day, watching television, playing video games, or spending most of their time on mobile devices. Nevertheless, the benefits outweigh the consequences of such unhealthy behaviors that put students at risk of becoming obese or developing diabetes, high blood pressure, depression, and heart disease. To put it simply, there are both mental and physical challenges to be met. How? Through a formula of careful lesson planning, physical acclimatization, conversation, and slow physical progression, students will adapt toward the expectations and requirements.

INCORPORATING CARDIORESPIRATORY FITNESS INTO ROUTINES AND CIRCUITS

Although cardiorespiratory fitness has been recognized as an important fitness component in several previous chapters, it is important to note that, through programs that address muscular strength and endurance as well as flexibility, you are also enhancing cardiorespiratory fitness. Remember, it is the teacher's responsibility to prepare students for all of the fitness evaluations throughout the school year, including the PACER and one-mile run and walk tests, as addressed in chapter 7. It is important for students to understand what this component of fitness is and how it is being measured. Once they understand why cardiorespiratory fitness is important, students will soon realize that they are enhancing their overall health and well-being, and not just a grade on their report card. Always keep in mind that cardiorespiratory activities should *never* be used for punishment.

Throughout the fitness methods of training described in this chapter, the cardiorespiratory portion of the workouts is well embedded and involves a locomotive element. For example, if both the warm-up and cool-down sum up to a half mile (0.8 km), between the rest of the workout, the teacher can be sure that the circuit workout covers another half mile through traveling from one cone to the next, in total, equaling one mile (1.6 km). This would be a more positive experience for students to experience than just running four laps around the track.

Be mindful that you are a teacher, not a coach. Emphasize that the goal is to complete the task safely, not compete as in an athletic competition. Always communicate with students and remind them that the activity is individualized and that there is no room for humility or shame toward this endeavor, only celebration of every accomplishment made, big or small. Positivity and encouragement are just two of the components that will motivate them to do more for themselves in and out of the classroom.

METHODS OF FITNESS TRAINING

Several methods of training can enhance student fitness levels while providing a variety of options to the physical education teacher. In this section, we'll briefly describe some of these methods: high-intensity interval training (HIIT); stacker; Tabata; circuits; and routines, or samples of full-body workouts. A sample workout is included for each method. Following these descriptions and sample workouts are two sample lesson plans to get you started on how to pull it all together.

High-Intensity Interval Training (HIIT)

As previously discussed in chapter 2, a high-intensity interval training (HIIT) workout is designed to increase the heart rate by repeated bursts of intense exercise followed by periods of rest or low-intensity exercise. This method enables accomplishing a number of movements within a short period of time. With the body-weight exercises explored in this book, HIIT is the perfect model that allows students to perform these same workouts at home. The workouts can be performed as part of a blended or flipped classroom model, implemented as a family fitness program, or maintained as a lifelong fitness plan.

HIIT Summary

- Quick, intense bursts of exercises, followed by short, low-intensity (sometimes active) recovery periods
- Keeps heart rate up and burns fat

HIIT Sample Lower-Body Routine

- 10 squats
- 10 high knees
- 10 curtsy squats
- 10 jump squats
- 10 alternate lunges
- 10 butt kicks
- 10 calf raises

Repeat two to three sets.

Stacker

This particular method is an interval routine beneficial for both strength and endurance while incorporating the cardiorespiratory component. This gives the teacher the freedom to adapt the exercises, making stackers suitable for the students. Stackers also allow for a full-body workout in a minimum period of time. A routine is made up of two to three sets, or stacks, of exercises based on the goals.

Stacker Summary

- Perform the first exercise for 30 seconds, then rest 30 seconds.
- Add an exercise and perform each for 30 seconds, then rest 30 seconds.
- Add third exercise and perform each for 30 seconds, then rest 30 seconds.
- Choose to replace the number of repetitions rather than seconds (one of each exercise, then two of each, then three, and so on).

- Complete all three sets in order to include the full body.

Sample Stacker Full-Body Routine

Set 1	Set 2	Set 3
Jumping jacks	Mountain climbers	Plank push-ups
Full burpees	Russian twisters	Shoulder taps
Ski jumps	Flutter kicks	Knee taps

Repeat two to three rounds.

Note: Caution to students that the words *stack, stacker,* and *stacked* take on a variety of definitions when researched. In the worlds of bodybuilding and weightlifting, the terms refer to the intake of sports nutrition supplements and how to group them.

Tabata

Originated in Japan by Dr. Izumi Tabata and his team of scientists from the National Institute of Fitness and Sports, Tabata is a high-intensity interval training that consists of eight sets of 20-second, fast-paced exercises followed by a rest period of 10 seconds. The difference from HIIT is the rest and work periods are generally shorter. If structured correctly and performed at maximum effort, this is only a four-minute session.

Tabata Summary

- High-intensity interval training with rest and work periods.
- Consists of eight rounds of high-intensity exercises.
- Specific ratio of 20 seconds of exercise and 10-second rest periods.

Sample Tabata Upper-Body and Core Routine

- Isometric presses: 20 seconds
- Rest: 10 seconds
- Full burpees: 20 seconds
- Rest: 10 seconds
- Swimmers arm jacks: 20 seconds
- Rest: 10 seconds
- Plank push-ups: 20 seconds
- Rest: 10 seconds
- Shoulder taps: 20 seconds
- Rest: 10 seconds
- Knee taps: 20 seconds
- Rest: 10 seconds
- Spiderman crunches: 20 seconds
- Rest: 10 seconds
- Superman: 20 seconds
- Rest: 10 seconds

Repeat two to three sets.

Circuits

A circuit is a completion of a set of exercises that aerobically and anaerobically targets the fitness components of muscular strength, muscular endurance, and cardiorespiratory endurance. This method gives the teacher the freedom to focus a workout on one section of the body or to integrate all of the body parts within one workout.

Circuits Summary

- Consecutive timed exercises are performed one after the other with rest time between each exercise.
- Five to 10 exercises target different muscle groups.
- Exercises are performed at each station.
- Students perform locomotive movement to travel to each cone (e.g., lunges, frog hops, crawls, skips, running).
- Students travel in groups, partners, or individually.
- Space awareness is important to avoid wait time.
- Set cones up in a traveling pattern. Designate the specific exercise at each cone.

Sample Circuits Full-Body Routine

- Jumping jacks
- Frog jump to next cone
- Plank push-ups
- High knee to next cone
- Full burpees
- Hop to next cone
- Mountain climbers
- Alternate lunges to next cone
- Curtsy squats
- Side shuffle to next cone
- Calf raises

Repeat rotation.

Routines

A routine is a plan of physical exercises to improve one's fitness performed through a pattern. An exercise routine is a series of physical activities that are performed in a fixed order. Each exercise session should follow the fixed order of warm-up, exercise, and cool-down. Within this generalized framework, the routine is also the order of each exercise performed within those three categories. Following a routine can reduce risk for injury because the routine progresses exercises in intensity. It can optimize the workout by making clear the expectations of what, when, and how for both the instructor and students since there is no stopping to think about what to do next. Exercises can address multiple components, such as cardiorespiratory endurance, muscular strength, flexibility, power, reaction time, coordination, speed, agility, and balance. This method allows for optimal instruction based on the environment and expectations of the lesson.

Routines Summary

- An overall exercise plan that incorporates several components.
- Space awareness.
- To be performed in seconds or repetitions.

Sample Full-Body Routine

- Sumo squats
- Curtsy squats
- Side lunges
- Swimmers arm jacks
- Plank push-ups
- Full burpees
- Mountain climbers
- Russian twists
- V sit-ups

Repeat two to three sets.

Note: Any exercise can be incorporated into the previously mentioned training methods found in the earlier chapters. Keep in mind that this is only part of a lesson depending on the objective. Be sure to include a warm-up and cool-down respectively to avoid injury.

SAMPLE LESSON PLANS

Following are two sample lesson plans designed to assist physical education teachers in getting started in developing and designing their fitness education class. The first lesson plan represents a traditional 50- to 60-minute class period, whereas the second lesson plan represents a 90- to 100-minute block class schedule. When designing a class that incorporates both health- and skill-related fitness teachers should refer back to table 2.1 in chapter 2 for additional ideas.

LESSON PLAN 1

Topic: Lower-Body Strengthening

Activity: Flexibility

Unit: Muscular strength and endurance

Lesson: Lower-body circuit routine

Lesson length: 50 to 60 minutes (traditional class period)

Grade level: 9th to 12th

National Standards and GLOs: S1.H3, S2.H2, S3.H8, S3.H9, S3.H12, S4.H5

Grade level: 6th to 8th

National Standards and GLOs: S3.M3, S3.M4, S3.M6, S3.M8, S3.M9, S3.M11, S3.M12, S3.M14, S3.M15, S3.M16

PHASE I: WARM-UP AND FLEXIBILITY EXPLANATION AND DEMONSTRATION

Setup: Students will line up in roll call for instructions.

Objective: Students will perform a warm-up routine through dynamic stretching showing ROM in preparation for the activity. Include a cardiorespiratory activity to prepare the body by raising body temperature and increasing blood flow to the muscles.

Activity: Warm up with a one-lap or five-minute jog. Then, repeat the following movements for 15 to 20 seconds:

- Arm circles (forward and backward)
- Arm swings (alternate arms)
- High kicks (alternate legs)
- Leg swings (forward and backward)
- Leg abduction and adduction swings
- Windmills

Focus: Body part + associated major muscle group + name of stretch = flexibility

PHASE II: MUSCULAR STRENGTH AND ENDURANCE EXPLANATION AND DEMONSTRATION

Setup: Students will form straight, even lines behind each cone.

Objective: Students will receive instruction on how to perform a lower-body muscular strength and endurance circuit (phase III) showing proper technique throughout each movement.

Activity: The teacher demonstrates each exercise in the lower-body muscular strength and endurance circuit, showing the proper technique and explaining the muscle groups targeted by the exercises.

Focus: Body part + associated major muscle group + name of exercise = muscular strength and endurance training

PHASE III: LOWER-BODY MUSCULAR STRENGTH AND ENDURANCE CIRCUIT

Setup: Students will be appropriately spaced behind cones to safely perform the exercises.

Objective: Students will perform a specific exercise at each cone (5 or 10 reps) and then perform a locomotor movement to travel to the next cone.

Activity: Students travel to a cone and do 5 or 10 reps of the designated exercise and then travel to the next cone using a designated locomotor movement. After a rest period, repeat sets as time and fitness levels allow. Complete the workout with a one-lap or five-minute jog.

- Jumping jacks
- Jog to next cone
- Squats
- Alternate lunges to next cone
- Jump squats
- Ski jumps to next cone
- Sumo squats
- Frog hops to next cone

- Curtsy squats
- High knees to next cone
- Alternate side kicks
- Butt kicks to next cone
- Calf raises
- Hops to next cone

Hydration: Take a water break!

Focus: Body part + associated major muscle group + name of exercise = muscular strength and endurance training

PHASE IV: COOL-DOWN AND FLEXIBILITY EXPLANATION AND DEMONSTRATION

Setup: Students will line up in roll call.

Objective: Students will perform a cool-down routine of static stretching showing ROM in preparation for the activity.

Activity: Hold each stretch for 15 to 20 seconds.

- Sumo squat stretch, crossover hamstring stretch
- Lunging stretch, kneeling hip-adductor stretch
- Seated knee-flexor stretch
- Calf stretch

Repeat each 3 to 4 times or as needed.

Hydration: Take a water break!

PHASE V: CLOSURE

Ask students the following:

- What is the difference between a warm-up and a cool-down?
- What is the difference between dynamic stretching and static stretching?
- What are the benefits of stretching?
- Which body parts and muscle groups did you work out?
- What is the difference between muscular strength and muscular endurance?
- What are the benefits of working out these muscles?
- How do you feel after the workout?

LESSON PLAN 2

Topic: Cardiorespiratory Endurance and Core Muscular Strength and Endurance

Activity: Flexibility

Unit: Cardiorespiratory fitness and muscular strength and endurance

Lesson: Aerobic fitness core routine

Lesson length: 90 to 100 minutes (block class period)

Grade level: 9th to 12th

National Standards and GLOs: S1.H3, S2.H2, S3.H8, S3.H9, S3.H12, S4.H5

Grade level: 6th to 8th

National Standards and GLOs: S3.M3, S3.M4, S3.M6, S3.M8, S3.M9, S3.M11, S3.M12, S3.M13, S3.M14, S3.M15, S3.M16

PHASE I: WARM-UP AND FLEXIBILITY EXPLANATION AND DEMONSTRATION

Setup: Students will line up in roll call for instructions.

Objective: Students will perform a warm-up routine through dynamic stretching showing ROM in preparation for the activity. Include a cardiorespiratory activity to prepare the body by raising body temperature and increasing blood flow to muscles.

Activity: Warm up with a one-lap or five-minute jog. Then repeat the following movements for 15 to 20 seconds:

- Arm circles (forward and backward)
- Arm swings (alternate arms)
- High kicks (alternate legs)
- Leg swings (forward and backward)
- Leg abduction and adduction swings
- Windmills

Focus: Body part + associated major muscle group + name of stretch = flexibility

PHASE II: COOPER TEST AND 12-MINUTE RUN-WALK PRE-EVALUATION OF AEROBIC FITNESS

Setup: Students will begin at a designated starting point. When using a track, teachers should place cones every quarter lap so that students can keep track of how many laps they run to the nearest quarter.

Objective: Students will be able to show their ability to complete a measured distance within 12 minutes by running or walking.

Activity: Cooper test and 12-minute run-walk pre-evaluation of aerobic fitness

Hydration: Take a water break!

Focus: Cardiorespiratory fitness; to measure the maximum distance covered by students during the 12-minute period.

PHASE III: WARM-UP AND FLEXIBILITY EXPLANATION AND DEMONSTRATION

Setup: Students will line up in roll call for instructions.

Objective: Students will perform a warm-up routine through dynamic stretching showing ROM in preparation for the activity.

Activity: Dynamic stretches: Repeat each movement for 15 to 20 seconds.

- Trunk lateral flexion
- Trunk rotations
- Windmills

Focus: Body part + associated major muscle group + name of stretch = flexibility

PHASE IV: MUSCULAR STRENGTH AND ENDURANCE EXPLANATION AND DEMONSTRATION

Setup: Students will line up in roll call for instructions.

Objective: Students will receive instruction on how to perform a core muscular strength and endurance routine (phase V) showing proper technique throughout each movement.

Activity: The teacher demonstrates each exercise in the core muscular strength and endurance routine, showing the proper technique and explaining the muscle groups targeted by the exercises.

Focus: Body part + associated major muscle group + name of exercise = muscular strength and endurance training

PHASE V: CORE MUSCULAR STRENGTH AND ENDURANCE ROUTINE

Setup: Students will be appropriately spaced to safely perform the exercises.

Objective: Students will perform a series of core exercises.

Activity: In the following core muscular strength and endurance routine, students will perform a series of core exercises for time of each exercise (10, 20, and 30 seconds at teacher's discretion and depending on fitness levels). Repeat 2 to 3 sets as time and fitness levels allow.

- Double straight-leg raises
- Alternate straight-leg raises
- Bicycles
- Heel taps
- Bridges
- Low planks
- Side planks
- Mountain climbers
- Spiderman crunches
- Superman

Focus: Body part + associated major muscle group + name of exercise = muscular strength and endurance training

PHASE VI: COOL-DOWN AND FLEXIBILITY EXPLANATION AND DEMONSTRATION

Setup: Students will line up in roll call for instructions.

Objective: Students will perform a cool-down routine through a static stretching routine showing ROM in preparation for the activity.

Activity: Hold each stretch for 15 to 20 seconds.

- Cobra stretch
- Child's pose
- Spinal stretch
- Single knee to chest
- Double knees to chest

Repeat each stretch 3 to 4 times or as needed.

Hydration: Take a water break!

PHASE VII: CLOSURE

Ask students the following:

- What is the difference between a warm-up and a cool-down?
- What is the difference between dynamic stretching and static stretching?
- What are the benefits of stretching?
- What is the objective of the Cooper test?
- What is the difference between muscular strength and muscular endurance?
- What are the benefits of working out these muscles?
- How do you feel after the workout?

Routines can be developed through modifications and accommodations for all students enrolled in your class. Sample routines can be seen in figures 15.1 and 15.2.

Chair Exercises
WORKOUT © darebee.com
3 sets | up to 2 minutes rest between sets
www.nhs.uk NHS choices
20 chest expansions
20 side arm raises
10 dives
10 raised arm circles
5 clockwise / 5 counterclockwise
20 overhead punches
20 punches

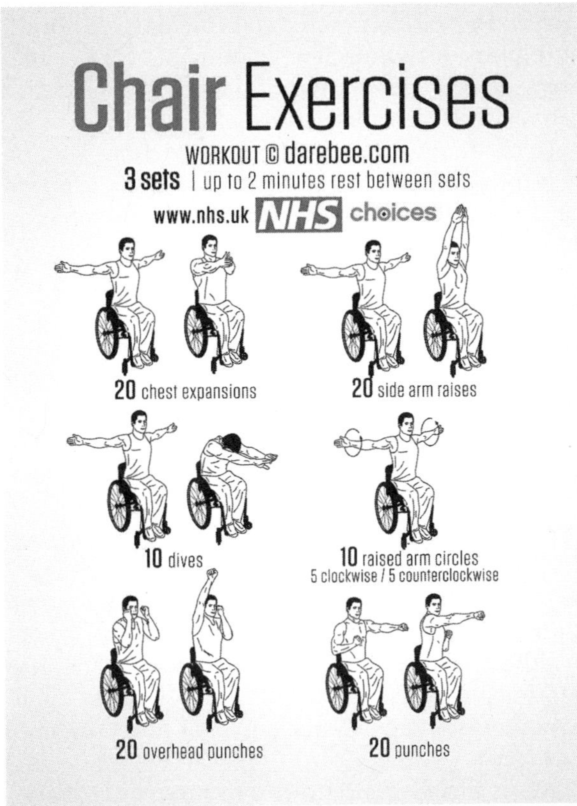

Figure 15.1 Chair exercise workout.

Use of the included DAREBEE illustrated workouts within this publication and attendant specified material with permission from the DAREBEE organization.

WORKOUT
© darebee.com
SUPER X
Level I 3 sets
Level II 5 sets
Level III 7 sets
Rest up to 2 minutes
20 chest expansions
20 side arm raises
10 chest squeezes
20 dives
20 twists
10 circles
20 overhead punches
20 punches
10 speed circles

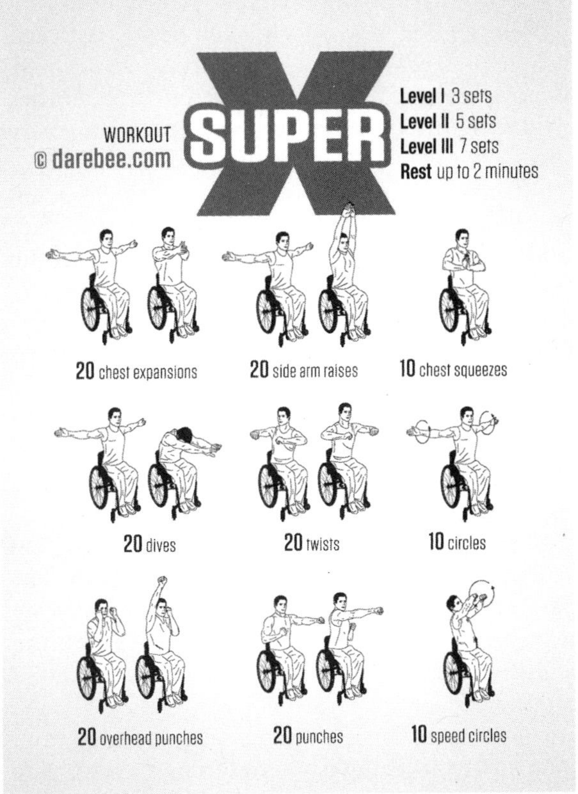

Figure 15.2 SuperX workout.

Use of the included DAREBEE illustrated workouts within this publication and attendant specified material with permission from the DAREBEE organization.

TEACHING TIPS

It's very important to keep things simple and fun. Start with the basics and associate everything done in class with prior lessons and prior knowledge, making connections of class activities to students' daily lives.

When preparing lesson plans, remember that any lesson is relevant to more than just that day, that hour, that moment; it is part of a series of lessons that will guide students on a road to success. A *plan* is a method of achieving something that you have worked out in detail beforehand with the intent to do it, so this suggests both intention and a long-term perspective for the teacher.

When designing a fitness plan, make the attempt to prescribe the workouts in such a way that each movement feeds off of the next one. Allow students to move seamlessly from one exercise to the other by placing the exercises in a sequence that easily flows.

Make sure students know what to expect when they come to class. Giving them an idea or peek of what is in store for the day will provide them the opportunity to prepare themselves both mentally and emotionally. This will set the stage and assist you, the teacher, as well. Simply writing the lesson on a whiteboard in the locker room will go a long way. You will find that this effortless task will result in better organization, time management, discipline, and direction of the class, leading to everyone's success.

As you begin to implement the class, consistency in delivery and constant motivation will encourage students to keep reaching higher levels. As long as students engage in the workouts and attain the cognitive knowledge within this book, they will continue to develop in some way, every day. As a teacher, you must embrace, acknowledge, and applaud their accomplishments. In most cases, they will ask for more, and you need to be prepared to offer that to them. Whether it is nutritional needs, weight management, or strength or endurance education, it is every teacher's obligation to listen to them and accommodate their needs in a safe manner. Positive motivation goes a long way in assisting students in developing their physical, social, and emotional development.

Last, but not least, the perception of the physical education class also needs to be a positive one. Learning needs to be everlasting; the atmosphere uplifting; the classroom setting exciting; and the mode of instruction an interactive experience, and always, an unforgettable one. More importantly, class needs to just be simple fun! Keeping students motivated, healthy, and active in every way possible is what this generation strives for, and they will want to return for more. All this will help them reach their individual goals now and throughout their lifetime.

CONCLUSION

Introducing each fitness component in a variety of ways through your fitness education course will help guide students to use these concepts, workouts, and principles outside the classroom and give them the confidence to partake in future fitness endeavors. Whichever method of fitness training chosen to be incorporated into the day's lesson is purely up to the teacher, making sure each and every student, no matter individual fitness levels, can relate to the exercises and attain achievement.

These daily routines will soon become part of students' practice, and little to no explanation will be necessary because the students know what to do and why.

Following the health recommendations of a minimum of 150 minutes per week of cardiorespiratory exercise, an activity that raises heart rate is a must to reduce health risks. When considering health risks that may affect the rest of our lives, such as cardiovascular disease, diabetes, obesity, and depression, versus the benefits of weight loss and building and strengthening of muscles and bones, the benefits of the latter outweigh the health risks. Constant reminders and reviews of the target heart rate are a great place to start. By knowing their resting heart rate and knowing their personal healthy target heart rate zone, the zone where they will burn the most fat and calories, students will have a personal challenge and goal to attain on a daily basis.

When incorporating cardiorespiratory exercise in the program, just about any movement will do, as long as it involves raising the heart rate into the heart rate zone. More importantly, how will it work with your class? Feel free to explain to students that cardiorespiratory endurance is not just running; it comes in many forms. We mimic cardiorespiratory exercise in several of our everyday activities, from walking, jogging, and swimming to biking, hiking, shopping, and dancing. Interpreting these simple activities as cardiorespiratory exercises may be baffling to students at first. To make the point clear, tell students that, when it comes to fitness, what counts is mainly how vigorously or intensely they take part in each exercise or activity.

Review Questions

1. How would you design a fitness circuit using exercises from each health-related fitness component?
2. Explain the importance of keeping a fitness log.
3. Describe what a stacker interval training would look like.
4. Explain a Tabata type of interval training.
5. Describe a method you would do to assist a peer who may need special accommodations.

Visit HK*Propel* for additional material related to this chapter.

Part III

Extending Fitness Education

CHAPTER 16

Extending Fitness Education Into the Community

Chapter Objective

After reading this chapter, you will understand how school-based physical education and fitness programs connect to the community; how to select appropriate community-based fitness programs; how to train for select races; understand the importance of group cohesion and exercise adherence; and how to ensure that all students enrolled in your physical education classes have an opportunity to be physically active for a lifetime through community engagement.

Key Concepts

- Community-based fitness programs serve as an extension to the school's fitness education program.
- Implementing a variety of fitness programs and opportunities will expand the fitness education program and keep students motivated.
- Training progressions should be followed to properly prepare for community fitness activities and competitions.
- Appropriate warm-up and cool-down activities should be performed before and after workouts.
- Accommodations and modifications should be implemented to provide for full inclusion in community activities.

INTRODUCTION

Participating in community-based fitness activities should be viewed as an extension of the physical education and fitness education program. Throughout this text, we have seen evidence of the immediate and long-term health benefits of participating in 60 or more minutes a day of physical activity, as well as the importance of being physically active across the lifespan. We've also seen how the physical education and fitness education guidelines are embedded in the National Standards for Physical Education and the Grade-Level Outcomes. This chapter will further convey how participating in community-based events, as an extension of the school physical education program, will align with the national framework for physical education and physical activity, the Comprehensive School Physical Activity Program (CSPAP), as well as the Whole School, Whole Community, Whole Child (WSCC) model. To make the connections in a collaborative manner, the overarching goal of this chapter is to provide innovative and creative ways for students to participate in community-based activities as a means of transitioning from senior high school physical education classes to physical activity for a lifetime.

CONNECTING COMMUNITY EVENTS TO SCHOOLS

Developing lifelong physical activity habits and maintaining a healthy lifestyle goes beyond the school doors. Introducing secondary school aged students to the opportunities that exist within their own communities is one way for them to continue on their journey for lifelong fitness.

The notion that the delivery of a comprehensive plan for fitness education and physical activity takes a coordinated approach is well researched and well embedded in national frameworks and models such as the CSPAP and WSCC model as described in the following sections. Both use a multifaceted and collaborative approach to promote and deliver physical activity, health, and wellness components to youth using the school as the hub.

Comprehensive School Physical Activity Plan (CSPAP)

As stated throughout this text and with the recommendations of several national and international reports, it is highly recommended that all children participate in 60 or more minutes of physical activity daily. Since over 95 percent of children spend between seven to nine hours a day at school, the school environment is uniquely positioned as the place for students to reach those activity minutes. However, it has become evident through the Shape of the Nation (2016) and School Health Policies and Practices Study (SHPPS) (2016) reports that nationwide physical education programs alone cannot provide the critical 60 minutes a day of physical activity, unless intentional minutes per day are provided and dedicated toward physical activity in the school environment. Building community and school capacity becomes a necessary component for expanding student physical activity to achieve the recommended goal.

CSPAP (see figure 16.1) has been recognized as the national framework for physical education and physical activity for young people (Centers for Disease Control and Prevention, 2014). The main goal of the CSPAP is to increase physical activity opportunities before, during, and after school and increase students' overall physical activity and health. More specifically, the goals of the CSPAP are the following (SHAPE America, 2013; Centers for Disease Control and Prevention, 2019; Carson & Webster, 2019):

- Provide a variety of physical activity opportunities throughout the school day, with a high-quality physical education program as the foundation.
- Provide physical activity opportunities both before and after school, so that all students can participate in at least 60 minutes of physical activity daily.
- Provide a variety of school-based physical activities to enable all students to participate in 60 minutes of moderate-to-vigorous physical activity each day.
- Incorporate physical activity opportunities for faculty and staff members, as well as for families.
- Encourage and reinforce physical activity opportunities in the community.
- Coordinate among the CSPAP components to maximize understanding, application, and practice of the knowledge and skills learned in physical education so that all students are physically educated and motivated to pursue a lifetime of physical activity.

CSPAP is a multicomponent framework that school districts and schools use to plan and organize opportunities for students to be physically active; meet the nationally recommended 60 min-

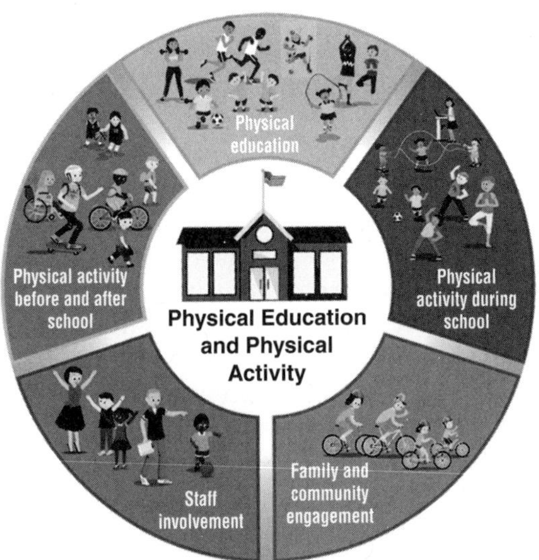

Figure 16.1 Comprehensive School Physical Activity Program.

Source: Comprehensive School Physical Activity Program (CSPAP). Cited in CDC Healthy Schools. https://www.cdc.gov/healthyschools/physicalactivity/index.htm

utes of physical activity each day; and develop the knowledge, skills, and confidence to be physically active for a lifetime (Carson & Webster, 2019). Through this model, there is coordination and synergy across all of its five components: physical education as the foundation of the program, physical activity during school, physical activity before and after school, staff involvement, and family and community engagement (Centers for Disease Control and Prevention, 2019). At the heart of the framework, physical education provides youth with the fundamental education and skills needed to make decisions regarding physical activity. Physical activity during the school day includes active recess and physical activity integrated into classroom lessons. Physical activity before and after school includes opportunities for physical activity through active transport, activity clubs, intramurals, interscholastic sports, and during before-school and extended day school programs. Staff involvement allows for staff members to become engaged as positive role models and support programs for school-based physical activity. Family and community engagement enables parents, staff, and community members to work together to increase physical activity opportunities before, during, and after the school day. Community organizations can establish shared-use agreements with schools that allow them to use school facilities for physical activity opportunities or events (Centers for Disease Control and Prevention, 2017, 2019).

Throughout this chapter, the focus will be on family and community engagement in providing opportunities for school-aged youth to be physically active in a variety of opportunities, which, in turn, will assist in developing and maintaining fitness levels as an extension of the school day. The CSPAP along with the WSCC model will further support the role of education and community partners in a collaborative effort to improve the health and learning outcomes for students.

Whole School, Whole Community, Whole Child (WSCC) Model

The Whole School, Whole Community, Whole Child (WSCC) model, in collaboration with key leaders from the fields of health, public health, education, and school health, expanded on the eight elements of the CDC's Coordinated School Health (CSH) approach and combined with the ASCD's Whole Child framework approach to strengthen a unified and collaborative approach designed to improve learning and health in our nation's schools and create a greater alignment between health and educational outcomes (Lewallen, Hunt, Potts-Datema, Zaza, & Giles, 2015).

The WSCC model depicted in figure 16.2 was designed to put the student at the center as the focal point, followed by the five tenets of the whole child:

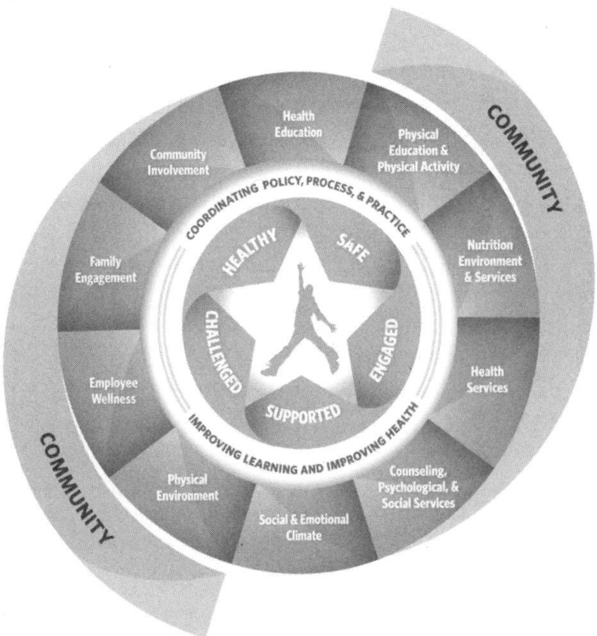

Figure 16.2 The Whole School, Whole Community, Whole Child (WSCC) model.

Reprinted from ASCD, *Whole School, Whole Community, Whole Child: A Collaborative Approach to Learning and Health*, 2014.

healthy, safe, engaged, supported, and challenged. The ring surrounding the student stresses the need for coordination among policy, process, and practice. The outer ring of the WSCC model reflects greater integration and alignment between health and education by incorporating the components of the CSH approach and emphasizing the school as an integral part of the community. The importance of sectors and individuals working together, with emphasis on the community, to implement policies, practice, and process is now prominent in this integrated approach that addresses health and learning. The 10 components of the outer ring are represented by the following:

- Health education
- Nutrition environment and services
- Employee wellness
- Social and emotional school climate
- Physical environment
- Health services
- Counseling, psychological, and social services
- Community involvement
- Family engagement
- Physical education and physical activity

As we focus on community involvement, with the support of family engagement, there are many opportunities to collaborate with community and organizational stakeholders to provide a wide range of physical activities in the communities where we live, work, and play. Schools often look to communities to garner support and leverage assistance in developing policies. There is great value in developing school and community partnerships. Programs through local running clubs; park and recreation departments; city councils; local businesses; and local colleges and universities are often available, are publicized locally, and encourage youth and adult participation.

This WSCC model further provides greater alignment, integration, and collaboration between health and education across the school setting to improve each child's cognitive, physical, and social and emotional development. The CSPAP provides a framework to implement the physical education and physical activity sector of the WSCC model to increase physical activity opportunities before, during, and after school to increase both physical activity and student health.

After-School Programs

After-school hours, the time spent outside of school, is a critical period for youth because many of them are unsupervised between the times when the school bell rings for dismissal and parents return home from work. The physical education teacher and school site administration are uniquely positioned to assist in developing onsite programs such as clubs, intramurals, and interscholastic sports that school site personnel conduct. District-wide contracts can also be activated to provide services at as many schools sites as possible that can be conducted on the school site but run by an external organization. Some of the most popular after-school programs are the After-School All-Stars, Kids on the Move, 100 Mile Club and Billion Mile Race, Boys and Girls Clubs, Police Athletic League (PAL), Marathon Kids, Alliance for a Healthier Generation, CATCH, and SPARK. There are many other after-school programs that are available in each community that the physical education teacher, counselor, activities director, athletic director, or night-school staff can assist in identifying.

Many community-based programs, such as the YMCA and local parks and recreation departments, conduct programs both at the school site after school or at their independent facility. Although most programs are fee based, they can provide a wide variety of activities for students to choose from. Other community-based programs offer activity or sport-specific activities such as karate or martial arts schools.

COMMUNITY-BASED PROGRAMS AND ACTIVITIES

Although most of this chapter focuses on preparing to participate in community-based road races, there are several other community-based fitness activities that students should explore. Not all community-based fitness activities need to be competitive in nature; many produce the same benefits, but they have the added value of fun attached. To mention just a few examples, many community-based programs offer a wide array of programs and activities such as tennis, basketball, softball, swimming, volleyball, beach volleyball, pickleball, geocaching, scavenger hunts, and many other fitness-related activities. Additionally, local event planners and directors will attest that bringing people from the community together for a common goal makes the community stronger and more cohesive.

Group Cohesion

Engaging in community-based physical activity often is easier for people when they can join with others in groups and support and motivate each other. According to the Office of Disease Prevention and Health Promotion (2012), "by engaging communities in physical activity, you can help people share knowledge about the benefits of physical activity, develop awareness about opportunities to be physically active, and overcome barriers and negative attitudes that may exist about exercise."

Carron, Widmeyer, and Brawley (1988; cited in Weinberg & Gould, 2019, p. 192) define group cohesion as a "dynamic process that is reflected in the tendency for a group to stick together and remain united in pursuit of its instrumental objectives and/or for the satisfaction of member affective needs." When the relationship of group cohesion to individual adherence to physical activity was examined, Carron, Widmeyer, and Brawley (1988) further concluded that group cohesiveness is related to individual adherence behavior. Group cohesion, as a social process, where group members interact with each other, bringing them closer together, is also associated with team satisfaction, conformity, adherence, social support, and stability.

Physical education teachers at the secondary school level have the opportunity to get their students involved with community-based group events, which could begin with school district–sponsored events and fundraisers. As students begin to engage in community-related events and become engaged in the activities with others who share the same interests, there would be a greater probability that students would continue these activities in postsecondary years into adulthood.

Exercise Adherence

Since starting and adhering to an exercise program alone is often difficult and requires great levels of motivation on the part of the individual, participating in community events with other students who share the same physical activity interests is a great way to stay motivated and continue with your exercise plan outside of the school environment.

Exercise adherence, in simple terms, is sticking to an exercise program after getting started. Cognitive factors such as internal and external motivation play a role as to whether a person sticks to the exercise program or decides to stop. Additionally, personal factors, such as self-efficacy, self-motivation, and self-monitoring; environmental factors, such as social support, convenience, and proximity; and physical activity characteristics, such as exercise intensity, frequency, and duration also contribute to exercise adherence. Since approximately 50 percent of people who start an exercise program do not stick with it (Weinberg & Gould, 2019), the Association for Applied Sport Psychology offers the following tips for exercise adherence:

- Keep it fun
- Work out with friends
- Choose an activity you like
- Begin easy and slowly increase your effort
- Set realistic, measureable goals
- Keep an exercise journal

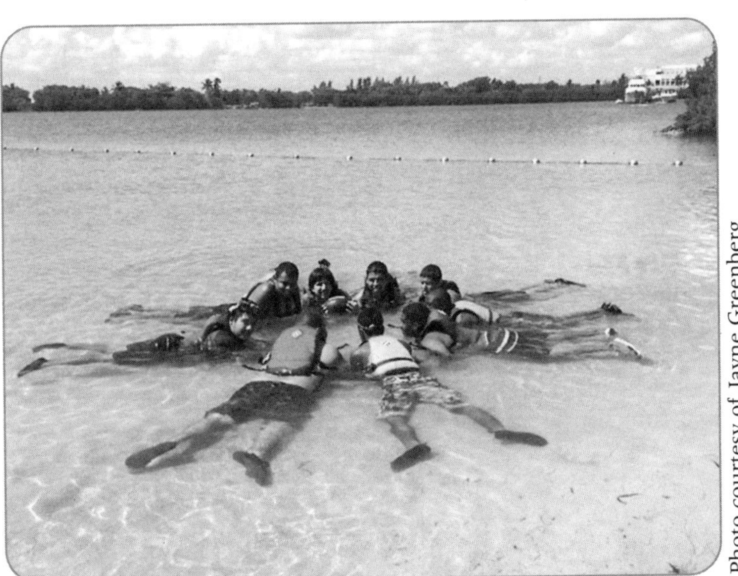

Photo courtesy of Jayne Greenberg

Physical activities are often more fun in groups.

- Establish a routine
- Make exercise a priority

Since regular exercise is necessary for the prevention of many chronic diseases such as diabetes, cardiovascular disease, and obesity, long-term adherence to physical activity is essential to facilitate and maintain the associated health benefits of being physically active. Being physically active further supports the social and emotional benefits of reducing stress and anxiety, increasing cognitive function, boosting mood, sleeping better, improving self-image, and increasing self-confidence.

Getting Started

When looking for a starting point, many community programs that are implemented through city or county offices, including parks and recreation departments, provide free, safe, and family-oriented activities such as walking and biking trails, community pools, and free exercise classes, which also include buddy systems and group walks.

When selecting a community-based program, be realistic about your needs, likes, and abilities. For example, if extreme weather conditions, such as it being too hot or too cold, bother you, selecting an indoor activity would be best; if you are looking for enjoyment, select an activity such as cycling or sports that you have always had fun participating in; if budget is a concern, select free activities as opposed to those which might be cost prohibitive; and if you are just beginning, select activities that you can progress through, rather than going on an all-out run. There is something for everyone in every community, so contact your local municipal office to determine what is available and meets your needs.

Community-Wide Fitness Challenges

There is no better way to bring a community together than to create an opportunity for some friendly competition among community members and families. Hosting a community-wide fitness challenge is a fun way to increase engagement while encouraging families, friends, and colleagues to participate for the first time, or on an ongoing basis.

These fitness challenges should have a set duration and feature a very specific goal with clear instructions; challenges could include a 30-day abs workout challenge, a distance run or walk challenge, or even a plank day challenge.

Fitness-related strength activities could also be conducted in local parks on playgrounds using equipment benches, hills, and other features for an intense body-weight workout session. No matter what the activity, make sure it can also be done at home so everyone can participate. It's up to you to log onto the website and choose an activity for your challenge that is fun and easy to track performance or progress and allows for recognition and incentives for the successful participants.

Boot Camps

In many communities, fitness clubs and local parks and recreation programs host after-school, evening, and weekend boot camps for those who really want a workout by pushing themselves to the limit. These may not be for everyone, depending on individual fitness levels, but boot camps will certainly be a way for the local clubs to grow their membership. Hosting these types of community-based programs allows participants to try different activities and avoid boredom by doing the same activity every day.

Running, Biking, Hiking, and Rolling Events

Getting back to the great outdoors brings a sense of calm and freedom to everyone who engages in outdoor activities, whether running, biking, walking, and rolling or skiing, snowboarding, and cross-country skiing. This feeling comes from the fresh air and connecting with the environment. A 5K fun run around the neighborhood, a hike on a natural trail, or a bike ride around the town are perfect ways to get people from the community outdoors and to mingle. These inclusive events attract individuals of a wide variety of fitness levels who are interested in challenging themselves with physical activity in a natural environment, with varying weather conditions. Many of these local events also provide participants with a "swag" bag filled with usable fitness materials, such as sweat bands, medals, workout towels, and even coupons for gym memberships, bike tune-ups, or other fitness-related services.

Such events are often hosted by running or biking clubs, which are great assets for the community. These clubs usually welcome participants of all abilities, from beginners to veteran competitors. Through participating in group-training activities, all participants receive support from each other by having buddies who keep them motivated; seek inspiration from someone who has already completed a 5K or 10K; find people with the same interests; and participate in other social activities as well.

There are many different types of running events that are popular today.

Color Runs

Color runs usually take place outdoors and are untimed, fun running events. Typically, they are 5K-runs for adults, but they also can be any distance for youth. Runners often start out wearing white T-shirts and are doused from head to toe in a different color at each kilometer. By the time runners cross the finish line, they are plastered in different colors. Once the event is over and the festivities begin, there are more massive color-throws that create a variety of color combinations. The color used during the Color Run is nontoxic, a combination of baking soda, cornstarch, and safe dyes. Even though it is safe, it may take a few washes to get the color completely out of your clothing. Some people wear glasses or goggles to keep the color away from their eyes and use a bandana to keep it out of their mouth, but you can enjoy being a "color runner" without the extra protection. Since no official times are kept and the event is fully accessible, it can be for fun or as a charity fundraiser.

Theme-Based Community Runs

Theme-based community runs draw runners from all ages and might be focused around holidays, special events, or just fun ideas that bring families out for a day of fitness and fun. Although the sky's the limit, here are some ideas to consider around the school-year calendar:

- September: Get acclimated: 1.5K walk or run
- October: Pumpkin run, goblin run, October feast (healthy snacks), costume runs
- November: Turkey trot
- December: Jingle run, Santa dash, reindeer run
- January: New Year's challenge, Super Bowl run
- February: Heart run, Valentine's Day run
- March: Scavenger hunt run, illuminated run (glow in the dark), shamrock run
- April: Bunny-hop run, April Fools' surprise run
- May: Color run
- June: Graduate to the next level: 3K to 5K
- July: Firecracker run
- August: Superhero run

The list can go on and on and the theme is up to the organizer's imagination. It is recommended, however, that the themes also are culturally sensitive so as not to exclude any group. As physical education teachers, you can also host these events at your school site and secure community business sponsorship so that the registration fees become a fundraiser for your program.

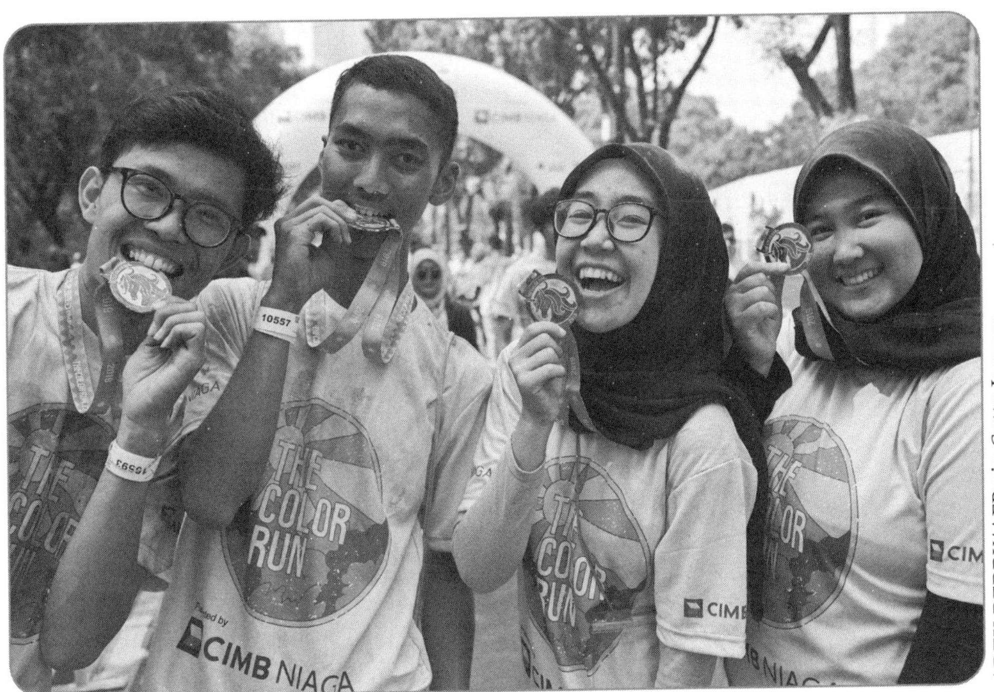

ADEK BERRY/AFP via Getty Images

Color runs are a popular type of community run.

Outdoor Obstacle Courses

With the popularity of adventure races and *American Ninja Warrior*, obstacle courses have become more prevalent in many communities and in various forms. What's unique about participating in an obstacle course outing is that community members and families can participate in courses with varying levels of difficulty from fun to challenging. While some obstacle courses comprise fixed equipment, other obstacle courses can be set up anywhere with predetermined stations and virtually no equipment if conducting the activity through a park or on a nature trail.

Group Cycling Events

Just as running clubs have been set up to bring community members together to participate in a variety of events, cycling clubs have also become a way for cycling or exercise enthusiasts to participate in events. These events can be theme based, competitive, for charitable causes, or just for fun. Depending on the type of event, they also range in varying distances from single-day to multiple-day rides. Additionally, specific cycling events can cater to those with road bikes, BMX, and mountain bikes for trail rides. Cycling events can be in-person rides, virtual rides, or even indoor cycling done as an individual or group challenge.

If cycling is part of your physical education curriculum, or if you are encouraging your students to become associated with cycling clubs or events, make sure that your students learn the rules of the road and safety measures and that they always wear helmets.

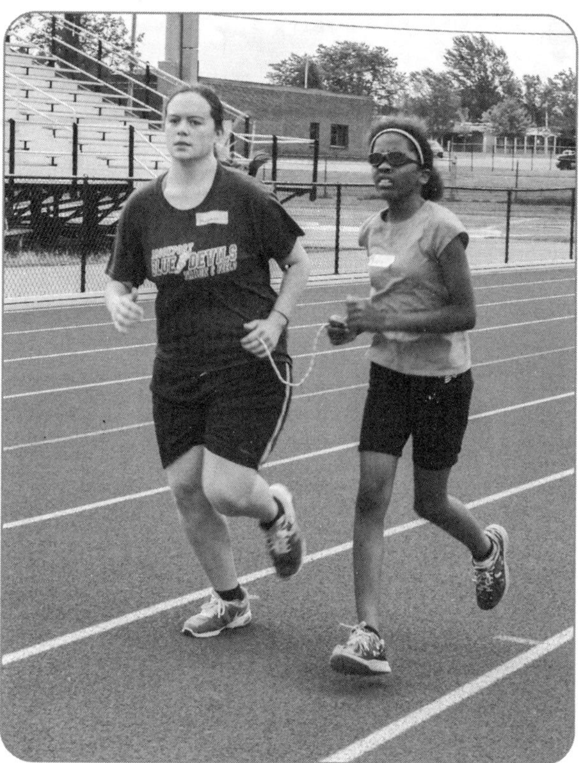

Students with and without disabilities benefit from community fitness events.

INCLUSION TIPS FOR COMMUNITY-BASED PROGRAMS

Students with disabilities receive the same benefits from being physically active as their peers without disabilities and should have the same opportunities to participate in community-based events and sports and fitness activities. Although several barriers exist, such as public attitudes, finances, lack of recreation, physical access, transportation, and assistance, the benefits of becoming physically fit and active, having an outlet to cope with stress and anxiety, building self-esteem, developing friendships, and becoming more self-sufficient and confident far outweigh the barriers (Bauman, n.d.). With proper planning and support from parents, teachers, community members, and leaders of parks and recreation and other organizations, activities and community sporting events can be made accessible for full inclusion.

With regards to road races, National Center on Health, Physical Activity and Disability (NCHPAD) provides the following tips, guidance, and valuable information for community participation in its "*Let's Race! Guidelines for Inclusive Road Racers*" brochure. See figure 16.3 for complete details.

Race Course Must-Haves

- Accessible bathrooms.
- Accessible parking.
- A firm smooth surface—concrete or pavement is best.
- A clearly marked course: Racing chairs will be much faster than runners, so make sure they know where to go.
- A safe route: Wheelchair racers may have a hard time making sharp turns particularly at higher speeds.
- Blocked roads: Often, wheelchair racers are much lower to the surface, and cars might not be able to see them as easily. Make sure cross traffic is well maintained.

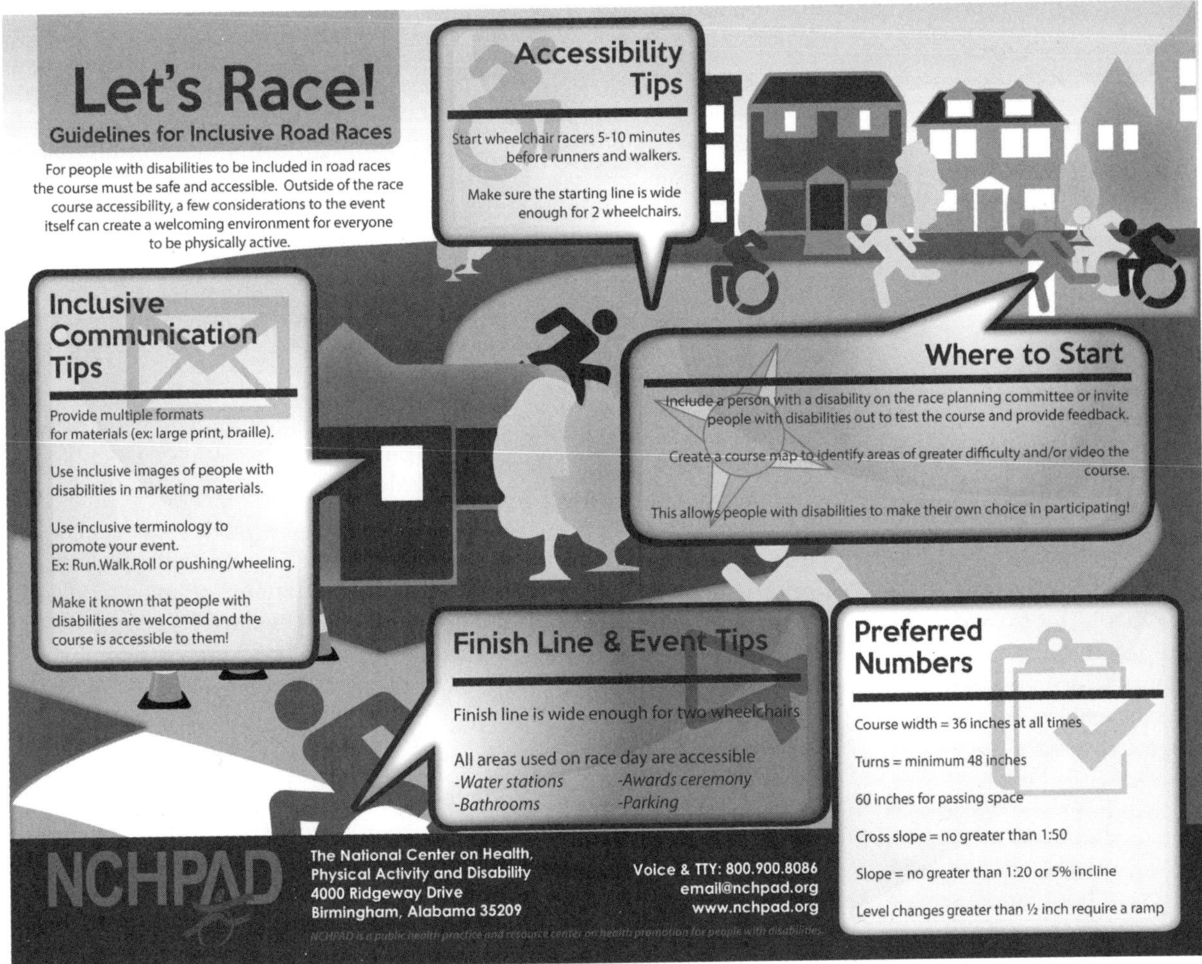

Figure 16.3 Tips for inclusion in race events.
Reprinted by permission from National Center on Health, Physical Activity and Disability.

- No steps or level changes.
- No grades or slopes too steep.

Race Course Checklist

- Is there enough space for a wheelchair plus at least one other person?
- Are there any uneven surfaces?
- Is there adequate passing room?
- Is the grade too steep?
- Are there any steps?
- Is the surface firm and smooth?
- Is there anything blocking the path?
- Is the route safe?
- Are there any dangerous curves?
- Is your course clearly marked?
- Is your finish line wide enough for two wheelchairs?

TRAINING FOR A ROAD RACE

When selecting community events to participate in, students must be realistic and determine what the purpose for participating is (fun or competition); what their level of readiness is for the activity they chose (3K, 5K, half marathon); how much time they are willing to commit to get ready; and are they really committed? Once students can answer these questions, they can begin training for their participation. Hopefully, as a physical education teacher, you have had these types of discussions with your students and incorporated their intent into their individualized fitness plans. Activities that students participate in outside of the school day should also be recorded in student portfolios and as part of their journaling.

Since there are many types of community-based events, the following examples are the most common events that secondary school students

Virtual Races

Whether it has been a weather situation, a pandemic, or just a new way of participating in community-based events, virtual running, biking, and swimming events have become popular ways of staying physically fit and active. A virtual running race is a competition that can be run, walked, or rolled from any location you choose, on a treadmill, at the gym, outside, or on the track. It can also be done alone or with a group of friends. Students get to run their own race, at their own pace, and time it themselves, either using their own fitness tracker or a fitness app such as RaceJoy. The major difference is that there are no street closures, no crowds, no parking issues, and no distance travel involved.

Virtual races work the same way as other in-person races. Share the following list with students, which provides some basic steps to follow when making the decision to become involved in a virtual race.

1. Select the community-based virtual race that you are interested in joining. Since many races have a fee attached, see if your school fundraisers or community partners can assist in paying the entry fee. Another option would be to look for races that are conducted at no cost as free community events.
2. Choose the distance that you are looking to run. Some races have set distances, where other organizations may offer 1K, 3K, 5K, 10K, half marathons, or full marathons.
3. Once you register, you have the option to get your race package sent to you. Race packages usually include your race medal, bib, and a race T-shirt. Otherwise, you can pick your race package up at a community location after you complete your race.
4. Set a time to run either during the race period or on your own schedule, depending on the rules of the race.
5. If outdoors, select a safe, lit path to run and if alone, always let someone know where you are running. Using a fitness tracker with a GPS will also be useful. Remember, it's all about setting your own personal goal and completing the race.
6. Once you complete your run, don't forget to log onto the race site and log your time.
7. At the end of the race, after you've received your race medal, take photos of yourself and share your accomplishments with your teachers, classmates, and families. Don't forget to put the photos in your portfolio!

Since virtual races are designed to inspire, challenge, and get students to their goal, these are exciting opportunities for physical education teachers to implement in their classes as either a class assignment or for extra credit.

can participate in. We begin with the one-mile (1.6 km) run, often an option in community-themed events, such as the turkey trot; the 5K run (3.1 miles), a common community-based run that usually happens throughout the year; and finally a half marathon, for students who are more serious about running activities.

One-Mile Run Training Schedule

As mentioned in chapter 8, cardiorespiratory endurance, one of the five fitness components, is part of every physical education class and fitness education program. The school-based goal has been the one-mile run or walk because, along with the PACER test, they are part of the FitnessGram test battery administered in schools. Table 16.1 features the steps for acclimating students when preparing for the one-mile run, as well as preparing to participate in community-based running events.

5K Training Schedule*

When training for your first 5K, first and foremost, make sure you are properly geared up. Consider a visit to a running specialty store to get properly fitted for running shoes, shirt, shorts, and running socks.

Start your workout with four to five minutes of brisk walking or jogging to warm up. Take a break for about two or three minutes, drink some water, and make sure those shoes are laced and ready.

Table 16.1 School-Based One-Mile Training Schedule*

Monday	Tuesday	Wednesday	Thursday	Friday
Week 1 (track equivalent: run 1/4 lap, walk 3/4 lap)				
• Jog or run 100 m (1/16 mile) • Walk 300 m • Repeat 3 times	Rest or cross-train	• Jog or run 100 m • Walk 300 m • Repeat 3 times	Rest: other class activities	• Jog or run 100 m • Walk 300 m • Repeat 3 times
Week 2 (track equivalent: run 1/2 lap, walk 1/2 lap)				
• Jog or run 200 m • Walk 200 m • Repeat 3 times	Rest or cross-train	• Jog or run 200 m • Walk 200 m • Repeat 3 times	Rest: other class activities	• Jog or run 200 m • Walk 200 m • Repeat 3 times
Week 3 (track equivalent: run 3/4 lap, walk 1/4 lap)				
• Jog or run 300 m • Walk 100 m • Repeat 3 times	Rest or cross-train	• Jog or run 300 m • Walk 100 m • Repeat 3 times	Rest: other class activities	• Jog or run 300 m • Walk 100 m • Repeat 3 times
Week 4				
Jog or run 800 m (1/2 mile) Track equivalent: 2 laps	Rest or cross-train	Jog or run 1,200 m (3/4 mile) Track equivalent: 3 laps	Rest: other class activities	Jog or run 1 mile Track equivalent: 4 laps

Next, you'll start that GPS watch (or smartphone) to help keep you inside a 21-minute time frame but not to monitor your pace. Instead, you'll monitor and adjust your pace based on your breathing effort. Start walking or jogging depending on your current state of fitness and pay special attention to your breathing. Once breathing becomes panting or excessively shallow, making it almost impossible to sing a song or have full sentence conversation, then it's time to walk very slowly.

Begin jogging or brisk walking again only after your breathing has returned to your calm breathing, as you might have when having a normal, easy conversation with someone. You'll then slow again once you've hit that heavy breathing again. Repeat this pattern until you've hit the 21-minute mark.

Always end each workout session with an easy five-minute cool-down walk or jog followed by a light static stretch routine of about five minutes as well. Examples of appropriate stretching can be found in chapters 9 through 11.

One way to route your course is to go out 10 minutes and return the same direction you came from to end back at your home or starting location. Do this same routine and don't add any time to the 21-minute goal until you are able to jog the entire 21 minutes straight without walking breaks and heavy breathing. Once you can do this for about seven consecutive days (with no more than a day of rest in between each session), then you can begin to add three minutes every five to seven days of consecutive running. Once you get over 40 minutes, you should be ready to comfortably complete your first 5K race. The important thing is to remember not to worry about how far you're running or how fast; instead, focus on your target, which is to run the entire length of time for that session and eventually for the race.

Don't forget to end each session with a five-minute easy walk or jog followed by a stretch routine to help you cool down and recover better between sessions. You always want to finish your sessions knowing you could have done more. Work hard but smart. There is no need to empty the effort tank. The old mantra, "no pain, no gain" doesn't apply to running. Be smart about the way you begin your run training so you'll learn to enjoy running for the rest of your life while staying injury-free.

Half-Marathon Training Schedule*

Are you ready to take on the half marathon distance (13.1 miles, or 21 km)? The following 12-week plan, shown in table 16.2, will help prepare your body so that you can enjoy your experience and perform at a higher level if you are a veteran of the distance. This plan is based on a 12-week schedule; however, depending on your current fitness level, this plan can vary by a few weeks. It is highly recommended that you be in shape to complete at least a 5K (or be able to run at minimum 15 minutes per mile for 45 minutes straight) before beginning to train for the half. For the days of the week that have been assigned, it is OK to shuffle the workouts, but keep at least 48 hours between the more intense workouts.

If you're looking to just complete the race and have fun doing it, the schedule provided will certainly help you achieve that. If you're a more seasoned veteran of running and are looking for a personal record (PR) or to compete, you can still follow the plan, but you should add more intensity and adjust your total volume accordingly.

Make sure you check with your doctor to be sure you're cleared to start your training, and visit a running store to get good shoes and other recommended gear. You should also have some kind of device that records distance and time, such as a wearable GPS-enabled watch or other smart watch. You could also take your smartphone with you and download any of the many running apps available.

Your training will include varied runs that are described by running jargon. Training jargon can be a bit confusing, and, in many cases, different terms mean different things to different runners. To provide the best understanding before you dive into the training, take a few moments to review the following list of terminology used for our training. Much like a recipe, each term has a purpose and a specific, recommended amount.

Within these assigned runs, you'll be running at different speeds and maintaining certain paces as you progress. Don't get ahead of yourself—this way, you are less likely to burn out and get injured.

- *Tempo run.* This type of workout is best described as sustained speed for a predetermined duration, usually no longer than about 40 minutes or so. For our purpose, this is another term for *quality running,* a pace that makes talking with a friend difficult or impossible because you will just grow too winded and have to slow down. It's a pace where you aren't too comfortable but one that you can handle steadily for a lengthy period of time.
- *Interval.* This type of workout is usually done on a track or an unimpeded, leveled path. The idea here is that you will run fast but for short distance bouts with rest between each repetition. Your form and strength are gaining the most from this type of workout. Here we think, "shorter distance but higher intensity."
- *Long run.* This is the one element of training for a half marathon you can't live without. As the term suggests, it is when we go longer and hold a pace that is usually conversational or at least comfortable; in other words, longer duration of runs but lower intensity. This is a distance we slowly progress to so that we can eventually come close to that coveted distance of 13.1 miles (21 km). The physical gains are tremendous, but equally important is the confidence you'll be building as you complete the increased distance each week. This is where the endurance is built, so you slowly build to push forth when you feel you can't, and, next time, that moment comes even later.
- *Fartlek.* This is a Swedish term for speed-play. When this is assigned, it means you will vary your speed within the run and use slower speeds to recover for an allotted time.
- *Strider.* While not a sprint, it is close to one. A strider is about 10 to 20 seconds long and used for helping with your form and promoting an efficient stride. The pace for striders is usually a gradual buildup to almost a sprint. This is a good time to run like the cameras are on you. You want to pay extra attention to your posture, your arm swing, and your leg turnover. Striders will be one of the more frequently assigned elements to your training. Following each strider, you can jog for about double the time it took you to do the strider to recover before your next bout. When the "+" symbol is in the assigned distance, it means striders are to be done within the distance. Striders should be done at any point after the midpoint of your run.
- *Recovery.* This is crucial for every athlete on this half-marathon training journey. The lowered intensity and reduced volume is where we give time to the body to adapt and repair itself. The greatest gains of the body and mind will come during the easy days. We still try to do some movement on these days labeled *recovery.* This will help us mix things up and avoid feeling the training has become stale. Recovery also helps us train the entire body as an overall athlete, not just our running legs. You can also use the recovery days to substitute the running for other exercise, such as cycling, swimming, or other cardiorespiratory activity.

*The 5K training schedule and half-marathon training schedule sections have been contributed by Frankie Ruiz, Run Coach, and International Race Events Director.

Table 16.2 12-Week Half-Marathon Training Plan

Monday	Tuesday	Wednesday	Thursday	Friday	Saturday	Sunday
Week 1						
20 min easy pace + 6 reps 100 m striders	30 min medium pace + 6 reps 100 m strid-ers	Recovery: 20 min easy pace	Tempo: 20 min tempo pace + 6 reps 100 m striders	Recovery: 20 min easy pace	Touchpoint Long run: 4 miles (6.4 km) or 30 min	Recovery: 30 min easy pace
Week 2						
Recovery: 20 min easy pace + 6 reps 100 m striders	30 min easy pace + 6 reps 100 m strid-ers	Recovery: 20 min easy pace + core workout	Tempo: 22 min tempo pace + 6 reps 100 m striders	Recovery: 20 min easy pace	Long run: 5 miles (8 km) or 35 min + 6 reps 100 m striders	Recovery: 20 min easy pace
Week 3						
Recovery: 22 min easy pace + 8 reps 100 m striders	Intervals: • 10 min easy run • 6 reps 400 m with 3 min jog or rest between each rep • 10 min easy run	Recovery: 20 min easy pace	Fartlek: 10 min easy run 8 reps (2 min fast, 1 min easy) 8 reps 100 m striders	Recovery: 22 min easy pace	Long run: 5 miles (8 km) or 35 minutes + 6 reps 100 m striders	Recovery or rest (optional): 25 min easy pace
Week 4						
Recovery: 30 min easy pace + 8 reps 100 m striders	Intervals: • 10 minute easy run • 4 reps 400 m with 3 min jog between each rep • 2 reps 800 m with 4-5 min jog between each rep • 2 reps 200 m with 2 min jog between each rep • 10 min easy run	Recovery: 22 min easy pace	Fartlek: 10 reps (2 min fast, 1 min easy) + 8 reps 100 m striders	Recovery: 22 min easy pace	Long run: 6 miles (9.7 km) or 40 min + 6 reps 100 m striders	Recovery: 25 min easy pace
Week 5						
Recovery: 35 min easy pace + 8 reps 100 m striders	Intervals: • 10 min easy run • 8 reps 400 m with 3 min jog or rest between each rep • 10 min easy run	Recovery: 25-30 min easy pace	Long intervals: • 15 min easy run • 3 reps 1 mile (1.6 km) • Rest between each rep should be half the time it took to complete • 15 min easy run	Recovery or rest (optional): 20-25 min easy pace	Long run: 7 miles (11 km) or 45 min + 6 reps 100 m striders	Recovery: 25 min easy pace

(continued)

Table 16.2 *(continued)*

Monday	Tuesday	Wednesday	Thursday	Friday	Saturday	Sunday
			Week 6			
Recovery: 35 min easy pace + 8 reps 100 m striders	Intervals: • 10 min easy run • 10 reps 400 m with 3 min jog or rest between each rep • 10 min easy run	Recovery: 25-30 min easy pace	Long intervals: • 10 min easy run • 4 reps 1 mile (1.6 km) • Rest between each rep should be half the time it took to complete • 15 min easy run	Recovery or rest (optional): 20-25 min easy pace	Long run: 8 miles (12.8 km) or 50 min + 6 reps 100 m striders	Recovery: 20-25 min easy pace
			Week 7			
Recovery: 35-40 min easy pace + 8 reps 100 m striders	Intervals: • 10 min easy run • 6 reps 1 km • 4 min jog or rest between each rep • 10 min easy run	Recovery: 25-30 min easy pace	Tempo: 25 min tempo pace + 8 reps 100 m striders	Tempo: 25 min tempo pace + 8 reps 100 m striders	Long run: 9 miles (14.5 km) or 60 min + 6 reps 100 m striders	Recovery: 20-25 min easy pace
			Week 8			
Recovery: 40 min easy pace + 10 reps 100 m striders	Intervals: • 1,200 m • 1,000 m • 800 m • 2 reps 400 m • 2 reps 200 m • 10 min easy run	Recovery: 25-30 min easy pace	Tempo: 25 min tempo pace + 10 reps 100 m striders	Recovery or rest (optional): 20-25 min easy pace	Long run: 6 miles (9.7 km) or 50 min + 6 reps 100 m striders	Recovery: 20-25 min easy pace
			Week 9			
Recovery: 40 min easy pace + 10 reps 100 m striders	Intervals: • 2 reps 400 m with • 3 min jog or rest between each rep • 4 reps 200 m with 2 min jog or rest between each rep • 10 min easy run	Recovery: 25-30 min easy pace	Fartlek: 12 reps 90 sec with 2 min break and easy jog between each rep + 10 reps 100 m striders	Recovery: 20-25 min easy pace	Long run: 10 miles (16 km) or 80 min + 6 reps 100 m striders	Recovery: 20-25 min easy pace
			Week 10			
Recovery: 40-45 min easy pace + 12 reps 100 m striders	Recovery: 25-30 min easy pace + 12 reps 100 m striders	Recovery: 25-30 min easy pace	Intervals: • 10 min easy run • 6 reps 1 km (progressively get faster with each rep) with 4 min jog or rest between each rep • 10 min easy run	Recovery: 20-25 min easy pace	Long run: 11 miles (17.7 km) or 95 min + 6 reps 100 m striders	Recovery: 20-25 min easy pace

Monday	Tuesday	Wednesday	Thursday	Friday	Saturday	Sunday
Week 11						
Recovery: 40-45 min easy pace + 12 reps 100 m striders	Intervals: • 1 mile (1.6 km), rest for total time it took to complete 1 mile • 2 reps 800 m with 4 min jog or rest between each rep • 2 reps 400 m with 4 min jog or rest between each rep • 4 reps 200 m with 2 min jog or rest between each rep • 5 min easy jog	Recovery: 20 min easy pace	Tempo: 30 min at tempo pace + 12 reps 100 m striders	Recovery: 20 min easy pace	Long run: 12 miles (19.3 km) or 95 min + 6 reps 100 m striders	Recovery: 20-25 min easy pace
Week 12						
Recovery: 25 min easy pace + 12 reps 100 m striders	Intervals: • 20 min medium pace • 4 reps 400 m with 3 min jog or rest between each rep • 5 min easy jog	Recovery: 20 min easy pace	Tempo: 20 min tempo pace + 6 reps 100 m striders	Recovery: 25 min easy pace	5K easy pace + 6 reps 100 m striders	**Race day**

Reprinted by permission from Frankie Ruiz.

- *Pace.* You'll see terms such as *easy, recovery, medium, moderate,* and so forth. These terms are relative to you, not to those around you. There are days where *easy* can feel easier than other days. You should also expect your pace to feel easier as you progress through the program. In sum, assigned pace description means different speeds for different days, uniquely defined to everyone.

Alright, let's get this show started. We know that the race is the focus, but the fun and the positive life impact are in the training itself. You can move the workouts around during the week, but don't do any of the workout days back to back. Instead, always insert a recovery day between workouts or a rest day if it is on the calendar for that particular week. Keep in mind that recovery always means we are still doing something. The word *rest* means you do no exercise that day. You can also use other local run groups or teams to do your weekday running.

Warming up properly is always important to help you accrue mileage volume and lessen the chance of injury. It also helps create the right mindset.

- 7- to 12-minute easy jog and appropriate stretching.
- Drink your fluids and tighten the laces right before you head out after warming up.
- Long static stretching should be done after the workout is complete, and those stretching holds should be for 20 to 30 seconds.

Reprinted by permission from Frankie Ruiz.

Touchpoints are opportunities to interact with other participants across multiple outlets such as the race website, email, social media, training groups, and other points of common interest. These can be built into the training program regularly if you like.

As you can see, based on your individual level of fitness and fitness goals, reaching beyond your present status is achievable if you develop a plan, train hard, and stick to the plan. There are several community-based running clubs and organizations available to assist you in reaching higher. The rest is up to you!

CONCLUSION

As physical educators, we teach students that being physically active and fit is a lifelong commitment to develop and maintain a healthy lifestyle. Reaping the health benefits associated with being physically active begins in childhood and extends into adulthood and well beyond the school walls. Fitness education, embedded in quality physical education programs, aligns with the Comprehensive School Physical Activity Program (CSPAP) and Whole School, Whole Community, Whole Child (WSCC) model. Through this framework and model, students are provided with opportunities to see how community and family engagement support physical activity and fitness programs beyond the school day.

Civic and municipal entities, local organizations, and business leaders in every community provide a variety of opportunities for physical activity, sports, and fitness that meets the needs of every ability, every level of interest, and every fitness and activity goal. Whether exercising with a buddy, running or cycling with a group, or just selecting your individual activity and routine, communities offer those options. It's now up to you and your students to take advantage of these opportunities and get started.

Review Questions

1. Explain the relationship between the CSPAP and WSCC with regards to being physically active for a lifetime.
2. Explain, based on your level of fitness, the steps that you would take to participate in either a mile run (1.6 km) or 5K run.
3. Identify the factors you would consider when selecting to participate in a community-based activity.
4. Describe the differences between a virtual race and an in-person race.
5. Develop an outdoor obstacle course and describe the steps you would incorporate to ensure that it is fully inclusive.

➤ Visit HK*Propel* for additional material related to this chapter.

CHAPTER 17

Pacing Guides for Semester Planning

Chapter Objective

After reading this chapter, you will understand how to use and develop a pacing guide, which will enable you to implement a fitness education course based on the information learned in previous chapters into a fitness education program during individual class sessions; ensure that a standards-based fitness education program is delivered; pace the activities so that students have an opportunity to improve their fitness levels through continuity of instruction; and identify resources to support and supplement the delivery of instruction.

Key Concepts

- Pacing guides provide an opportunity to ensure that the standards are being implemented across the semester.
- Pacing guides provide the teacher the opportunity to plan for a semester to ensure that all content is covered.
- Pacing guides ensure curricular continuity across schools in the same district.
- Pacing guides are aligned with grade-level outcomes and benchmarks for assessment.
- Pacing guides provide recommendations for delivering instruction and are not prescriptive.

INTRODUCTION

As we learned throughout this book, regardless of whether you are implementing a fitness education course at the beginning of the school year or during the second semester, the physical education teacher must know how to develop the course curriculum using a scope and sequence; how to identify the standards that all students should know or be able to do at the end of the course; which essential questions should be asked and answered; which course materials will assist students in understanding the course content to meet the intended objectives; and which assessments should be administered to determine student achievement of the course content and objectives. Both beginning and veteran teachers who develop and use pacing guides can effectively employ a strategy to ensure that all of the course objectives are implemented and that expected student learning outcomes are achieved.

Pacing guides are guidance documents that assist teachers in planning their instructional program by emphasizing the main curriculum points and related topics derived from each chapter. They further provide a road map for taking the central ideas and offering recommendations for activities, materials, assessment, and instructional strategies from the first week of the course to the last. Additionally, pacing guides provide the physical education teacher the opportunity to structure the course in a sensible manner, determining what standards should be taught as well as how long it will take to ensure student attainment of each learning outcome through a self-determined time line. By customizing their pacing guide, teachers can also build in time to account for some predictable delays, such as the administration using the gymnasium for class pictures or testing, as well as unpredictable factors, such as inclement weather or facility repair issues. Pacing guides are *not* prescriptive, and teachers should view them as an asset to delivering instruction rather than a hindrance to the teacher's (or student's) creativity. Pacing guides should be reviewed and modified throughout the course as needed.

In large, urban school districts, where there is often a high student-mobility rate, pacing guides are used to ensure curricular continuity across schools in the district so that when students transfer schools, they are relatively within a few pages of instruction from their previous school. Pacing guides further ensure *equity of instruction*, requiring all schools in a district to deliver the same quality instruction to all students. This serves further importance in school districts that require standardized, end-of-course exams in physical education.

HOW TO USE THE PACING GUIDES

To provide assistance in implementing the fitness education course described in this book, we have provided pacing guides for the full 18-week semester for both a daily physical education schedule and a two to three days per week block schedule. The physical education teacher is reminded that this is just a guidance document with recommendations, and the pacing guides in HK*Propel* appear in a Word document, which will enable you to revise and customize to meet your instructional delivery preferences. Physical education teachers should also review the content in the chapters and HK*Propel* to ensure that the material is approved, based on your district standards and requirements, as well as the maturity of the students in your class.

The pacing guides provided are developed by week, and include eight categories:

1. Topics and chapters: This section provides the recommended order for the delivery of chapter and topic content.
2. Standards and grade-level outcomes: Standards and GLOs are based on the National Standards from SHAPE America. It is strongly recommended that you add your own state and district standards to the pacing guides to provide local alignment for your course.
3. Objectives: The objectives provide some ideas of what instructional expectations will be achieved that week.
4. Class discussion topics: The main discussion topics provide some recommended content that should be covered and are key to the individual chapter topics.
5. Activities: Recommended activities are provided to assist students in achieving the intended outcomes for the standards covered in that week. They also coincide with HK*Propel* and student handouts, assignments, and assessments provided.
6. Assessments: It is recommended that assessments be both formal, such as FitnessGram and Brockport assessments and written tests, as well as informal, such as class participation, and alternative assessments, such as student journals and portfolios.
7. Teaching strategies and tips: This section offers suggestions that physical education teachers can use to implement the course content for that day or week. It also includes lesson closure ideas.

8. Instructional tools, vocabulary, and HK*Propel*: In a comprehensive manner, this section begins with vocabulary words and terms that students should be knowledgeable about from the instructional objectives for the week; it then provides the list of content from HK*Propel*, which should be used to assist in delivering the instruction and to support student learning outcomes; and in some weeks, it provides links to helpful online resources. It should be noted that online resources are also embedded in each chapter.

CONCLUSION

This book was developed to provide theoretical constructs and content on topics related to fitness education as well as innovative ideas and practical solutions for teaching a fitness education course to students in secondary schools, grades 6 through 12. The online resources in HK*Propel* were developed to provide teachers with valuable instructional materials to deliver the fitness education course. On HK*Propel* you will find all of the 18-week Pacing Guides; PowerPoint presentations with photos and videos embedded for ease of instruction; and handouts to support each chapter's instructional materials, student assignments, projects, and assessments. It should also be noted that the Pacing Guides in HK*Propel* were designed to allow you to modify them in order to meet your preferences and individual state and local instructional standards. The ancillary HK*Propel* materials are separated by chapters and weeks allowing for greater flexibility in the way you design your courses.

We hope that you find these resources helpful as you design and implement your fitness education course. Keeping students motivated to participate on a daily basis in physical education class and to embrace physical activity for a lifetime will take innovative ideas and practical solutions on your part! Embrace it! Deliver it! And they will succeed!

Pacing Guide: Week 1

<table>
<tr><th>Topics and chapters</th><th>Standards and GLOs</th><th>Objectives</th><th>Class discussion topics</th></tr>
<tr>
<td>Orientation
• Lock and uniform distribution
• Classroom expectations
• Health forms
• Provide first couple of days for administrative schedule changes and class size leveling
Chapter 1: Introduction to Fitness Education
• Benefits of physical activity
• Introduction to fitness education
• Learning domains in fitness education
Chapter 4: Classroom Considerations and Teaching Tips (Sections 1 and 2)</td>
<td>Middle school
• S4.M1.6
• S4.M1.7
• S4.M2.8
• S4.M7.6
• S4.M7.7
• S4.M7.8
• S5.M6.6
• S5.M6.7
• S5.M6.8
High school
• S3.H5.L1
• S4.H1.L1
• S4.H1.L2
• S4.H2.L1
• S4.H2.L2
• S4.H3.L1
• S4.H3.L2
• S4.H4.L1
• S4.H4.L2
• S4.H5.L1</td>
<td>• Develop responsible personal and social behaviors in physical activity settings
• Describe how to create a safe, inclusive, and motivational class climate
• Demonstrate knowledge of rules and safety procedures for participating in an active environment
• Explain the main goal of a fitness education course
• Describe the physical activity guidelines to reduce the risk for chronic diseases</td>
<td>Course orientation
Class expectations
• Attendance
• Arriving to class on time
• Following policies and procedures
• Assignments
• Respectful and supportive behavior
• Classroom management routines and discipline
• Class participation and engagement
• Safety protocols
• Student interests:
– Physical activity preferences
– Physical activity habits
– Fitness goals
Chapter 1
• What is fitness education?
• Common barriers to high-quality fitness education
• Learning domains and assessments in fitness education
• Benefits of physical activity
• Common barriers to achieving physical fitness
• Physical activity vs. exercise
• Physical activity guidelines
Chapter 4
• Safety considerations
• Class climate
• Exercise safety protocols</td>
</tr>
</table>

Pacing Guide: Week 1

Activities	Assessments	Teaching strategies and tips	Instructional tools, vocabulary, and HK*Propel*
• Icebreakers to have students introduce themselves • Surveys to gather information on students, such as physical activity habits and student interests • Tour of facilities, gym spaces, locker rooms • Behavioral norms discussions—what helps make a positive classroom environment, what *respect* means • Introduction of course objectives	• Participation in discussion topics and icebreaker activities • Student assignments: Benefits of Regular Physical Activity, Student Interest Questionnaire • Signed code of student conduct for parent and student	• Build rapport with students by introducing yourself and sharing your teaching philosophy; let students know what they can expect from you as a teacher • Focus on creating a safe, inclusive, and motivational class climate by providing students with opportunities to connect with their classmates and establishing behavioral norms • Explain the purpose of the course and provide a rationale for why the course is structured the way it is • Focus on the importance of following safety protocols throughout the course **Lesson closure** • Review the daily topic and key points • Review the lesson objectives and assess to what extent students met the objectives • Give reminders and prepare for the next class	**Vocabulary** • Class climate • Communication (verbal, written, nonverbal, active listening) • Hydration • Heat illness • Physical literacy **HK*Propel*** • Chapter 1 Course Introduction PowerPoint • Chapter 4 Class Considerations and Student Safety PowerPoint • Student Interest Questionnaire • Icebreaker Ideas • Benefits of Regular Physical Activity • Physical Activity Log • Fitness Class Journal **Online resources** www.shapeamerica.org/ www.cdc.gov/disasters/extremeheat/warning.html www.cdc.gov/physicalactivity/basics/pa-health/index.htm www.hhs.gov/fitness/resource-center/physical-activity-resources/index.html

From J.D. Greenberg, N.D. Calkins, and L.S. Spinosa, *Designing and Teaching Fitness Education Courses.* (Champaign, IL: Human Kinetics, 2022)

Pacing Guide: Week 2

Topics and chapters	Standards and GLOs	Objectives	Class discussion topics
Fitness pre-assessments **Chapter 1:** Continue **Chapter 2:** Fitness Components and Training Principles Benefits of physical fitness **Chapter 7:** Standards, Grade-Level Outcomes, and Assessment • Fitness assessment protocols • Best practices for assessing fitness	**Middle school** • S3.M1.7 • S3.M1.8 • S3.M7.6 • S3.M7.7 • S3.M7.8 • S3.M10.6 • S3.M11.6 • S3.M11.7 • S3.M11.8 • S3.M13.6 • S3.M13.7 • S3.M13.8 • S3.M14.6 • S3.M14.7 • S4.M1.6 • S4.M1.7 • S4.M2.8 • S5.M1.6 • S5.M1.7 • S5.M1.8 **High school** • S1.H3.L1 • S1.H3.L2 • S2.H2.L1 • S3.H1.L1 • S3.H3.L2 • S3.H8.L2 • S3.H9.L1 • S3.H9.L2 • S3.H10.L1 • S3.H10.L2 • S3.H11.L2 • S3.H12.L1 • S3.H12.L2 • S5.H1.L1 • S5.H1.L2	• Demonstrate knowledge of the principles of training for all components of health-related fitness • Differentiate between health- and skill-related fitness • Describe the benefits associated with achieving health-enhancing fitness for all of the health-related components of fitness • Describe the importance of self-assessing personal fitness • Assess current fitness status by comparing personal fitness assessment scores to nationally recognized fitness standards	**Chapter 1:** Continue with chapter concepts **Chapter 2** • Components of physical fitness in relationship to disease prevention and athletic performance • Difference between health- and skill-related fitness • Benefits of health-enhancing physical fitness • Principles of training • FITT framework • Physiology of exercise • Functional training • HIIT and interval training **Chapter 7** • Fitness assessment protocols • Purpose of fitness assessment • FitnessGram and Brockport Physical Fitness Test protocols

Pacing Guide: Week 2

<table>
<tr><th>Activities</th><th>Assessments</th><th>Teaching strategies and tips</th><th>Instructional tools, vocabulary, and HKPropel</th></tr>
<tr><td>Through lecture and discussions, students will learn and understand the importance of evaluating the following:
Health-related fitness tests
• One-mile (1.6 km) run or walk, PACER
• Body fat composition
• Curl-ups
• Trunk lifts
• Push-ups
• Back saver sit and reach
Skill-related fitness tests
• Agility: Illinois agility run
• Balance: one foot stand
• Coordination: alternate hand wall toss test
• Power: standing long jump
• Reaction time: yardstick test
• Speed: 50-yard dash</td><td>• Begin FitnessGram and Brockport Physical Fitness Test assessment for pretest
• Ensure that test items are performed correctly
• Student assignments: Components of Physical Fitness
• Engagement in class discussion topics
• Engagement in skill-related fitness assessments</td><td>• Explain the purpose of fitness assessments and provide an opportunity for students to practice the tests before performing pre-assessments
• Follow the best practices for fitness assessments such as not grading performance and emphasizing personal improvement
• Lead students through a proper warm-up and cool-down before and after fitness assessments
Lesson closure
• Review the daily topic and key points
• Review the lesson objectives and assess to what extent students met the objectives
• Give reminders and prepare for the next class</td><td>Vocabulary
• Health-related fitness
– Cardiorespiratory endurance
– Muscular strength and endurance
– Flexibility
– Body composition
• Skill-related fitness
– Agility
– Balance
– Coordination
– Power
– Reaction time
– Speed
HKPropel
• Chapter 2 Components of Physical Fitness PowerPoint
• Chapter 7 Fitness Assessments PowerPoint
• Components of Physical Fitness Assignment
• Components of Physical Fitness Handout
• Assessing Physical Fitness Assignment
• School-Based One-Mile (1.6 km) Training Plan
• Physical Activity Log
• Fitness Class Journal
• Skill-Related Fitness Assessment Student Handout
• Skill-Related Fitness Assessment Score Sheet
• Student Fitness Portfolio and Grading Rubric
Online resources
www.pyfp.org
https://fitnessgram.net/</td></tr>
</table>

From J.D. Greenberg, N.D. Calkins, and L.S. Spinosa, *Designing and Teaching Fitness Education Courses.* (Champaign, IL: Human Kinetics, 2022)

Pacing Guide: Week 3

Topics and chapters	Standards and GLOs	Objectives	Class discussion topics
Fitness pre-assessments: Continue Skill-related fitness assessments **Chapter 2:** Fitness Components and Training Principles • Principles of training • FITT framework • Resting heart rate • Target heart rate zone • Personal fitness planning **Chapter 6:** Social and Emotional Learning Setting SMART goals **Chapter 7:** Standards, Grade-Level Outcomes, and Assessment • Fitness assessment protocols • Developing fitness plans	**Middle school** • S3.M7.6 • S3.M7.7 • S3.M7.8 • S3.M8.6 • S3.M8.7 • S3.M10.6 • S3.M10.8 • S3.M15.6 • S3.M15.7 • S3.M15.8 • S3.M16.6 • S3.M16.7 • S3.M16.8 • S4.M1.6 • S4.M1.7 • S4.M2.8 **High school** • S2.H2.L1 • S3.H3.L2 • S3.H8.L2 • S3.H9.L1 • S3.H10.L1 • S3.H10.L2 • S3.H11.L2 • S3.H12.L1 • S5.H1.L1	• Demonstrate knowledge of training for all components of health-related fitness • Describe how training for different components of fitness can improve athletic performance and reduce the risk of chronic diseases • Analyze current fitness status using fitness assessment data and set personal fitness goals to achieve and/or maintain a health-enhancing level of physical fitness • Develop and implement a personal fitness plan to achieve fitness goals • Explain the components of an effective goal • Demonstrate how to calculate target heart rate zone	**Chapter 2** • Principles of training • FITT framework • Physiology of exercise • Training progressions • HIIT and interval training • Functional training • Rate of perceived exertion • Barriers and solutions to fitness • Fitness program planning **Chapter 6** • Types of goals • Setting SMART goals for fitness **Chapter 7** • Developing individual fitness plans based on fitness assessments

Pacing Guide: Week 3

Activities	Assessments	Teaching strategies and tips	Instructional tools, vocabulary, and HK*Propel*
• Completing the health- and skill-related fitness pre-assessments • Creating fitness goals based on fitness assessment scores • Designing personal fitness plans • Calculating resting heart rates • Calculating target heart rate zones • Instruction on training principles • Discussions on SMART goals and what are not SMART goals	Health- and skill-related fitness tests **Student assignments** • FITT framework, principles of training, target heart rate calculation, assessing skill-related fitness assignment • Engagement in class discussion topics	• Have students reflect on their fitness assessment scores and explain the why behind their scores; if students did not give a good effort during the assessments, ask them to explain why they did not perform well • Provide examples of effective SMART goals and non-examples of goals that do not meet the SMART criteria **Lesson closure** • Review the daily topic and key points • Review the lesson objectives and assess to what extent students met the objectives • Give reminders and prepare for the next class	**Vocabulary** • Training principles: – Specificity – Individuality – Overload – Progression – Variation – Regularity • Strength and power • Static, dynamic, and ballistic stretching • Training adaptations • Functional training • HIIT training • SMART goals • Process goals • Performance goals • Outcome goals **HK*Propel*** • Chapter 2 Components of Physical Fitness PowerPoint • Chapter 2 Principles of Training PowerPoint • Chapter 6 Setting SMART Goals for Fitness and Increasing Motivation PowerPoint • Chapter 7 Assessments and Fitness Components PowerPoint • FITT Framework Student Assignment • FITT Framework Handout • Principles of Training Student Assignment • Principles of Training Handout • Calculating Resting Heart Rate Assignment • Calculating Target Heart Rate Assignment • Skill-Related Fitness Assessment Assignment • Skill-Related Fitness Assessment Score Sheet • Physical Activity Log • Fitness Class Journal • Personalized Fitness Plan (Weeks 1 Through 6) **Online resources** PYFP: www.pyfp.org FitnessGram: https://fitnessgram.net

Pacing Guide: Week 4

Topics and chapters	Standards and GLOs	Objectives	Class discussion topics
Chapter 8: Cardiorespiratory Fitness **Chapter 9:** Upper-Body Stretching Exercises **Chapter 12:** Upper-Body Muscular Strength and Endurance Exercises	**Middle school** • S3.M3.7 • S3.M3.8 • S3.M4.7 • S3.M4.8 • S3.M6.6 • S3.M6.7 • S3.M6.8 • S3.M7.6 • S3.M7.8 • S3.M8.8 • S3.M9.6 • S3.M9.7 • S3.M9.8 • S3.M10.6 • S3.M10.8 • S3.M12.6 • S3.M12.7 • S3.M12.8 • S3.M14.6 • S3.M14.7 • S4.M1.6 • S4.M1.7 • S4.M2.8 • S4.M4.6 • S4.M4.8 • S4.M7.6 • S4.M7.7 • S4.M7.8 • S5.M6.6 • S5.M6.7 • S5.M6.8 **High school** • S2.H2.L1 • S3.H3.L2 • S3.H6.L1 • S3.H7.L2 • S2.H2.L1 • S3.H9.L1 • S3.H9.L2 • S3.H10.L1 • S3.H10.L2	**Chapter 8** • Take part in a discussion and lecture session on cardiorespiratory fitness • Calculate THR • Practice taking THR before warm-up • Practice taking THR after a 400 m walk **Chapters 9 and 12** • Identify the following muscles and exercises for each flexibility and muscular strength and endurance exercise: – Body part – Muscle group – Exercise • Perform and execute the flexibility and muscular strength and endurance exercises for the upper body • Identify specific sports that use the muscle groups of the upper body	**Cardiorespiratory fitness** • Briefly review principles of training: – Overload, progression, specificity, individuality, variation, and regularity – FITT and HIIT – Benefits – Breathing – Warm-ups and cool-downs – Jogging training – THRZ – Taking pulse – Safety – Types of assessment technology **Stretching** • Dynamic • Static • Ballistic • Proprioceptive neuromuscular facilitation (PNF) **Muscle movements** • Upper-body flexibility and muscular strength and endurance exercises • Understand the biomechanics of select exercises

Pacing Guide: Week 4

Activities	Assessments	Teaching strategies and tips	Instructional tools, vocabulary, and HK*Propel*

Completing their THR calculations (MHR, RHR, HRR, THRZ)
Completing a 400-meter walk
After viewing the PowerPoint or class instructions, students will do the following:
• Follow and copy the teacher routine of a warm-up and a cool-down
• Follow and copy the teacher routine of dynamic, static, ballistic, and PNF stretches
• Participate in daily cardiorespiratory activities
• Apply basic muscular strength and endurance principles to upper-body exercises
• Properly execute upper-body exercises
	• Preparation for class
	• Participation and engagement in activities and discussion
	• Following teacher commands through routine
	• Applying appropriate warm-up and cool-down techniques while participating in a variety of activities
	• Staying on task
	• Supporting and assisting classmates
	• Knowledge of vocabulary
	• Completing THR calculation
	  – THR log
	  – PA log
		• Emphasize that the lesson is designed to help them learn about the health-related fitness components of cardiorespiratory, flexibility, and muscular strength of the upper body
		• Emphasize that improving the components of fitness will assist them in performing daily activities and specific sports
		• Stress the importance of performing each stretch accurately
		• Briefly review and explain how fitness assessment items can be improved through participation in cardiorespiratory, flexibility, and muscular strength and endurance activities
		Lesson closure
		• Review the daily topic and key points
		• Review the lesson objectives and assess to what extent students met the objectives
		• Give reminders and prepare for the next class
			Vocabulary
			• MVPA
			• Anaerobic
			• Aerobic
			• Interval training
			• Continuous training
			• Fartlek training
			• Circuit training
			• Muscles
			• Tendons
			• Ligaments
			• Joints
			• Range of motion
			HK*Propel*
			• Chapter 8 Cardiorespiratory Fitness PowerPoint
			• Chapter 9 Upper-Body Stretching Part 1 PowerPoint
			• Chapter 9 Upper-Body Stretching Part 2 PowerPoint
			• Chapter 12 Upper-Body Muscular Strength and Endurance Part 1 PowerPoint
			• Chapter 12 Upper-Body Muscular Strength and Endurance Part 2 PowerPoint
			• Calculating Target Heart Rate Assignment
			• Calculating Resting Heart Rate Assignment
			• Physical Activity Log
			• Fitness Class Journal
			• Personalized Fitness Plan (Weeks 1 Through 6)
			• Student Fitness Portfolio and Grading Rubric
			• STRAVA Challenge Data Chart Cardio and THR
			• Circuits Alphabet Warm-Up
			• Circuits Locomotive Circuit
			• Hands-Only CPR Poster
			Online resources
			PYFP: www.pyfp.org
			FitnessGram: https://fitnessgram.net
			SHAPE America: https://shapeamerica.org
			American Heart Association: www.heart.org

Pacing Guide: Week 5

Topics and chapters	Standards and GLOs	Objectives	Class discussion topics
Chapter 10: Core Stretching Exercises **Chapter 13:** Core Muscular Strength and Endurance Exercises Cardiorespiratory activities are performed daily	**Middle school** • S3.M4.7 • S3.M14.6 • S3.M4.8 • S3.M14.7 • S3.M6.6 • S3.M14.8 • S3.M6.7 • S4.M1.6 • S3.M6.8 • S4.M1.7 • S3.M7.6 • S4.M2.8 • S3.M7.8 • S4.M7.6 • S3.M9.6 • S4.M7.7 • S3.M9.7 • S4.M7.8 • S3.M9.8 • S5.M6.6 • S3.M10.6 • S5.M6.7 • S3.M10.8 • S5.M6.8 • S3.M12.8 **High school** • S2.H2.L1 • S3.H6.L1 • S3.H7.L2 • S3.H9.L1 • S3.H9.L2	**Chapters 10 and 13** • Identify the following muscles and exercises for each flexibility and muscular strength and endurance exercise: – Body part – Muscle group – Exercise • Perform and execute the flexibility and muscular strength and endurance exercises for the core • Identify specific sports that use the core muscle groups	**Core muscles** • Torso • Stomach • Lower back **Major muscle groups** • Abdominals • Obliques • Erectors • Execution **Stretching** • Dynamic • Static • Ballistic • Proprioceptive neuromuscular facilitation (PNF) **Muscle movements** • Core exercises for flexibility and muscular strength and endurance • Understand the biomechanics of select exercises

Pacing Guide: Week 5

Activities	Assessments	Teaching strategies and tips	Instructional tools, vocabulary, and HK*Propel*
After viewing the PowerPoint or class instructions, students will do the following: • Follow the teacher routine of a warm-up and a cool-down • Follow the teacher routine of dynamic, static, ballistic, and PNF stretches • Participate in daily cardiorespiratory activities • Apply basic muscular strength and endurance principles to core exercises • Properly execute core exercises	• Preparation for class • Participation and engagement in activities and discussions • Following teacher commands through routine • Applying appropriate warm-up and cool-down techniques while participating in a variety of activities • Staying on task • Supporting and assisting classmates • Knowledge of vocabulary • Execution of exercises	• Emphasize that the lesson is designed to help them learn about the health-related fitness components of cardiorespiratory, flexibility, and muscular strength and endurance of the core • Emphasize that improving on the components of fitness will assist them in performing daily activities and specific sports • Stress the importance of performing each stretch accurately • Briefly review and explain how fitness assessment items can be improved through participation in cardiorespiratory, flexibility, and muscular strength and endurance activities **Lesson closure** • Review the daily topic and key points • Review the lesson objectives and assess to what extent students met the objectives • Give reminders and prepare for the next class	**Vocabulary** • Muscles • Tendons • Ligaments • Joints • Range of motion • Circuit training **HK*Propel*** • Chapter 10 Core Stretching Part 1 PowerPoint • Chapter 10 Core Stretching Part 2 PowerPoint • Chapter 13 Core Muscular Strength and Endurance Part 1 PowerPoint • Chapter 13 Core Muscular Strength and Endurance Part 2 PowerPoint • Physical Activity Log • Fitness Class Journal • Personalized Fitness Plan (Weeks 1 Through 6)

From J.D. Greenberg, N.D. Calkins, and L.S. Spinosa, *Designing and Teaching Fitness Education Courses.* (Champaign, IL: Human Kinetics, 2022)

Pacing Guide: Week 6

Topics and chapters	Standards and GLOs	Objectives	Class discussion topics
Chapter 11: Lower-Body Stretching Exercises **Chapter 14:** Lower-Body Muscular Strength and Endurance Exercises Cardiorespiratory activities are performed daily	**Middle school** • S3.M4.7 • S3.M14.6 • S3.M4.8 • S3.M14.7 • S3.M6.6 • S3.M14.8 • S3.M6.7 • S4.M1.6 • S3.M6.8 • S4.M1.7 • S3.M7.6 • S4.M2.8 • S3.M7.8 • S4.M7.6 • S3.M9.6 • S4.M7.7 • S3.M9.7 • S4.M7.8 • S3.M9.8 • S5.M6.6 • S3.M10.6 • S5.M6.7 • S3.M10.8 • S5.M6.8 • S3.M12.8 **High school** • S2.H2.L1 • S3.H6.L1 • S3.H7.L2 • S3.H9.L1 • S3.H9.L2	**Chapters 11 and 14** • Identify the following muscles and exercises for each flexibility and muscular strength and endurance exercise: – Body part – Muscle group **Exercise** • Perform and execute the flexibility and muscular strength and endurance exercises for the core • Identify specific sports that use the muscle groups of the lower body	**Core muscles** • Hips • Buttocks • Thighs • Calves **Major muscle groups** • Quadriceps • Hamstrings • Gluteals • Gastrocnemius **Stretches** • Dynamic • Static • Ballistic • Proprioceptive neuromuscular facilitation (PNF) **Muscle movements** • Lower-body exercises for flexibility and muscular strength and endurance • Understand the biomechanics of select exercises

Pacing Guide: Week 6

Activities	Assessments	Teaching strategies and tips	Instructional tools, vocabulary, and HK*Propel*
After viewing the PowerPoint or class instructions, students will do the following: • Follow the teacher routine of a warm-up and a cool-down • Follow the teacher routine of dynamic, static, ballistic, and PNF stretches • Participate in daily cardiorespiratory activities • Apply basic muscular strength and endurance principles to lower-body exercises • Properly execute lower-body exercises	• Preparation for class • Participation and engagement in activities and discussion • Following teacher commands through routine • Applying appropriate warm-up and cool-down techniques while participating in a variety of activities • Staying on task • Supporting and assisting classmates • Knowledge of vocabulary • Execution of exercises	• Emphasize that the lesson is designed to help them learn about the health-related fitness components of cardiorespiratory, flexibility, and muscular strength and endurance of the lower body • Emphasize that improving on the components of fitness will assist them in performing daily activities and specific sports • Stress the importance of performing each stretch accurately • Briefly review and explain how fitness assessment items can be improved through participation in cardiorespiratory, flexibility, and muscular strength and endurance activities **Lesson closure** • Review the daily topic and key points • Review the lesson objectives and assess to what extent students met the objectives • Give reminders and prepare for the next class	**Vocabulary** • Muscles • Tendons • Ligaments • Joints • Range of motion • Circuit training **HK*Propel*** • Chapter 11 Lower-Body Stretching Part 1 PowerPoint • Chapter 11 Lower-Body Stretching Part 2 PowerPoint • Chapter 14 Lower-Body Muscular Strength and Endurance Part 1 PowerPoint • Chapter 14 Lower-Body Muscular Strength and Endurance Part 2 PowerPoint • Physical Activity Log • Fitness Class Journal • Personalized Fitness Plan (Weeks 1 Through 6)

Pacing Guide: Week 7

Topics and chapters	Standards and GLOs	Objectives	Class discussion topics
Chapter 15: Implementing the Fitness Education Program • Continue emphasizing warm-up and cool-down techniques while participating in a variety of activities • Continue emphasizing correct techniques for implementing exercises in chapters 9 through 14 Cardiorespiratory activities are performed daily Provide instruction in American Heart Association's hands-only CPR	**Middle school** • S3.M6.6 • S3.M6.7 • S3.M6.8 • S3.M7.6 • S3.M7.8 • S3.M12.8 • S3.M14.6 • S4.M1.6 • S4.M1.7 • S4.M2.8 • S4.M7.6 • S4.M7.7 **High school** • S2.H2.L1 • S3.H3.L2 • S3.H6.L1 • S3.H9.L1 • S3.H9.L2 • S3.H10.L1 • S3.H10.L2	• Participate in a variety of workouts, routines, and circuits to help improve fitness level • Continue to improve techniques for flexibility exercises in chapters 9 through 11 • Continue to improve their techniques for strength exercises in chapters 12 through 14 • Continue practicing exercises in weeks 4-6 • Receive hands-only CPR training (American Heart Association program will be implemented) • Receive instruction in the use of an AED	**Methods of training** • HIIT • Routines • Stackers • Tabata • Circuits Learn how to administer hands-only CPR through the American Heart Association training protocols; follow up from chapter 8

Pacing Guide: Week 7

Activities	Assessments	Teaching strategies and tips	Instructional tools, vocabulary, and HK*Propel*
Receive instruction on the different types of fitness activities: • Routines • Stackers • Tabata • Circuits Participating and engaging throughout class time Following teacher commands Supporting and assisting classmates in performing activities Properly executing exercises and routines Execute proper techniques of performing hands-only CPR	Students will be assessed on: • Preparation for class • Participation and engagement in activities and discussion • Following teacher commands through routine • Applying appropriate warm-up and cool-down techniques while participating in a variety of activities • Staying on task • Supporting and assisting classmates • Knowledge of vocabulary • Execution of exercises • Perform proper techniques of hands-only CPR	• Emphasize that the lesson is designed to help them learn about the health-related fitness components of cardiorespiratory, flexibility, and muscular strength • Emphasize that participation in these activities will improve their components of skill-related fitness • Emphasize that improving on the components of fitness will assist them in performing daily activities and specific sports • Stress the importance of performing each exercise, routine, and circuit accurately • Emphasize the importance of using proper techniques when performing hands-only CPR **Lesson closure** • Review the daily topic and key points • Review the lesson objectives and assess to what extent students met the objectives • Emphasize that students should continue doing their assigned workout outside of class • Give reminders and prepare for the next class	**Vocabulary** • HIIT training • Routines • Stackers • Tabata • Circuits **HK*Propel*** • Chapter 15 Implementing Fitness Education PowerPoint • Physical Activity Log • Fitness Class Journal • Tabata #1 • Tabata #2 • Circuit: Did You Forget Something? • Circuit: Follow the Leader • Circuit: Take the Challenge • Hands-Only CPR Resources • Personalized Fitness Plan (Weeks 1 Through 6) **Online resources** https://cpr.heart.org

Pacing Guide: Week 8

Topics and chapters	Standards and GLOs	Objectives	Class discussion topics
Chapter 4: Classroom Considerations and Teaching Tips Section 3 • Equity, diversity, inclusion, and social justice • Class climate considerations **Chapter 6:** Social and Emotional Learning • Types of motivation • Creating a mastery-oriented environment • Developing social-awareness skills • Developing responsible decision-making skills • Becoming culturally competent **Chapter 15:** Continue	**Middle school** • S3.M7.6 • S4.M1.6 • S4.M1.7 • S4.M2.8 • S5.M3.6 • S5.M3.7 • S5.M3.8 • S5.M6.7 • S5.M6.8 **High school** • S3.H6.L1 • S4.H1.L1 • S4.H1.L2 • S4.H2.L1 • S4.H2.L2 • S4.H3.L1 • S4.H3.L2 • S4.H4.L1 • S4.H4.L2 • S4.H5.L1 • S5.H4.L1 • S5.H5.L2	**Chapter 4** • Differentiate between equity, equality, and social justice • Explain the importance of creating an inclusive environment in physical education **Chapter 6** • Self-assess social and emotional competencies • Describe how social and emotional competencies can influence physical activity habits • Assess class climate • Differentiate between extrinsic and intrinsic motivation in physical activity • Describe how social-awareness and responsible decision-making skills impact the class climate • Explain how culture can influence physical activity behavior • Discuss ways to enhance motivation to remain physically active	**Chapter 4** • Class climate • Appreciating diversity • Creating an inclusive environment – Diversity – Inclusion – Equity – Equality – Social justice **Chapter 6** • Intrinsic and extrinsic motivation • Mastery-oriented climate • CASEL's SEL competencies • Developing social-awareness skills – Perspective-taking – Showing empathy in overcoming barriers – Showing respect for others – Becoming culturally competent – Developing responsible decision-making skills – Ethical responsibility in health and fitness

Pacing Guide: Week 8

Activities	Assessments	Teaching strategies and tips	Instructional tools, vocabulary, and HK*Propel*
• Instruction on how equity, equality, and social justice play a role in physical education opportunities • Discussions on how to stay motivated to achieve goals and remain physically active • Completing a self-assessment of social-awareness skills and reflection on how to respect others and appreciate diversity • Completing a class climate survey to examine the current state of motivation and engagement in the course • Participating in a perspective-taking activity such as performing fitness activities from a seated position to simulate the experience one has in a wheelchair	• Class climate survey • Social-emotional competencies self-assessment and reflection • Responsible decision-making skills reflection • Engagement in class discussion topics	• Have students reflect on their use of social and emotional competencies and how they contribute to an inclusive, motivational climate; then have students set behavioral goals for social and emotional competence • Provide opportunities for students to share their barriers to being physically active outside of school • Take information from the class climate eight weeks into the course to assess how students perceive the climate of the class; then identify any issues with creating a positive learning environment that may need attention or start conversations with students who are not feeling connected or engaged **Lesson closure** • Review the lesson objectives and assess to what extent students met the objectives • Give reminders and prepare for the next class	**Vocabulary** • Diversity • Inclusion • Equity • Equality • Social justice • Intrinsic motivation • Extrinsic motivation • Empathy • Cultural competency **HK*Propel*** • Chapter 4 Equity, Diversity, Inclusion, and Social Justice PowerPoint • Chapter 6 Setting SMART Goals for Fitness and Increasing Motivation PowerPoint • Chapter 6 Social and Emotional Learning Competencies PowerPoint • SEL: Social and Emotional Competencies Self-Assessment and Reflection • Class Climate Survey • Responsible Decision-Making Skills Reflection • Physical Activity Log • Fitness Class Journal • Personalized Fitness Plan (Weeks 1 Through 6) **Online resources** https://casel.org/

Pacing Guide: Week 9

Topics and chapters	Standards and GLOs	Objectives	Class discussion topics
Midterm assessment Review status of fitness plans **Chapter 6:** Social and Emotional Learning • Social and emotional learning • Developing self-awareness skills **Chapter 16:** Extending Fitness Education Into the Community	**Middle school** • S3.M7.6 • S3.M7.7 • S3.M7.8 • S3.M12.8 • S3.M14.6 • S4.M1.6 • S4.M1.7 • S4.M2.8 **High school** • S3.H3.L2 • S3.H6.L1 • S3.H6.L2 • S3.H9.L1 • S3.H10.L1 • S3.H10.L2 • S3.H11.L2 • S5.H1.L1	Review and administer midterm exam covering topics in weeks 1 through 8 Review the status of individual student fitness plans through student conferences **Chapter 6** • Describe how a growth mindset or a fixed mindset can influence physical activity goals and behavior • Self-assess physical activity habits to identify personal strengths and where improvement is needed **Chapter 16** • Discuss how school-based physical education and activity programs connect to the community • Discuss the role of group cohesion and exercise adherence in community events • Discuss tips on inclusion for community-based events	**Chapter 6** • CASEL's SEL competencies • Developing self-awareness skills – Growth mindset versus fixed mindset – Developing self-efficacy in physical activity – Accurate self-perception **Chapter 16** • Discuss various community events • Venues for participation • Bike and running clubs • Inclusion opportunities • Virtual races – Training progression – One-mile (1.6 km) run or walk – PACER – 5K training schedule – Half marathon training schedule

Pacing Guide: Week 9

Activities	Assessments	Teaching strategies and tips	Instructional tools, vocabulary, and HK*Propel*
• Researching a community-based event • Choosing the appropriate activity for that event: students should select an event that they are physically able to participate in based on their realistic level of fitness • Evaluating level of fitness needed, if running • Setting a time line for preparation: students should select a community-based activity that they can participate in, and complete, **by week 15** • Participating in the event; training and preparing properly by using fitness exercises learned in the course • Completing the Personal Fitness Plan Progress Reflection to identify their areas of strength and improvement	• Investigate and use local fitness community resources and organizations • Research available community events • Participate in a community fitness program • Identify participation experience and share that opportunity and experience with the class through an oral presentation in **week 15** • Design outdoor fitness obstacle course or fitness scavenger hunt in a local park or safe, enclosed environment for portfolio	• Encourage students to continue enrolling in school-site physical education classes • Encourage students to continue to participate in daily physical activity • Encourage students to continue to seek out community-based physical activity opportunities • Have students self-reflect on their physical activity habits to determine areas of strength and improvement **Lesson closure** • Review the lesson objectives and assess to what extent students met the objectives • Give reminders and prepare for the next class	**Vocabulary** • Exercise adherence • Group cohesion • Self-efficacy • Self-perception **HK*Propel*** • Chapter 6 Setting SMART Goals for Fitness and Increasing Motivation PowerPoint • Chapter 6 Social and Emotional Learning Competencies PowerPoint • Chapter 16 Community Events PowerPoint • Physical Activity Log • Fitness Class Journal • Student Fitness Portfolio and Grading Rubric • 12-Week Half-Marathon Training Plan • Personalized Fitness Plan (Weeks 1 Through 6) • Community-Based Participation Handout

Pacing Guide: Week 10

Topics and chapters	Standards and GLOs	Objectives	Class discussion topics
Chapter 6: Social and Emotional Learning • Developing relationship skills • Developing self-management skills • Managing stress **Chapter 15:** Continue	**Middle school** • S3.M4.7 • S3.M4.8 • S3.M6.6 • S3.M6.7 • S3.M6.8 • S4.M1.6 • S4.M1.7 • S4.M2.8 • S5.M2.6 • S5.M2.7 • S5.M2.8 **High school** • S2.H2.L1 • S3.H6.L1 • S3.H6.L2 • S4.H1.L1 • S4.H1.L2 • S4.H2.L1 • S4.H2.L2 • S4.H3.L1 • S4.H3.L2 • S4.H4.L1 • S4.H4.L2	• Describe how developing relationship skills can enhance physical activity behavior • Identify ways to offer support to others in achieving physical activity and fitness goals • Describe characteristics of effective communication in a group setting • Collaborate with others to create a group goal to work toward • Describe how to give effective feedback • Identify ways to constructively resolve conflict • Summarize Maslow's hierarchy and how it relates to creating a positive class climate • Discuss how to effectively manage stress	• Maslow's hierarchy • CASEL's SEL competencies • Developing self-management skills – Managing stress – Impulse control – Mental imagery • Developing relationship skills – Effective communication in teams – Collaborative problem-solving – Seeking or offering support – Group dynamics – Providing and accepting feedback – Conflict resolution

Pacing Guide: Week 10

Activities	Assessments	Teaching strategies and tips	Instructional tools, vocabulary, and HK*Propel*
• Have students set a group-based fitness goal to work toward • Create opportunities for students to work together in teams to accomplish goals and then discuss effective communication strategies • Discuss how managing stress and controlling impulses impacts one's overall health • Provide examples of how mental imagery can be used in a physical activity setting to relieve stress and enhance performance • Provide activities for students to provide corrective feedback to a peer • Students continue to work on their fitness circuit group project and activities	• Engagement in class discussion topics • Engagement in class activities for group-based fitness goal activities • Stress Management Handout • Stress Management Assignment	• After students have taken the mid-semester fitness assessments, have them vote on a group fitness goal that all students will pursue over a set period of time • Collectively track the class progress and encourage students to seek and offer support for accomplishing the group goal **Lesson closure** • Review the lesson objectives and assess to what extent students met the objectives • Give reminders and prepare for the next class	**Vocabulary** • Stress management • Corrective feedback • Communication • Impulse control • Conflict resolution **HK*Propel*** • Chapter 15 Implementing Fitness Education PowerPoint • Creating a Group-Set Fitness Goal (Teacher Resource) • Stress Management Handout • Stress Management Assignment • Designing a Fitness Circuit Group Project • Physical Activity Log • Fitness Class Journal

From J.D. Greenberg, N.D. Calkins, and L.S. Spinosa, *Designing and Teaching Fitness Education Courses.* (Champaign, IL: Human Kinetics, 2022)

Pacing Guide: Week 11

Topics and chapters	Standards and GLOs	Objectives	Class discussion topics
Chapter 5: Nutrition, Wellness, and Consumer Issues • Nutritional needs of adolescents • Caloric intake • Weight management • Dieting and eating disorders • Macronutrients and micronutrients • Hydration • Vitamins and minerals • Wellness (stress, sleep, alcohol) • Healthy meals and snacks **Chapter 15:** Continue with student daily activities, routines, and circuits	**Middle school** • S3.M4.7 • S3.M4.8 • S3.M6.6 • S3.M6.7 • S3.M6.8 • S3.M10.7 • S3.M16.7 • S3.M17.6 • S3.M17.7 • S3.M17.8 • S3.M18.6 • S3.M18.7 • S3.M18.8 **High school** • S2.H2.L1 • S3.H1.L2 • S3.H2.L1 • S3.H6.L1 • S3.H6.L2 • S3.H8.L1 • S3.H8.L2 • S3.H13.L1 • S3.H13.L2 • S3.H14.L1 • S3.H14.L2 • S4.H5.L1	• Identify and reinforce healthy nutritional habits • Adopt healthy eating habits which promote positive dietary changes • Identify various macronutrients and micronutrients and food sources • Describe the relationship between proper diets and good health • Describe and categorize foods according to food groups (plant, animal, and processed) • Explain the benefits of drinking water and proper nutrition during physical activity • Explain how culture, media, peers, family, and other factors influence eating behaviors • Differentiate between a nutritious meal or snack versus an unhealthy meal or snack	• Adolescent and teen nutrition • Calories and weight management – BMI – Exercise • Dieting and eating disorders – Anorexia nervosa – Bulimia nervosa – Binge-eating – Muscle dysmorphia • Macronutrients • Micronutrients (vitamins and minerals) • Sugars • Hydration • Skin health • Supplements • Steroids • Wellness • Influence of media • Sample menus

Pacing Guide: Week 11

Activities	Assessments	Teaching strategies and tips	Instructional tools, vocabulary, and HK*Propel*
• Through lecture and discussions, learning and understanding the importance of evaluating the components of nutrition • Participating in the topics for discussion at the end of each section • Responding verbally or in writing to the questions at the end of each section • Writing their responses to the journal prompts at the end of each section • Continuing with daily fitness activities • Continuing group project work for designing individual fitness circuits	• Develop a three-day nutrition log • Physical activity logs • Journal entries • Participation in class discussions and daily fitness activities	• Explain the importance of proper nutrition and provide opportunities for students to develop their own nutritional plan • Emphasize the dangers inherent in fad diets or consumer supplements • Provide opportunities for students to explore food labels online to ensure that they understand the nutritional value of select food items **Lesson closure** • Review the daily topic and key points • Review the lesson objectives and assess to what extent students met the objectives • Give reminders and prepare for the next class	**Vocabulary** • Nutrition • Metabolism • Anorexia nervosa • Bulimia nervosa • Binge-eating • Muscle dysmorphia • Macronutrients • Carbohydrates • Proteins • Fats • Sugars • Hydration • Micronutrients • Vitamins • Minerals • Diets • Supplements • Steroids **HK*Propel*** • Chapter 5 Nutrition, Wellness, and Consumer Issues PowerPoint • Three-Day Nutrition Log • Physical Activity Log • Fitness Class Journal • Personalized Fitness Plan (Weeks 7 Through 12) • Designing a Fitness Circuit Group Project • Daily Nutritional Goals for Age-Sex Groups (Females and Males Ages 9-13 and 14-18) • Calculating Daily Caloric and Macronutrient Needs • Calculating Sweat Rate **Online resources** www.eatright.org/ www.sportsrd.org/ https://kidshealth.org/en/teens/eat-disorder.html?WT.ac=t-ra www.fda.gov/food/nutrition-education-resources-materials/health-educators-nutrition-toolkit-setting-table-healthy-eating https://kidshealth.org/en/teens/triad.html https://theicn.org/icn-resources-a-z/food-allergy-fact-sheets www.gssiweb.org/education-resources/all https://kidshealth.org/en/teens/nutrition-fitness-center/nutrition/?WT.ac=en-t-fitness-nutrition-center-b https://nnlm.gov/psr/guides/nutrition-information-resources/websites-and-tools https://nnlm.gov/classes/nutrition https://schoolnutrition.org/ www.nal.usda.gov/fnic/teen-nutrition www.commonthreads.org/ www.usda.gov www.dietaryguidelines.gov/sites/default/files/2020-12/Dietary_Guidelines_for_Americans_2020-2025.pdf

From J.D. Greenberg, N.D. Calkins, and L.S. Spinosa, *Designing and Teaching Fitness Education Courses.* (Champaign, IL: Human Kinetics, 2022)

Pacing Guide: Week 12

Topics and chapters	Standards and GLOs	Objectives	Class discussion topics
Chapter 15: Implementing the Fitness Education Program • Continue emphasizing warm-up and cool-down techniques while participating in a variety of activities • Continue emphasizing correct techniques for implementing exercises in chapters 9 through 14 • Continue with implementing routines and circuits • Introduce group project Cardiorespiratory activities are performed daily	**Middle school** • S3.M4.7 • S3.M4.8 • S3.M6.6 • S3.M6.7 • S3.M6.8 • S3.M7.6 • S3.M7.8 • S3.M9.6 • S3.M9.7 • S3.M9.8 • S3.M12.8 • S3.M14.6 • S4.M1.6 • S4.M1.7 • S4.M2.8 • S4.M7.6 • S4.M7.7 • S4.M7.8 • S5.M6.6 • S5.M6.7 • S5.M6.8 **High school** • S2.H2.L1 • S3.H3.L2 • S3.H6.L1 • S3.H9.L1 • S3.H9.L2 • S3.H10.L1 • S3.H10.L2	• Participate in a variety of workouts, routines, and circuits to help improve their fitness level • Continue to improve on their techniques for flexibility exercises in chapters 9 to 11 • Continue to improve on their techniques for strength exercises in chapters 12 to 14 **Group project** Divide into working groups for group project to develop original exercise circuits and routines	**Methods of training** • Routines and flow • HIIT • Routines • Stackers • Tabata • Circuits Teacher provides instructions for and discussion of the group project: • Students will break into groups of three to four • Students will use the activities learned in weeks 4 through 6 (chapters 9 through 14) and develop their original exercise routines and circuits • Students will present their work to the class during **weeks 14 through 15**

Pacing Guide: Week 12

Activities	Assessments	Teaching strategies and tips	Instructional tools, vocabulary, and HK*Propel*
• Receive continued instruction on the different types of fitness activities: – Routines – Stackers – Tabata – Circuits • Participating and engaging throughout class time • Following teacher commands • Supporting and assisting classmates in performing activities • Properly executing exercises and routines • Breaking into groups for their group project	• Preparation for class • Participation and engagement in activities and discussion • Following teacher commands through routine • Applying appropriate warm-up and cool-down techniques while participating in a variety of activities • Supporting and assisting classmates • Knowledge of vocabulary • Execution of exercises • Expedience in developing own groups for group project	• Emphasize that the lesson is designed to help them learn about the ***health-related fitness*** components of flexibility and muscular strength • Emphasize that participation in these activities will improve components of *skill-related fitness* • Emphasize that improving on the components of fitness will assist them in performing daily activities and specific sports • Stress the importance of performing each exercise, routine, and circuit accurately **Lesson closure** • Review the daily topic and key points • Review the lesson objectives and assess to what extent students met the objectives • Emphasize that students should continue doing their assigned workout outside of class • Give reminders and prepare for the next class	**Vocabulary** • HIIT training • Routines • Stackers • Tabata • Circuits **HK*Propel*** • Chapter 15 Implementing Fitness Education PowerPoint • Physical Activity Log • Fitness Class Journal • Tabata #1 • Tabata #2 • Circuit: Did You Forget Something? • Circuit: Follow the Leader • Circuit: Take the Challenge • Personalized Fitness Plan (Weeks 7 Through 12) • Designing a Fitness Circuit Group Project

From J.D. Greenberg, N.D. Calkins, and L.S. Spinosa, *Designing and Teaching Fitness Education Courses*. (Champaign, IL: Human Kinetics, 2022)

Pacing Guide: Week 13

Topics and chapters	Standards and GLOs	Objectives	Class discussion topics
Chapter 15: Implementing the Fitness Education Program • Continue emphasizing warm-up and cool-down techniques while participating in a variety of activities • Continue emphasizing correct techniques for implementing exercises in chapters 9 through 14 • Continue with implementing routines and circuits **Chapter 6:** Social and Emotional Learning • Self-awareness • Social awareness • Responsible decision-making • Self-management • Relationship skills	**Middle school** • S3.M4.7 • S3.M14.6 • S3.M4.8 • S4.M1.6 • S3.M6.6 • S4.M1.7 • S3.M6.7 • S4.M2.8 • S3.M6.8 • S4.M7.6 • S3.M7.6 • S4.M7.7 • S3.M7.8 • S4.M7.8 • S3.M9.6 • S5.M6.6 • S3.M9.7 • S5.M6.7 • S3.M9.8 • S5.M6.8 • S3.M12.8 **High school** • S2.H2.L1 • S3.H3.L2 • S3.H6.L1 • S3.H9.L1 • S3.H9.L2 • S3.H10.L1 • S3.H10.L2	• Participate in a variety of workouts, routines, and circuits to help improve their fitness level • Continue to improve on their techniques for flexibility exercises in chapters 9 through 11 • Continue to improve on their techniques for strength exercises in chapters 12 through 14 • Continue working in groups for group project in developing original exercise circuits and routines • Through group project participation, practice SEL skills: – Self-awareness – Social awareness – Responsible decision-making – Self-management – Relationship skills	**Methods of training** • Routines and flow • HIIT • Routines • Stackers • Tabata • Circuits Teacher provides further assistance and support for the group project: • Students continue working with their groups in individual areas of the class space • Students will use the activities learned in weeks 4 through 6 (chapters 9 through 14) and develop their original exercise routines and circuits • Students will present their work to the class during **weeks 14 through 15** Continue practicing SEL skills from chapter 6

Pacing Guide: Week 13

Activities	Assessments	Teaching strategies and tips	Instructional tools, vocabulary, and HK*Propel*
• Receive continued instruction on the different types of fitness activities: – Routines – Stackers – Tabata – Circuits • Participating and engaging throughout class time • Following teacher commands • Supporting and assisting classmates in performing activities • Properly executing exercises and routines • Breaking into groups for group project and continuing work on their routines and circuits • Emphasize SEL skills	• Preparation for class • Participation and engagement in activities and discussion • Following teacher commands through routine • Applying appropriate warm-up and cool-down techniques while participating in a variety of activities • Supporting and assisting classmates • Knowledge of vocabulary • Execution of exercises • Expedience in developing own groups for group project	• Emphasize that the lesson is designed to help them learn about the ***health-related fitness*** components of flexibility and muscular strength • Emphasize that participation in these activities will improve their components of ***skill-related fitness*** • Emphasize that improving on the components of fitness will assist them in performing daily activities and specific sports • Stress the importance of performing each exercise, routine, and circuit accurately • Emphasize SEL skills and strategies **Lesson closure** • Review the daily topic and key points • Review the lesson objectives and assess to what extent students met the objectives • Emphasize that students should continue doing their assigned workout outside of class • Give reminders and prepare for the next class	**Vocabulary** • HIIT training • Routines • Stackers • Tabata • Circuits **HK*Propel*** • Chapter 15 Implementing Fitness Education PowerPoint • Physical Activity Log • Fitness Class Journal • Personalized Fitness Plan (Weeks 7 Through 12) • Tabata #1 • Tabata #2 • Circuit: Did You Forget Something? • Circuit: Follow the Leader • Circuit: Take the Challenge • CASEL's SEL Competencies • Student Fitness Portfolio and Grading Rubric • Group Project: Designing a Fitness Circuit

From J.D. Greenberg, N.D. Calkins, and L.S. Spinosa, *Designing and Teaching Fitness Education Courses.* (Champaign, IL: Human Kinetics, 2022)

Pacing Guide: Week 14

Topics and chapters	Standards and GLOs	Objectives	Class discussion topics
Chapter 15: Implementing the Fitness Education Program • Continue emphasizing warm-up and cool-down techniques while participating in a variety of activities • Continue emphasizing correct techniques for exercises in chapters 9 through 14 • Group project presentations begin **Chapter 6:** Social and Emotional Learning • Self-awareness • Social awareness • Responsible decision-making • Self-management • Relationship skills	**Middle school** • S3.M4.7 • S3.M14.6 • S3.M4.8 • S4.M1.6 • S3.M6.6 • S4.M1.7 • S3.M6.7 • S4.M2.8 • S3.M6.8 • S4.M7.6 • S3.M7.6 • S4.M7.7 • S3.M7.8 • S4.M7.8 • S3.M9.6 • S5.M6.6 • S3.M9.7 • S5.M6.7 • S3.M9.8 • S5.M6.8 • S3.M12.8 **High school** • S2.H2.L1 • S3.H3.L2 • S3.H6.L1 • S3.H9.L1 • S3.H9.L2 • S3.H10.L1 • S3.H10.L2	• Participate in a variety of workouts, routines, and circuits to help improve their fitness level • Continue to improve on their techniques for flexibility exercises in chapters 9 through 11 • Continue to improve on their techniques for strength exercises in chapters 12 through 14 • Present group project for developing original exercise circuits and routines • Through group project participation, students will practice SEL skills: – Self-awareness – Social awareness – Responsible decision-making – Self-management – Relationship skills	**Methods of training** • Routines and flow • HIIT • Routines • Stackers • Tabata • Circuits Teacher provides further assistance and support for the group project: • Students in their groups present their original routines and circuits to the class • Students will use the activities learned in weeks 4 to 6 (chapters 9 through 14) and develop their original exercise routines and circuits • Students will present their work to the class during **weeks 14 through 15** Continue practicing SEL skills from chapter 6

Pacing Guide: Week 14

Activities	Assessments	Teaching strategies and tips	Instructional tools, vocabulary, and HK*Propel*
• Receive continued instruction on the different types of fitness activities: – Routines – Stackers – Tabata – Circuits • Participating and engaging throughout class time • Following teacher commands • Supporting and assisting classmates in performing activities • Properly executing exercises and routines • Presenting for group project and continuing to work on their routines and circuits • Emphasize SEL skills	• Preparation for class • Participation and engagement in activities and discussion • Following teacher commands through routine • Apply appropriate warm-up and cool-down techniques while participating in a variety of activities • Supporting and assisting classmates • Knowledge of vocabulary • Execution of exercises • Cooperative learning in groups for group project • Group project presentation	• Emphasize that the lesson is designed to help them learn about the ***health-related fitness*** components of flexibility and muscular strength • Emphasize that participation in these activities will improve components of ***skill-related fitness*** • Emphasize that improving on the components of fitness will assist them in performing daily activities and specific sports • Stress the importance of performing each exercise, routine, and circuit accurately • Emphasize SEL skills and strategies **Lesson closure** • Review the daily topic and key points • Review the lesson objectives and assess to what extent students met the objectives • Emphasize that students should continue doing their assigned workout outside of class • Give reminders and prepare for the next class	**Vocabulary** • HIIT training • Routines • Stackers • Tabata • Circuits **HK*Propel*** • Chapter 15 Implementing Fitness Education PowerPoint • Physical Activity Log • Fitness Class Journal • Personalized Fitness Plan (Weeks 7 Through 12) • Tabata #1 • Tabata #2 • Circuit: Did You Forget Something? • Circuit: Follow the Leader • Circuit: Take the Challenge • CASEL's SEL Competencies • Student Fitness Portfolio and Grading Rubric • Group Project: Designing a Fitness Circuit

From J.D. Greenberg, N.D. Calkins, and L.S. Spinosa, *Designing and Teaching Fitness Education Courses*. (Champaign, IL: Human Kinetics, 2022)

Pacing Guide: Week 15

Topics and chapters	Standards and GLOs	Objectives	Class discussion topics
Chapter 15: Implementing the Fitness Education Program • Continue emphasizing warm-up and cool-down techniques while participating in a variety of activities • Continue emphasizing correct techniques for exercises in chapters 9 through 14 • Student group project presentations are finalized **Chapter 6:** Social and Emotional Learning • Self-awareness • Social awareness • Responsible decision-making • Self-management • Relationship skills	**Middle school** • S3.M4.7 • S3.M14.6 • S3.M4.8 • S4.M1.6 • S3.M6.6 • S4.M1.7 • S3.M6.7 • S4.M2.8 • S3.M6.8 • S4.M7.6 • S3.M7.6 • S4.M7.7 • S3.M7.8 • S4.M7.8 • S3.M9.6 • S5.M6.6 • S3.M9.7 • S5.M6.7 • S3.M9.8 • S5.M6.8 • S3.M12.8 **High school** • S2.H2.L1 • S3.H3.L2 • S3.H6.L1 • S3.H9.L1 • S3.H9.L2 • S3.H10.L1 • S3.H10.L2	• Participate in a variety of workouts, routines, and circuits to help improve their fitness level • Continue to improve on their techniques for flexibility exercises in chapters 9 through 11 • Continue to improve on their techniques for strength exercises in chapters 12 through 14 • Present group project for developing original exercise circuits and routines • Through group project participation, practice the following SEL skills: - Self-awareness - Social awareness - Responsible decision-making - Self-management - Relationship skills	**Methods of training** • Routines and flow • HIIT • Routines • Stackers • Tabata • Circuits Teacher provides further assistance and support for the group project: • Students in their groups present their original routines and circuits to the class • Students will use the activities learned in weeks 4 through 6 (chapters 9 through 14) and develop their original exercise routines and circuits • Student work will be presented to class during **weeks 14 through 15** Continue practicing SEL skills from chapter 6

Pacing Guide: Week 15

Activities	Assessments	Teaching strategies and tips	Instructional tools, vocabulary, and HK*Propel*
• Receive continued instruction on the different types of fitness activities: - Routines - Stackers - Tabata - Circuits • Participating and engaging throughout class time • Following teacher commands • Supporting and assisting classmates in performing activities • Properly executing exercises and routines • Student presentations for group project and continue working on their routines and circuits • Emphasize SEL skills	• Preparation for class • Participation and engagement in activities and discussion • Following teacher commands through routine • Applying appropriate warm-up and cool-down techniques while participating in a variety of activities • Supporting and assisting classmates • Knowledge of vocabulary • Execution of exercises • Cooperative learning in groups for group project • Group project presentation	• Emphasize that the lesson is designed to help them learn about the ***health-related fitness*** components of flexibility and muscular strength • Emphasize that participation in these activities will improve their components of ***skill-related fitness*** • Emphasize that improving on the components of fitness will assist them in performing daily activities and specific sports • Stress the importance of performing each exercise, routine, and circuit accurately • Emphasize SEL skills and strategies **Lesson closure** • Review the daily topic and key points • Review the lesson objectives and assess to what extent students met the objectives • Give reminders and prepare for next class • Emphasize that students should continue doing their assigned workout outside of class	**Vocabulary** • HIIT training • Routines • Stackers • Tabata • Circuits **HK*Propel*** • Chapter 15 Implementing Fitness Education PowerPoint • Physical Activity Log • Fitness Class Journal • Personalized Fitness Plan (Weeks 7 Through 12) • Tabata #1 • Tabata #2 • Circuit: Did You Forget Something? • Circuit: Follow the Leader • Circuit: Take the Challenge • CASEL's SEL Competencies • Student Fitness Portfolio and Grading Rubric • Designing a Fitness Circuit Group Project

From J.D. Greenberg, N.D. Calkins, and L.S. Spinosa, *Designing and Teaching Fitness Education Courses*. (Champaign, IL: Human Kinetics, 2022)

Pacing Guide: Week 16

Topics and chapters	Standards and GLOs	Objectives	Class discussion topics
Fitness assessment posttest **Chapter 2:** Fitness Components and Training Principles **Chapter 7:** Standards, Grade-Level Outcomes, and Assessment • One-mile (1.6 km) run or walk, PACER • Body composition • Curl-ups • Trunk lifts • Push-ups • Back saver sit and reach **Chapter 15:** Continue **Chapter 16:** Extending Fitness Education Into the Community Student community event participation presented to class	**Middle school** • S3.M7.6 • S3.M7.8 • S3.M12.8 • S3.M14.6 • S4.M1.6 • S4.M1.7 • S4.M1.8 • S4.M2.7 • S4.M2.8 **High school** • S3.H3.L2 • S3.H6.L1 • S3.H9.L1 • S3.H9.L2 • S3.H10.L1 • S3.H10.L2 • S3.H11.L2	• Assess current fitness status by comparing personal fitness assessment scores to nationally recognized fitness standards • Compare pre- and posttest FitnessGram and Brockport Physical Fitness Test assessment scores • Make a determination based on the FitnessGram and Brockport Physical Fitness Test of whether or not they met their goals on their individual fitness plan • Present to the class their community event participation	**Chapter 2** Components of physical fitness **Chapter 7** • Fitness assessment protocols • Purpose of fitness assessment • FitnessGram and Brockport Physical Fitness Test protocols **Chapter 16** Presentation of community event participation to class (chapter 16, week 9)

Pacing Guide: Week 16

Activities	Assessments	Teaching strategies and tips	Instructional tools, vocabulary, and HK*Propel*
• Participating and engaging throughout class time • Participating in posttest of FitnessGram and Brockport Physical Fitness Test assessment • Presenting community event participation to class (chapter 16, week 9)	• Preparation for class • Participation and engagement in activities and discussion • Supporting and assisting classmates • Knowledge of vocabulary • Execution of exercises • Class presentation of community event participation	• Remind students of the purpose of posttest fitness assessments and provide an opportunity for students to practice the tests before performing pre-assessments • Follow the best practices for fitness assessments such as not grading performance and emphasizing personal improvement • Lead students through a proper warm-up and cool-down before and after fitness assessments • Review student pre- and posttest fitness scores in their personalized fitness plan **Lesson closure** • Review the daily topic and key points • Review the lesson objectives and assess to what extent students met the objectives • Emphasize that students continue to do assigned workout outside of class • Give reminders and prepare for the next class	**Vocabulary** • Cardiorespiratory • Muscular strength • Muscular endurance • Flexibility • Body composition **HK*Propel*** Chapter 2 Components of Physical Fitness PowerPoint Chapter 7 Fitness Assessments PowerPoint Physical Activity Log Fitness Class Journal FitnessGram Student Score Sheet Personalized Fitness Plan (Weeks 7 Through 12) Student Fitness Portfolio and Grading Rubric Community-Based Participation Handout **Online resources** www.pyfp.org https://fitnessgram.net/

Pacing Guide: Week 17

Topics and chapters	Standards and GLOs	Objectives	Class discussion topics
Fitness assessment posttest **Chapter 2:** Fitness Components and Training Principles **Chapter 7:** Standards, Grade-Level Outcomes, and Assessment • One-mile (1.6 km) run or walk, PACER • Body composition • Curl-ups • Trunk lifts • Push-ups • Back saver sit and reach	**Middle school** • S3.M7.6 • S3.M7.8 • S3.M12.8 • S3.M14.6 • S4.M1.6 • S4.M1.7 • S4.M1.8 • S4.M2.7 • S4.M2.8 **High school** • S3.H3.L2 • S3.H6.L1 • S3.H9.L1 • S3.H9.L2 • S3.H10.L1 • S3.H10.L2 • S3.H11.L2	Assess current fitness status by comparing personal fitness assessment scores to nationally recognized fitness standards Compare pre- and posttest FitnessGram and Brockport Physical Fitness Test assessment scores Make a determination based on the FitnessGram and Brockport Physical Fitness Test of whether or not they met their goals on their individual fitness plan	**Chapter 2** Components of physical fitness **Chapter 7** Fitness assessment protocols Purpose of fitness assessment FitnessGram and Brockport Physical Fitness Test protocols **Finalize projects and presentations** Designing a Fitness Circuit Group Project Community-Based Participation Event Student Fitness Portfolio Personalized Fitness Plan (Weeks 1 Through 6 and 7 Through 12)

Pacing Guide: Week 17

Activities	Assessments	Teaching strategies and tips	Instructional tools, vocabulary, and HK*Propel*
• Participating and engaging throughout class time • Participating in posttest FitnessGram and Brockport Physical Fitness Test assessment • Reviewing personal fitness plan **Students will finalize all outstanding assignments and assessments**	• Preparation for class • Participation and engagement in activities and discussion • Supporting and assisting classmates • Knowledge of vocabulary • Execution of exercises **Finalizing projects and presentations** • Designing a Fitness Circuit Group Project • Community-Based Participation Event • Student Fitness Portfolio • Personalized Fitness Plan (Weeks 1 Through 6 and Weeks 7 Through 12) • Physical Activity Log • Fitness Class Journal	• Remind students of the purpose of posttest fitness assessments and provide an opportunity for students to practice the tests before performing pre-assessments • Follow the best practices for fitness assessments such as not grading performance and emphasizing personal improvement • Lead students through a proper warm-up and a cool-down before and after fitness assessments • Review student pre- and posttest fitness scores in their personal fitness plans **Lesson closure** • Review the daily topic and key points • Review the lesson objectives and assess to what extent students met the objectives • Give reminders and prepare for next class • Emphasize that students should continue doing their assigned workout outside of class	**Vocabulary** • Cardiorespiratory • Muscular strength • Muscular endurance • Flexibility • Body composition **HK*Propel*** • Physical Activity Log • Fitness Class Journal • FitnessGram Student Score Sheet • Personalized Fitness Plan (Weeks 1 Through 6 and Weeks 7 Through 12) • Student Fitness Portfolio and Grading Rubric • Community-Based Participation Handout • Designing a Fitness Circuit Group Project **Online resources** www.pyfp.org https://fitnessgram.net/

From J.D. Greenberg, N.D. Calkins, and L.S. Spinosa, *Designing and Teaching Fitness Education Courses*. (Champaign, IL: Human Kinetics, 2022)

Pacing Guide: Week 18

Topics and chapters	Standards and GLOs	Objectives	Class discussion topics
Course closure • Review for course final exam • Collect students' Physical Activity Log • Review students' Fitness Class Journal • Collect finalized Student Fitness Portfolios • Collect students' Personalized Fitness Plan (Weeks 1 through 6 and Weeks 7 through 12) • Have students complete and submit all outstanding assignments **Administer final exam** **Managerial duties** • Collect locks • Have students clean out their physical education lockers	**Middle school** • S3.M7.6 • S3.M7.7 • S3.M7.8 • S3.M12.8 • S3.M14.6 • S4.M1.6 • S4.M1.7 • S4.M2.8 **High school** • S3.H6.L1 • S3.H6.L2 • S5.H1.L1	The teacher will: • Bring class to closure • Review major components and concepts for final exam • Discuss class objectives and overall impact on students	• What students have learned from this class • Student reflections on their accomplishments • Review of Student Interest Questionnaires and whether or not students' opinions regarding physical education and fitness education, in particular, have changed

Pacing Guide: Week 18

Activities	Assessments	Teaching strategies and tips	Instructional tools, vocabulary, and HK*Propel*
• Review with students their original questionnaires reflecting physical activity habits and individual interests • Students submit any outstanding assignments • Review for final exam **Final exam**	Collect all assignments and assessments from students: • Final exam • Fitness Portfolio • Physical Activity Log • Fitness Class Journal • Individual and group projects: – Community-Based Participation Event – Designing a Fitness Circuit Group Project • Personalized Fitness Plan (Weeks 1 Through 6 and Weeks 7 Through 12)	**Lesson closure** • Encourage students to continue enrolling in school-site physical education classes • Encourage students to continue to participate in daily physical activity • Encourage students to continue to seek out community-based physical activity opportunities	**Vocabulary:** Review all vocabulary for final exam **HK*Propel*** • Student Interest Questionnaire • Student Fitness Portfolio and Grading Rubric • Physical Activity Log • Fitness Class Journal • Personalized Fitness Plan (Weeks 1 Through 6 and Weeks 7 Through 12) • Community-Based Participation Handout • Designing a Fitness Circuit Group Project

Visit HK*Propel* for additional material related to this chapter.

REFERENCES

Chapter 1

Ahmed, M.D., Walter, K.Y., Rudolph, L.V., Morris, T., Elayaraja, M., Lee, K., & Randles, E. (2017). The self-esteem, goal orientation, and health-related physical fitness of active and inactive adolescent students. *Cogent Psychology, 4*(1), 1-14. https://doi.org/10.1080/23311908.2017.1331602

American College of Cardiology. (2019, March). *Heart attacks increasingly common in young adults: Youngest heart attack survivors have same likelihood of dying as survivors 10+ years older; substance abuse may be contributing to trend.* Retrieved from www.sciencedaily.com/releases/2019/03/190307081026.htm

Bandura, A. (1977). Self-efficacy: Toward a unifying theory of behavioral change. *Psychological Review, 84*(2), 191-215.

Belanger, K., Barnes, J.D., Longmuir, P.E., Anderson, K.D., Bruner, B., Copeland, J.L., Gregg, M.J., Hall, N., Kolen, A.M., Lane, K.N., Law, B., MacDonald, D.J., Martin, L.J., Saunders, T.J., Sheehan, D., Stone, M., Woodruff, S.J., & Tremblay, M.S. (2018). The relationship between physical literacy scores and adherence to Canadian physical activity and sedentary behavior guidelines. *BMC Public Health, 18*(Suppl 2), 113-121. https://doi.org/10.1186/s12889-018-5897-4

Bernstein, E., Phillips, S.R., & Silverman, S. (2011). Attitudes and perceptions of middle school students toward competitive activities in physical education. *Journal of Teaching in Physical Education, 30*, 69-83.

Bejerot, S., Edgar, J., & Humble, M.B. (2011). Poor performance in physical education - a risk factor for bully victimization. A case-control study. *Acta Paediatrica, 100*(3), 413-419. https://doi.org/10.1111/j.1651-2227.2010.02016.x

Biddle, S.J., Bennie, J.A., Bauman, A.E., Chau, J.Y., Dunstan, D., Owen, N., Stamatakis, E., & van Uffelen, J.G. (2016). Too much sitting and all-cause mortality: Is there a causal link? *BMC Public Health, 16*, 635. https://doi.org/10.1186/s12889-016-3307-3

Bland, H.W., Melton, B.F., Bigham, L.E., & Welle, P.D. (2014). Quantifying the impact of physical activity on stress tolerance in college students. *College Student Journal, 48*(4), 559-568.

Booth, F.W., Roberts, C.K., & Laye, M.J. (2012). Lack of exercise is a major cause of chronic diseases. *Comprehensive Physiology, 2*(2), 1143-1211. https://doi.org/10.1002/cphy.c110025

Bryan, C. L., & Solmon, M. A. (2012). Student motivation in physical education and engagement in physical activity. *Journal of Sport Behavior, 35*(3), 267–285.

Budde, H., Voelcker-Rehage, C., Pietrabyk-Kendziorra, S., Ribeiro, P., & Tidow, G. (2008). Acute coordinative exercise improves attentional performance in adolescents. *Neuroscience Letters, 441*(2), 219-223. https://doi.org/10.1016/j.neulet.2008.06.024

California State University San Marcos (n.d.). *Teaching Online.* Retrieved from www.csusm.edu/ats/idesign/coursedesign/teachingonline/index.html

Capel, S. & Blair, R. (2007). Making physical education relevant: increasing the impact of initial teacher training. *London Review of Education*, 5(*1*), 15-34.

Centers for Disease Control and Prevention. (2020, June). *Physical activity: How much physical activity do children need?* Retrieved from www.cdc.gov/physicalactivity/basics/children/index.htm#:~:text=Children%20and%20adolescents%20ages%206,doing%20push%2Dups)%20%E2%80%93%203

Centers for Disease Control and Prevention. (2020, April). *Physical activity: Measuring physical activity intensity.* Retrieved from www.cdc.gov/physicalactivity/basics/measuring/index.html

Centers for Disease Control and Prevention. (2017, February). *National center for health statistics.* Retrieved from www.cdc.gov/nchs/nhis/physical_activity/pa_glossary.htm

Centers for Disease Control and Prevention. (2020, June). *Heart disease facts.* Retrieved from www.cdc.gov/heartdisease/facts.htm

Centers for Disease Control and Prevention. (2010). *The association between school based physical activity, including physical education, and academic performance.* Atlanta, GA: U.S. Department of Health and Human Services.

Chaddock-Heyman, L., Erickson, K.I., Voss, M., Knecht, A., Pontifex, M.B., Castelli, D., Hillman, C., and Kramer, A. (2013). The effects of physical activity on functional MRI activation associated with cognitive control in children: A randomized controlled intervention. *Frontiers in Human Neuroscience, 72*(7). https://doi.org/10.3389/fnhum.2013.00072

Corbin, C., Kulinna, P., & Yu, H. (2019). Conceptual physical education: A secondary innovation. *Quest, 72*(10), 1-24. https://doi.org/10.1080/00336297.2019.1602780

Corbin, C., Kulinna, P., & Sibley, B. (2020). A dozen reasons for including conceptual physical education in quality secondary school programs. *Journal of Physical Education, Recreation & Dance. 91*(3), 40-49. https://doi.org/10.1080/07303084.2019.1705211

Corbin, C.B., Castelli, D.M., Sibley, B.A., & Le Masurier, G.C. (2022). *Fitness for life (7th ed.).* Champaign, IL: Human Kinetics.

DePaul University. (n.d.). *Teaching commons: Course objectives & learning outcomes.* Retrieved from https://resources.depaul.edu/teaching-commons/teaching-guides/course-design/Pages/course-objectives-learning-outcomes.aspx

Donnelly, J.E., Hillman, C.H., Castelli, D., Etnier, J.L., Lee, S., Tomporowski, P., Lambourne, K., & Szabo-Reed, A.N. (2016). Physical activity, fitness, cognitive function, and academic achievement in children: A systematic review. *Medicine and Science in Sports and Exercise, 48*(6), 1197-1222. https://doi.org/10.1249/MSS.0000000000000901

Ennis, C. (2014). What goes around comes around . . . Or does it? Disrupting the cycle of traditional, sport-based physical education. *Kinesiology Review, 3*(1), 63-70. https://doi.org/10.1123/kr.2014-0039

Fedewa, A.L., & Ahn, S. (2011). The effects of physical activity and physical fitness on children's achievement and cognitive outcomes: A meta-analysis. *Research Quarterly for Exercise and Sport, 82*(3), 521-535.

Frazier, P., Gabriel, A., Merians, A., & Lust, K. (2019). Understanding stress as an impediment to academic performance. *Journal of American College Health,67*(6), 562-570. https://doi.org/10.1080/07448481.2018.1499649

Graham, D.J., Sirard, J.R., & Neumark-Sztainer, D. (2011). Adolescents' attitudes toward sports, exercise, and fitness predict physical activity 5 and 10 years later. *Preventive Medicine, 52*(2), 130-132. https://doi.org/10.1016/j.ypmed.2010.11.013

Greenberg, J.D., and LoBianco, J.L. (2020). *Organization and administration of physical education: Theory and practice.* Champaign, IL: Human Kinetics.

Guthold, R., Stevens, G. Riley, L., & Bull, F. (2019). Global trends in insufficient physical activity among adolescents: A pooled analysis of 298 population-based surveys with 1·6 million participants. *The Lancet Child & Adolescent Health, 4*(1), 23-35. https://doi.org/10.1016/S2352-4642(19)30323-2

Haidar, A.H. (1997). Prospective chemistry teachers' conceptions of the conservation matter and related concepts. *Journal of Research in Science Teaching, 34,* 181-197.

Hallal P.C, Victora C.G, Azevedo M.R, & Wells, J.C. (2006). Adolescent physical activity and health: A systematic review. *Sports Medicine, 36,* 1019-1030. https://doi.org/10.2165/00007256-200636120-00003

Hillman, C. H., Pontifex, M. B., Castelli, D. M., Khan, N. A., Raine, L. B., Scudder, M. R., Drollette, E. S., Moore, R. D., Wu, C. T., & Kamijo, K. (2014). Effects of the FITKids randomized controlled trial on executive control and brain function. *Pediatrics, 134*(4), e1063–e1071. https://doi.org/10.1542/peds.2013-3219

Hruby, A., & Hu, F.B. (2015). The epidemiology of obesity: A big picture. *PharmacoEconomics, 33*(7), 673-689. https://doi.org/10.1007/s40273-014-0243-x

Iowa Department of Education Guidance. (2019, October). *Guidance for physical education standards.* Retrieved from https://educateiowa.gov/sites/files/ed/documents/Guidance%20for%20Physical%20Education%20Standards.pdf

Integrated Benefits Institute (2018). Press release: Poor health costs US employers $530 billion and 1.4 billion work days of absence and impaired performance according to Integrated Benefits Institute. Retrieved from www.ibiweb.org/poor-health-costs-us-employers-530-billion-and-1-4-billion-work-days-of-absence-and-impaired-performance

Institute of Medicine. (2013). *Educating the student body: Taking physical activity and physical education to school.* Washington, DC: The National Academies Press. https://doi.org/10.17226/18314

Jenkinson, K.A. & Benson, A.C. (2010). Barriers to providing physical education and physical activity in Victorian State secondary schools. *Australian Journal of Teacher Education, 35*(8), 1-17. http://ro.ecu.edu.au/ajte/vol35/iss8/1

Kirk, D. (2013). Educational value and models-based practice in physical education. *Educational Philosophy and Theory, 45*(9), 973-986. https://doi.org/10.1080/00131857.2013.785352

Kulinna, P.H., Corbin, C.B., & Yu, H. (2018). Effectiveness of secondary school conceptual physical education: A 20-year longitudinal study. *Journal of Physical Activity & Health, 15*(12),1-6. https://doi.org/10.1123/jpah.2018-0091

Lieberman, L., Grenier, M., Brian, A., & Arndt, K. (2020). *Universal design for learning in physical education* (1st ed.). Champaign IL: Human Kinetics.

Logan, N., Raine, L., Drollette, E., Castelli, D., Khan, N., Kramer, A., & Hillman, C. (2020). The differential relationship of an afterschool physical activity intervention on brain function and cognition in children with obesity and their normal weight peers. *Pediatric Obesity.* https://doi.org/10.1111/ijpo.12708

Lonsdale, C., Rosenkranz, R.R., Peralta, L. R., Bennie, A., Fahey, P., & Lubans, D. R. (2013). A systematic review and meta-analysis of interventions designed to increase moderate-to-vigorous physical activity in school physical education lessons. *Preventive Medicine, 56*(2), 152-161.

Lou, D. (2014). *Sedentary behaviors and youth: Current trends and the impact on health.* Retrieved from www.activelivingresearch.org

MacDonald, L. (2015). Moving high school students toward physical literacy. *Journal of Physical Education, Recreation & Dance, 86* (7), 23-27.

Mandigo, J., Francis, N., Lodewyk, K., & Lopez, R. (2012). Physical literacy for educators. *Physical Education and Health Journal, 75*(3), 27-30.

Master, L., Nye, R. T., Lee, S., Nahmod, N. G., Mariani, S., Hale, L., & Buxton, O. M. (2019). Bidirectional, daily temporal associations between sleep and physical activity in adolescents. *Scientific Reports, 9*(1), 7732. https://doi.org/10.1038/s41598-019-44059-9

Mattke, S., Liu, H., Caloyeras, J., Huang, C.Y., Van Busum, K.R., Khodyakov, D., & Shier, V. (2013). Workplace wellness programs study: Final report. *Rand Health Quarterly, 3*(2), 7.

Patel, A.V., Maliniak, M.L., Rees-Punia, E., Matthews, C.E., & Gapstur, S.M. (2018). Prolonged leisure time spent sitting in relation to cause-specific mortality in a large US cohort. *American Journal of Epidemiology, 187*(10), 2151–2158. https://doi.org/10.1093/aje/kwy125

Pfeifer, C.E., Sacko, R.S., Ortaglia, A., Monsma, E.V., Beattie, P.F., Goins, J., & Stodden, D.F. (2019). Fit to play? Health-related fitness levels of youth athletes: A pilot study. *Journal of Strength and Conditioning Research.* Advance online publication. https://doi.org/10.1519/JSC.0000000000003430

Philippot, A., Meerschaut, A., Danneaux, L., Smal, G., Bleyenheuft, Y., & De Volder, A. G. (2019). Impact of physical exercise on symptoms of depression and anxiety in pre-adolescents: A pilot randomized trial. *Frontiers in Psychology, 10*(1820). https://doi.org/10.3389/fpsyg.2019.01820

Quay, J., & Peters, J. (2008). Skills, strategies, sport, and social responsibility: Reconnecting physical education. *Journal of Curriculum Studies, 40*(5), 601-626. https://doi.org/10.1080/00220270801886071

Raghuveer ,G., Hartz, J., Lubans, D. R., Takken, T., Wiltz, J. L., Mietus-Snyder, M., . . . Edwards, N. M. (2020). Hypertension and obesity in the young committee of the council on lifelong congenital heart disease and heart health in the young. Cardiorespiratory fitness in youth: An important marker of health: A scientific statement from the American Heart Association. *Circulation, 142(*7), e101-e118. https://doi.org/10.1161/CIR.0000000000000866

Reilly, J.J., & Kelly, J. (2011). Long-term impact of overweight and obesity in childhood and adolescence on morbidity and premature mortality in adulthood: Systematic review. *International Journal of Obesity, 35*(7), 891-898. https://doi.org/10.1038/ijo.2010.222

Ross, S.M., Smit, E., Yun, J., Bogart, K., Hatfield, B., & Logan, S.W. (2020). Updated national estimates of disparities in physical activity and sports participation experienced by children and adolescents with disabilities: NSCH 2016-2017. *Journal of Physical Activity & Health,* 17(4), 443-455. https://doi.org/10.1123/jpah.2019-0421

Sanyaolu, A., Okorie, C., Qi, X., Locke, J., & Rehman, S. (2019). Childhood and adolescent obesity in the United States: A public health concern. *Global Pediatric Health, 6,* 1-11. https://doi.org/10.1177/2333794X19891305

Salvy, S.J., Roemmich, J.N., Bowker, J.C., Romero, N.D., Stadler, P.J., & Epstein, L.H. (2009). Effect of peers and friends on youth physical activity and motivation to be physically active. *Journal of Pediatric Psychology, 34*(2), 217–225. https://doi.org/10.1093/jpepsy/jsn071

SHAPE America. (2012). *Instructional framework for fitness education in physical education. Guidance document.* Reston, VA: Society of Health and Physical Educators.

SHAPE America. (2014). *National standards & grade-level outcomes for K-12 physical education.* Champaign IL: Human Kinetics.

SHAPE America. (2015). *The essential components of physical education (guidance document).* Reston, VA: Society of Health and Physical Educators.

SHAPE America. (2017). *Appropriate and inappropriate practices related to fitness testing.* Reston, VA: Society of Health and Physical Educators.

Siedentop, D., Hastie, P.A., & van der Mars, H. (2019). Complete guide to sport education. Champaign, IL: Human Kinetics.

Shulman, L.S. (1986). Those who understand: Knowledge growth in teaching. *Educational Researcher, 67,* 4-14.

Teixeira, P.J., Carraça, E.V., Markland, D. Silva, M., & Ryan, R.l. (2012). Exercise, physical activity, and self-determination theory: A systematic review. *International Journal of Behavioral Nutrition and Physical Activity, 9*(78). https://doi.org/10.1186/1479-5868-9-78

Thompson, A., & Hannon, J. (2012). Health-related fitness knowledge and physical activity of high school students. *Physical Educator, 69*(1), 71-88.

U.S. Department of Health and Human Services. (2018). *Physical activity guidelines for Americans* (2nd ed.). Washington, DC: U.S. Department of Health and Human Services.

Ward, W., & Ayvazo, S. (2016). Pedagogical content knowledge: Conceptions and findings in physical education. *Journal of Teaching in Physical Education, 35*(3), 194-207. https://doi.org/10.1123/jtpe.2016-0037

Wiggins, G., & McTighe, J. (2005). *Understanding by design* (2nd ed.). Alexandria, VA: Association for Supervision and Curriculum Development.

Williams, S. Phelps, D., Laurson, K., Thomas, D., & Brown, D. (2013). Fitness knowledge, cardiorespiratory endurance and body composition of high school students. *Biomedical Human Kinetics, 5*(1), 17-21. https://doi.org/10.2478/bhk-2013-0004

World Health Organization. (⊠2009)⊠. Global health risks: Mortality and burden of disease attributable to selected major risks. World Health Organization. Retrieved from https://apps.who.int/iris/handle/10665/44203

World Health Organization. (2018). *More active people for a healthier world.* Geneva: World Health Organization.

World Health Organization. (⊠2021, February 23)⊠. Physical activity. https://www.who.int/health-topics/physical-activity#tab=tab_2

Yun, J., & Beamer, J. (2018). Promoting physical activity in adapted physical education. *Journal of Physical Education, Recreation & Dance, 89*(4), 7-13. https://doi.org/10.1080/07303084.2018.1430628

Zhu, X., Haegele, J.A., & Sun, H. (2019). Health-related fitness knowledge growth in middle school years: Individual-and school-level correlates. *Journal of Sport and Health Science, 9*(6), 664-669. https://doi.org/10.1016/j.jshs.2019.04.005

Chapter 2

Al-Hamad, D., & Raman, V. (2017). Metabolic syndrome in children and adolescents. *Translational Pediatrics, 6*(4), 397–407. https://doi.org/10.21037/tp.2017.10.02

Athletics for All. (n.d.) *Wheelchair basketball.* Retrieved from http://assets.ngin.com/attachments/document/0117/2211/A4A_Wheelchair_Basketball.pdf

American College of Sports Medicine. (2018). *ACSM's guidelines for exercise testing and prescription, (10th ed.).* Philadelphia, PA: Wolters Kluwer.

American College of Sports Medicine. (2013). *ACSM's guide to exercise prescription and testing.* Philadelphia, PA: Lippencott, Williams, and Williams.

Batista M.B., Romanzini C.L., Castro-Piñero, J., & Vaz Ronque, E.R. (2017). Validity of field tests to estimate cardiorespiratory fitness in children and adolescents: A systematic review. *Revista Paulista de Pediatria, 35*(2), 222-233. https://doi.org/10.1590/1984-0462/;2017;35;2;00002

Biology. (n.d.) Authored by: OpenStax. Provided by: OpenStax College. Retrieved from http://cnx.org/contents/185cbf87-c72e-48f5-b51e-f14f21b5eabd@9.44:1/Biology

Boyle, M. (2016). *New functional training for sports* (2nd ed.). Champaign, IL: Human Kinetics.

Buchheit, M., & Laursen, P.B. (2013). High-intensity interval training, solutions to the programming puzzle. Part I: Cardiopulmonary emphasis. *Sports Medicine, 43,* 313-338.

Centers for Disease Control and Prevention. (2020, April). *Physical activity: Measuring physical activity intensity.* Retrieved from www.cdc.gov/physicalactivity/basics/measuring/index.html

Corbin, C.B. & LeMasurier, G.C. (2014). *Fitness for life.* (6th ed.). Champaign. IL: Human Kinetics.

Delgado-Floody, P., Espinoza-Silva, M., García-Pinillos, F., & Latorre-Román, P. (2018). Effects of 28 weeks of high-intensity interval training during physical education classes on cardiometabolic risk factors in Chilean schoolchildren: A pilot trial. *European Journal of Pediatrics, 177*(7), 1019-1027. https://doi.org/10.1007/s00431-018-3149-3

Faigenbaum, A. (2012). Dynamic warm-up. In J.R. Hoffman (Ed.), *NSCA's guide to program design* (pp. 51-70). Champaign, IL: Human Kinetics.

Faigenbaum, A., Lloyd, R., Oliver, J., & American College of Sports Medicine. (2020). *Essentials of youth fitness.* Champaign, IL: Human Kinetics.

Garber, C.E., Blissmer, B., Deschenes, M.R., Franklin, B.A., Lamonte, M.J., Lee, I.M., . . . American College of Sports Medicine (2011). American College of Sports Medicine position stand. Quantity and quality of exercise for developing and maintaining cardiorespiratory, musculoskeletal, and neuromotor fitness in apparently healthy adults: guidance for prescribing exercise. *Medicine and Science in Sports and Exercise, 43*(7), 1334–1359. https://doi.org/10.1249/MSS.0b013e318213fefb

García-Hermoso, A., Cerrillo-Urbina, A. J., Herrera-Valenzuela, T., Cristi-Montero, C., Saavedra, J.M., & Martínez-Vizcaíno, V. (2016). Is high-intensity interval training more effective on improving cardiometabolic risk and aerobic capacity than other forms of exercise in overweight and obese youth? A meta-analysis. *Obesity Reviews: An Official Journal of the International Association for the Study of Obesity, 17*(6), 531-540. https://doi.org/10.1111/obr.12395

Going, S., & Hingle, M. (2020). Body composition. In J. Conkle (Ed.), Physical best (4th ed., p.147). Champaign, IL: Human Kinetics.

Going, S.B., Lohman, T.G., & Eisenmann, J.C. (2013). Body Composition Assessments. In S.A. Plowman & M.D. Meredith (Eds.), *Fitnessgram/Activitygram Reference Guide (4th ed.)* (pp. 7-1-7-12). The Cooper Institute.

Hedrick, A. (2012). Flexibility, body weight, and stability ball exercises. In J. W. Coburn & M. H. Malek (Eds.), *NSCA's essentials of personal training* (2nd ed., pp. 251-286). Champaign, IL: Human Kinetics.

Henriksson, H., Henriksson, P., Tynelius, P., Ekstedt, M., Berglind, D., Labayen, . . . Ortega, F.B. (2020). Cardiorespiratory fitness, muscular strength, and obesity in adolescence and later chronic disability due to cardiovascular disease: A cohort study of 1 million men. *European Heart Journal, 41*(15), 1503-1510. https://doi.org/10.1093/eurheartj/ehz774

Institute of Medicine. (2010). *Fitness measures and health outcomes in youth.* Washington, D.C.: National Academies Press.

Jeffreys, I. (2016) Warm-up and flexibility training. In G.G. Haff & N.T. Triplett (Eds.), *Essentials of strength training and conditioning* (4th ed., pp. 317-350). Champaign, IL: Human Kinetics.

Jemni, M., Prince, M.S., & Baker, J.S. (2018). Assessing cardiorespiratory fitness of soccer players: Is test specificity the issue?-A review. *Sports Medicine-Open, 4*(28). https://doi.org/10.1186/s40798-018-0134-3

Jouven, X., Empana, J.P., Escolano, S., Buyck, J.F., Tafflet, M., Desnos, M., Ducimetiére, P. (2009). Relation of heart rate at rest and long-term (>20 years) death rate in initially healthy middle-aged men. *The American Journal of Cardiology, 103*(2), 279-283. https://doi.org/10.1016/j.amjcard.2008.08.071

Kato, E., Oda, T., Chino, K., Nagayoshi, T., Fukunaga, T., & Kawakami, Y. (2005). Musculoteninous factors influencing difference in ankle joint flexibility between women and men. *International Journal of Sport and Health Science,* 3, 218-225.

Klavora, P. (2018). Foundations of kinesiology: Studying human movement and health (3rd ed.). Toronto, ON: Kinesiology Book Publisher.

Laurson, K.R., Eisenmann, J.C., & Welk, G.J. (2011). Body Mass Index standards based on agreement with health-related body fat. *American Journal of Preventive Medicine,* 41(4 Suppl 2), S100-105. https://doi.org/10.1016/j.amepre.2011.07.004

Lloyd, R. et al. (2012). UKSCA Position Statement: Youth Resistance Training. UK Strength and Conditioning Association, 26, 26-39.

McMaster, D.T., Gill, N., Cronin, J., & McGuigan, M. (2013). The development, retention and decay rates of strength and power in elite rugby union, rugby league and American football. *Sports Medicine, 43,* 367-384. https://doi.org/10.1007/s40279-013-0031-3

National Strength and Conditioning Association. Haff, G.G., & Triplett, N.T. (Eds.) (2016). *Essentials of strength and conditioning* (4th ed.). Champaign, IL: Human Kinetics.

Neufer, P.D. (1989). The effect of detraining and reduced training on the physiological adaptations to aerobic exercise training. *Sports Medicine, 8*(5),302-320. https://doi.org/10.2165/00007256-198908050-00004

Ostchega, Y., Porter, K.S., Hughes, J., Dillon, C. F., & Nwankwo, T. (2011). Resting pulse rate reference data for children, adolescents, and adults: United States, 1999-2008. *National Health Statistics Report, 41,* 1-16.

Page, P. (2012). Current concepts in muscle stretching for exercise and rehabilitation. *International Journal of Sports Physical Therapy,* 7(1), 109-119.

Parrott, J., & Zhu, X. (2013). A critical view of static stretching and its relevance in physical education. *The Physical Educator, 70*(4), 395-412.

Pavlovic, A. (2018). *Power training is for everyone.* Dallas, TX: Cooper Institute.

Plowman, S.A. & Meredith, M.D. (Eds.) (2013). *Fitnessgram/Activitygram Reference Guide* (4th ed). The Cooper Institute.

Quinn, E. Verywell Fit. (2019, November). How to do a shoulder flexibility test. Retrieved from www.verywellfit.com/shoulder-flexibility-test-3120278

Reuter, B.H., & Dawes, J.J. (2016). Program design and technique for aerobic endurance training. In G.G. Haff & N.T. Triplett (Eds.), *Essentials of strength training and conditioning* (4th ed., pp. 317-350). Champaign, IL: Human Kinetics.

Schroeder, J., & Alencar, M.K. (2017). Increasing your flexibility. In B. Bushman (Ed.), American College of Sports Medicine complete guide to fitness and health (2nd ed., pp. 147-180). Champaign, IL: Human Kinetics.

SHAPE America. Conkle, J. (Ed.). (2020). *Physical best: Physical education for lifelong fitness and health* (4th ed.). Champaign, IL: Human Kinetics.

U.S. Department of Health and Human Services. (2010, December). Definitions: Health, fitness, and physical activity. President's Council on Physical Fitness and Sports Research Digest. Retrieved from https://static1.squarespace.com/static/572a208737013b7a93cf167e/t/57898e918419c2c106a0cef3/1468632721790/Digest+2000_Definitions-Health%252C+Fitness%252C+and+Physical+Activity_Series+3+Number+9+%2528March%2529.pdf

U.S. Department of Health and Human Services. (2018). *Physical activity guidelines for Americans* (2nd ed.). Washington, DC: U.S. Department of Health and Human Services. https://health.gov/sites/default/files/2019-09/Physical_Activity_Guidelines_2nd_edition.pdf

Winnick, J.P., & Poretta, D.L. (2017). *Adapted physical education and sport* (6th ed.). Champaign, IL: Human Kinetics

Chapter 3

Ayvazo, S., & Ward, P. (2011). Pedagogical content knowledge of experienced teachers in physical education: Functional analysis of adaptations. *Research Quarterly for Exercise and Sport, 82*(4), 675-684.

Brookhart, S.M. (2017). *How to give effective feedback to your students* (2nd ed.). ASCD.

Corbin, C.B., Hodges Kulinna, P., & Sibley, B. A. (2020). A dozen reasons for including conceptual physical education in quality secondary school programs. *Journal of Physical Education, Recreation & Dance. 91*(3), 40-49. https://doi.org/10.1080/07303084.2019.1705211

Donnelly, F.C., Mueller, S.S., & Gallahue, D.L. (2017). *Developmental physical education for all children. Theory into practice* (5th ed.). Champaign, IL: Human Kinetics.

Ellison, D.W., Walton-Fisette, J.L., & Eckert, K. (2019). Utilizing the teaching personal and social responsibility (TPSR) model as a trauma-informed practice (TIP) tool in physical education. *Journal of Physical Education, Recreation & Dance, 90*(9), 32-37. https://doi.org/10.1080/07303084.2019.1657531

Greenberg, J.D., & LoBianco, J.L. (2020). *Organization and administration of physical education: Theory and practice.* Champaign, IL: Human Kinetics.

Guo, P., Kim, J., & Rubin, R. (2014). How video production affects student engagement: An empirical study of MOOC videos. *Proceedings of the first ACM conference on Learning @ scale conference.* Association for Computing Machinery, New York, NY, 41-50. https://doi.org/10.1145/2556325.2566239

Hannon, J.C., Holt, B.J., & Hatten, J.D. (2008). Personalized system of instruction model: Teaching health-related fitness content in high school physical education. *Journal of Curriculum and Instruction, 2*(2), 20-33.

Hattie, J., & Timperley, H. (2007). The power of feedback. *Review of Educational Research, 77*(1), 81-112. https://doi.org/10.3102/003465430298487

Haywood & Getchell (2020). *Life Span Motor Development* (7th ed). Champaign, IL: Human Kinetics.

Hellison, D. (2011). *Teaching personal and social responsibility through physical activity* (3rd ed.). Champaign, IL: Human Kinetics.

Lieberman, L.J., & Houston-Wilson, C. (2018). *Strategies for inclusion* (3rd ed.). Champaign IL: Human Kinetics.

Lieberman, L., Grenier, M., Brian, A., & Arndt, K. (2020). *Universal design for learning in physical education* (1st ed.). Champaign IL: Human Kinetics.

Metzler, M. (2011). *Instructional models for physical education* (3rd ed.). Scottsdale, AZ: Holcomb Hathaway.

Moss, C.M., & Brookhart, S.M. (2015). *Formative classroom walkthroughs: How principals and teachers collaborate to raise student achievement.* ASCD.

Ntuli, E. (2018). Seven characteristics (and six tools) that support meaningful feedback. *ASCD Express, 13*(9). http://www.ascd.org/ascd-express/vol13/1309-ntuli.aspx

Prewitt, S., Hannon, J.C., Colquitt, G., Brusseau, T.A., Newton, M., & Shaw, J. (2015). Effect of personalized system of instruction on health-related fitness knowledge and class time physical activity. *The Physical Educator, 72*, 23-39.

Prewitt, S., Hannon, J.C., Colquitt, G., Brusseau, T.A., Newton, M., & Shaw, J. (2015). Implementation of a personal fitness unit using the personalized system of instruction model. *The Physical Educator, 72*, 382-402.

Rink, J. (2020). *Teaching physical education for learning* (8th ed.). McGraw-Hill Education.

Schinske, J. & Tanner, K. (2014). Teaching more by grading less (or differently). *CBE Life Sciences Education, 13*(2), 159-166. doi: 10.1187/cbe.CBE-14-03-0054

Schmidt, R.A., Lee, T.D., Winstein, C., Wul, G., & Zelaznik, H. (2019). *Motor control and learning: A behavioral emphasis* (6th ed.). Champaign, IL: Human Kinetics.

Chapter 4

Active Living Research. (2010, February). *Parks, playgrounds, and active living research synthesis.* Retrieved from www.activelivingresearch.org/ files/Synthesis_Mowen_Feb2010.pdf

Active Living Research. (2011, November). *Do all children have places to be active? Disparities in access to physical activity environments in racial and ethnic minority and low-income communities.* Retrieved from http://activelivingresearch.org/sites/default/files/Synthesis_Taylor-Lou_Disparities_Nov2011_0.pdf

Adams, M., Bell, L.A., Goodman, D.J., & Joshi, K.Y. (2016). *Teaching for diversity and social justice* (3rd ed.). p.1. New York, NY: Routledge

Allensworth, E.M., Farrington, C.A., Gordon, M.F., Johnson, D.W., Klein, K., McDaniel, B., & Nagaoka, J. (2018, November). *Supporting social, emotional, and academic development: Research implications for educators.* Retrieved from https://consortium.uchicago.edu/sites/default/files/2019-01/Supporting%20Social%20Emotional-Oct2018-Consortium.pdf

American Academy of Pediatrics (2011). Sports drinks and energy drinks for children and adolescents: Are they appropriate? *Pediatrics*, 127, 1182-1189.

American Heart Association. (2014). Staying hydrated – Staying Healthy. Retrieved from www.heart.org/en/healthy-living/fitness/fitness-basics/staying-hydrated-staying-healthy

American Library Association. (2001). Imagining fairness: Equality and equity of access in search of democracy. In N. Kranich, *Libraries and democracy* (pp. 15-27). Chicago, IL: American Library Association. Retrieved from www.ala.org/aboutala/offices/oitp/publications/infocommons0204/schement; library-science.weebly.com/uploads/4/1/3/2/4132239/libraries__democracy.pdf

American Library Association. (2007). "Equality and Equity of Access: What's the Difference?", American Library Association, May 29, 2007. Retrieved from www.ala.org/advocacy/intfreedom/equalityequity

Americans with Disability Act Accessibility Guidelines, Federal Register July 23, 2004 and Amended August 5, 2005. Retrieved from: www.federalregister.gov/documents/2004/07/23/04-16025/americans-with-disabilities-act-accessibility-guidelines-for-buildings-and-facilities

Aspen Institute (2019). *State of play: Trends and developments in youth sports.* Retrieved from www.aspeninstitute.org/wp-content/uploads/2019/10/2019_SOP_National_Final.pdf

Aspen Institute (2019). *From a nation at risk to a nation at hope: Recommendations from the National Commission on Social, Emotional, and Academic Development.* Retrieved from http://nationathope.org/report-from-the-nation/

Aspen Institute (2020). The recovery we need now. July 15, 2020. Retrieved from: www.aspenprojectplay.org/summit/summer-conversation-series/event/the-recovery-we-need-now

The Australian Council for Health, Physical Education and Recreation, Victorian Branch (2009). *Physical activity and fitness education.* Retrieved from www.education.vic.gov.au/Documents/school/teachers/teachingresources/social/physed/phasephys.pdf

Bell, L. (2013). Theoretical foundations. In M. Adams, W.J. Blumenfield, C. Castaneda, H.W. Hickman, M.L. Peters & X. Zuniga. (Eds.) *Readings for diversity and social justice.* p. 21. New York, NY: Routledge.

Benes, S., & Alperin, H. (2016). *Essentials of teaching health education: Curriculum, instruction, and assessment.* SHAPE America. Champaign, IL: Human Kinetics.

Bowes, M., & Tinning, R. (2015). Productive pedagogies and teachers' professional learning in physical education. *Asia-Pacific Journal of Health, Sport and Physical Education*, 6:1, 93-109. https://doi.org/10.1080/18377122.2014.997863

Bushman, B. (Ed.) (2017). *American College of Sports Medicine complete guide to fitness and health* (2nd ed.). Champaign, IL: Human Kinetics.

Castelli, D., Glowacki, E., Barcelona, J., Calvert, H., & Hwang, J. (2015). *Active education: Growing evidence on physical activity and academic performance.* Retrieved from https://activelivingresearch.org/sites/activelivingresearch.org/files/ALR_Brief_ActiveEducation_Jan2015.pdf. pp 1-5.

Centers for Disease Control and Prevention (2019). *Increasing physical education and physical activity: A framework for schools.* Retrieved from www.cdc.gov/healthyschools/physicalactivity/pdf/2019_04_25_PE-PA-Framework_508tagged.pdf

Centers for Disease Control and Prevention (2020). *Whole school, whole community, whole child (WSCC).* Retrieved from www.cdc.gov/healthyschools/wscc/index.htm

Council of Chief State School Officers (2017). *Leading for equity: Opportunities for state education chiefs.* Retrieved from https://ccsso.org/sites/default/files/2018-01/Leading%20for%20Equity_011618.pdf

Donnelly, F.C., Mueller, S.S., & Gallahue, D. (2017). *Developmental physical education for all children: Theory into practice.* Champaign, IL: Human Kinetics.

Durlak, J.A., Weissberg, R.P., Dymnicki, A.B., Taylor, R.D. & Schellinger, K.B. (2011). The impact of enhancing students' social and emotional learning: A meta-analysis of school-based universal interventions. *Child Development, 82*(1), 405-432.

Equality and Human Rights Commission (2018). Scotland, London, UK. Retrieved from https://equalityhumanrights.com/en

Farrey, T. (2020, June 1). How sports can help rebuild America [Web log post]. Retrieved from www.aspeninstitute.org/blog-posts/how-sports-can-help-rebuild-america/

French, R., Henderson, H., Kinnison, L., & Sherrill, C. (1998). Revisiting Section 504, physical education and sport. *Journal of Physical Education, Recreation & Dance, 69*(7), 57-63.

Gagen, L., & Getchell, N. (2004). Combining theory and practice in the gymnasium. "Constraints" within an ecological perspective. *Journal of Physical Education, Recreation & Dance, 75*(5), 25-30.

Greenberg, J.D., & LoBianco, J.L. (2020). *Organization and administration of physical education: Theory and practice.* Champaign, IL: Human Kinetics.

Grenier, M., Miller, N., & Black, K. (2017). Applying universal design for learning and the inclusion spectrum for students with severe disabilities in general physical education. *Journal of Teaching in Physical Education, 88*(6), 51-56.

Grube, D., Ryan, S., Lowell, S., & Stringer, A. (2018). Effective classroom management in physical education: Strategies for beginning teachers. *JOPERD, 89*(8) pp 47-52.

LA84 Foundation (2018). P.E. is a social justice issue. Retrieved from la84.org/play-equity/

Lieberman, L.J., & Houston-Wilson, C. (2018). *Strategies for inclusion: Physical education for everyone* (3rd ed.). Champaign, IL: Human Kinetics.

Lynch, S., & Landi, D. (2018, September 26). Social justice in physical education [Web log post]. Retrieved from https://blog.shapeamerica.org/2018/09/

Lynch, S., Sutherland, S., Walton-Fisette, J. (2020). The A-Z of social justice physical education: Part 1. *JOHPERD, 91*(4), 8-13.

Lynch, S., Sutherland, S., Walton-Fisette, J. (2020). The A-Z of social justice physical education: Part 2. *JOHPERD, 91*(5), 20-27.

MacNeil, A.J., Prater, D.L., & Busch, S. 2009. The effects of school culture and climate on student achievement. *International Journal of Leadership in Education, 12*(1), 73-84.

Morgan, K., & Carpenter, P.J. (2002). Effects of manipulating the motivational climate in physical education lessons. *European Physical Education Review,* 28(3), 207-229.

National Center for Education Statistics. (2016, August). *Digest of education statistics.* Retrieved from https://nces.ed.gov/fastfacts/display.asp?id=64

National Education Association (n.d.). *Diversity toolkit: Social justice.* Retrieved from http://ftp.arizonaea.org/tools/diversity-toolkit.html

Ntoumanis, N., & Biddle, S.J.H. (1999). A review of motivational climate in physical activity. *Journal of Sports Science,* 17(8), 643-665.

Ommundsen, Y., & Kvalo, S.E. (2007). Autonomy-mastery supportive or performance focused? Different teacher behaviors and pupils' outcomes in physical education. *Scandinavian Journal of Educational Research,* 51(4), 385-413.

Organization for Economic Co-Operation and Development (2008, January). *Ten steps to equity in education.* Retrieved from www.oecd.org/education/school/39989494.pdf

Powell, L., Slater, S., & Chaloupka, F. (2004). The relationship between community physical activity settings and race, ethnicity and socioeconomic status. *Evidence-Based Preventive Medicine, 1*(2), 135-144.

Qi, J. & Ha, A.S. (2012). Inclusion in physical education: A review of literature. *International Journal of Disability, Development and Education, 59*(3), 257-281. https://doi.org/10.1080/1034912X.2012.697737

Rasberry, C., Lee, S., Robin, L., Laris, B., & Russell, L. (2011). The association between school-based physical activity, including physical education, and academic performance: A systematic review of the literature. *Preventive Medicine, 52*(Suppl. 1), S10-S20.

Reid, M.A., MacCormack, J., Cousins, S., & Freeman, J.G. . (2015). Physical activity, school climate, and the emotional health of adolescents: Findings from 2010 Canadian health behaviour in school-aged children (HBSC) study. *School Mental Health, 7,* 224-234. https://doi.org/10.1007/s12310-015-9150-3

Rink, J. (2014). *Teaching physical education for learning* (7th ed.). New York, NY: McGraw Hill.

Roman, C.G., & Taylor, C.J. (2013). A multilevel assessment of school climate, bullying victimization, and physical activity. *Journal of School Health, 83*(6), 400-407.

Schweig, J., Hamilton, L.S., & Baker, G. (2019). *School and classroom climate measures: Considerations for use by state and local education leaders.* Retrieved from www.rand.org/pubs/research_reports/RR4259.html

SHAPE America. (2009). *Appropriate instructional practice guidelines, K-12: A side-by-side comparison society of health and physical educators.* Retrieved from www.shapeamerica.org/uploads/pdfs/Appropriate-Instructional-Practices-Grid.pdf

Shindler, J., Jones, A., Williams, D., Taylor, C., &Cardenas, H. (2016). The school climate-student achievement connection: If we want achievement gains, we need to begin by improving the climate. *Journal of School Administration Research and Development,* (1), 9-16.

Sng, B.B. (2012). The Impact of Teachers' Communication Skills on Teaching: Reflections of Pre-service Teachers on Their Communication Strengths and Weaknesses. *Humanising Language Teaching. 14*(1). Retrieved from: http://old.hltmag.co.uk/feb12/mart.htm

Spengler, J.O., Anderson, P.M., Connaughton, D.P., and Baker, T.A. (2016). *Introduction to sport law* (2nd ed.). Champaign, IL: Human Kinetics.

Sproule, J., Wang, C.K., Morgan, K., McNeill, M., & McMorris, T. (2003). Effects of motivational climate in Singaporean physical education lessons on intrinsic motivation and physical activity intention. *Personality and Individual Differences,* 43(5), 1037-1049.

Standage, M., Duda, J.L., & Ntoumanis, N. (2003). A model of contextual motivation in physical education: Using constructs and tenets from self-determination and goal theories to predict leisure-time exercise intentions. *Journal of Educational Psychology,* 95(1), 97-110.

Stuart-Cassel, V. (2015). *In brief: School-based physical fitness and the link to student academic outcomes and improved school climate.* Retrieved from https://safesupportivelearning.ed.gov/sites/default/files/InBrief_Physical%20Fitness%20Brief_10.27.15%20FINAL_0.pdf

United Nations World Food Programme. (2021). What does equality mean to me? Retrieved from: https://www.wfp.org/stories/what-does-equality-mean-me

United States Congress. (1973). PL 93-112—Rehabilitation Act.

United States Department of Education. (1995). The Civil Rights of Students with Hidden Disabilities Under Section 504 of the Rehabilitation Act of 1973. Retrieved from: https://www2.ed.gov/about/offices/list/ocr/docs/hq5269.html

Wadsworth, D.D., Robinson, L.E., Rudisill, M.E., & Gell, N. (2013). The effect of physical education climates on elementary students' physical activity behaviors. *Journal of School Health, 83*(5), 306-313. https://doi.org/10.1111/josh.12032

Wolfram, T. (2018). *Eat right, hydrate right.* Chicago, IL: Academy of Nutrition and Dietetics.

Women's Sports Foundation. (2021). The equity project. Retrieved from: https://www.womenssportsfoundation.org/the-equity-project/

Yelm, M.L. (1998). The legal basis of inclusion. *Educational Leadership, 56*(2), 70-73.

Chapter 5

Ackerman, K.E., Holtzman, B., Cooper, K.M., Flynn, E.F., Bruinvels, G., Tenforde, A.S., & Popp, K.L.. (2019). Low energy availability surrogates correlate with health and performance consequences of relative energy deficiency in sport. *British Journal of Sports Medicine, 53*(10), 628-633. https://doi.org/10.1136/bjsports-2017-098958

American Psychiatric Association. (n.d.) *What are eating disorders?* Retrieved from www.psychiatry.org/patients-families/eating-disorders/what-are-eating-disorders

Armstrong, L.E., Johnson, E.C., Kunces, L.J., Ganio, M.S., Judelson, D.A., Kupchak, B.R., & Vingren, J.L. (2014) Drinking to thirst versus drinking ad libitum during road cycling. *Journal of Athletic Training, 49*(5), 624-31. https://doi.org/10.4085/1062-6050-49.3.85

Arnett, J.J. (1999). Adolescent storm and stress, reconsidered. *American Psychology, 54*(5), 317-26.

Avery, A., Anderson, C., & McCullough, F. (2017). Associations between children's diet quality and watching television during meal or snack consumption: A systematic review. *Maternal & Child Nutrition, 13*(4). https://doi.org/10.1111/mcn.12428

Bingham, M.E., Borkan, M., & Quatronmoni, P. (2015) Sports nutrition advice for adolescent athletes: A time to focus on food. *American Journal of Lifestyle Medicine, 9*(6), pp. 398-402. https://doi.org/10.1177/1559827615598530

Bould, H., De Stavola, B., Lewis, G., & Micali, N. (2018). Do disordered eating behaviours in girls vary by school characteristics? A UK cohort study. *European Child & Adolescent Psychiatry, 27*(11), 1473-1481. https://doi.org/10.1007/s00787-018-1133-0

Casa, D., Cheuvront S., Galloway S., & Shirreffs, S. (2019). Fluid Needs for Training, Competition, and Recovery in Track-and-Field Athletes. *International Journal of Sport Nutrition and Exercise Metabolism. 29*(2):175-180.

Celiac Disease Foundation. (2020). *Non-celiac gluten/wheat sensitivity.* Retrieved from https://celiac.org/about-celiac-disease/related-conditions/non-celiac-wheat-gluten-sensitivity/

Celiac Disease Foundation. (n.d.) *What is celiac disease?* Retrieved from https://celiac.org/about-celiac-disease/what-is-celiac-disease/

Cerea S., Bottesi G., Pacelli Q.F., Paoli A., Ghisi M. (2018). Muscle Dysmorphia and its Associated Psychological Features in Three Groups of Recreational Athletes. *Scientific Reports. 8*, 8877. https://doi.org/10.1038/s41598-018-27176-9

Cullen, K., Thompson, D., Boushey, C., Konzelmann, K., & Chen, T. (2013). Evaluation of a web-based program promoting healthy eating and physical activity for adolescents: Teen choice: Food and fitness. *Health Education Research, 28*(4), 704-14. https://doi.org/10.1093/her/cyt059

Danby, F.W. (2010). Nutrition and acne. *Clinics in Dermatology, 28*(6), 598-604. https://doi.org/10.1016/j.clindermatol.2010.03.017

Das, J.K., Salam, R.A., Thornburg, K.L., Prentice, A.M., Campisi, S., Lassi, Z.S., & Koletzko, B, (2017). Nutrition in adolescents: Physiology, metabolism, and nutritional needs. *The New York Academy of Sciences, 1393*(1), 21-33. https://doi.org/10.1111/nyas.13330

Desbrow, B., McCormack, J., Burke, L.M., Cox, G.R., Fallon, K., Hislop, M., & Logan, R. (2014). Sports Dietitians Australia position statement: Sports nutrition for the adolescent athlete. *International Journal of Sport Nutrition and Exercise Metabolism, 24*(5), 570-84. https://doi.org/10.1123/ijsnem.2014-0031

De Souza, M.J., Williams, N., Nattiv, A., Joy, E., Misra, M., Loucks, A.B., & Matheson, G. (2014). Misunderstanding the female athlete triad: Refuting the IOC consensus statement on relative energy deficiency in sport (RED-S). *British Journal of Sports Medicine, 48*(20), 1461-1465. https://doi.org/10.1136/bjsports-2014-093958

Donglikar, C. (2020). Socio-economic impact on dietary intake patterns of adolescents: A study. *University Grants Commission Care Journal, 40*(38), pp. 51-61.

Dorfman, L. (2019). Nutrition for exercise and sports performance. In J.L. Raymond & K. Morrow (Eds.), *Krause's Food & The Nutrition Care Process* (15th ed.) (pp. 441-470). Philadelphia, PA: W.B. Saunders.

Dorfman, L. (2010). *Performance nutrition for football: How diet can provide the competitive edge.* Ithaca, NY: Momentum Media.

Elliott, T. (2019). Identifying food marketing to teenagers: A scoping review. *International Journal of Behavioral Nutrition and Physical Activity, 16*(1), 67. https://doi.org/10.1186/s12966-019-0833-2

Engeln, R., Sladek, M., & Waldron, H. (2013). Body talk among college men: Content, correlates, and effects. *Body Image, 10*(3).

Ferdowsian, H., & Levin, S. (2010). Does diet really affect acne? *Skin Health Letter, 15*(3). Retrieved from www.skintherapyletter.com/acne/diet-role/

Freisling H., Haas, K., & Elmadfa, I. (2010). Mass media nutrition information sources and associations with fruit and vegetable consumption among adolescents. *Public Health Nutrition, 13*(2), 269-75.

Food Marketing Institute. (n.d.). *Why family meals matter?* Retrieved from www.fmi.org/family-meals-movement/meals-matter

Frühauf, P., Nabil El-Lababidi, N., & Szitányi, P. (2018). Celiac disease in children and adolescents. *Journal of Czech Physicians, 157*(3), 117-121.

Fulkerson, J.A., Farbakhsh, K., Lytle, L., Hearst, M.O., Dengel, D.R., & Pasch, K.E. (2011). Away-from-home family dinner sources and associations with weight status, body composition, and related biomarkers of chronic disease among adolescents and their parents. *Journal of the American Dietetic Association, 111*(12), 1892-1897.

Gibbs, J.C., Williams, N., & De Souza, M.J. (2013). Prevalence of individual and combined components of the female athlete triad. *Medicine & Science in Sports & Exercise, 45*(5), 985-96. https://doi.org/10.1249/MSS.0b013e31827e1bdc

Glazer, K.B., Sonneville, K.R., Micali, N., Swanson, S.A., Crosby, R., Horton, N.J., & Eddy, K.T. (2019). The course of eating disorders involving bingeing and purging among adolescent girls: Prevalence, stability, and transitions. *Journal of Adolescent Health, 64*(2), 165-171. https://doi.org/10.1016/j.jadohealth.2018.09.023

Grant, R., Becnel, J.N., Giano, Z.D., Williams, A.L., & Martinez, D. (2019). A latent profile analysis of young adult lifestyle behaviors. *American Journal of Health Behavior, 43*(6), 1148-1161. https://doi.org/10.5993/AJHB.43.6.12

Grave, R., & Calugi, S. (2020). *Cognitive behavior therapy for adolescents with eating disorders.* New York, NY: The Guilford Press.

Haynos, A.F., Wall, M.M., Chen, C., Wang, S.B., Loth, K., & Neumark-Sztainer, D. (2018)

Patterns of weight control behavior persisting beyond young adulthood: Results from a 15-year longitudinal study. *International Journal of Eating Disorders, 51*(9), 1090-1097. https://doi.org/10.1002/eat.22963

Hughes, E.K., Kerr, J.A., Patton, G.C., Sawyer, S.M., Wake, M., Le Grange, D., & Azzopardi P. (2019). Eating disorder symptoms across the weight spectrum in Australian adolescents. *International Journal of Eating Disorders, 52*(8), 885-894. https://doi.org/10.1002/eat.23118

Juhl, C.R., Bergholdt, H.K., Miller, I.M., Jemec, G.B., Kanters, J.K., & Ellervik, C. (2018). Dairy intake and acne vulgaris: A systematic review and meta-analysis of 78,529 children, adolescents, and young adults. *Nutrients, 10*(8), 1049. https://doi.org/10.3390/nu10081049

Lapierre, M., Fleming-Milici, F., Rozendaal, E., McAlister A., & Castonguay, J. (2017). The effect of advertising on children and adolescents. *Pediatrics, 140*(Suppl 2), S152-S156. https://doi.org/10.1542/peds.2016-1758V

Larson, N., Miller, J.M., Eisenberg, M.A., Watts, A.V., Story, M., & Neumark-Sztainer, D. (2017). Multicontextual correlates of energy-dense, nutrient-poor snack food consumption by adolescents. *Appetite,* 112, 23-34. https://doi.org/10.1016/j.appet.2017.01.008

Larson N., Neumark-Sztainer, D., Laska, M.N., & Story M. (2011). Young adults and eating away from home: associations with dietary intake patterns and weight status differ by choice of restaurant. *Journal of the American Dietetic Association, 111*(11), 1696-1703.

Lis, D.M. (2019). Exit Gluten-Free and Enter Low FODMAPs: A Novel Dietary Strategy to Reduce Gastrointestinal Symptoms in Athletes. *Sports Medicine, 49*(Suppl 1), 87-97.

Lis D., Stellingwerff T., Shing C.M., Ahuja K.D., Fell J. (2015). Exploring the popularity, experiences, and beliefs surrounding gluten-free diets in nonceliac athletes. *International Journal of Sport Nutrition and Exercise Metabolism, 25*(1), 37-45.

Lisha, N.E., & Sussman, S. (2010). Relationship of high school and college sports participation with alcohol, tobacco, and illicit drug use: A review. *Addictive Behaviors, 35*(5), 399-407. https://doi.org/10.1016/j.addbeh.2009.12.032

Mahmood, S.N., & Bowe, W.P. (2014). Diet and acne update: Carbohydrates emerge as the main culprit. *Journal of Drugs in Dermatology, 13*(4), 428-35.

Manore, M., Patton-Lopez, M., Meng, Y., & Wong, S. (2017). Sport nutrition knowledge, behaviors and beliefs of high school soccer players. *Nutrients, 9*(4), 350. https://doi.org/10.3390/nu9040350

Manore, M.M. (2005). Exercise and the Institute of Medicine recommendations for nutrition. *Current Sports Medicine Reports. 4*(4),193-8.

Marra, M., & Bailey, R. (2018). Position of the academy of nutrition and dietetics: Micronutrient supplementation. *Journal of the Academy of Nutrition Dietetics, 118*(11), 2162-2173. https://doi.org/10.1016/j.jand.2018.07.022

Martinsen M., & Sundgot-Borgen, J. (2014). Adolescent elite athletes' cigarette smoking, use of snus, and alcohol. *Scandinavian Journal of Medicine & Science in Sports, 24*(2), 439-46. https://doi.org/10.1111/j.1600-0838.2012.01505.x

McHugh, C., Hurst, A., Bethel, A., Lloyd, J., Logan, S., & Wyatt, K. (2020). The impact of the World Health Organization Health Promoting Schools framework approach on diet and physical activity behaviours of adolescents in secondary schools: A systematic review. *Public Health, 182,* 116-124. https://doi.org/10.1016/j.puhe.2020.02.006

Medina-Caliz, I., Garcia-Cortes, M., Gonzales-Jimenez, Lucen, M.I., & Andrade, R.J. (2018). Herbal and dietary supplement-induced liver injuries in the Spanish DILI Registry. *Clinical Gastroenterology and Hepatology, 16*(9), 1495-1502. https://doi.org/10.1016/j.cgh.2017.12.051

Mountjoy, M., Sundgot-Borgen, J., Burke, L., Carter, S., Constantini, N., Lebrun, C., & Meyer, N. (2014). The IOC consensus statement: Beyond the Female Athlete Triad—Relative Energy Deficiency in Sport (RED-S). *British Journal of Sports Medicine, 48*(7), 491.

Murray G. (2019). Child Eating Disorders in Males. *Child and Adolescent Psychiatric Clinics of North America. 28*(4), 641-651.

Nagata, J.M., Garber, A.K., Tabler, J., Murray, S.B., Vittinghoff, E., & Bibbins-Domingo, K. (2018). Disordered eating behaviors and cardiometabolic risk among young adults with overweight or obesity. *International Journal of Eating Disorders, 51*(8), 931-941. https://doi.org/10.1002/eat.22927

National Center for Health Statistics. (2017). *Health, United States, 2017: With special feature on mortality.* Retrieved from https://www.cdc.gov/nchs/data/hus/2017/053.pdf

Partida, S., Marshall, A., Henry, R., Townsend, J., & Toy, A. (2018). Attitudes toward nutrition and dietary habits and effectiveness of nutrition education in active adolescents in a private school setting: A pilot study. *Nutrients, 10*(9), 1260. https://doi.org/10.3390/nu10091260

Pujalte, G.G., & Benjamin, H.J. (2018). Sleep and the athlete. *Current Sports Medicine Report, 17*(4), 109-110. https://doi.org/10.1249/JSR.0000000000000468

Perreault-Briere, M., Beliveau, J., Jeker, D., Deshayes, T.A., Duran, A., & Goulet, E.D. (2019). Effect of thirst-driven fluid intake on 1 H cycling time-trial performance in trained endurance athletes. *Sports,* 7(10), 223. https://doi.org/10.3390/sports7100223

Rogerson, D. (2017). Vegan diets: practical advice for athletes and exercisers. *Journal of the International Society of Sports Nutrition.* 14, 36.

Sadegholvad, S., Yeatman, H., Parrish, A.M., & Worsley, A. (2017). What should be taught in secondary schools' nutrition and food systems education? Views from prominent food-related professionals in Australia. *Nutrients, 9*(11), 1207. https://doi.org/10.3390/nu9111207

Santos, I., Sniehotta, F.F., Marques, M.M., Carraça, E.V., & Teixeira, P.J. (2017). Prevalence of personal weight control attempts in adults: A systematic review and meta-analysis. *Obesity Reviews, 18*(1), 32-50.

Silvia C., Bottesi,G., Pacelli,F., Paoli, A., & Ghisi, M. (2018). Muscle Dysmorphia and its Associated Psychological Features in Three Groups of Recreational Athletes. *Scientific Reports,* 8, 8877.

Singh, P., Arora, A., Strand, T., Leffler, D., Catassi, C., Green, P., Kelly, C., Ahuja, V., & Makharia, G. (2018). Global

Prevalence of Celiac Disease: Systematic Review and Meta-analysis. *Clinical Gastroenterology and Hepatology, 16*(6), 823-836.e2.

Sobal, J., & Hanson, K. (2014). Family dinner frequency, settings and sources, and body weight in US adults. *Appetite, 78*, 81-88. https://doi.org/10.1016/j.appet.2014.03.016

Solmi, F., Sonneville, K.R., Easter, A., Horton, N.J., Crosby, R.D., Treasure, J., & Rodrigez, A. (2015). Prevalence of purging at age 16 and associations with negative outcomes among girls in three community-based cohorts. *Journal of Child Psychology and Psychiatry, 56*(1), 87-96. https://doi.org/10.1111/jcpp.12283

Stok, F.M., Renner, B., Clarys, P., Lien, N., Lakerveld, J., & Deliens, T. (2018). Understanding eating behavior during the transition from adolescence to young adulthood: A literature review and perspective on future research directions. *Nutrients, 10*(6), 667. https://doi.org/10.3390/nu10060667

Swanson, S., Crow, S., & Le Grange, D. (2011). Prevalence and correlates of eating disorders in adolescents: Results from the National Comorbidity Survey Replication Adolescent Supplement. *Archives of General Psychiatry, 68*(7), 714-723. https://doi.org/doi:10.1001/archgenpsychiatry.2011.22

Tarokh, L., Saletin, J.M., & Carskadon, M.A. (2016). Sleep in adolescence: Physiology, cognition and mental health. *Neuroscience & Biobehavioral Reviews, 70*, 182-188. https://doi.org/10.1016/j.neubiorev.2016.08.008

Taylor Hooton Foundation. (n.d.) *Anabolic steroids*. Retrieved from https://taylorhooton.org/anabolic-steroids/

Turpin, C. (2014). *Grocery shopping on a budget for athletes*. Retrieved from www.mysportsd.com/myathleteseatingonabudget

Ulvestad, M., Bjertness, E., Dalgard, F., & Halvorsen, J.A. (2017). Acne and dairy products in adolescence: Results from a Norwegian longitudinal study. *Journal of the European Academy of Dermatology Venereology, 31*(3), 530-535. https://doi.org/10.1111/jdv.13835

Vanderlee, L., Hobin, E.P., White, C.M., & Hammond, D. (2018). Grocery shopping, dinner preparation, and dietary habits among adolescents and young adults in Canada. *Canadian Journal of Dietetic Practice and Research, 79*(4), 157-163. https://doi.org/10.3148/cjdpr-2018-025

Walton, K., Horton, N.J., Rifas-Shiman, S.L., Field, A.E., Austin, S.B., Haycraft, E., & Breen, A. (2018). Exploring the role of family functioning in the association between frequency of family dinners and dietary intake among adolescents and young adults. *JAMA Network Open, 1*(7), e185217. https://doi.org/10.1001/jamanetworkopen.2018.5217

Ward, Z., Rodriguez, P., Wright, D., Austin, A., & Long, W. (2019). Estimation of eating disorders prevalence by age and associations with mortality in a simulated nationally representative US cohort. *JAMA Network Open, 2*(10), e1912925. https://doi.org/10.1001/jamanetworkopen.2019.12925

West, C., Goldschmidt, A., Mason, S., & Neumark-Sztainer, D. (2019). Differences in risk factors for binge eating by socioeconomic status in a community-based sample of adolescents: Findings from Project EAT. *International Journal of Eating Disorders*. *52*(6), 659–668.

Wilksch, S.M., O'Shea, A., Ho, P., Byrne, S., & Wade, T.D. (2020). The relationship between social media use and disordered eating in young adolescents. *International Journal of Eating Disorders, 53*(1), 96-106. https://doi.org/10.1002/eat.23198

Winpenny, E.M., Penney, T.L., Corder, K., White, M., & van Sluijs, E.M. (2017). Change in diet in the period from adolescence to early adulthood: A systematic scoping review of longitudinal studies. *International Journal of Behavioral Nutrition and Physical Activity, 14*(1), 60. https://doi.org/10.1186/s12966-017-0518-7

Worsley, A. Nutrition knowledge and food consumption: can nutrition knowledge change food behaviour? *Asia Pacific Journal of Clinical Nutrition, 11*(Suppl 3), S579-S585.

Zuromski, K.L., & Witte, T.K. (2015). Fasting and acquired capability for suicide: A test of the interpersonal-psychological theory of suicide in an undergraduate sample. *Psychiatry Research, 226*(1), 61-67. https://doi.org/10.1016/j.psychres.2014.11.059

Chapter 6

Alesi, M., Gómez-López, M., Chicau Borrego, C., Monteiro, D., & Granero-Gallegos, A. (2019). Effects of a motivational climate on psychological needs satisfaction, motivation and commitment in teen handball players. *International Journal of Environmental Research and Public Health, 16*(15), 2702. https://doi.org/10.3390/ijerph16152702

Ames, C., & Archer, J. (1988). Achievement goals in the classroom: Students' learning strategies and motivation processes. *Journal of Educational Psychology, 80*, 260-267.

Bandura, A. (1997). *Self-efficacy: The exercise of control*. New York, NY: W.H. Freeman and Company.

Bortoli, L., Bertollo, M., Comani, S. & Robazza, C. (2011). Competence, achievement goals, motivational climate, and pleasant psychobiosocial states in youth sport. *Journal of Sports Sciences, 29*(2), 171-80. https://doi.org/10.1080/02640414.2010.530675

Burton, D., & Raedeke, T.D. (2008). *Sport psychology for coaches*. Champaign, IL: Human Kinetics.

Calkins, N.D. (2015). The impact of self-regulation strategy training on secondary physical education students' physical fitness performance (Publication No. 3664363). [Doctoral dissertation, Seattle Pacific University]. ProQuest Dissertations Publishing.

Castillo, I., Molina-García, J., Estevan, I., Queralt, A., & Álvarez, O. (2020). Transformational teaching in physical education and students' leisure-time physical activity: The mediating role of learning climate, passion and self-determined motivation. *International Journal of Environmental Research and Public Health, 17*(13), 4844. https://doi.org/10.3390/ijerph17134844

Center for the Study of Social Policy. (2015). *Core meanings of the strengthening families protective factors*. Retrieved from https://cssp.org/wp-content/uploads/2018/10/Core-Meanings-of-the-SF-Protective-Factors-2015.pdf

Centers for Disease Control and Prevention. (2014, August). *The relationship between bullying and suicide: What we know and what it means for schools*. Retrieved from www.cdc.gov/violenceprevention/pdf/bullying-suicide-translation-final-a.pdf

Collaborative for Academic, Social, and Emotional Learning. (2015). *CASEL schoolkit: A guide for implementing schoolwide academic, social, and emotional learning*. Chicago, IL, CASEL.

Collaborative for Academic, Social, and Emotional Learning. (2021). *SEL: What are the core competence areas and where are they promoted?* Retrieved from https://casel.org/core-competencies/

Council of Chief State School Officers. (2017, December). *Leading for equity: Opportunities for State Education Chiefs*. Retrieved from https://ccsso.org/sites/default/files/2018-01/Leading%20for%20Equity_011618.pdf

de Bruin, M., Sheeran, P., Kok, G., Hiemstra, A., Prins, J.M., Hospers, H.J., & van Breukelen, G.J. (2012). Self-regulatory processes mediate the intention-behavior relation for adherence and exercise behaviors. *Health Psychology, 31*(6), 695-703. https://doi.org/10.1037/a0027425

DeMink-Carthew, J., Olofson, M.W., LeGeros, L., Netcoh, S. & Hennessey, S. (2017). An analysis of approaches to goal setting in middle grades personalized learning environments. *RMLE Online: Research in Middle Level Education, 40(*10), 1-11. https://doi.org/10.1080/19404476.2017.1392689

Dweck, C. (2007). *Mindset: The new psychology of success.* New York, NY: Ballantine Books.

Edmunds, J., Ntoumanis, N., & Duda, J.L. (2006). A test of self-determination theory in the exercise domain. *Journal of Applied Social Psychology, 36*(9), 2240-2265. https://doi.org/10.1111/j.0021-9029.2006.00102.x

Ellison, D., Walton-Fisette, J., & Eckert, K. (2019). Utilizing the Teaching Personal and Social Responsibility (TPSR) model as a trauma-informed practice (TIP) tool in physical education. *Journal of Physical Education, Recreation & Dance, 90*(9) 32-37. https://doi.org/10.1080/07303084.2019.1657531

Fisher, D., & Frey, N. (2016). Show & tell: A video column/Two times ten conversations. *Educational Leadership, 74*(1); 84-85.

García-González, L., Sevil-Serrano, J., Abós, Á., Aelterman, N., & Haerens, L. (2019). The role of task and ego-oriented climate in explaining students' bright and dark motivational experiences in physical education. *Physical Education & Sport Pedagogy, 24*(4), 344-358. https://doi.org/10.1080/17408989.2019.1592145

Gerstein, J. (2014, August 28). The educator with a growth mindset: A staff workshop [Web log post]. Retrieved from https://usergeneratededucation.wordpress.com/2014/08/29/the-educator-with-a-growth-mindset-a-staff-workshop.

Giri, V.N. (2006). Culture and communication style. *The Review of Communication, 6*(1), 124-130.

Graham, D.J., Sirard, J.R., & Neumark-Sztainer, D. (2011). Adolescents' attitudes toward sports, exercise, and fitness predict physical activity 5 and 10 years later. *Preventive Medicine, 52*(2), 130-132. https://doi.org/10.1016/j.ypmed.2010.11.013

Greenberg, J.D., & LoBianco, J.L. (2020). *Organization and administration of physical education: Theory and practice.* Champaign, IL: Human Kinetics.

Hansen, K. (2014). The importance of ethnic cultural competency in physical education. *Strategies: A Journal for Physical and Sport Educations, 27*(3), 12-16. https://doi.org/10.1080/08924562.2014.900462

Harwood, C.G., Keegan, R.J., Smith, J.M., & Raine, A.S. (2015). A systematic review of the intrapersonal correlates of motivational climate perceptions in sport and physical activity. *Psychology of Sport and Exercise, 18,* 9-25. https://doi.org/10.1016/j.psychsport.2014.11.005

Hortz, B., & Petosa, R.L. (2008). Social cognitive theory variables mediation of moderate exercise. *American Journal of Health Behavior, 32*(3), 305-314.

Jago, R., Brockman, R., Fox, K.R., Cartwright, K., Page, A.S., & Thompson, J.L. (2009). Friendship groups and physical activity: Qualitative findings on how physical activity is initiated and maintained among 10-11 year old children. *International Journal of Behavioral Nutrition and Physical Activity, 6*(4), 1-9. Retrieved from www.ijbnpa.org/content/6/1/4

Jefferies, P., Ungar, M., Aubertin, P., & Kriellaars, D. (2019). Physical literacy and resilience in children and youth. *Frontiers in Public Health,* 7(346), 1-7. https://doi.org/10.3389/fpubh.2019.00346

Keels, M. (2018, March 23). *Supporting students with chronic trauma.* Retrieved from www.edutopia.org/article/supporting-students-chronic-trauma

Ladwig, M.A., Vazou, S., & Ekkekakis, P. (2018). "My best memory is when I was done with it": PE memories are associated with adult sedentary behavior, *Translational Jouranl of the ACSM, 3*(16), 119-129. https://doi.org/10.1249/TJX.0000000000000067

Laird, Y., Fawkner, S., Kelly, P., McNamee, L., & Niven, A. (2016). The role of social support on physical activity behaviour in adolescent girls: a systematic review and meta-analysis. *International Journal of Behavioral Nutrition and Physical Activity, 13*(79), 1-14.

LaMorte, W.W. (2019, September). *The social cognitive theory.* Retrieved from https://sphweb.bumc.bu.edu/otlt/MPH-Modules/SB/BehavioralChangeTheories/BehavioralChangeTheories5.html

Loades, M.E., Chatburn, E., Higson-Sweeney, N., Reynolds, S., Shafran, R., Brigden, A., & Linney, C. (2020). Rapid systematic review: The impact of social isolation and loneliness on the mental health of children and adolescents in the context of COVID-19. *Journal of the American Academy of Child & Adolescent Psychiatry, 59*(11), 1218-1229. https://doi.org/10.1016/j.jaac.2020.05.009

Matthews, J., & Moran, A. (2011). Physical activity and self-regulation strategy use in adolescents. *American Journal of Health Behavior, 35*(6), 807-814.

Minahan, J. (2019). Trauma-informed teaching strategies. *Educational Leadership,* 77(2), 30-35. Retrieved from www.ascd.org/publications/educational_leadership/oct19/vol77/num02/Trauma-Informed_Teaching_Strategies.aspx

Morisano, D. (2013). Goal setting in the academic arena. In E.A. Locke & G. Latham (Eds.), *New Developments in Goal Setting and Task Performance,* (pp. 495-506). New York, NY: Routledge.

National Association of Social Workers. (2015*). Standards and indicators for cultural competence in social work practice.* Retrieved from www.socialworkers.org/LinkClick.aspx?fileticket=PonPTDEBrn4=&portalid=0

National Center for Educational Statistics. (2019, July). *Student reports of bullying: Results from the 2017 School Crime Supplement To The National Crime Victimization Survey.* Retrieved from https://nces.ed.gov/pubs2019/2019054.pdf

Pratt-Johnson, Y. (2006). Communicating cross-culturally: What teachers should know. *The Internet TESL Journal, 12*(2). In http://iteslj.org/Articles/Pratt-Johnson-CrossCultural.html

Reuter, B.H. & Dawes, J. (2016). Program design and technique for aerobic endurance training. In Haff, G.G. & Triplett, N.T. (Eds.), *Essentials of strength training and conditioning (4th ed.)* (pp. 559-581). Champaign, IL: Human Kinetics.

Rose, T., Barker, M., Maria Jacob, C., Morrison, L., Lawrence, W., Strömmer, S., & Vogel, C. (2017). A systematic review of digital interventions for improving the diet and physical activity behaviors of adolescents. *Journal of Adolescent Health, 61*(6), 669-677. https://doi.org/10.1016/j.jadohealth.2017.05.024

SHAPE America. (2013). *Grade-level outcomes for K-12 physical education.* Reston, VA: Author.

Saunders, S.A. (2013). *The impact of a growth mindset intervention on the reading achievement of at-risk adolescent students* (Publication No. 3573523). [Doctoral dissertation, University of Virginia]. ProQuest Dissertations Publishing.

SHAPE America. (2012). *Instructional framework for fitness education in physical education. Guidance document.* Reston, VA: Society of Health and Physical Educators.

Sherwood, N., & Jeffery, R. (2000). The behavioral determinants of exercise: Implications for physical activity interventions. *Annual Review of Nutrition, 20*(1), 21-44. https://doi.org/10.1146/annurev.nutr.20.1.21

Shilts, M.K., Horowitz, M., & Townsend, M.S. (2004). Goal setting as a strategy for dietary and physical activity behavior change: a review of the literature. *American Journal of Health Promotion, 19*(2), 81-93. https://doi.org/10.4278/0890-1171-19.2.81

Shimon, J.M., & Petlichkoff, L.M. (2009). Impact of pedometer use and self-regulation strategies on junior high school physical education students' daily step counts. *Journal of Physical Activity and Health, 6*, 178-184.

Smith, D., Fisher, D., & Frey, N. (2015). *Better than carrots or sticks: Restorative practices for positive classroom management.* Alexandria, VA: Association for Supervision and Curriculum Development.

Souers, K.V., & Hall, P. (2019). *Relationship, responsibility, and regulation: Trauma-invested practices for fostering resilient learners.* Alexandria, VA: Association for Supervision and Curriculum Development.

Spencer-Cavaliere, N., & Rintoul, M.A. (2012). Alienation in physical education from the perspectives of children. *Journal of Teaching in Physical Education, 31*(4), 344-361, https://doi.org/10.1123/jtpe.31.4.344

Standage, M., Curran, T., & Rouse, P.C. (2019). Self-determination-based theories of sport, exercise, and physical activity motivation. In T.S. Horn & A.L. Smith (Eds.), *Advances in sport and exercise psychology* (4th ed.). (pp. 289-304). Champaign, IL: Human Kinetics.

Stokes, R., & Schultz, S.L. (2007). *Personal fitness for you.* Winston-Salem, NC: Hunter Textbooks.

Substance Abuse and Mental Health Services Administration. (2020, April). *Recognizing and treating child trauma.* Retrieved from www.samhsa.gov/child-trauma/recognizing-and-treating-child-traumatic-stress

Swearer, S.M., & Cary, P.T. (2007). Perceptions and attitudes toward bullying in middle school youth: A developmental examination across the bullying continuum. In J.E. Zins, M.J. Elias, & C.A. Maher (Eds.), *Bullying, victimization, and peer harassment* (pp. 67–83). New York, NY: Haworth Press.

Terrasi, S., & de Galarce, P.C. (2017). Trauma and learning in America's classrooms. *Phi Delta Kappan, 98*(6), 35-41.

Teixeira, P.J., Carraça, E.V., Markland, D., Silva, M.N., & Ryan, R.M. (2012). Exercise, physical activity, and self-determination theory: A systematic review. *The International Journal of Behavioral Nutrition and Physical Activity, 9*, 78. https://doi.org/10.1186/1479-5868-9-78

Thomason, D.L., Lukkahatai, N., Kawi, J., Connelly, K., & Inouye, J. (2016). A systematic review of adolescent self-management and weight loss. *Journal of pediatric health care: Official publication of National Association of Pediatric Nurse Associates & Practitioners, 30*(6), 569-582. https://doi.org/10.1016/j.pedhc.2015.11.016

Trudeau F., & Shephard R. (2008). Is there a long-term health legacy of required physical education? *Sports Medicine, 38*(4), 265-270. https://doi.org/10.2165/00007256-200838040-00001

Weissberg, R.P., Durlak, J.A., Domitrovich, C.E., & Gullotta, T.P. (2015). Social and emotional learning: Past, present, and future. In J.A. Durlak, C.E. Domitrovich, R.P. Weissberg, & T.P. Gullotta (Eds.), *Handbook of social and emotional learning. Research and practice* (pp. 3-19). New York, NY: The Guilford Press.

World Athletics. (2020, September 7). *World records.* Retrieved from www.worldathletics.org/records/by-category/world-records

Vogel, S., & Schwabe, L. (2016). Learning and memory under stress: implications for the classroom. *npj Science Learn, 1.* https://doi.org/10.1038/npjscilearn.2016.11

Young, J. (2014). *Encouragement in the classroom.* Alexandria, VA: Association for Supervision and Curriculum Development.

Zook, K.R., Saksvig, B.I., Wu, T.T., & Young, D.R. (2014). Physical activity trajectories and multilevel factors among adolescent girls. *Journal Of Adolescent Health, 54*(1), 74-80. https://doi.org/10.1016/j.jadohealth.2013.07.015

Chapter 7

American Heart Association. (2020). Nearly 60% of American children lack healthy cardiorespiratory fitness, American Heart Association Scientific Statement, July 20, 2020. Retrieved from: https://newsroom.heart.org/news/nearly-60-of-american-children-lack-healthy-cardiorespiratory-fitness

American Institutes of Research. (2016). Hard to Measure Content Areas: Training Materials. Washington, DC.

Andrade, H.G. (2014, June). *Understanding rubrics.* Retrieved from www.saddleback.edu/uploads/goe/understanding_rubrics_by_heidi_goodrich_andrade.pdf

Chepko, S., Holt/Hale, S., Doan, R.J., & MacDonald, L.C. (2019). *PE metrics: Assessing student performance using the National Standards & Grade-Level Outcomes for K-12 physical education* (3rd ed.). Champaign, IL: Human Kinetics.

Clark, M., Lucett, S., & Sutton, B. (2014). *NASM essentials of corrective exercise training.* Burlington, MA: Jones & Bartlett Publishing.

Cooper Institute (2017). *FittnessGram administration manual* (5th ed.). Champaign, IL: Human Kinetics.

Fisher, M.R., Jr. (2020). *Student assessment in teaching and learning.* Retrieved from https://cft.vanderbilt.edu/student-assessment-in-teaching-and-learning.

Greenberg, J.D., & LoBianco, J.L. (2020) *Organization and administration of physical education: Theory and practice.* Champaign, IL: Human Kinetics.

Herman, J., Aschbacher, P., & Winters, L. (1992). *A practical guide to alternative assessment.* Alexandria, VA: Association for Supervision and Curriculum Development.

Hoeger W., & Hoeger S. (2018). *Principles and labs for fitness and wellness.* Boston, MA: Cengage Learning.

Lund, J., & Veal, M.L. (2013). *Assessment-driven instruction in physical education: A standards-based approach to promoting and documenting learning.* Champaign, IL: Human Kinetics.

McKenzie, T.L. (2009). *SOFIT, System for Observing Fitness Instruction Time: General description and procedures manual.* San Diego, CA: San Diego State University.

McKenzie, T.L. (2012). *Tools and measures, SOFIT: System For Observing Fitness Instruction Time.* San Diego, CA: University of California, San Diego.

McKenzie, T.L. (2016). Context matters: Systematic observation of place-based physical activity. *Research Quarterly for Exercise and Sport, 87*(4), 334-341. https://doi.org/10.1080/02701367.2016.1234302

McKenzie, T.L., & van der Mars, H. (2015). Top 10 research questions related to assessing physical activity and its contexts using systematic observation. *Research Quarterly for Exercise and Sport, 86*(1), 13-29. https://doi.org/10.1080/02701367.2015.991264

Mitchell, S.A., & Walton-Fisette, J.L. (2016). *The essentials of teaching physical education: Curriculum, instruction, and assessment.* Champaign, IL: Human Kinetics.

Mueller, J. (2018). *Authentic assessment toolbox.* Naperville, IL: North Central College.

Pate, R., Oria, M., & Pillsbury, L. (Eds.). (2012). *Fitness measures and health outcomes in youth.* Retrieved from https://www.ncbi.nlm.nih.gov/books/NBK241315/

Phillips, S., Marttinen, R., & Mercier, K. (2017). Fitness assessment: Recommendations for an enjoyable student experience. *Strategies, 30*(5), 19-24. https://doi.org/10.1080/08924562.2017.1344168

Presidential Youth Fitness Program. (2017). *Presidential Youth Fitness program physical educator resource*. Retrieved from www.pyfp.org/storage/app/media/documents/teacher-guide.pdf

SHAPE America. (2012). *Instructional framework for fitness education in physical education*. Retrieved from www.shapeamerica.org/upload/Instructional-Framework-for-Fitness-Education-in-Physical-Education.pdf

SHAPE America. (2013). *Grade-level outcomes for K-12 physical education*. Retrieved from www.shapeamerica.org/standards/pe/upload/Grade-Level-Outcomes-for-K-12-Physical-Education.pdf

SHAPE America. (2017). *Appropriate and inappropriate practices related to fitness testing*. Retrieved from www.shapeamerica.org/advocacy/positionstatements/pe/upload/Appropriate-and-Inappropriate-Uses-of-Fitness-Testing-FINAL-3-6-17.pdf

Tankersley, K. (2007). *Tests that teach: Using standardized tests to improve instruction*. Alexandria, VA: Association for Supervision and Curriculum Development.

Temertzoglou, C. (n.d.). *Quality assessment practices for PE* [Web log post]. Retrieved from www.gophersport.com/blog/quality-assessment-practices-for-pe/

U.S. Department of Health and Human Services. (2018). *Physical activity guidelines for Americans* (2nd ed.). Washington, DC: U.S. Department of Health and Human Services.

Winnick, J.P., & Short, F.X. (2014). Brockport physical fitness test manual: A health-related assessment for youngsters with disabilities (2nd ed.). Champaign, IL: Human Kinetics.

Chapter 8

American Lung Association (2016, January 19). Breathing basics for runners [Web log post]. Retrieved from www.lung.org/blog/breathing-basics-for-runners

Armstrong N., & McManus, A.M. (2011). Endurance training and elite young athletes. *Medicine and Sport Science, 56*, 59-83. https://doi.org/10.1159/000320633

Armstrong, N., & Weisman, J. (2019). Youth cardiorespiratory fitness: Evidence, myths and misconceptions. *Bulletin of the World Health Organization, 97*(11), 777-782. https://doi.org/10.2471/BLT.18.227546

Bushman, B.A. (Ed.). (2017). *ACSM's complete guide to fitness and health* (2nd ed.). Champaign, IL: Human Kinetics.

Carlisle A.J., & Sharp, N.C. (2001). Exercise and outdoor ambient air pollution. British Journal of Sports Medicine, *35*(4), 214-222.

Centers for Disease Control and Prevention. (2020). *Increasing physical activity among adults with disabilities*. Retrieved from www.cdc.gov/ncbddd/disabilityandhealth/materials/infographic-increasing-physical-activity.html

Corbin, C.B., & LeMasurier, G.C. (2014). *Fitness for life* (6th ed.). Champaign, IL: Human Kinetics.

Faigenbaum, A., Lloyd, R., & Oliver, J. (2020). *Essentials of youth fitness*. Champaign, IL: Human Kinetics.

Foster, C., & Porcari, J.P. (n.d.). Ace-sponsored research: Validating the talk test as a measure of exercise intensity. Retrieved from www.acefitness.org/certifiednewsarticle/888/ace-sponsored-research-validating-the-talk-test-as-a-measure-of-exercise-intensity/

Harvard Health Publishing. (2016, July). *Does regular exercise reduce cancer risk?* Retrieved from www.health.harvard.edu/exercise-and-fitness/does-regular-exercise-reduce-cancer-risk

Healthwise Staff. (2018, December 8). Pulse measurement. Retrieved from www.uofmhealth.org/health-library/hw233473

Hildebrand, M., & Ekelund, U. (2017). Assessment of physical activity. In: N. Armstrong N & W. van Mechelen (Eds.), *Oxford textbook of children's sport and exercise medicine* (3rd ed.) (pp. 303-314). Oxford: Oxford University Press.

LaComb, C.O., Tandy, R.D., Lee, S.P., Young, J.C., & Navalta, J.W. (2017). Oral versus nasal breathing during moderate to high intensity submaximal aerobic exercise. International Journal of Kinesiology and Sports Science, *5*(1), 9-16.

Lang, J.J., Tomkinson, G.R., Janssen, I., Ruiz, J.R., Ortega, F.B., Léger L, & Tremblay, M.S. (2018). Making a case for cardiorespiratory fitness surveillance among children and youth. *Exercise and Sport Science Reviews, 46*(2), 66-75. https://doi.org/10.1249/JES.0000000000000138

Martinez, A. (2018, December 4). Inclusive physical education fitness stations. Retrieved from www.nchpad.org/1711/6830/Inclusive~Physical~Education~Fitness~Stations

McGill, E.A., & Montel, I.N. (Eds.). (2017). NASM essentials of personal fitness training. Burlington, MA: Jones & Bartlett Learning.

McKinney, J., Lithwick, D.J., Morrison, B.N., Nazzari, H., Isserow, S.H., Heilbron, B., & Krahn, A.D. (2016). The health benefits of physical activity and cardiorespiratory fitness. *British Columbia Medical Journal, 58*(3). Retrieved from www.sportscardiologybc.org/wp-content/uploads/2016/03/BCMJ_Vol58_No_3_cardiorespiratory_fitness.pdf

National Institutes of Health. (n.d.). Physical activity and your heart. Retrieved from https://www.nhlbi.nih.gov/health-topics/physical-activity-and-your-heart

Pangrazi, R.P., Beighle, A., & Sidman, C.L. (2009). *Pedometer power*. Champaign, IL: Human Kinetics.

Powell, K. (2019, August 16). High-intensity interval training: For fitness, for health or both? [Web log post]. Retrieved from www.acsm.org/blog-detail/acsm-blog/2019/08/16/high-intensity-interval-training-for-fitness-for-health-or-both

Raghuveer, G., Hartz, J., Lubans, D.R., Takken, T., Wiltz, J.L., Mietus-Snyder, M., . . . Edwards, N.M. (2020). Cardiorespiratory fitness in youth: An important marker of health: A scientific statement from the American Heart Association. *Circulation, 142*, e101-e118. https://doi.org/10.1161/CIR.0000000000000866

Recinto, C., Efthemeou, T., Boffelli, P.T., & Navalta, J.W. (2017). Effects of nasal or oral breathing on anaerobic power output and metabolic responses. *International Journal of Exercise Science, 10*(4), 506-514. Retrieved from www.ncbi.nlm.nih.gov/pmc/articles/PMC5466403/

Ruiz, J.R., Ortega, F.B., Rizzo, N.S., Villa, I., Hurtig-Wennlöf, A., Oja, L., & Sjöström, M. (2007). High cardiovascular fitness is associated with low metabolic risk score in children: The European youth heart study. Pediatric Research, *61*(3), 350-355. Retrieved from www.nature.com/articles/pr200769

SHAPE America. Conkle, J. (Ed.). (2020). *Physical best: Physical education for lifelong fitness and health* (4th ed.). Champaign, IL: Human Kinetics.

Strain, T., Brage, S., Sharp, S.J., Richards, J., Tainio, M., Ding, D., Benichou, J., & Kelly, P. (2020). Use of the prevented fraction for the population to determine deaths averted by existing prevalence of physical activity: a descriptive study. *The Lancet Global Health, 8*(7), E920-E930. https://doi.org/10.1016/S2214-109X(20)30211-4

Strand, B.N., Scantling, E., & Johnson, M. (1997). Fitness education: Teaching concept-based fitness in schools. Scottsdale, AZ: Gorsuch Scarisbrick.

Thygerson, A.L., & Thygerson, S.M. (2019). Fit to be well: Essential concepts (5th ed.). Burlington, MA: Jones & Bartlett Learning.

Tudor-Locke, C., Craig, C.L., Beets, M.W, Belton, S., Cardon, G.M., Duncan, S., . . . Blair, S.N. (2011). How many steps/day are enough? for children and adolescents. *International Journal of Behavioral Nutrition and Physical Activity, 8*(78). https://doi.org/10.1186/1479-5868-8-78

U.S. Department of Health and Human Services. (2018). *Physical activity guidelines for Americans* (2nd ed.). Retrieved from https://health.gov/sites/default/files/2019-09/Physical_Activity_Guidelines_2nd_edition.pdf

Williams, H., Ball, L., Lieberman, L.J., & Pierce, T. (2020). Running strategies for individuals with visual impairments. *Journal of Physical Education, Recreation, & Dance, 91*(6), 41-45. https://doi.org/10.1080/07303084.2020.1770521

Wittfeld, K., Jochem, C., Dörr, M., Schminke, U., Glaser, S., Bahls, M., . . . Grabe, H.J. (2020). Cardiorespiratory fitness and gray matter volume in the temporal, frontal, and cerebellar regions in the general population. *Mayo Clinic Proceedings, 95*(1), 44-56. https://doi.org/10.1016/j.mayocp.2019.05.030

World Health Organization (2019). Risk reduction of cognitive decline and dementia: WHO guidelines. Retrieved from https://apps.who.int/iris/bitstream/handle/10665/312180/9789241550543-eng.pdf?ua=1

Zschucke, E., Gaudlitz, K., & Ströhle, A. (2013). Exercise and physical activity in mental disorders: Clinical and experimental evidence. *Journal of Preventive Medicine & Public Health, 46*(Suppl 1): S12-S21. https://doi.org/10.3961/jpmph.2013.46.S.S12

Chapter 9

Bushman, B. (2016). Flexibility exercises and performance. *ACSM's Health & Fitness Journal, 5*(20), 5-9. https://doi.org/10.1249/FIT.0000000000000226

Bushman, B. (Ed.). (2017). *American College of Sports Medicine complete guide to fitness and health* (2nd ed.). Champaign, IL: Human Kinetics.

Cooper Institute. (n.d.). *FitnessGram assessment*. Retrieved from https://fitnessgram.net/assessment

Corbin, C.B., & LeMasurier, G.C. (2014). *Fitness for life* (6th ed.). Champaign, IL: Human Kinetics.

Cronkleton, E. (2019, September). *12 stretches to help relieve tight shoulders*. Retrieved from www.healthline.com/health/tight-shoulders - stretches

Delavier, F., Clémenceau, J.P., & Gundill, M. (2011). *Delavier's stretching anatomy*. Champaign, IL: Human Kinetics.

Harvard Health Publishing. (2015, April). *Benefits of flexibility exercises*. Retrieved from www.health.harvard.edu/staying-healthy/benefits-of-flexibility-exercises

Harvard Health Publishing. (2019, September 25). *The importance of stretching*. Retrieved from www.health.harvard.edu/staying-healthy/the-importance-of-stretchingh

McGill, E.A., & Montel, I.N. (Eds.). (2017). *NASM essentials of personal fitness training* (2nd ed.). Burlington, MA: Jones & Bartlett Learning.

Morrison, W., & Frothingham, S. (2019, May). *How many joints are in the human body?* Retrieved from www.healthline.com/health/how-many-joints-in-human-body

Nelson, A.G., & Kokkonen, J. (2014). *Stretching anatomy*. Champaign, IL: Human Kinetics.

Physiofitness Physical Therapy. (2014, August 19). *5 exercises you can do on the road*. Retrieved from https://physiofitness.com/2014/08/19/5-exercises-you-can-do-on-the-road

SHAPE America. Conkle, J. (Ed.). (2020). *Physical best: Physical education for lifelong fitness and health* (4th ed.). Champaign, IL: Human Kinetics.

Thielen, S. (2015, September 15). 5 chest stretch variations [Web log post]. Retrieved from www.acefitness.org/education-and-resources/lifestyle/blog/5657/5-chest-stretch-variations

Thygerson, A.L. & Thygerson, S.M. (2019). *Fit to be well: Essential concepts* (5th ed.). Jones & Bartlett Learning.

Winslow, V.L. (2015). *Classic human anatomy in motion: The artist's guide to the dynamics of figure drawing*. (pp. 50-51). Penguin Random House.

Chapter 10

Bushman, B. (Ed.). (2017). *American College of Sports Medicine complete guide to fitness and health* (2nd ed.). Champaign, IL: Human Kinetics.

Cooper Institute. (n.d.). *FitnessGram assessment*. Retrieved from https://fitnessgram.net/assessment

Corbin, C.B., & LeMasurier, G.C. (2014). *Fitness for life* (6th ed.). Champaign, IL: Human Kinetics.

Cronkleton, E. (2019, May). *Why being flexible is great for your health*. Retrieved from www.healthline.com/health/benefits-of-flexibility

Cronkleton, E. (2019, February). *7 lower back stretches to reduce pain and build strength*. Retrieved from www.healthline.com/health/lower-back-stretches

Delavier, F., Clémenceau, J.P., & Gundill, M. (2011). *Delavier's stretching anatomy*. Champaign, IL: Human Kinetics.

Harvard Health Publishing. (2015, April). *Benefits of flexibility exercises*. Retrieved from www.health.harvard.edu/staying-healthy/benefits-of-flexibility-exercises

Harvard Health Publishing. (2019, September). *The importance of stretching*. Retrieved from www.health.harvard.edu/staying-healthy/the-importance-of-stretching

Harvard Health Publishing. (2012, May). *Core conditioning—It's not just about abs*. Retrieved from www.health.harvard.edu/healthbeat/core-conditioning-its-not-just-about-abs

Kaminoff, L., & Matthews, A. (2012). *Yoga anatomy* (2nd ed.). Champaign, IL: Human Kinetics.

KD Smart Chair (2019). Stretching exercises for wheelchair users. Retrieved from: https://www.pinterest.com/pin/761319511994111130/

Lindberg, S. (2019, August). *How to stretch your abs and why it matters*. Retrieved from www.healthline.com/health/exercise-fitness/how-to-stretch-abs

McGill, E.A., & Montel, I.N. (Eds.). (2017). *NASM essentials of personal fitness training* (2nd ed.). Burlington, MA: Jones & Bartlett Learning.

Morrison, W., & Frothingham, S. (2019, May). *How many joints are in the human body?* Retrieved from www.healthline.com/health/how-many-joints-in-human-body

Nelson, A.G., & Kokkonen, J. (2014). *Stretching anatomy*. Champaign, IL: Human Kinetics.

Physiofitness Physical Therapy. (2014, August 19). *5 exercises you can do on the road*. Retrieved from https://physiofitness.com/2014/08/19/5-exercises-you-can-do-on-the-road

SHAPE America. Conkle, J. (Ed.). (2020). *Physical best: Physical education for lifelong fitness and health* (4th ed.). Champaign, IL: Human Kinetics.

Thielen, S. (2015, September 15). 5 chest stretch variations [Web log post]. Retrieved from www.acefitness.org/education-and-resources/lifestyle/blog/5657/5-chest-stretch-variations

Chapter 11

Bushman, B. (Ed.). (2017). *American College of Sports Medicine complete guide to fitness and health* (2nd ed.). Champaign, IL: Human Kinetics.

Cooper Institute. (n.d.). *FitnessGram assessment*. Retrieved from https://fitnessgram.net/assessment

Corbin, C.B., & LeMasurier, G.C. (2014). *Fitness for life* (6th ed.). Champaign, IL: Human Kinetics.

Cronkleton, E. (2019, May). *Why being flexible is great for your health*. Retrieved from www.healthline.com/health/benefits-of-flexibilityh

Delavier, F., Clémenceau, J.P., & Gundill, M. (2011). *Delavier's stretching anatomy*. Champaign, IL: Human Kinetics.

Harvard Health Publishing. (2015, April). *Benefits of flexibility exercises*. Retrieved from www.health.harvard.edu/staying-healthy/benefits-of-flexibility-exercises

Harvard Health Publishing. (2019, September 25). *The importance of stretching*. Retrieved from www.health.harvard.edu/staying-healthy/the-importance-of-stretchingh

Kirkendall, D.T., & Sayers, A.L. (2021). *Soccer anatomy* (2nd ed.). Champaign, IL: Human Kinetics.

McGill, E.A., & Montel, I.N. (Eds.). (2017). *NASM essentials of personal fitness training* (2nd ed.). Burlington, MA: Jones & Bartlett Learning.

Morrison, W., & Frothingham, S. (2019, May). *How many joints are in the human body?* Retrieved from www.healthline.com/health/how-many-joints-in-human-body

Nelson, A.G., & Kokkonen, J. (2014). *Stretching anatomy*. Champaign, IL: Human Kinetics.

Physiofitness Physical Therapy. (2014, August). *5 exercises you can do on the road*. Retrieved from https://physiofitness.com/2014/08/19/5-exercises-you-can-do-on-the-road

SHAPE America. Conkle, J. (Ed.). (2020). *Physical best: Physical education for lifelong fitness and health* (4th ed.). Champaign, IL: Human Kinetics.

Thielen, S. (2015, September 15). 5 chest stretch variations [Web log post]. Retrieved from www.acefitness.org/education-and-resources/lifestyle/blog/5657/5-chest-stretch-variations

Winslow, V.L. (2015). Classic human anatomy in motion: The artist's guide to the dynamics of figure drawing. (pp. 59, 60, & 62). Penguin Random House.

Chapter 12

Allgood, K. (n.d.) *3 upper-body strength and flexibility exercises*. Retrieved from www.active.com/fitness/articles/3-upper-body-strength-and-flexibility-exercises

Bauer, A. (n.d.). *Why runners need upper body strength*. Retrieved from www.active.com/running/articles/why-runners-need-upper-body-strength

Capritto, A. (2020). 3 big benefits of a strong lower body. Retrieved from: https://www.livestrong.com/article/13724107-benefits-lower-body-strength/

Contreras, B. (2014). *Bodyweight strength training anatomy*. Champaign, IL: Human Kinetics.

Cooper Institute. (n.d.). *FitnessGram assessment*. Retrieved from https://fitnessgram.net/assessment

Delavier, F., Clémenceau, J.P., & Gundill, M. (2011). *Delavier's stretching anatomy*. Champaign, IL: Human Kinetics.

Iacono, D.A., Padula, J., & Ayalon, M. (2016). Core stability on lower limb balance and strength. *Journal of Sports Science, 34*(7), 671-678. https://doi.org/10.1080/02640414.2015.1068437

Jonaitis, J. (2020, April). *These 12 exercises will help you reap the benefits of good posture*. Retrieved from www.healthline.com/health/fitness-exercise/posture-benefits

McLeod, I. (2010). *Swimming anatomy*. Champaign, IL: Human Kinetics.

Nelson, A.G., & Kokkonen, J. (2014). *Stretching anatomy*. Champaign, IL: Human Kinetics.

Physiofitness Physical Therapy. (2014, August 19). *5 exercises you can do on the road*. Retrieved from https://physiofitness.com/2014/08/19/5-exercises-you-can-do-on-the-road

Salyer, J. (2015, July). *The top 5 muscular endurance exercises*. Retrieved from www.healthline.com/health/fitness-exercise/muscular-endurance-exercises- plank

Thielen, S. (2015, September 15). 5 chest stretch variations [Web log post]. Retrieved from www.acefitness.org/education-and-resources/lifestyle/blog/5657/5-chest-stretch-variations

Chapter 13

Bushman, B. (Ed.). (2017). *American College of Sports Medicine complete guide to fitness and health* (2nd ed.). Champaign, IL: Human Kinetics.

Cleveland Clinic (2020, May). *Planning to start exercising? Start with your core first*. Retrieved from https://health.clevelandclinic.org/planning-to-start-exercising-start-with-your-core-first/

Cleveland Clinic (2020, May). *Why a strong core can help reduce low back pain*. Retrieved from https://health.clevelandclinic.org/strong-core-best-guard-back-pain/

Contreras, B. (2014). *Bodyweight strength training anatomy*. Champaign, IL: Human Kinetics.

Cooper Institute. (n.d.). *FitnessGram assessment*. Retrieved from https://fitnessgram.net/assessment

Corbin, C.B., & LeMasurier, G.C. (2014). *Fitness for life* (6th ed.). Champaign, IL: Human Kinetics.

Delavier, F., Clémenceau, J.P., & Gundill, M. (2011). *Delavier's stretching anatomy*. Champaign, IL: Human Kinetics.

Dweck, C. (2007). *Mindset: The new psychology of success*. New York, NY: Ballantine Books.

Hibbs, A.E., Thompson, K.G., French, D., Wrigley, A., & Spears, I. (2008). Optimizing performance by improving core stability and core strength. *Sports Medicine, 38*(12), 995-1008. https://doi.org/10.2165/00007256-200838120-00004

Jonaitis, J. (2020, April). *These 12 exercises will help you reap the health benefits of good posture*. Retrieved from www.healthline.com/health/fitness-exercise/posture-benefits

Mayo Clinic Staff. (n.d.). *Core exercises: Why you should strengthen your core muscles*. Retrieved from www.mayoclinic.org/healthy-lifestyle/fitness/in-depth/core-exercises/art-20044751

McGill, E.A., & Montel, I.N. (Eds.). (2017). NASM essentials of personal fitness training. Burlington, MA: Jones & Bartlett Learning.

Nelson, A.G., & Kokkonen, J. (2014). *Stretching anatomy*. Champaign, IL: Human Kinetics.

Nunez, K. (2019, June). *The best core exercises for all fitness levels*. Retrieved from https://www.healthline.com/health/best-core-exercises

Salyer, J. (2015, July). *The top 5 muscular endurance exercises*. Retrieved from www.healthline.com/health/fitness-exercise/muscular-endurance-exercises - plank

SHAPE America. Conkle, J. (Ed.). (2020). *Physical best: Physical education for lifelong fitness and health* (4th ed.). Champaign, IL: Human Kinetics.

SHAPE America. (2014). *National standards & grade-level outcomes for K-12 physical education*. Champaign IL: Human Kinetics.

Thielen, S. (2015, September 15). 5 chest stretch variations [Web log post]. Retrieved from www.acefitness.org/education-and-resources/lifestyle/blog/5657/5-chest-stretch-variations

United States Tennis Association. Roetert, P., & Kovacs, M. (Eds.). (2020). *Tennis anatomy* (2nd ed.). Champaign, IL: Human Kinetics.

Chapter 14

Capritto, A. (2020). *3 big benefits of a strong lower body*. Retrieved from www.livestrong.com/article/13724107-benefits-lower-body-strength/

Cronkleton, E. (2019, September). *How to get a full-body strength training workout at home*. Retrieved from www.healthline.com/health/exercise-fitness/strength-training-at-home - bodyweight-exercises.

Contreras, B. (2014). *Bodyweight strength training anatomy*. Champaign, IL: Human Kinetics.

Cooper Institute. (n.d.). *FitnessGram assessment*. Retrieved from https://fitnessgram.net/assessment

Delavier, F., Clémenceau, J.P., & Gundill, M. (2011). *Delavier's stretching anatomy*. Champaign, IL: Human Kinetics.

Iacono, D.A., Padulo, J., & Ayalon, M. (2016). Core stability on lower limb balance and strength. *Journal of Sports Sciences, 34*(7), 671-678. https://doi.org/10.1080/02640414.2015.1068437

Jonaitis, J. (2020, April). *These 12 exercises will help you reap the health benefits of good posture*. Retrieved from www.healthline.com/health/fitness-exercise/posture-benefits

Lloyd R.S., Faigenbaum, A.D., Stone, M.H., Oliver, J.L., Jeffreys, I., Moodym J.A., . . . Myer, G.D. (2014). Position statement on youth resistance training: The 2014 International Consensus. *British Journal of Sports Medicine, 48*, 498-505. https://doi.org/10.1136/bjsports-2013-092952

National Strength and Conditioning Association. Haff, G.G., & Triplett, N.T. (Eds.) (2016). *Essentials of strength and conditioning* (4th ed.). Champaign, IL: Human Kinetics.

Nelson, A.G., & Kokkonen, J. (2014). *Stretching anatomy*. Champaign, IL: Human Kinetics.

Physiofitness Physical Therapy. (2014, August). *5 exercises you can do on the road*. Retrieved from https://physiofitness.com/2014/08/19/5-exercises-you-can-do-on-the-road

Salyer, J. (2015, July). *The top 5 muscular endurance exercises*. Retrieved from www.healthline.com/health/fitness-exercise/muscular-endurance-exercises - plank

Sovndal, S. (2020). *Cycling anatomy* (2nd ed.). Champaign, IL: Human Kinetics.

Thielen, S. (2015, September 15). 5 chest stretch variations [Web log post]. Retrieved from www.acefitness.org/education-and-resources/lifestyle/blog/5657/5-chest-stretch-variations

Chapter 15

Bushman, B. (Ed.). (2017). *American College of Sports Medicine complete guide to fitness and health* (2nd ed.). Champaign, IL: Human Kinetics.

Beckham, S. (2012, November). *Top fitness trends for 2013*. Retrieved from www.cooperinstitute.org/2012/11/top-fitness-trends-for-2013/

Bowling, N. (2016, December). *Aerobic vs. anaerobic exercise: Which is best for weight loss?* Retrieved from www.healthline.com/health/fitness-exercise/aerobic-vs-anaerobic

Corbin, C.B., & LeMasurier, G.C. (2014). *Fitness for life* (6th ed.). Champaign, IL: Human Kinetics.

Delavier, F., Clémenceau, J.P., & Gundill, M. (2011). *Delavier's stretching anatomy*. Champaign, IL: Human Kinetics.

Eddolls, W.T, McNarry, M.A., Stratton, G., Winn, C.O., Mackintosh, K.A. (2017). High-intensity interval training interventions in children and adolescents: A systematic review. *Sports Medicine, 47*(11), 2363-2374. https://doi.org/10.1007/s40279-017-0753-8

Faigenbaum, A. (2015). *Physical activity in children and adolescents*. Retrieved from https://www.acsm.org/docs/default-source/files-for-resource-library/physical-activity-in-children-and-adolescents.pdf?sfvrsn=be7978a7_2

Faigenbaum, A., & Micheli, L. (2017). *Youth strength training*. Retrieved from https://www.acsm.org/docs/default-source/files-for-resource-library/smb-youth-strength-training.pdf?sfvrsn=85a44429_2

Harvard Health Publishing. (n.d.). *Exercise and fitness*. Retrieved from www.health.harvard.edu/topics/exercise-and-fitness

McGill, E.A., & Montel, I.N. (Eds.). (2017). *NASM essentials of personal fitness training* (2nd ed.). Burlington, MA: Jones & Bartlett Learning.

Nelson, A.G., & Kokkonen, J. (2014). *Stretching anatomy*. Champaign, IL: Human Kinetics.

SHAPE America. Conkle, J. (Ed.). (2020). *Physical best: Physical education for lifelong fitness and health* (4th ed.). Champaign, IL: Human Kinetics.

Chapter 16

Association for Applied Sport Psychology. (n.d.). *Exercise adherence tips*. Retrieved from https://appliedsportpsych.org/resources/health-fitness-resources/exercise-adherence-tips/

Bauman, J. (n.d.). *Benefits and barriers to fitness for children with disabilities*. Retrieved from https://www.nchpad.org/173/1308/Benefits~and~Barriers~To~Fitness~For~Children~With~Disabilities

Carron, A.V., Brawley, L.R., & Widmeyer, W.N. (1998). The measurement of cohesion in sport groups. In J.L. Duda (Ed.), *Advances in sport and exercise psychology measurement* (pp. 213-226). Morgantown, WV: Fitness Information Technology.

Carron, A.V., Widmeyer, W.N., & Brawley. L.R. (1988). Group cohesion and individual adherence to physical activity. *Journal of Sport and Exercise Psychology, 10*(2), 127-138. https://doi.org/10.1123/jsep.10.2.127

Centers for Disease Control and Prevention. (2014). *School health policies and practices study*. Atlanta, GA: United States Department of Health and Human Services.

Centers for Disease Control and Prevention. (2016). *School health policies and practices study*. Atlanta, GA: United States Department of Health and Human Services.

Centers for Disease Control and Prevention. (2017). *Increasing physical education and physical activity: A framework for schools*. Atlanta, GA: United States Department of Health and Human Services.

Centers for Disease Control and Prevention. (2019). *Increasing physical education and physical activity: A framework for schools*. Atlanta, GA: United States Department of Health and Human Services.

Lewallen, T.C., Hunt, H., Potts-Datema, W., Zaza, S., & Giles, W. (2015). The whole school, whole community, whole child model: A new approach for improving educational attainment and healthy development for students. *Journal of School Health, 85*(11), 729-739.

National Commission on Certification of Physician Assistants. (2012, June 7). Engaging fitness in the community [Web log post]. Retrieved from https://health.gov/news-archive/blog/2012/06/engaging-fitness-in-the-community/index.html

SHAPE America. Carson, R.L., & Webster, C.A. (Eds.). (2019). *Comprehensive school physical activity programs: Putting research into evidence-based practice.* Champaign, IL: Human Kinetics.

SHAPE America, American Heart Association, & Voices for Healthy Kids. (2016). *Shape of the nation report.* Reston, VA: SHAPE America.

Weinberg, R.S., & Gould, D. (2019). *Foundations of sport and exercise psychology.* Champaign, IL: Human Kinetics.

INDEX

A

B

C

D

E

F

U

V

W

Z

ABOUT THE AUTHORS

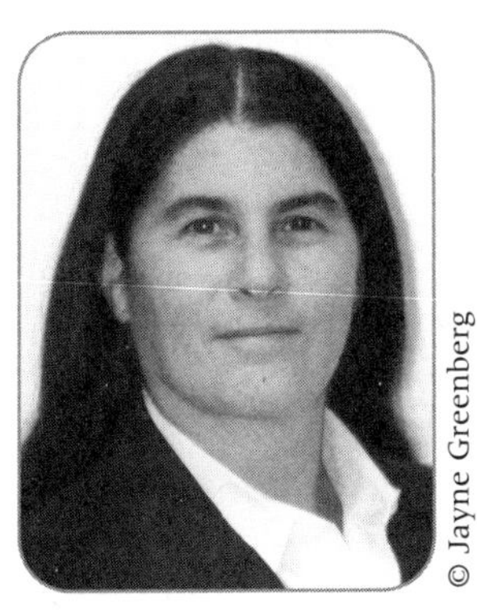
© Jayne Greenberg

Jayne Greenberg, EdD, has served as program director for the I Can Do It! program for the U.S. Department of Health and Human Services. Prior to that position, Dr. Greenberg served as the district director of physical education and health literacy for Miami-Dade County Public Schools from 1995 to 2017. During her career in education, she has worked as an elementary, middle, and high school physical education teacher in both public and private schools; a region physical education coordinator; a high school and middle school administrator; and an adjunct professor teaching both undergraduate and graduate courses in teaching methods, sport psychology, and research.

Dr. Greenberg has served as president of the Florida Association of Health, Physical Education, Recreation and Dance. She also has chaired the Sport Development Committee for the United States Olympic Committee and USA Field Hockey. She assisted the U.S. Department of Health and Human Services in the development of the I Can Do It, You Can Do It! program, a national initiative to address the physical activity levels of youth with disabilities. Dr. Greenberg was named the 2005 National Physical Education Administrator of the Year by the National Association for Sport and Physical Education and received the 2005 Highest Recognition Award from the U.S. Secretary of Health and Human Services, Michael Leavitt. In 2009, she received the Point of Light Award from Florida Governor Charlie Crist and was appointed to the Governor's Council on Physical Fitness. In 2011, Dr. Greenberg was appointed by President Barack Obama to serve on the President's Council on Sports, Fitness, and Nutrition. In 2015, she was named as the North America chair for the International Sport and Culture Association. In 2016, she was named as an Aspen Institute Scholar and received the 2016 North America Society of HPERD Professionals Award. In 2017, she received the Lifetime of Giving Award from Delta Psi Kappa and was named as the education sector chair for the National Physical Activity Plan. Dr. Greenberg was inducted into the SHAPE America Hall of Fame in 2019.

Dr. Greenberg serves as an international consultant in many capacities. She coordinated Olympic education programs in Canada; developed the sport science curriculum at the University of Malaya in Kuala Lumpur, Malaysia; and developed a math and science sailing curriculum for the National Maritime Museum and Royal Observatory in London and Sydney, Australia.

Dr. Greenberg coauthored the Human Kinetics text *Organization and Administration of Physical Education* and the handbook *Developing School Site Wellness Centers* and has published numerous articles. She also has been a featured speaker at several state, national, and international conventions and meetings. In the past 12 years, Dr. Greenberg has secured more than $39 million in federal and foundation grants for educational programs.

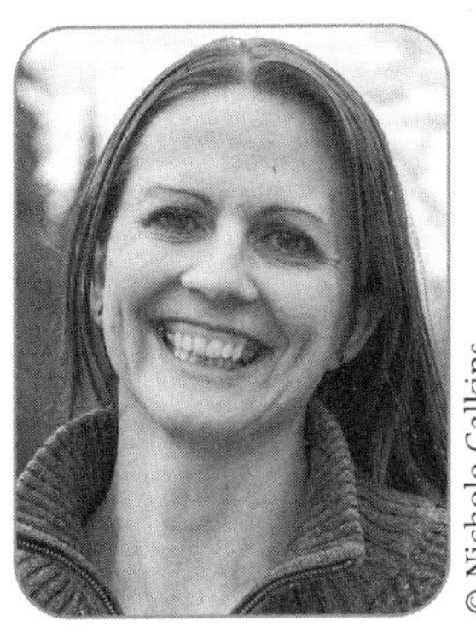
© Nichole Calkins

Nichole Calkins, EdD, is an assistant professor of physical education pedagogy and the program director of the kinesiology department at Gonzaga University in Spokane, Washington. She was a high school health and physical education teacher and a sports coach in the public school system for more than 14 years, and she was a district health and physical education instructional specialist for two years. Dr. Calkins is a curriculum writer and works with various school districts and organizations as a consultant on curriculum design and instructional practices. She is certified by the NSCA as Certified Strength and Conditioning Specialist.

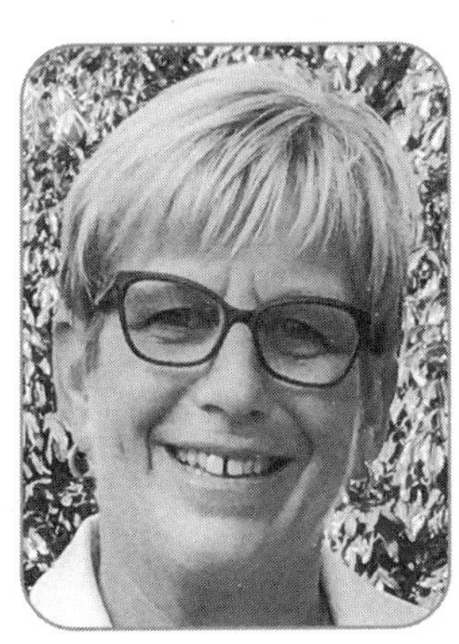
© Lisa Spinosa

Lisa S. Spinosa, MSEd, is a physical education teacher for Miami-Dade County Public Schools. She received both her bachelor's and master's of education from Florida International University, where she was part of the women's basketball team. She later pursued her leadership degree from Nova University. In addition to being a physical education teacher, Spinosa has worked in many capacities, including as a girls' and boys' high school basketball coach, athletic trainer, assistant athletic director, and athletic business manager. She was recruited to open a new high school, where she later became the athletic director and department chair. Ms. Spinosa presently has returned to the classroom to further pursue her goal of finding and implementing new, innovative, and motivating ways to transform children's ways of thinking regarding health and fitness.

ABOUT THE CONTRIBUTOR

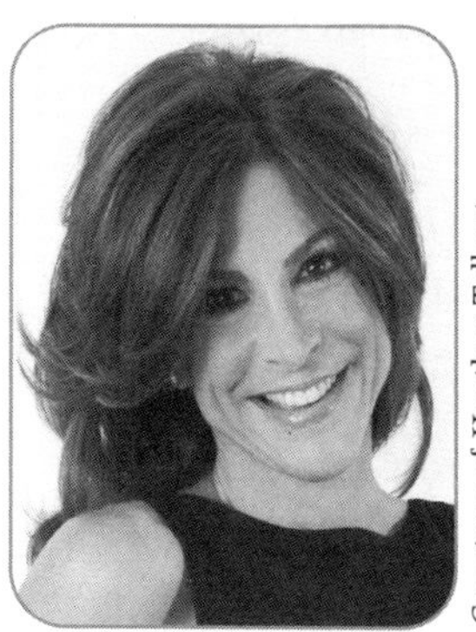

Courtesy of Heather Talbert.

Lisa Dorfman, known internationally as *the Running Nutritionist*, is an award-winning health expert and consultant. She was the *2019 recipient of the President's Council on Sports, Fitness, and Nutrition (PCSFN) Community Leadership Award and the 2017 recipient of the Dietitians in Integrative and Functional Medicine (DIFM) Excellence in Practice Award.* Lisa is a licensed nutritionist/registered dietitian, board certified specialist in sports dietetics, board certified professional counselor, certified chef, certified USA track and field and USA triathlon coach, certified Reiki practitioner, certified horticulturist, and fellow of the Academy of Nutrition and Dietetics. She was previously the director of the graduate nutrition program at the University of Miami (UM) and served as the UM athletic team sports nutritionist. She was the sports nutritionist for the 2008 U.S. Olympic and Paralympic sailing team and nutrition expert for the Plate by Zumba and Strong by Zumba programs. The author of eight books, Lisa has appeared on *20/20*, *Dateline*, *Good Morning America Health*, Fox News, CNN, MSNBC, and ESPN. She has been featured in numerous publications, including *USA Today*, *Newsweek*, *Wall Street Journal*, *New York Times*, *Men's Fitness*, *Outside*, and *Runner's World*. She has held many professional board positions on the local, national, and international levels and speaks worldwide on sports and performance nutrition. She resides in Miami, Florida, and is wife and mother to three children.